ORTHOPEDIC EXAM REVIEW
A Comprehensive Manual for Postgraduates

[For MS, DNB & Diploma Students]

ORTHOPEDIC EXAM REVIEW

A Comprehensive Manual for Postgraduates

[For MS, DNB & Diploma Students]

Second Edition

Ashraf Shaikh
MBBS MS DNB MNAMS MRCS(England)
Assistant Professor
Department of Orthopedics
Seth GS Medical College and KEM Hospital
Mumbai, Maharashtra, India

Foreword

Mohan Desai

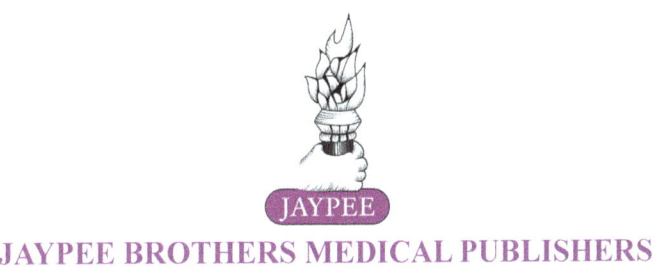

JAYPEE BROTHERS MEDICAL PUBLISHERS
The Health Sciences Publisher
New Delhi | London

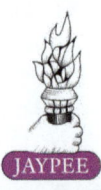 **Jaypee Brothers Medical Publishers (P) Ltd**

Headquarters
EMCA House
23/23-B, Ansari Road, Daryaganj
New Delhi 110 002, India
Landline: +91-11-23272143, +91-11-23272703
+91-11-23282021, +91-11-23245672
E-mail: jaypee@jaypeebrothers.com

Overseas Office
JP Medical Ltd.
83, Victoria Street, London
SW1H 0HW (UK)
Phone: +44-20 3170 8910
E-mail: info@jpmedpub.com

Corporate Office
Jaypee Brothers Medical Publishers (P) Ltd.
4838/24, Ansari Road, Daryaganj
New Delhi 110 002, India
Phone: +91-11-43574357
Fax: +91-11-43574314
E-mail: jaypee@jaypeebrothers.com

EU GPSR Authorised Representative
Logos Europe, 9 rue Nicolas Poussin
17000, La Rochelle, France
Phone: +33 (0) 6 67 93 73 78
E-mail: Contact@logoseurope.eu

Website: www.jaypeebrothers.com
Website: www.jaypeedigital.com

© 2024, Jaypee Brothers Medical Publishers

The views and opinions expressed in this book are solely those of the original contributor(s)/author(s) and do not necessarily represent those of editor(s) or publisher of the book.

All rights reserved. No part of this publication may be reproduced, stored or transmitted in any form or by any means, electronic, mechanical, photocopying, recording or otherwise, without the prior permission in writing of the publishers.

All brand names and product names used in this book are trade names, service marks, trademarks or registered trademarks of their respective owners. The publisher is not associated with any product or vendor mentioned in this book.

Medical knowledge and practice change constantly. This book is designed to provide accurate, authoritative information about the subject matter in question. However, readers are advised to check the most current information available on procedures included and check information from the manufacturer of each product to be administered, to verify the recommended dose, formula, method and duration of administration, adverse effects and contraindications. It is the responsibility of the practitioner to take all appropriate safety precautions. Neither the publisher nor the author(s)/editor(s) assume any liability for any injury and/or damage to persons or property arising from or related to use of material in this book.

This book is sold on the understanding that the publisher is not engaged in providing professional medical services. If such advice or services are required, the services of a competent medical professional should be sought.

Every effort has been made where necessary to contact holders of copyright to obtain permission to reproduce copyright material. If any have been inadvertently overlooked, the publisher will be pleased to make the necessary arrangements at the first opportunity.

Inquiries for bulk sales may be solicited at: jaypee@jaypeebrothers.com

Orthopedic Exam Review: A Comprehensive Manual for Postgraduates / Ashraf Shaikh

First Edition: 2023

Second Edition: **2024**

ISBN: 978-93-5696-854-7

DEDICATED TO

*My parents for their constant love and support,
Dr Fazal Shaikh (Consultant Pediatrician) and
Dr Parveen Shaikh (Consultant Dermatologist)*

From the Desks of My Mentors

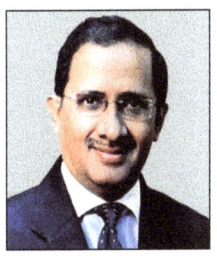

Shrinand V Vaidya MBBS MS FACS(USA)
Consultant and Head, Department of Joint Reconstruction Surgery
Global Hospital, Mumbai, Maharashtra, India
Former Professor and Head of Unit, King Edward Memorial Hospital, Mumbai, Maharashtra, India
Fellow, Ranawat Orthopaedic Research Foundation, USA
Past President, Indian Society of Hip and Knee Surgeons

I am aware of Dr Ashraf's penchant for publishing right from his residency days. Being one of our star students, he has compiled a narrative that fills the gap for what is required as a necessary support for MS and DNB examinations. Being an examiner for 30 years myself, I must admit that Dr Ashraf's *"Orthopedic Exam Review"* fits in well for examinees. If used together with major textbooks, it will make the art of writing the postgraduate examinations extremely effective and impactful.

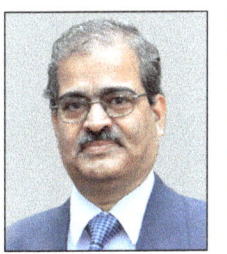

Sudhir K Srivastava MBBS MS Fellowship in Spine Surgery(UK, Germany)
Consultant Spine Surgeon
Dr LH Hiranandani Hospital, Mumbai, Maharashtra, India
Professor, Department of Orthopedics
KJ Somaiya Hospital and Research Centre, Mumbai, Maharashtra, India
Former Professor and Head, Department of Orthopedics
King Edward Memorial Hospital, Mumbai, Maharashtra, India

As Dr Shaikh's postgraduate guide, I have seen him evolve from a House Surgeon to an Assistant Professor at the Department of Orthopedics, KEM Hospital. His manual is an excellent resource that provides students with simple and easy-to-follow summaries of the most important concepts in Orthopedics.

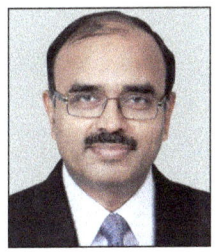

Shubhranshu S Mohanty MBBS(Distn) MS(Orthopedics) FASIF(Swiss) FRCS(Edinburgh) FICS(USA) FACS(USA)
Consultant Orthopedics and Joint Replacement Surgeon
Jaslok, Shushrusha and Nanavati Hospitals
Mumbai, Maharashtra, India
Professor and Unit Head in Orthopedics, King Edward Memorial Hospital
Mumbai, Maharashtra, India
President, Indian Arthroplasty Association (IAA) 2019–21
President, Bombay Orthopaedic Society (BOS) 2020–21
BOS Vice-President (2011–12); Secretary and Treasurer (2006–08);
IAA Joint Secretary (2013–15); ISHKS Fellowship Chair (2015–17); Education Chair (2018–21)

Having taught Orthopedics for many years, I have seen numerous students struggle with their theory examinations. That is why I highly recommend this manual to any student who wants to excel in their postgraduate examination. It offers comprehensive guidance, making it easier for students to understand complex concepts. I commend Dr Ashraf for his dedication in creating this valuable resource, and I wish him all the very best for his book.

Foreword

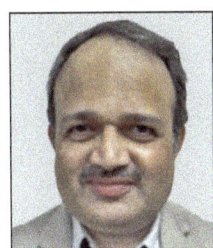

Mohan Desai
Professor and Head
Department of Orthopedics
Seth GS Medical College and KEM Hospital
Medical Superintendent, KEM Hospital
Mumbai, Maharashtra, India
President, Bombay Orthopaedic Society

Having served as an examiner for two decades, I have seen countless students struggle with theory papers. One of the main reasons for this is their vague and imprecise writing, which often results in a significant reduction in their scores. As examiners, we require specific points and terminologies on a given topic, and once we have assessed them, we mark accordingly.

In Dr Shaikh's manual, the answers are crisp and to the point, almost knowing what the examiner wants to read. The use of numbered points, flowcharts, and diagrams makes an examiner's job easier and helps students present their ideas more cohesively.

I have known and mentored Dr Shaikh since his residency days and can vouch for his unwavering commitment to academia and his meticulous attention to detail. This book is a reflection of those traits.

I extend my best wishes to Dr Shaikh for his work in helping postgraduate trainees around the country with their theory examinations.

Preface

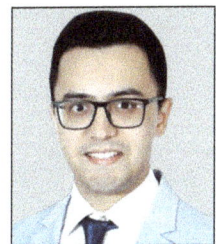

Orthopedics is a vast field with complex concepts that require comprehensive and deep understanding of subject matter. While textbooks and reference materials provide a wealth of knowledge, it is extremely challenging to condense all the information into concise and effective examination answers. This is exactly where the *Orthopedic Exam Review* comes in.

During my final year of residency, I began compiling notes from multiple resources to gain a thorough understanding of each topic. Whether it is a blessing or a curse, my obsessive-compulsive disorder (OCD) tendencies drove me to meticulously scour all available material on a given topic and ensure that there were no lacunae left by individual sources, thus creating the Orthopedic Exam Review.

In this second edition, I have added the recently asked important topics and corrected some errors of the previous edition.

Please remember that **this manual is not a replacement for textbooks**. It is just to make your life easy. It is a culmination of the most important points on a topic from multiple sources to help you review topics rapidly, months, days, hours and even minutes before the examinations.

Understanding core concepts in Orthopedics remains irreplaceable and you must read the recommended textbooks for that. This manual serves as a supplementary tool to aid your understanding and preparation. My recommendation is to read each topic in this manual after studying the corresponding topic in the textbook of your choice.

As someone who has recently been on both sides of a theory examination, I understand how examiners frame their questions and the responses they seek. Thus, I have organized the answers in a structured format with headings, subheadings, and numerical points to aid your memorization and retention. Additionally, I have drawn the figures by hand in most cases, which the publishers have digitally replicated, allowing students to recreate them with ease.

Your paper will be checked for a very brief amount of time and within that you have to convince the examiner that you know, and know well. For this reason, presentation in these examinations is of significant importance. Therefore, incorporating diagrams and flowcharts from this manual would be an asset to your answers.

Lastly, despite my rigorous efforts to minimize errors, I am only human and may have missed some. Please do not hesitate to contact me at *ashrafshaikh123@gmail.com* if you spot any.

Ashraf Shaikh

Acknowledgments

I would like to express my heartfelt gratitude to *Dr Chandan Mehta* for his invaluable contributions to various topics covered in this manual, as well as to Dr Kunal Chaudhari and Dr Swapnil Chitnavis for their input in enhancing its content. I would also like to thank my friend and undergrad batchmate, Dr Aishwarya Sankhe, who undertook the monumental task of deciphering my illegible handwriting and transforming it into a digital format.

I am grateful to Ms Chetna Malhotra (Senior Director—Professional Publishing, Marketing and Business Development), Ms Asmi Bharati (Development Editor), Mr CS Gawde (Regional Business Manager, West), and Mr Sameer S Mulla (Business Manager Channel Sales) from M/s Jaypee Brothers Medical Publishers (P) Ltd, New Delhi, India, for their exceptional work and patience with my semi-unrealistic expectations and tight deadlines. The designers also deserve recognition for their work in converting the hand-drawn diagrams into digital figures.

I would like to acknowledge my professors and teachers from *KEM Hospital*, who have always encouraged me to strive for excellence.

Finally, I would like to express gratitude to my family for their unwavering support and invaluable inputs in conceptualizing this book—to my parents *Dr Fazal Shaikh* and *Dr Parveen Shaikh* along with my brothers and their partners—*Dr Ahmed Shaikh* and *Dr Sanobar Jaka*, and *Dr Altaf Shaikh* and *Dr Adiba Shaikh*.

Contents

1. BASIC AND APPLIED SCIENCES 1

Calcium Metabolism 1
Rickets 2
Osteomalacia 4
Osteoporosis 5
Bisphosphonates (BP) 9
Denosumab 10
Parathyroid Hormone and Disorders 11
Brown Tumor 12
Scurvy 12
Skeletal Fluorosis 14
Development of Skeleton – Principles and Application 15
Collagen 18
Bone Healing 18
Cartilage 20
Cartilage Injuries and Defects 21
Autologous Chondrocyte Implantation (ACI) 23
Synovial Fluid Analysis 24
Gait 27
Blood Components 30
Hazards of Blood Transfusion 32
Autologous Transfusion 33
DVT And Pulmonary Embolism 34
Thromboprophylaxis/New Anticoagulants/LMWH 35
Fat Embolism 36
Tourniquet 37
Compartment Syndrome 38
Stress and Strain 41

2. PEDIATRIC ORTHOPEDICS 44

Proximal Femoral Focal Deficiency (PFFD) 44
Perthes Disease 47
DDH 50
Slipped Capital Femoral Epiphysis 56
Coxa Vara 59
Angular Deformities of LL in Children 60
Congenital Pseudoarthrosis of Tibia (CPT) 64
Tibia Vara 65
CTEV 67
Congenital Vertical Talus (CVT) 69
Calcaneovalgus Foot 70
Torticollis 71
Congenital Radio-ulnar Synostosis 72
Polydactyly 73
Congenital Trigger Thumb 74
Limping Child 74
Spina Bifida 74
Trash Lesions (The Radiographic Appearance Seemed Harmless) 75

3. HIP 77

Hip Biomechanics 77
Approaches to Hip Joint 79
Osteonecrosis (HIP)/AVN/Chandler's Disease 81
Femoroacetabular Impingement 84
Hip Arthroscopy 87
Hip Resurfacing Arthroplasty (HRA) 89
Femoral Neck Fracture Nonunion 90
Evolution of THR 92
Bearing Surfaces in Total Hip Arthroplasty 92
Tribology 93
Complications of THR and Periprosthetic Hip Fractures 94
Osteoarthritis Hip 99
Safe Surgical Dislocation of Hip/Ganz Surgical Dislocation of Hip 100

4. KNEE 103

Knee Arthroscopy 103
Anterior Cruciate Ligament Tear 105
Posterior Cruciate Ligament Injuries 109
Posterolateral Corner (PLC) Injury 110
Meniscus 112
Discoid Meniscus 115
Meniscal Cysts 116
Synovial Plicae/Plica Syndrome 116
Recurrent Dislocation of Patella 117
Osteochondritis Dissecans 120
Osteoarthritis of Knee 121
High Tibial Osteotomy 123
Unicompartmental Knee Replacement 125
Total Knee Replacement 126

5. SPINE 130

Anatomy of Vertebral Column 130
Spinal Approaches 134
Intervertebral Disc: Anatomy, Physiology and Prolapse 137
Cervical Spondylosis 138
Spondylolysis and Spondylolisthesis 142
Lumbar Canal Stenosis 144
Cauda Equina Syndrome 145
Scoliosis 146
Pedicle Screw 150
Lateral Mass Fixation for Cervical Spine 151
Vertebroplasty and Kyphoplasty 152
Video-assisted Thoracic Surgery 154
Minimally Invasive Spine Surgery 155
Dural Tear 156
Somatosensory–Evoked Potentials 157
Nerve Root Blocks/Epidural Steroids 158
Spinal Fusion Methods 159
Role of Physiotherapy in Low Back Pain 160
Failed Back Syndrome 161

6. SHOULDER 163

Shoulder Instability/Recurrent Shoulder Dislocation 163
Frozen Shoulder 168
Rotator Cuff Disease 169
Long Head of Biceps Brachii Rupture 171
Reverse Shoulder Arthroplasty 172

7. FOOT AND ANKLE 175

Arches of The Foot 175
Blood Supply of Talus 176
Tarsal Tunnel Syndrome 177
Tarsal Coalition 178
Flat Foot 180
Hallux Valgus (Bunion) 181
Retrocalcaneal Bursitis/Haglund 183
Post-polio Residual Paralysis 184
Claw Toes 185
Triple Arthrodesis 187

8. ORTHOPEDIC DISEASES 189

Osteogenesis Imperfecta 189
Cerebral Palsy (Static Encephalopathy) 190
Cleidocranial Dysostosis 195
Achondroplasia 196
Sprengel Deformity 197
Klippel-Feil Syndrome 198
Duchenne Muscular Dystrophy 198
Gout 200
Hemophilia 202
Paget's Disease (Osteitis Deformans) 204
Osgood-Schlatter Disease 206
Carpal Tunnel Syndrome 206
Tennis Elbow/Lateral Epicondylitis 208
Dupuytren's Contracture 209
Madelung Deformity 210
Klippel-Feil Syndrome 198
Dequervain's Tenosynovitis 211
Wrist Arthrodesis 213
Kienbock's Disease 214
Thoracic Outlet Syndrome 215
Cervical Rib 216

Rheumatoid Arthritis *217*
Rheumatoid Hand *221*
Pigmented Villonodular Synovitis (PVNS) *222*

9. BONE TUMORS 225

Introduction to Bone Tumors—Classification, Benign vs Malignant *225*
Bone Biopsy *227*
Aneurysmal Bone Cyst *227*
Giant Cell Tumor *229*
Osteoid Osteoma *231*
Chondroblastoma *232*
Chondrosarcoma *233*
Osteosarcoma *235*
Fibrous Dysplasia *236*
Ewing's Sarcoma *238*
Osteochondroma *239*
Amputation vs Limb Salvage/Principles of Surgery in Bone Tumors *241*
Multiple Myeloma *243*
Metastatic Bone Disease and Differentials *245*
Synovioma/Synovial Cell Sarcoma *247*
Muscle Biopsy *248*

10. BONE AND JOINT INFECTION 249

Osteomyelitis–Acute and Chronic *249*
Types of Sequestrum *253*
Septic Arthritis *253*
Tuberculosis of Hip *256*
TB Spine *258*
Psoas Abscess *263*
Mycetoma/Madura Foot *264*

11. TRAUMA 266

Monteggia Fracture–Dislocation *266*
Pelvis Fractures *268*
Acetabular Fractures *271*
Hip Dislocation *274*
Spinal Cord Injuries *276*
Hangman's Fracture *284*
Odontoid Fracture *285*
Canadian C-Spine Rule *286*
Morel Lavallee Lesion *286*
Scaphoid Non-union *288*
Terrible Triad of Elbow *290*
TFCC Injury *291*
Bennet and Rolando Fractures *292*
Carpal Instability *293*
Lunate Dislocation (Perilunate Dissociation) *294*
Flexor Tendon Injuries – Hand *295*
Game Keeper's Thumb *298*
Paediatric Fractures – Principles and Management *299*
Lateral Condyle of Humerus Fracture – Paediatrics *301*
Supracondylar Fracture Humerus – Paediatrics *302*
Paediatric Diaphyseal Forearm Fractures *304*
Pediatric Neck of Femur Fractures *305*
Complications of Colles' Fracture *307*
Ankle Sprain *308*
Ankle Injuries *309*
Lisfranc Injury *311*
Talus Neck Fractures *313*
Calcaneal Fractures *314*
Jones Fracture/5th Metatarsal Base *317*
Tendoachilles Tendon Rupture *318*
Chest Injuries *319*
Polytrauma *323*
Gas Gangrene *325*
Dynamization of Fractures *326*
Stress Fracture *326*

12. ORTHOPEDIC RADIOLOGY ... 329

Image Intensifier 329
MRI 330
CT Scan 333
Nuclear Medicine Scans 333
Ultrasound (US) 334

13. OTHER TOPICS ... 337

Bone Cement 337
Bone Bank 339
Amputation 340
Peripheral Nerve Injuries and
    Nerve Conduction Studies 343
Brachial Plexus 346
Obstetric Paralysis 349
Median Nerve 350
Ulnar Nerve 352
Radial Nerve 353
Nonunion (NU) 354
Lld/Limb Lengthening/Ilizarov 358
Masquelet Technique 364
Volkmann Ischemic Contracture 365
Chronic Regional Pain Syndrome (CRPS) 367
Heterotopic Ossification 368
Neurogenic Bladder 370
Obturator Neurectomy 371
Prosthesis 372
Myoelectric Prosthesis 373
Jaipur Foot 374
Spinal Orthoses 374
PTB Cast 374
Traction in Orthopedics 375
Gallow's/Bryant's Traction 376
Thomas Traction Splint 377
Skull Traction 377
Bone Plates 378
Tension Band Principles 380
Locking Plate 381
External Fixator 382
Implant Removal 383
Preoperative Preparation of Patient 384
Rehabilitation of a Paraplegic Patient 385

14. RECENT ADVANCES ... 387

Bone Substitutes 387
Orthobiologics and BMP 389
BMP (Bone Morphogenic Protein) 389
Laminar Air Flow 390
Reamer Irrigator Aspirator 391
Fibrin Gel 392
Lasers 393
Gene Therapy 394
Short Wave Diathermy 395
Interferential Therapy 396
Negative Pressure Wound Therapy (NPWT) 397
Radiofrequency Ablation 397
Ozone Therapy 398
Vascularized Fibula Graft 399
Intramedullary Nailing–Recent Advances 400
Recent Advances in THR 402
Viscosupplementation 402
Stem Cells 404
Bioabsorbable Implants 405
Tranexamic Acid in Orthopedics 406
Day Care Surgery 407
Navigation and Robotics 408
Isokinetic Exercises 409
Tens Therapy (Transcutaneous Electrical
    Nerve Stimulation) 410
OT Lights 411
Evidence-based Medicine 413

Index ... 415

Secrets of Writing a Successful Theory Exam

1. Write your answers point-wise, not in paragraphs.
2. Ensure that your handwriting is the best in the first two pages of your answer sheet. Remember, first impression is the last impression.
3. Divide your answers into headings and subheadings and underline them.
4. When space permits, leave a line between two points to improve the presentation.
5. Use flowcharts to represent sequences of events, such as pathophysiology.
6. Include diagrams in every answer and label them neatly.
7. Make sure your diagrams are large (half a page) and, if time and university rules permit, use colors. If using colors, avoid wasting time by drawing with a pencil/pen first; draw directly with colored pencils.
8. Underline all the most important words and salient specific features of an answer (e.g., in AVN-Sectoral sign).
9. If running short on time, it is better to write two shorter answers than to write more about one answer and completely skip the last one.
10. When making tables during the exam, create borders with a scale.

SECTION 1

Basic and Applied Sciences

CALCIUM METABOLISM

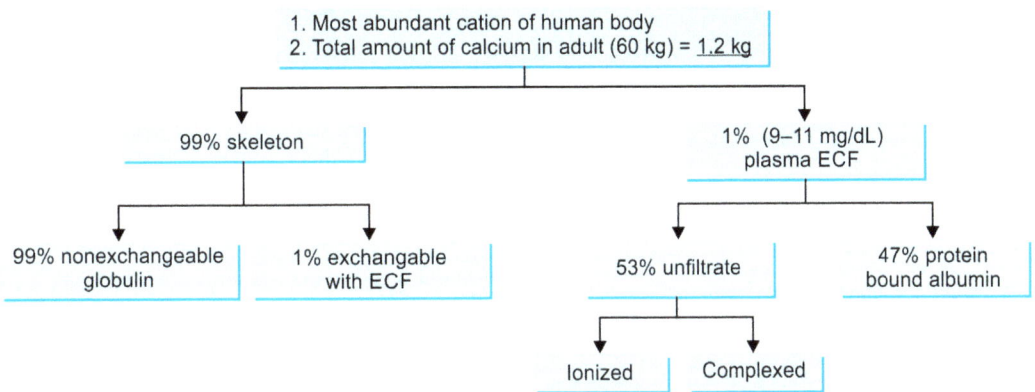

I. DAILY REQUIREMENTS

1. Adult = 1,000 mg/day
2. Pregnant = 1,200–1,500 mg/day
3. Lactating = 2,000 mg/day
4. Infants = 500 mg/day

II. CALCIUM PREPARATIONS

1. Ca gluconate
2. Ca lactate
3. Ca carbonate

III. SOURCES

1. Milk
2. Green leafy vegetables
3. Drinking water
4. Fish
5. Fruits: Sitaphal
6. Dry fruits: Dates
7. Ragi
8. Egg yolk

IV. CALCIUM ABSORPTION AND EXCRETION

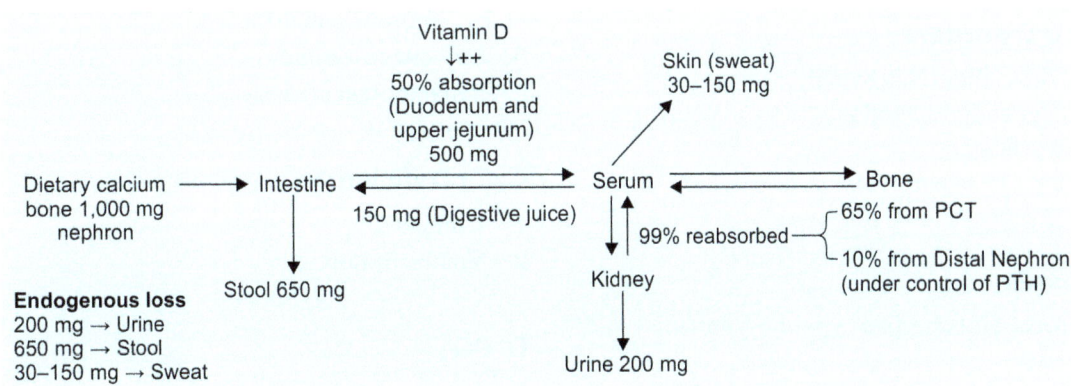

Functions of Calcium in Body

1. Forms major part of bone → takes part in formation and resorption of bone
2. Blood coagulation
3. Neuromuscular excitation
4. Transmission of nerve impulses
5. Cellular adhesiveness
6. Maintenance and functions of cell membranes
7. Activation of certain enzymes
8. Helps in synthesis of nucleic acids and proteins.

RICKETS

I. DEFINITION

Metabolic bone disease caused by a defect in mineralization of osteoid matrix due to inadequate Ca and phosphorus that occurs prior to closure of the physis.

II. VITAMIN-D METABOLISM (FIG. 1)

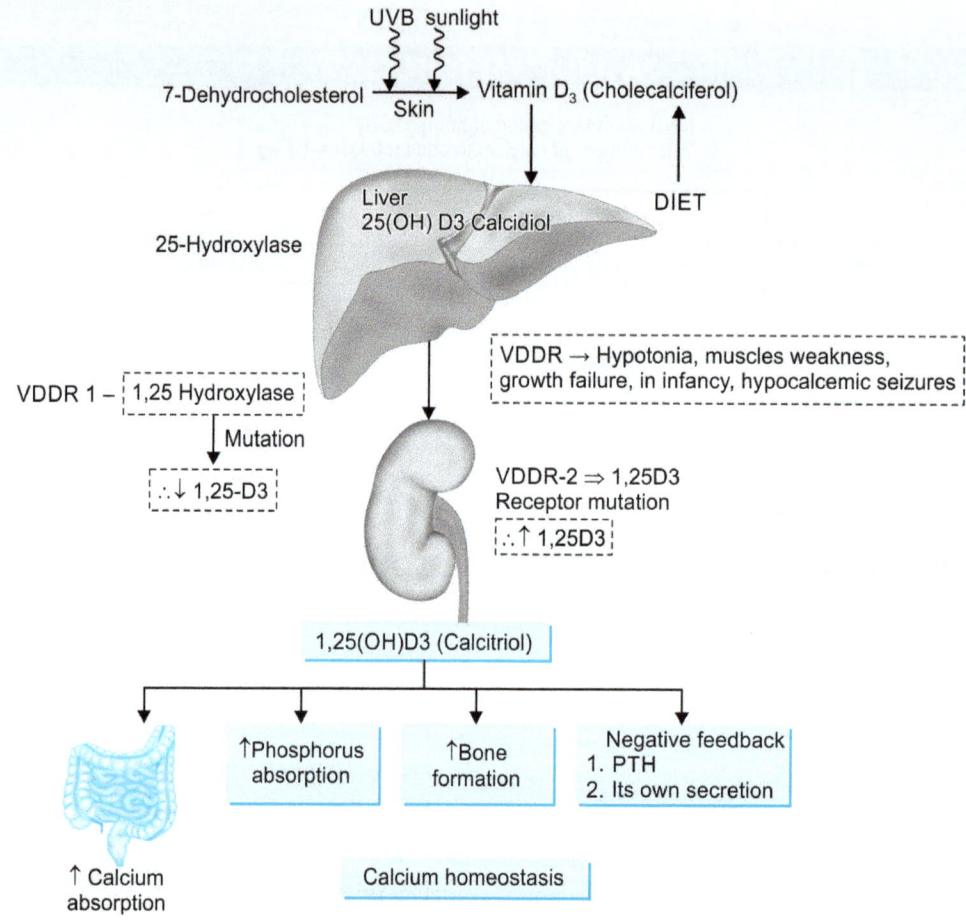

III. ETIOLOGICAL CLASSIFICATION

A. Vitamin D Disorders

1. Vitamin D deficiency (Nutritional)
2. Vitamin D dependent: 1 and 2
3. Congenital deficiency
4. 2° deficiency = Malabsorption
5. CRF

B. Renal Losses

1. Vitamin D-resistant (familial hypophosphatemic) → AD, AR, X-linked
2. ↑ Production of phosphatonins
   i. McCune Albright syndrome
   ii. Tumor induced
   iii. Neurofibromatosis
3. Fanconi syndrome
4. Renal tubular acidosis.

C. Ca Deficiency

1. ↓ Intake
2. Malabsorption.

D. PO_4^{2-}

1. Premature infant
2. Aluminum containing antacids.

IV. PATHOPHYSIOLOGY

i. *Nutritional*

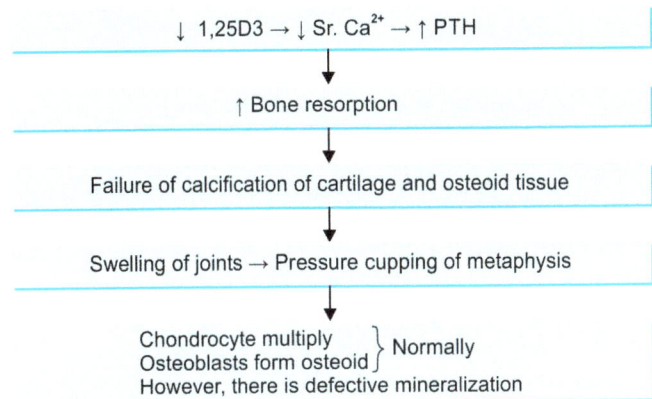

ii. *Vitamin D-resistant rickets*:
1. MC heritable rickets
2. Presents → 1–2 years of age
3. Cause → Inability of renal tubules to absorb phosphate

Types

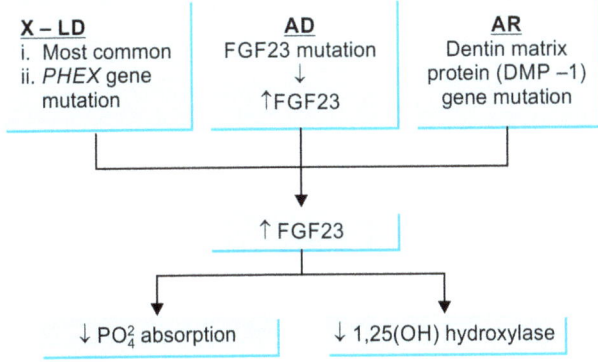

V. CLINICAL FEATURES

A. General
1. Failure to thrive
2. Irritability
3. Listlessness
4. Generalized muscle weakness
5. Protuberant abdomen
6. Ligament laxity
7. Hypocalcemic tetany.

B. Head
1. Craniotabes
2. Frontal bossing
3. Delayed dentition
4. Delayed frontal closure.

C. Spine
1. Kyphosis – Rachitic Cat back
2. Scoliosis
3. ↑ Lumbar lordosis.

D. Chest
1. Rachitic rosary
2. Harrison's sulcus
3. Pectus carinatum
4. Respiratory infections.

E. Limb and Joints
1. Bone pain and tenderness
2. Coxa vara
3. Genu varum > Genu valgus
4. Windswept deformity
5. Bowing of tibia, femur, radius, ulna
6. Widening of wrist, elbow, knee, ankle
7. Sausage enlargement of phalanges
8. Double malleoli sign → Enlarged ankle epiphysis

VI. RADIOLOGY (FIG. 2)

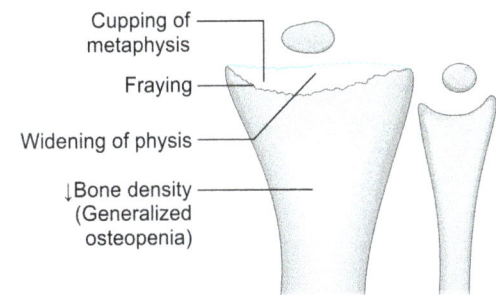

1. Cupping of metaphysis
2. Fraying
3. Widening of physis
4. ↓ Bone density (Generalized osteopenia)
5. Looser's zones: Pulsatile artery against soft bone
   ↓
   Sharply defined radiolucent transverse zones
6. Deformities.

VII. HISTOLOGY
1. Disordered and elongated zone of proliferation
2. Poorly defined zone of calcification.
3. "Swiss cheese" trabeculae
4. Abnormally arranged collagen fibers → perpendicular to haversian canals
5. Widened osteoid seams

VIII. LABORATORY INVESTIGATION

Types	Ca^{2+}	PO_4^{2-}	ALP	PTH	25–OH–D3	1,25–OH D3
Nutritional	N, ↓	↓	↑	↑	↓↓	↓↓
VD-resistant rickets	N	↓	↑	N	N	N
VDDR-1	↓	↓	↑	↑	↑↑	↓↓
VDDR-2	↓	↓	↑	↑	↑	↑↑
Renal osteodystrophy (CRF)	N, ↓	↑	↑	↑	N	↓↓

IX. TREATMENT

A. Goals
1. Restoration of metabolic abnormality by medications
2. Prevention of deformity
3. Correction of established deformity

B. Nutritional Rickets

STOSS therapy	60,000 IU weekly
3,00,000–6,00,000 IU over	↓
1–5 day oral/IM →→	Followed by 800 IU/day

Calcium → 500 mg/day

C. Hypophosphatemic (VDRR)
↓
Oral phosphorus

D. VDDR
VDDR I: Calcitriol
VDDR II: High dose vitamin D_3

E. Deformities
→ May resolve after treatment with vitamin D_3
If they don't, then

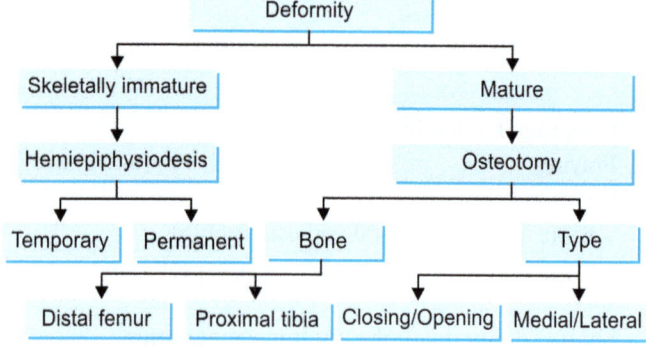

X. MONITORING
1. ALP → Normal → 6 months
2. X-ray → Dense line at the end of metaphysis
3. Epiphyseal shadow clearly defined
4. Transverse bands of calcification
5. Correction of deformities.

OSTEOMALACIA

I. INTRODUCTION
1. Metabolic bone disease seen in adult characterized by defective mineralization resulting in accumulation of unmineralized osteoid tissue.
2. Bone catabolism (osteoclastic resorption) and anabolism are normal.

II. ETIOLOGY
1. *Vitamin D deficiency*:
    i. Pregnancy
    ii. Antiepileptic drugs
    iii. Poor nutrition
    iv. Low socioeconomic status
2. *Gastrointestinal disorders*:
    i. Post-gastrectomy
    ii. Celiac disease
    iii. Hepatobiliary and pancreatic disease
3. Long-term use of anticonvulsant drugs
4. *Phosphate depletion*:
    i. Renal phosphate leak
    ii. Hyperparathyroidism
    iii. Chronic use of antacids

III. CLINICAL FEATURES
1. Bone pain and tenderness
2. Proximal muscular weakness
3. Pathological fractures → compression of fracture of vertebrae
4. Lower limb deformities → due to bending with weight-bearing pressures
5. Waddling gait: Weakness of hip adductors
6. Scoliosis
7. Kyphosis
8. Coxa vara
9. Protrusio acetabuli

IV. RADIOGRAPH
1. Generalized demineralization with loss of transverse trabeculae
2. Osteomalacia may be present without X-ray evidence
3. *Looser zones: Pseudofractures* (Fig. 3)

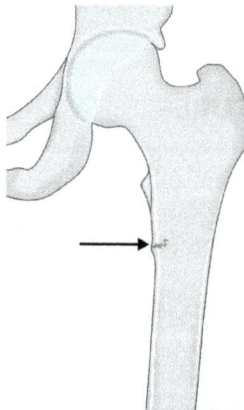

   i. Transverse bilateral symmetrical lines of rarefraction extending incompletely across the bone
   ii. The looser zones may occur as a single sign without evidence of other manifestation
   iii. *Occurs at*:
      1. Neck of femur
      2. Pubic rami
      3. Ischium
      4. Ribs
      5. Scapula
   iv. Disappears when cause can be corrected.

4. Cod-fish spine: Nucleus pulposus expands the discs and indents the end plates of the vertebral bodies.

V. LABORATORY FINDINGS

1. Always rule liver and kidney disease
2. *Calcium studies*:
   a. Sr. Ca^{++} ↓
   b. Urinary Ca^{++}
3. *Phosphorus studies*:
   a. Serum ↓
   b. Urinary
4. Alkaline phosphatase ↑
5. Vitamin D_3 ↓↓
6. PTH ↑

VI. DIFFERENTIAL DIAGNOSIS

1. Osteoporosis
2. Osteitis fibrosa generalisata

VII. TREATMENT

1. Calcium: Oral tablets 1,000 mg/day OD or BD
2. Vitamin D_3: 1,000 IU/day
3. Protein supplementation: 1 g/kg body weight.

OSTEOPOROSIS

I. INTRODUCTION

1. Diffuse reduction in bone density that results when the rate of bone resorption exceeds the rate of bone formation.
2. Most associated with the aging process in which bone formation is normal, but resorption occurs at higher rate.
3. WHO → Bone mineral density 2.5 SD below the mean for young adults of the same sex **(T-score)**.

II. ETIOPATHOGENESIS (FIG. 4)

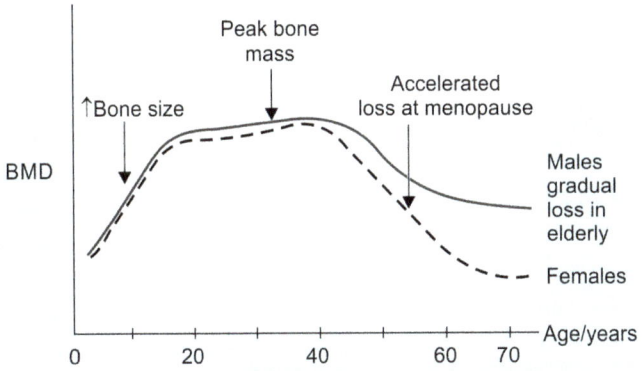

1. The increase in bone mass continues till 25–30 years.
2. Up to 45 years, bone mass is maintained due to similar rate of bone formation and bone loss (bone remodeling).
3. >45 years → Resorption exceeds formation. Exaggerated in women due to menopause.
4. Loss of cancellous bone is more rapid than cortical bone.
5. After 70 years, both men and women have rapid decline in bone density.
6. Predisposes them to low BMD and ↑ fractures.

III. RISK FACTORS

A. Nonmodifiable

1. Advanced age
2. Frailty
3. Parental history of fragility fracture
4. Early menopause (<45 years)
5. Primary estrogen (F) and androgen (M) deficiency
6. Hypogonadal states: Androgen insensitivity, anorexia nervosa, hyperprolactinemia, Turners and Klinefelter's syndrome.
7. Ethnicity
8. Genetic factors: Cystic fibrosis, Marfan's and Ehler Danlos syndrome, OI, glycogen storage diseases.
9. Small stature
10. Rheumatologic and autoimmune diseases → RA, AS, SLE
11. Gastrointestinal disorders: Peptic ulcers disease, IBD, pancreatic disease
12. Endocrine disorders: DM 1 and 2, central obesity, Cushing's syndrome, hyperparathyroidism
13. Hematological disorders: Hemophilia, leukemia, lymphoma, multiple myeloma
14. Neurological: Spinal cord injury, MS, stroke
15. Chronic liver and renal disease
16. Epidermolysis bullosa

B. Modifiable

1. BMI < 20 kg/m^2 in females, <25 in males
2. Low body weight
3. Hyperthyroidism and hyperparathyroidism
4. Glucocorticoid intake
5. Smoking
6. Alcohol
7. Caffeine intake >4 cups/day
8. Inadequate Ca and vitamin D intake
9. Prolonged immobilization
10. Lack of sunlight exposure
11. Sedentary lifestyle
12. Medications: Chemotherapy, PPIs, methotrexate
13. Space travel and prolonged low gravity exposure.

IV. CLASSIFICATION

Riggs and Melton

OSTEOPOROSIS	
Primary (1°)	**Secondary (2°)**
Type 1: Postmenopausal	• Hormonal
Type 2: Senile/involutional	• Drugs
	• Nutritional
	• Metabolic
	• Chronic liver and kidney disease

Postmenopausal	Senile osteoporosis
1. Age >50 years	1. Age >75 years
2. Only in Females	2. M:F = 2:1
3. Mainly trabecular bone	3. Both trabecular and cortical bone
4. High turnover osteoporosis	4. Low turnover osteoporosis
5. Vertebral fracture more common	5. Proximal femur fracture
6. PTH normal or decreased	6. PTH ↑
7. Estrogen withdrawal is the etiology	7. Age-related reduced bone turnover

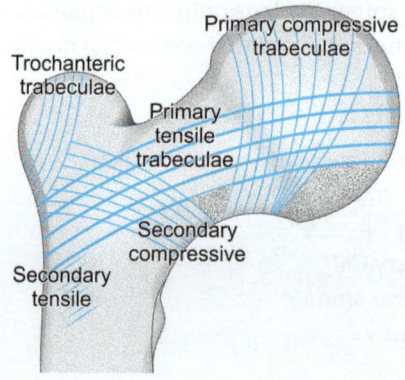

Fig. 5: Normal trabeculae of proximal femur.

V. CLINICAL PRESENTATION

1. Nonspecific, nonlocalized and mild bone pains mainly in the axial skeleton.
2. Slowly progressing in intensity and distribution.
3. Back pain: Due to microfractures.
4. Paraspinal muscle spasm and soreness.
5. Kyphosis → earliest sign associated with loss of height.
6. Stooped habitus.

VI. DIFFERENTIAL DIAGNOSIS

1. Multiple myeloma
2. Metastasis
3. Paget's disease
4. Pott's spine
5. Traumatic fracture earlier in life
6. Histiocytosis
7. Bone cyst
8. Brown tumor
9. Osteomyelitis
10. Gaucher's disease
11. Osteogenesis imperfecta
12. Osteomalacia.

VII. RADIOLOGICAL EXAMINATION

1. ↓ Cortical thickness
2. Loss of bony trabeculae
3. X-ray not sensitive as >30% bone loss needed to appreciate ↓ bone density
4. *Vertebral osteoporosis*:
    i. Penciling of vertebrae
    ii. Ghost vertebra: Loss of cortical and trabecular bone
    iii. Compression fracture and vertebra plana
    iv. Prominent vertical trabeculae (1°) with thinning of horizontal ones in vertebral body.
5. Cortical thickness <25% of the whole thickness of metacarpals
6. *Singh's index*: Loss of trabeculae in the proximal femoral area **(Fig. 5)**.

   i. Grade 6: All normal trabeculae visible.
   ii. Grade 5: Prominent wards triangle. Secondary compressive and 1° tensile attenuated.
   iii. Grade 4: 1° tensile trabeculae markedly reduced, but continuous.
   iv. Grade 3: Definite osteoporosis, break in continuity of 1° tensile.
   v. Grade 2: 1° tensile only at lateral cortex.
   vi. Grade 1: 1° Compressive trabeculae attenuated.
7. **DEXA = Dual-energy X-ray absorptiometry (SAQ)**
   1. Means of measuring bone mineral density using spectral imaging.
   2. Two X-ray beams, with different energy levels are aimed at patient's bones.
      ↓
      Soft tissue absorption is subtracted out.
      ↓
      BMD determined from absorption of each beam by bone.
   3. Fast, reliable and accurate measurement of bone mass → Used in screening population and also defining osteoporosis by WHO criteria.
   4. Gold standard for diagnosis, evaluation and follow-up of osteoporosis patients.
   5. Two types of beams:
      i. Pencil beam
      ii. Fan–Beam (cone)
   6. Pencil beam:
      i. Less scatter
      ii. Requires less dose (1 μSv)
      ↓
      iii. Reduces operator and patient radiation
   7. Fan–beam:
      i. Dose = 18 μSv
      ii. Higher dose → ↑ Radiation
      iii. However:
         a. Improved image quality
         b. ↑ accuracy of measurement
   8. DEXA gives a two-dimensional measure of BMD. Does not measure true volume density.

9. Bone mass is reported as an absolute value in g/cm² and presented as:
    i. Z-score
    ii. T-score
10. Z-score: Patient's value compared to an age-matched and sex-matched reference range.
    → Less clinical value
    → Used in young adults and postmenopausal females < 50 years of age
11. T-score:
    i. BMD relative to normal young, matched controls (30 years women)
    ii. Use:
        a. Predict fracture risk
        b. Classify disease status (WHO definition)
12. Performed in:
    i. Lumbar spine: BMD measured from L_2 to L_4
    ii. Hip: BMD from femoral neck, trochanter, intertrochanter
13. Measured from hip and spine because:
    i. Higher precision
    ii. Quality of trabecular bone at axial sites → Indicative of osteoporotic, burden (Fracture risk)
    iii. Bone loss begins early in trabecular bone as it is highly metabolically active compared to cortical bone and predominant in axial skeleton.
14. **Indications (Fig. 6):**

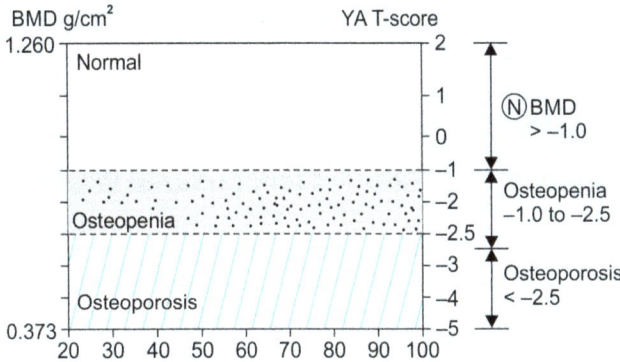

    i. >65 years women, >70 regardless of clinical risk factors.
    ii. Young menopausal women and 50–69 men and women with risk factors for fracture.
    iii. Adults having fracture at or >50 years
    iv. Adults with a condition (RA) or taking medication (Steroids) which decreases bone mass.
15. **Pitfalls:**
    i. Osteophytes due to high prevalence of facet and posterior element spinal OA in elderly → Falsely elevated bone mass.
    ii. OP though systemic occurs inhomogeneously across the body with discordance between sites. Can be misleading.

VIII. LABORATORY INVESTIGATIONS

1. Primarily used for excluding secondary causes of OP.
2. Protein electrophoresis. BJP (urine) → Multiple myeloma
3. Serum calcium, phosphorus, PTH
4. Sr. Calcium also advised before administering zoledronic acid → to exclude hypocalcemia that may precipitate tetany.
5. ↑ Ca, normal PTH → Metastasis
6. To rule out endocrine pathology: TSH, T3, T4, testosterone, cortisol.
7. ↓ IGF → ↑ Risk of ↓ BM
8. Vitamin D deficiency
9. **Bone turnover markers:**
    i. Used to assess effectiveness of therapy.
    ii. **Bone formation:**
        1. Procollagen I carboxy and amino terminal propeptide (PICP, PINP)
        2. Bone specific alkaline phosphatase
        3. Serum osteocalcin
    iii. **Bone resorption:**
        1. Plasma tartarate resistant acid phosphatase (TRAP)
        2. Urinary pyridinoline and deoxypyridinoline
        3. Urinary calcium
        4. Urinary hydroxyproline
        5. Urinary N-telopeptide
    iv. **Utility:**
        1. Predict rapidity to bone loss in untreated patients
        2. Predict fracture risk, independent of BMD
        3. Categorizes individuals as fast or slow bone turnovers. ↑ Fracture risk → fast.
        4. Follow-up → ↓ in markers of bone resorption leads to ↓ bone turnover with antiresorptive therapy.
        5. ↓ Urinary pyrrolidine and deoxypyrrolidine crosslinks after 6 months on alendronate therapy.
        6. Determine duration of "drug holiday"

IX. TREATMENT

Principles
1. Management of underlying etiology.
2. Prevention of fractures ⎯→ Reduction of RF
                          ⎯→ Pharmacological treatment
3. Management of fractures ⎯→ Supportive
                           ⎯→ Operative

A. Reduction of Risk Factors and Nutritional Modifications

1. Patient education and counseling
2. Early diagnosis → H/O, physical exam and radiological evaluation
3. Lifestyle modifications: Brisk walking for 1 hour × 3 times/week
4. Smoking and alcohol cessation

B. Pharmacological Treatment

a. Indications

1. Postmenopausal women and men >50 years with
   i. Hip/vertebral fracture
   ii. Other prior fracture and low bone mass (T-score = −1 to −2.5)
2. T-score < −2.5
3. Low bone mass (T-score −1 to −2.5) and risk factors for fracture (Glucocorticoids)
4. 10-year risk of hip fracture ≥3%
5. 10-year risk major osteoporosis-related fracture ≥20% by FRAX calculation.

b. Drugs

1. **Calcium and vitamin D:**
   i. Prophylactic in all patients, best for type II OP.
   ii. Dose: Ca → 1,200–1,500 mg/d: Postmenopausal women not on HRT.
   1,000–1,200 mg/d: Men, premenopausal, post-menopausal on HRT
   iii. Vitamin D_3 daily requirements 800–1,000 IU/day. Treatment for ↓D_3 → 60 k IU 1 cap/week × 8 weeks
   iv. Reduce fracture risk – hip and nonvertebral
2. **Bisphosphonates:**
   i. T-score <2.5 SD and fragility fracture of hip.
   ii. 1st line through for prevention and treatment of OP.
   iii.

Non-nitrogen containing	Nitrogen containing
↓	↓
Produce toxic ATP analog	Inhibit farnesyl pyrophosphate synthase

   ↓
   Osteoclast apoptosis
   ↓
   ↓↓ Bone resorption
   iv. Side effects → Esophagitis, dysphagia, gastric ulcers, ONJ, atypical subtrochanteric fracture.
3. **Calcitonin:**
   i. Women >5 years postmenopause
   ii. ↓ Pain in acute vertebral compression fracture
   iii. Binds to the membrane receptors on osteoclasts to inhibit resorption
   iv. Nasal spray or injection as it is destroyed by gastric acid
   v. Side effects → Transient rhinitis, nausea/vomiting, flushing, hypersensitivity reaction.
4. **Teriparatide:**
   i. Severe OP and high fracture risk
   ii. Receptors on osteoblasts → Activates them
   iii. Renal tubules and Intestine → ↑Ca^{2+} absorption
   iv. Daily SC injection (20 μg) × 3 months
   v. Side effects → Transient hypercalcemia, dizziness
   vi. Contraindication: in Paget's → Osteosarcoma risk
5. **Denosumab:**
   i. Monoclonal Ig2 against RANKL
   ii. SC injection in arm, thigh, abdomen
   iii. ONJ, arthralgia, nasopharyngitis
   iv. C/I → Severe hypocalcemia
6. **Hormone replacement therapy:**
   i. Indicated in type I OP ≤ 6 years of menopause
   ii. Two types:
      a. Conjugated estrogen: Progestin HRT
         ↓
         ↓ Risk of hip fracture but
         ↑ Risk of breast Ca, MI, stroke, Alzheimer's.
      b. Estrogen – only HRT: For women with prior hysterectomy as estrogen alone ↑ risk of uterine cancer.
7. **Romosozumab:**
   i. Postmenopausal women with prior fracture
   ii. Multiple risk factors of fracture
   iii. Failed Rx
   iv. Intolerant to other Rx
   v. Humanized Ig2 (Monoclonal) that activates Wnt pathway by binding to sclerostin. (Sclerostin inhibits Wnt pathway)
   vi. Promotes bone formation and inhibits resorption
   vii. SC injection monthly
   viii. Side effects → Hyperostosis, CVS ⊗, OA and Ca, ONJ, atypical subtrochanteric fracture
8. **Raloxifene:**
   i. Selective estrogen receptor modulator (SERM) indicated in female patients.
   ii. Agonist on estrogen receptor in bone. Antagonist – Breast, ↓ Ca.
   iii. ↓ Bone resorption
   iv. Side effect: Hot flashes, leg cramps C/I: DVT

C. Supportive Treatment for Fractured Patients

↓
Pain control and bracing

1. NSAIDs, low dose TCA and other neurotropic drugs
2. Transcutaneous electric nerve stimulation, fomentation – hot and cold, therapeutic USG
3. Calcitonin and some bisphosphonates relieve pain of compression fracture
4. Bracing → OP pain control. Can lead to muscle weakness and loss of postural control
5. Weight bearing exercises
6. Spinal extension exercises

D. Surgical Management of Fractures (Osteoporotic)

1. Geriatric patient as a whole is managed not just the fracture.
2. Quick and precise surgery by experienced surgeon.
3. Modalities offering quickest mobilization must be used. (Bipolar hemiarthroplasty over ORIF in old patients.)
4. Locked screw plate constructs rather than DCP.
5. IMN → Diaphyseal fracture: Biology preservation, dynamic load sharing, relative stability, less invasive nature.

6. Augmentation with bone cement.
7. Vertebral wedge compression fracture → Not managed conservatively → Vertebroplasty and kyphoplasty.

BISPHOSPHONATES (BP)

I. INTRODUCTION
1. Current first-line drugs for prevention and treatment of osteoporosis.
2. Analogs of pyrophosphates.
   ↓
   Phosphorus–carbon–phosphorus bond (P–C–P)
3. Prevents bone mass loss by inhibiting osteoclast resorption

II. CLASSIFICATION

A. Based on Route of Administration
1. *Oral*:
   i. Alendronate
   ii. Risedronate
   iii. Tiludronate
2. *IV*: i. Pamidronate; ii. Zoledronic acid
3. *Both*:
   i. Ibandronate
   ii. Clodronate

B. Presence/absence of Nitrogen

Nitrogen containing	Non-nitrogen
1. Alendronate	1. Tiludronate
2. Pamidronate	2. Clodronate
3. Risedronate	3. Etidronate
4. Zoledronic acid	

Zoledronic acid
↓
Appealing to patients as it is IV once a year.

III. MECHANISM OF ACTION
1. Accumulate in high concentration in bone due to binding affinity to Ca.
2. Ingested by osteoclasts and then work by 2 separate mechanisms based on presence or absence of nitrogen.
3. Nitrogen containing:

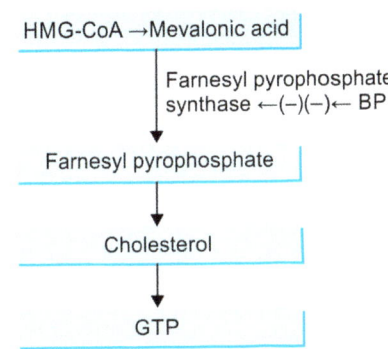

i. Thus, by inhibiting farnesyl pyrophosphate synthase, N-BP prevent the formation of guanosine triphosphate.
ii. GTP is required for formation, function and survival of osteoclasts.
iii. Thus, N-BP lead to cytoskeletal alterations, disappearance osteoclast cell death, ↓ resorptive capacity.
4. Non-nitrogen containing:
   ↓
   Form toxic ATP analog
   ↓
   Osteoclast premature death and apoptosis (**Fig. 7**).

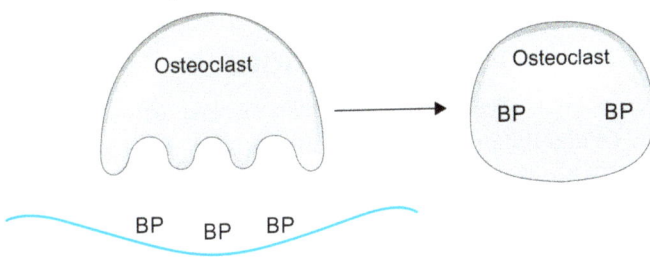

5. Main effect of BP → ↓ Bone resorption and born turnover.
6. 2° → Reduction of angiogenesis by depression of blood flow and ↓ VEGF
7. Net effect of these actions → **"Metabolic freeze"**
   ↓ healing capacity
   Bone metabolically inactive.

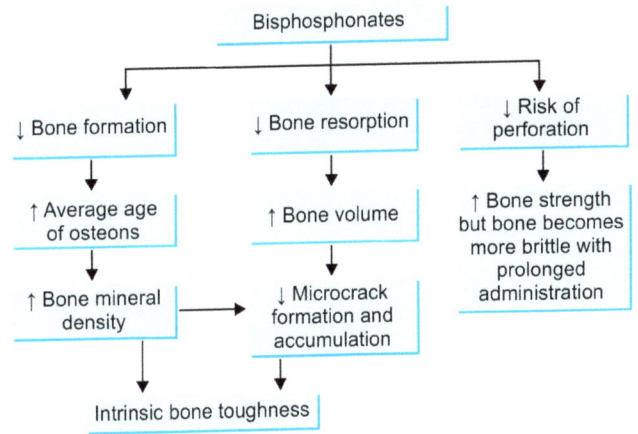

IV. INDICATIONS
1. Osteoporosis:
   i. 1st DOC
   ii. Zoledronate (3rd Gen) IV, yearly
   iii. Oral → up to 5 years
   iv. IV → up to 3 years
2. Multiple myeloma
3. Metastasis from breast ca:
   i. ↓ Pain
   ii. Prevents pathological fracture
4. Paget's disease
5. Early stage of osteonecrosis
6. Hypercalcemia of malignancy
7. Polyostotic fibrous dysplasia
8. Osteogenesis imperfecta

9. Total joint arthroplasty:
   i. To prevent osteolysis
   ii. To prevent heterotopic ossification

V. CONTRAINDICATIONS
1. Severe renal disease: Mechanism of excretion: Renal
2. Following lumbar fusion
3. Pregnancy
4. Achalasia
5. Esophageal strictures

VI. ADVERSE DRUG REACTIONS
1. Influenza like illness: Fever, chills, myalgia, arthralgia (30%)
2. Ocular inflammation: Conjunctivitis, uveitis, iritis
3. GI: Esophageal ulceration, gastritis
4. Atrial fibrillation
5. Bone joint and muscle pains
6. B–P related ON of jaw (BRONJ):
   i. Osteopetrosis like picture (freeze)
      ↓
      ON
   ii. As BP get concentrated in jaws.
7. Atypical insufficiency fracture (Fig. 8):

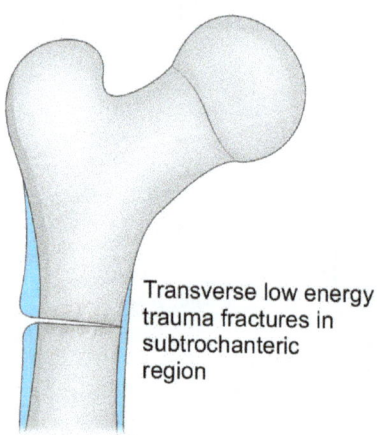

   i. Proximal femur (often B/L), femur shaft, sacrum
   ii. Micro-cracks accumulate, no remodeling

DENOSUMAB

I. INTRODUCTION
1. Recombinant human monoclonal Ig2 against receptor activator of nuclear factor kappa-B ligand.
2. It is functionally like osteoprotegerin – which inhibits osteoclast differentiation, fusion and activation.

II. MECHANISM OF ACTION
1. RANKL/RANK pathway (Fig. 9):

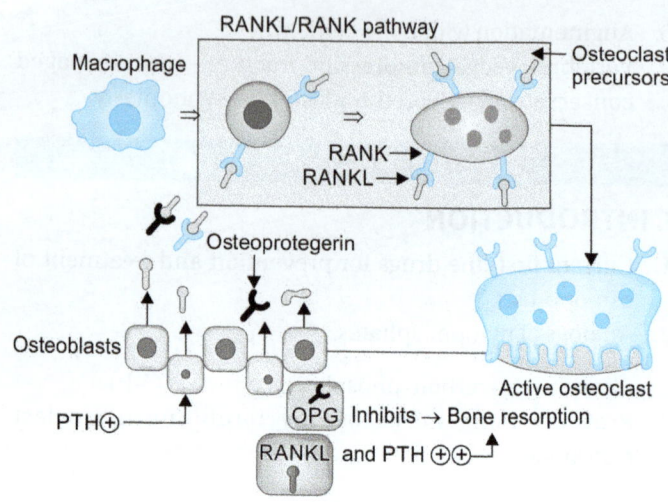

2. Denosumab (Fig. 10):

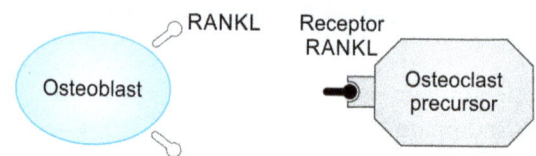

3. RANKL produced by osteoblasts and osteocytes regulates osteoclast number and activity.
4. Inhibitory effect of denosumab on RANKL/RANK pathway
   ↓
   i. ↑ in bone mass
   ii. Strength in both cortical and trabecular bone.
5. Suppression of bone resorption is seen within 24 hours
6. Decreases fracture risk: Hip, vertebral and nonvertebral fracture. (Freedom trial)

III. INDICATIONS
1. Men
2. Postmenopausal women } at high risk of fracture
3. Multiple risk factors for fracture
4. Intolerant to other therapies
5. Other therapies have failed
6. Autoimmune and inflammatory arthropathy →
   ↓
   Develop OP due to overactivity of RANKL
7. GCT

IV. DOSE
1. 60 mg SC/6 months
2. Not metabolized by kidney, ∴ good alternative in CKD patients.

V. SIDE EFFECTS
1. ON jaw
2. Hypocalcemia
3. ↑ Risk of infections
4. Delayed fracture healing
5. Atypical fracture

6. Pancreatitis
7. Neoplasia of breast, GI. (Controversial)

PARATHYROID HORMONE AND DISORDERS

1. Polypeptide hormone.
2. Maintains calcium homeostasis by stimulating bone resorption.
3. Low Sr. Ca^{2+} is the strongest stimulation for PTH secretion from parathyroid glands.

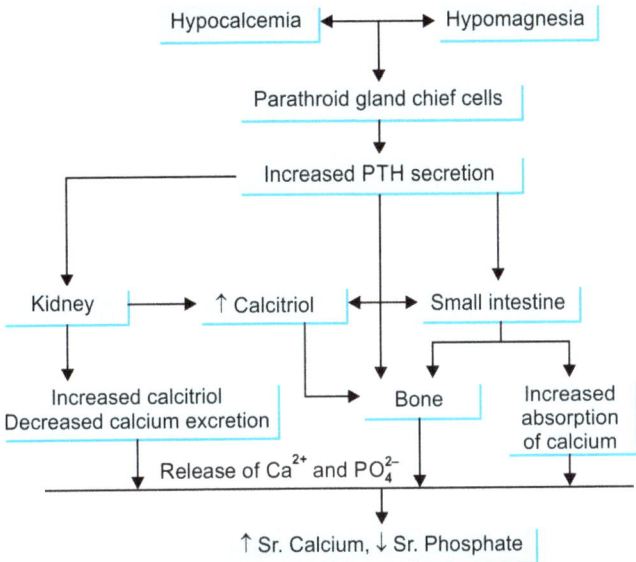

4. PTH bone resorption is mediated through the osteoblast. It has receptors on osteoblasts but not osteoclasts.
RANKL (OB) —+→ RANK (OC): Bone resorption (Receptor activator of Nuclear factor Kappa B)

I. CLASSIFICATION

1. *Primary (Most common):*
   (Osteitis fibrosa cystica, von Recklinghausen's disease, Parathyrotoxicosis)
   Hypersecretion of PTH due to:
   i. Parathyroid adenoma > Hyperplasia
   ii. Rarely parathyroid carcinoma as a part of MEN syndrome
2. *Secondary:*
   Hypersecretion of PTH in response to hypocalcemia or hyperphostemia
   Causes:
   i. Chronic renal failure (Most common cause)
   ii. Calcium malabsorption:
      1. Malabsorption syndrome
      2. Bariatric surgery
      3. Chronic pancreatitis
   iii. Osteomalacia
3. *Tertiary:*
   i. Long-standing secondary hyperparathyroidism eventually leads to hyperplasia of PTH gland and loss of response to Sr. calcium levels.
   ii. Most commonly seen in end-stage kidney disease.

4. *Pseudohyperparathyroidism:*
   i. Malignant tumors of non-PTH origin secrete PTH-like polypeptides
   ii. *Features*:
      a. Persistent hypercalcemia
      b. Hypophosphatemia
      c. Absence of bone metastasis
      d. PTH gland atrophy
   iii. Rx.: Resolution of hypercalcemia on removal of tumor.

II. CLINICAL FEATURES

1. Age group = 50–60 years
2. M:F = 1:3
3. 75% asymptomatic
4. Classic presentation "Stones, groans, bones and psychiatric moans"
5. *Renal*:
   a. Nephrocalcinosis
   b. Diabetes insipidus
   c. Renal failure
6. *Abdominal groans*:
   a. Constipation
   b. Vomiting
   c. Peptic ulcer disease (ZES)
   d. Acute pancreatitis
7. *Psychiatric moans*:
   a. Memory loss
   b. Fatigue
   c. Depression
   d. Delirium
8. Bones:
   a. Severe pain and tenderness in lower limb and back
   b. Generalized muscle weakness and hypotonia
   c. Pathologic fractures
   d. Delayed union
   e. Deformities of limb and spine

III. RADIOGRAPHY

1. Early finding: Generalized deossification
2. Trabeculae become thinned, transverse trabeculae disappear
3. Narrowing of cortices
4. As disease progresses → Cysts appear throughout skeleton
5. Bending deformities
6. Renal calculi
7. Diffuse osteoporosis seen in skull → "Pinhead stippling"
8. Vertebrae → Porotic and deeply indented by ballooned discs (codfish spine)
9. Collapse of vertebral bodies of lamina dura
10. Marrow fibrosis on MRI
11. Brown tumors (lytic lesions)

IV. INVESTIGATIONS

1.

	Ca^{2+}	PO_4^{2-}	PTH
1°	↑	↓	↑
2°	Normal or ↓	↑	↑
3°	↑	↑	↑

2. Increased alkaline phosphatase
3. Increased hydroxyproline in urine
4. *Cortisone suppression:* 150 mg/day × 10 days
   Hypercalcemia of sarcoidosis, thyrotoxicosis, MM, malignancy, hypervitaminosis D = reduced.

   Cortisone does not affect ↑ Ca^{2+} due to PTH.

V. TREATMENT

1°

1. Asymptomatic → Conservative management → Reduced calcium take and adequate hydration.
2. Annual follow up for Sr. Ca^{2+}, BMD and Sr. creatinine.
3. CVS, neuropsychiatric dysfunction, adverse effects of osteoporosis favor early surgery.
4. All symptomatic patients → Parathyroidectomy
5. Indications of parathyroidectomy in asymptomatic patients:
   i. Sr. Ca^{2+} >1 mg/dL above normal
   ii. Urinary Calcium >400 mg/24 hours
   iii. Bone density T-score <2.5
   iv. Age <50 years
6. Neck and mediastinum should be explored (1/4th tumors found in mediastinum)
7. Large amount of Ca^{2+} leaves the blood stream rapidly after PTHectomy = **dangerous hypocalcemic tetany**.
8. Therefore give adequate quantity of calcium and phosphorus till ALP normalizes
9. Extensive bone lesion, increased ALP = remove only portion of hyperfunctioning PTH tissue

2°

1. Treat the underlying cause
2. Hyperplasia of gland → suppressed by appropriate therapy
3. Calcitriol (2 µg/day)
4. Phosphate restricted diet
5. Cinacalcet (calcimimetics) for patients on dialysis
   ↓
   Allosteric activation of calcium sensitive PTH receptors
6. Long term management and maintenance of normocalcemia depends on renal transplantation.

BROWN TUMOR

1. Brown tumor (osteitis fibrosa cystica) is a bone lesion seen as a manifestation of hyperparathyroidism.
2. Reparative cellular progress → **not neoplastic**. Seen in 1° as well as 2°
3. ↓ Ca^{2+}/PTH adenoma
   ↓
   ↑PTH
   ↓
   Osteoclastic bone resorption to maintain Ca^{2+}
   ↓
   Localized regions where bone loss rapid
   ↓
   Hemorrhage and reparative granulation tissue with vascular, proliferating fibrous tissue replaces normal marrow contents
   ↓
   Brown tumor (Hemosiderin imparts brown color)

I. HISTOLOGY

1. Multinucleated giant cells (osteoclasts) in scalloped areas on the surface of the bone. (Howship's lacunae)
2. Normal cellular and marrow elements replaced by fibrous tissue.

II. RADIOGRAPHY

1. Well defined, purely lytic lesions
2. Cortex thinned and expanded, but not penetrated
   DSA = Hypervascular
   MRI = Solid, cystic or mixed
   Bone scan = Increased uptake.

III. TREATMENT

1. Treat Hyper-PTH
2. Parathyroidectomy = Spontaneous healing
3. Calcitriol and cinacalcet.

SCURVY

I. INTRODUCTION

1. Nutritional disorder caused by severe vitamin C deficiency.
2. Clinically characterized by a general hemorrhagic tendency.
3. Primarily affects tissues of mesodermal origin, mainly the skeletal system.

II. EPIDEMIOLOGY

1. M:F – 4:3

2. Bimodal age group:
    i. Artificially fed infants 5–10 months (Most commonly affected)
    ii. Elderly >60 years

III. PATHOPHYSIOLOGY

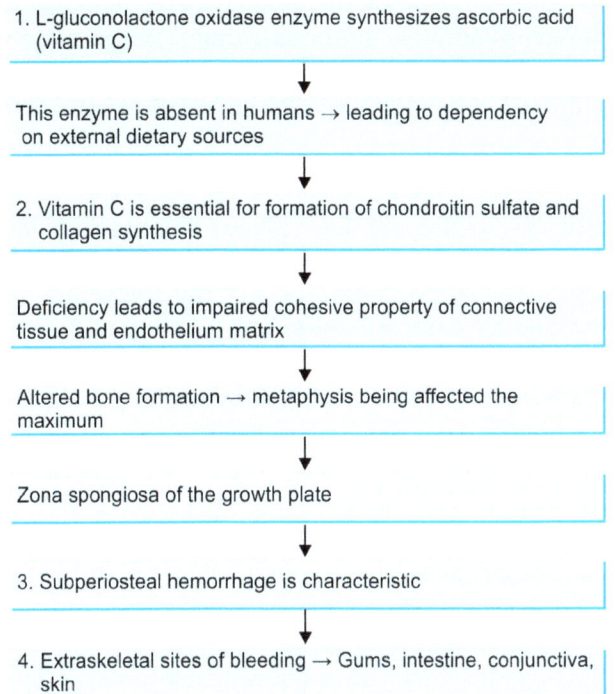

1. L-gluconolactone oxidase enzyme synthesizes ascorbic acid (vitamin C)

This enzyme is absent in humans → leading to dependency on external dietary sources

2. Vitamin C is essential for formation of chondroitin sulfate and collagen synthesis

Deficiency leads to impaired cohesive property of connective tissue and endothelium matrix

Altered bone formation → metaphysis being affected the maximum

Zona spongiosa of the growth plate

3. Subperiosteal hemorrhage is characteristic

4. Extraskeletal sites of bleeding → Gums, intestine, conjunctiva, skin

IV. CLINICAL FEATURES

A. Symptoms

1. Infant → Restless, pale, febrile
2. Pseudoparalysis → Voluntary immobilization of the extremities.
3. Malaise and fatigue
4. Myalgia and bone pain.

B. Physical Examination

1. Petechiae and ecchymosis
2. Extremely tender, palpable, non-mobile swelling over the growing end of bone → Subperiosteal hemorrhage.
3. Joint effusion
4. Bleeding and swollen gums
5. Loose and brittle teeth
6. Hematemesis and hematuria
7. Scorbutic rosary → Costochondral separation

Scorbutic rosary	Rickets rosary
Tender	Non-tender
Angular step-off	Rounded and nodular

V. RADIOLOGY (FIG. 11)

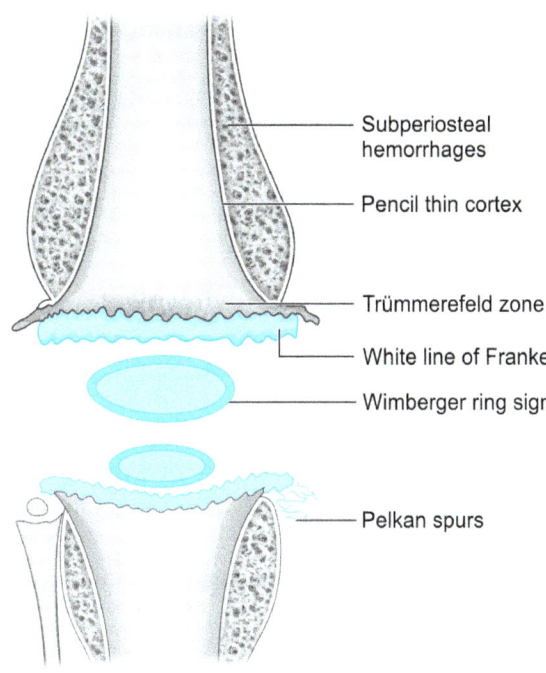

1. Areas of rapid growth are affected mainly → Knee, wrist, sternal end of ribs → X-ray.
2. **White line of Frankel** → Broadened zone of provisional calcification between epiphysis and metaphysis.
3. **Trummerfeld zone** (scurvy line) → Transverse zone of radiolucency adjacent to the white line of Frankel → as a result of bone resorption
4. **Wimberger ring** → Epiphysis encircling dense ring of calcified cartilage.
5. **Pelkan spur** → metaphyseal spurs and fractures
6. **Corner sign of Park** → Metaphyseal clefts
7. Pencil thin cortex
8. Ground-glass osteopenia with decreased trabeculae
9. Subperiosteal elevation
10. Epiphyseal separation
11. Fractures and dislocations

VI. DIFFERENTIAL DIAGNOSIS

1. Rickets. (Rickets + Scurvy together → Barton's disease)
2. Osteogenesis imperfecta
3. Acute osteomyelitis
4. Poliomyelitis
5. Luetic osteochondritis

VII. MANAGEMENT

1. Vitamin C therapy
2. Oral tablets → 500 mg twice a day for 1 month

3. Fruit juices → Orange, lemon, amla, guava
4. Artificial processed milk contraindicated in affected infants.
5. Fractures immobilized without an attempt at reduction.

SKELETAL FLUOROSIS

I. INTRODUCTION
1. Chronic metabolic bone disease caused by the ingestion of large amounts of fluoride → from drinking water and food.
2. The optimum upper safe limit is not more than 6 mg/day.

II. PATHOGENESIS
1. Inorganic fluoride replaces the hydroxyl groups of calcium hydroxyapatite and forms calcium fluorapatite which gets deposited in bone.
2. Osteons → irregular in size, shape and distribution in compact bone
3. Gross reduction in spongiosa.
4. The Haversian canals are enlarged and associated with irregular osteocyte distribution and ↑ irregular interstitial lamellae.
5. Bone invasion by capillaries is ↓ due to excess fluoride forming uneven paths and leading to isolated cartilage islands.
6. Bone marrow → fibrous and hypocellular.
7. Secondary hyperparathyroidism due to ↓ systemic calcium, leading to a high bone turnover state.

III. CLINICAL FEATURES
1. Fluorosis in humans is predominantly dental and skeletal.
2. Dental fluorosis occurs early in the disease process followed by a prolonged symptom free period of nearly 10–30 years which is ultimately followed by a crippling skeletal fluorosis and neurologic abnormalities.
3. During the apparent symptom free stage, the body keeps on accumulating excess fluoride and the patient suffers from vague gastrointestinal symptoms.
4. The neurological manifestations → Radiculomyelopathy: mainly due to mechanical compression of the nerve roots and also the spinal cord from sclerosed vertebral column, osteophytes, and ossified ligaments.
5. The cervical cord is involved earlier than the dorsal cord. The lumbar spine is the first to show skeletal changes, but the involvement of cauda equina is rare.
6. Minor trauma may precipitate neurologic deficits.
7. Spinal motion is restricted.
8. Bone and joint pains
9. Kyphosis

IV. DIAGNOSIS
1. Urinary and bone fluoride
2. Urinary fluoride levels → best indicators of fluoride intake.
3. Fluoride excretion is not constant throughout the day → 24-hour samples of urine.
4. Retention of fluoride is measured by the bone fluoride levels → monitors fluoride treatment of osteoporosis. The value varies from 6,000 to 8,400 ppm in bone ash in fluorosis, normal between 500 and 1,000 ppm or mg/kg.

V. RADIOLOGY
1. The radiographic findings are parallel to pathological changes.
2. Bone formation continues, but the trabeculae thus formed have uncalcified borders and are resistant to reabsorption by osteoclasts.
3. Radiological stages of skeletal fluorosis:
    i. Stage I: Axial skeleton involvement and ground glass appearance of cancellous bone.
    ii. Stage II: Thick primary trabeculae merge with sclerotic secondary trabeculae to make bone homogeneously dense, bone contours become uneven and calcification of paraspinous, sacrospinous and sacrotuberous ligaments is seen.
    iii. Stage III: Axial skeletal bones demonstrate the typical radiological features, marked calcification at the insertion of muscles and tendons.
4. Osteosclerosis (dense bone) is the typical feature of involved axial skeleton (spine, pelvis and ribs), whereas osteoporosis → appendicular skeleton.
5. Osteoporosis, exostoses, osteomalacia, changes resulting from secondary hyperparathyroidism and their combination.
6. Imaging: The best imaging modality to appreciate bony pathology is CT.
7. Calcified ligaments, spinal canal stenosis and root canal stenosis are also better appreciated.
8. MRI: A fluorotic vertebrae appears hypointense in both T1- and T2-weighted images.
9. Interosseous membrane ossification: Both bone forearm
10. Trabecular blurring or haziness
11. Compact bone thickening
12. Irregular periosteal bone formation
13. Ossification of the attachments of tendons, ligaments, and muscles.

VI. MANAGEMENT
1. Best prevented
2. Providing safe drinking water
3. Difficult to manage fractures → Bones are brittle
4. Spinal cord compression → Decompression and fixation

5. Bone mesenchymal stem cell (BMSC) transplantation holds promise in restoring osteoblast viability and bone turnover balance in bone lesions induced by fluoride.

DEVELOPMENT OF SKELETON – PRINCIPLES AND APPLICATION

I. INTRODUCTION

Fertilization → Embryo → 3 Germinal layers
↓
Endoderm, mesoderm, ectoderm **(Fig. 12)**

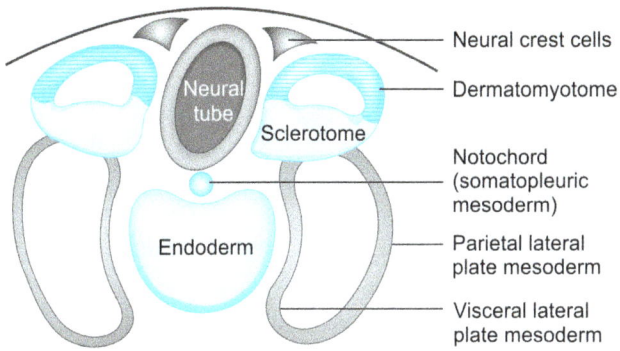

Musculoskeletal system develops from:

Paraxial mesoderm	Parietal layer of lateral mesoderm	Neutral crest cells
↓	↓	↓
Forms segmented blocks on either side of neural tube: Somites	Shoulder and pelvic girdle, limbs, sternum	Bones of skull and face
1. Ventromedial → Sclerotome → Mesenchymal cells → Fibroblasts, Chondroblasts, Osteoblasts. → Vertebral column		
2. Dorsolateral → Dermatomyotome		

II. DEVELOPMENT OF BONE

Two types:
i. Intramembranous
ii. Endochondral

i. Intramembranous Ossification

Development of bone directly from the membranous sheets laid down by the mesenchyme.
1. The mesenchymal connective tissue forms an original membrane model of the bones (e.g., cranial, facial).
2. An ossification center appears around the center of the membrane → characterized by osteoblasts **(Fig. 13A)**.

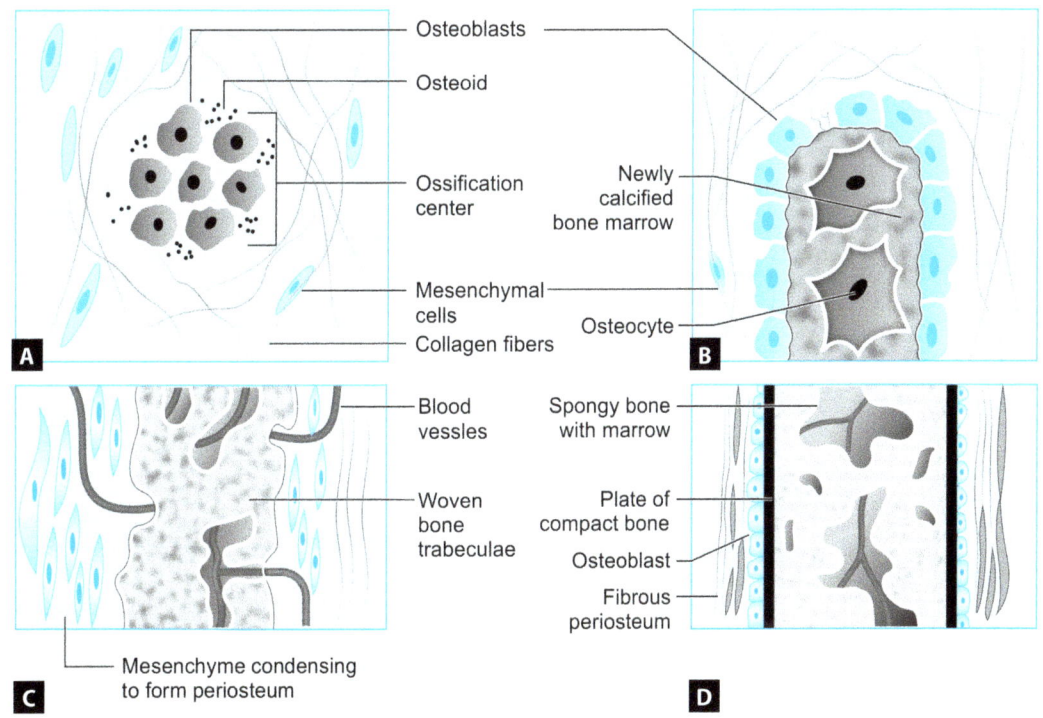

3. Osteoblasts lay down a meshwork of bony trabeculae spread radially in all directions
   ↓
   Trapped osteoblasts → osteocytes **(Fig. 13B)**
4. The mesenchyme at the periphery differentiates to form → fibrous sheath (periosteum)
5. The undersurface of this differentiates into osteoblasts.
   ↓
6. Deposit parallel plates of compact bone (lamellae) (periosteal ossification) **(Fig. 13C)**
7. The trabecular bone persists internally, and its vascular tissue becomes BM **(Fig. 13D)**.

Clinical Application and Examples

1. Cleidocranial dysostosis: Defective membranous ossification
2. Embryonic flat bone formation
3. Distraction osteogenesis
4. Blastem bone → In children after amputation
5. Fracture healing with rigid fixation and no gap.

ii. Endochondral Ossification (Fig. 14)

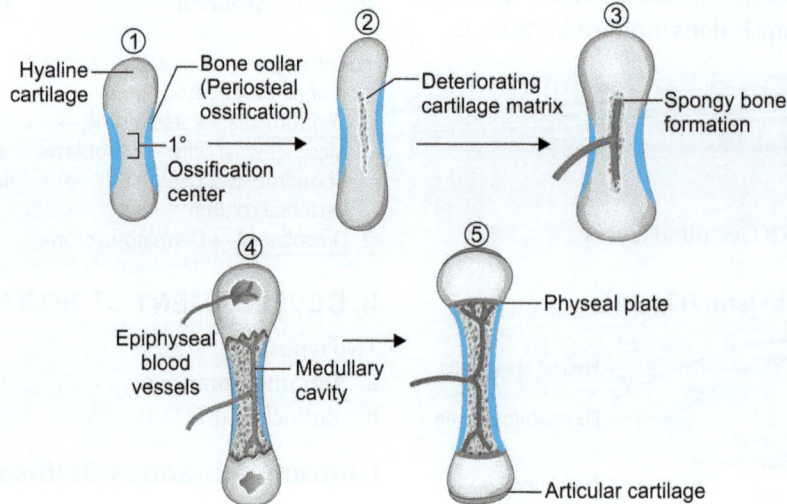

A cartilage model is formed which is subsequently replaced by bone.

1. Mesenchymal cells closely pack to form condensation at site of bone formation
2. Some mesenchymal cells become chondroblasts and lay down hyaline cartilage
3. Others form a membrane on the surface of the cartilage→ perichondrium
4. Perichondrium is vascular and has osteogenic cells (periosteum)
5. Inner layer of perichondrium is differentiated into osteoblasts
6. Formation of bone collar around the hyaline cartilage analage
7. Cartilage in center of diaphysis calcifies thus blocking nutrition
8. Chondrocytes die leaving behind empty cavities→primary areolae
9. Vessels and osteogenic cells (blasts and clasts) invade the cartilage matrix (periosteal bud)
10. Further resorb cartilage matrix to form larger cavities→secondary areolae
11. Ossification begins and continues to form medullary cavity
12. Secondary ossification centers → Epiphysis
13. Ossification extends in longitudinal direction hyaline cartilage remains only in the physeal plates and articular cartilage

17. Clinical application:
    i. Embryonic long bone formation
    ii. Longitudinal physeal growth.
    iii. Nonrigid fracture healing (2°) → Casting, IMN.

III. DEVELOPMENT OF JOINTS

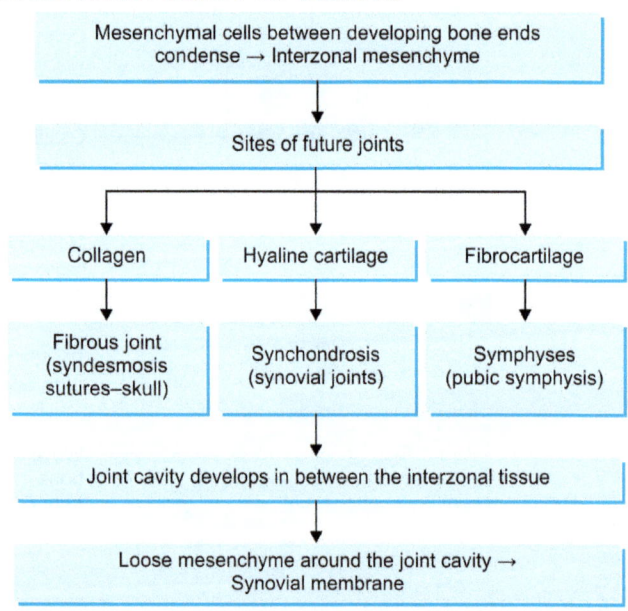

IV. AXIAL SKELETON

A.

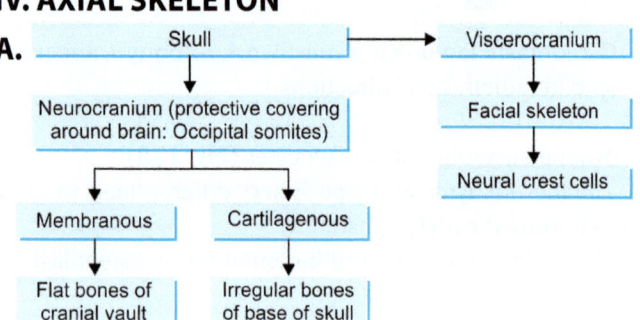

Clinical Application

1. Craniosynostosis: Premature closure of more than one sutures of skull.
   i. Scaphocephaly: Boat-shaped (sagittal sutures)
   ii. Acrocephaly: Short, high skull (coronal)
   iii. Plagiocephaly: Asymmetrically flattened skull (coronal and lambdoid)
2. Anencephaly: Vault missing. Not viable
3. Microcephaly: MR, small.
4. Congenital hydrocephalus: Widely separated.

B. Vertebral Column (Fig. 15)

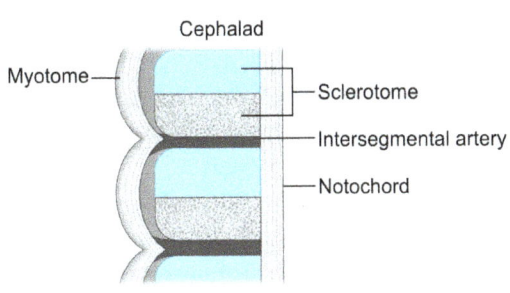
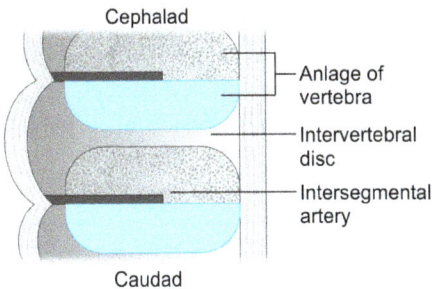

1. Notochord → Primitive axial support
2. Vertebral column is formed from sclerotomes of somites
3. Each sclerotome is separated from each other supero-inferiorly by the intersegmental artery.
   ↓
4. Caudal part of superior sclerotome unites with cranial part of inferior sclerotome.
   ↓
5. Dorsal extension of mesenchymal cells pass around the neural tube to form the vertebral arch.
6. Lateral extensions → Transverse process
7. Ventrally into the body wall → Ribs
8. Intervertebral tissue: Intervertebral disc
   Central part formed by → Notochord → Nucleus pulposus.
9. **Clinical application:**
   i. *Hemivertebra:* Only one side of vertebra is formed → Scoliosis
   ii. *Klippel–Feil syndrome:* Cervical vertebral fused.
   iii. *Spina bifida occulta:* Non-union of vertebral arches.
   iv. *Meningocele:* Protrusion of meninges through defect in vertebral arches.
   v. *Myelomeningocele:* Spinal cord protrudes.

C. Sternum and Ribs

1. Sternum: Parietal layer of lateral plate mesoderm.
2. Two mesenchymal sternal plates are formed on either side of ventral midline and these fuse to form cartilagenous sternum → ossify.
3. Ribs - costal element → sclerotomic cells of paraxial mesoderm
4. Clinical application:
   i. Pectus carinatum
   ii. Pectus excavatum
   iii. Cervical rib – C7 – Elongated costal element.

V. APPENDICULAR SKELETON

1. Derived from parietal layer of lateral plate mesoderm.
2. Limb buds → outpocketings from ventrolateral body all in the 5th week (UL just before LL)
3. Mesenchymal core covered by a layer of ectoderm.
4. Ectoderm thickens → Apical ectodermal ridge
   ↓
   Initiates and promotes growth of limb bud.
5. 6th week IU life → Outline of digits (Fig. 16)

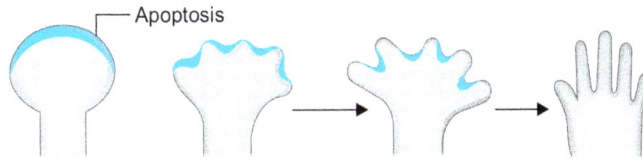

Interdigital areas → Cell death
6. 7th week: UL rotates 90° laterally
   : LL rotates 90° medially
7. 8th week: Subdivided by constrictions into arm, forearm and wrist (Fig. 17).
8. 12th week: 1° centers of ossification

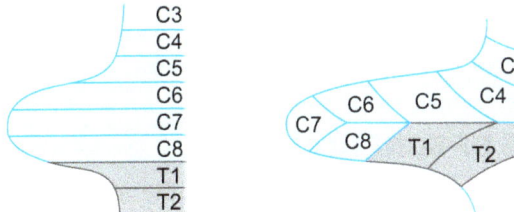
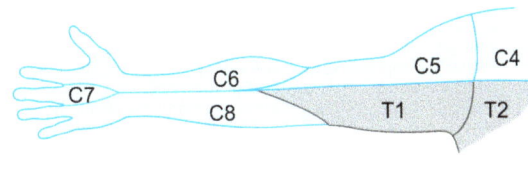

Fig. 17: Dermatomes of upper limb.

9. **Clinical application:**
   i. Teratogens → Extremities most susceptible during 4–7 week.
   ii. Amelia → complete absence of limb
   iii. Meromelia → partial absence of limb
   iv. Phocomelia → hand attached to trunk.
   v. Syndactyly → ≥fingers/toe fused
   vi. Polydactyly → ≥fingers/toes
   vii. Cleft hand/foot → fusion of 1st with 2nd and 4th with 5th and absence of 3rd digit.
   viii. Hand foot genital syndrome : fusion of carpal bones and small short digits + hypospadias
   ix. Marfan's syndrome: chr. 15q21 – Long slender limbs, hyperflexible joints.
   x. CTEV.

COLLAGEN

Most abundant protein in human body.

I. STRUCTURE

1. **Triple helix** → 2 α1 chains
                    1 α2 chains
2. Common amino acid sequence = Glycine-Proline-X
                                Glycine-Hydroxyproline-X
3. Collagen made up of elongated fibrils formed by fibroblasts.
4. Peculiarity → Formed both → Intracellularly
                               Extracellularly

II. FORMATION (FIG. 18)

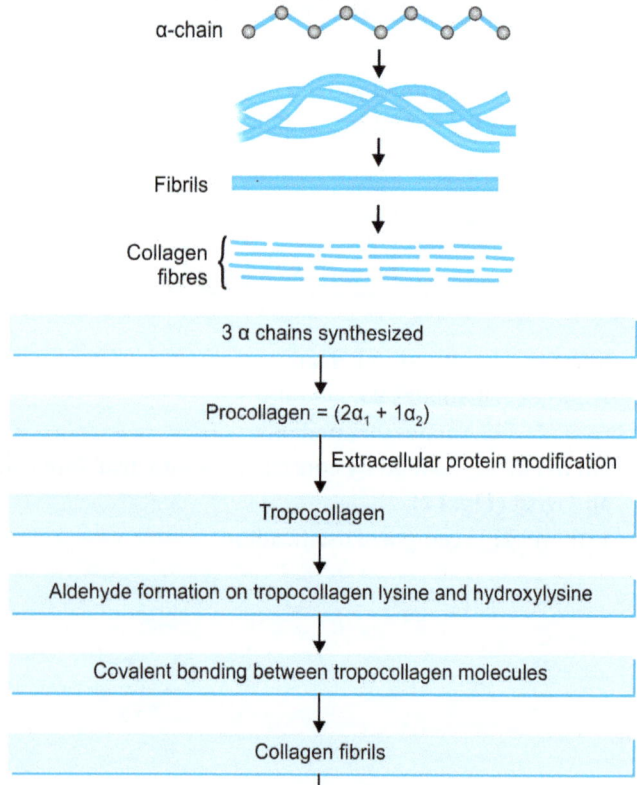

III. TYPES (> 25 types discovered)

I. Bone, ligament, tendon, meniscus
   Annulus fibrosus: Disc, reparative cartilage
II. Articular cartilage, NP – disc
III. Skin and blood vessels
IV. Cartilage basement membrane

IV. FUNCTION

1. Major constituent of most connective tissues
2. Strength and structural integrity
3. Good tensile strength
4. Skin and tendon: 70% collagen by dry weight
5. Bone: 23% dry weight
         90% organic matrix

V. DISORDERS

1. Osteogenesis imperfecta: Collagen I ⊗
2. Ehlers-Danlos syndrome: I and IV
3. Dupuytren's contracture: III
4. Scurvy: Vitamin C deficiency → Defective collagen production → Bleeding gums and bony abnormality.
5. CTEV → Collagen "crimps"
6. Autoimmune disorders → Autoantibodies to collagen → Erosive arthritis.
   i. RA
   ii. Psoriatic arthritis
   iii. SLE arthritis
7. Infantile cortical hyperostosis: Caffey's disease
8. Chondrodysplasias.

VI. APPLICATIONS

1. Wound healing: Open fracture dressing
2. Bone substitutes
3. Scaffold for delivery of growth factors → BMP, PRP
4. Helps in blood coagulation
5. Artificial temporary skin covering
6. Burns

VII. ADVANTAGES

Biocompatible, nontoxic, biodegradable.

BONE HEALING

Bone healing refers to complex and sequential events that occur to restore injured bone to preinjury state.

TYPES OF BONE HEALING

I. Healing with callus formation (2°, Indirect, endochondral)
II. Intramembranous repair (1°, Direct)
III. Healing by "Creeping substitution"

I. INDIRECT

→ MC, typical of diaphyseal fracture
Stages:
1. Hematoma formation
2. Inflammation
3. Granulation tissue formation
4. Soft callus formation
5. Hard callus formation
6. Remodeling

1. **Hematoma formation (Fig. 19):**

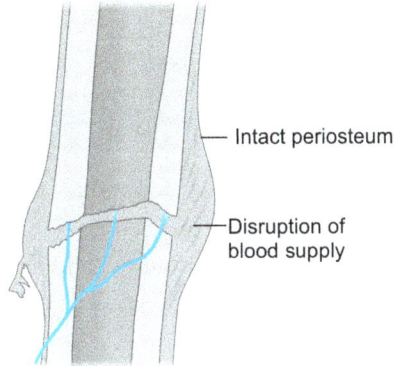

   i. Begins immediately (Day 1)
   ii. Disruption of blood vessels → hematoma
   iii. Soft tissue trauma.
   iv. Necrosis of 1-2 mm of bone due to loss of blood supply.
   v. Hematoma stabilized by fibrin fibers.

2. **Inflammation** (Day 1-5) **(Fig. 20):**

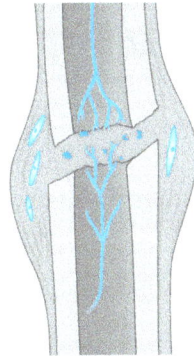

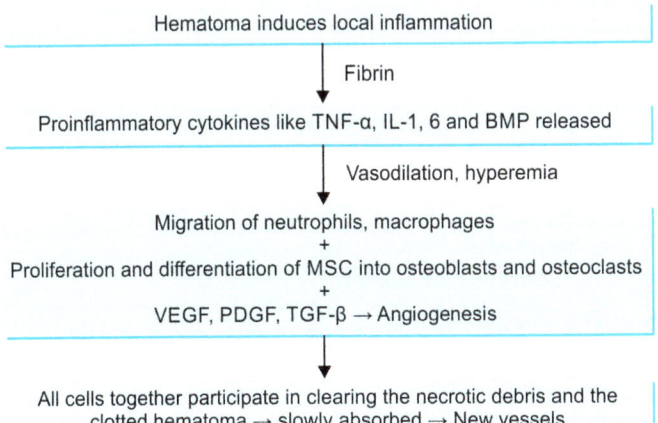

3. **Granulation tissue formation** (Day 5-14)

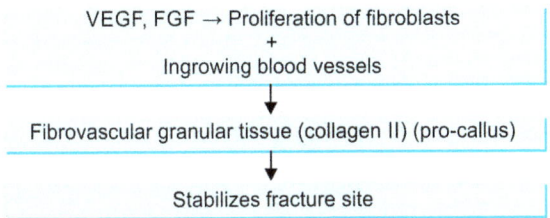

4. **Soft callus** (2-4 weeks) 1° callus **(Fig. 21):**

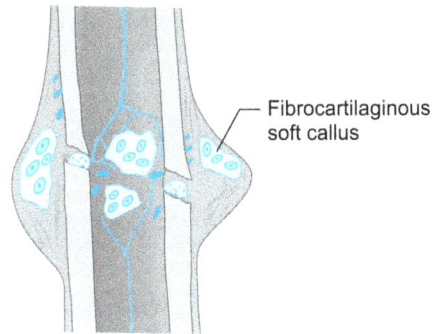

   a. Formation of callus → combined effect of four distinct healing responses
      i. Periosteum (most important)
      ii. Bone marrow
      iii. Bone cortex
      iv. External soft tissue
   b. Three types of callus:
      i. Periosteal bridging
      ii. Intramedullary
      iii. Intercortical
   c. Fibroblasts and chondroblasts form → Fibrocartilaginous soft callus
      ↓
      Anchorage to fracture ends.

5. **Hard callus** (4-16 weeks) **(Fig. 22):**

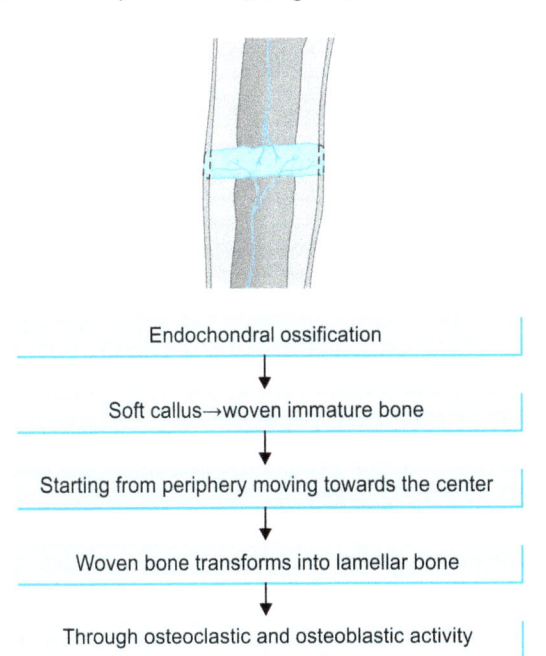

6. **Remodeling** (16 weeks–years) **(Fig. 23):**

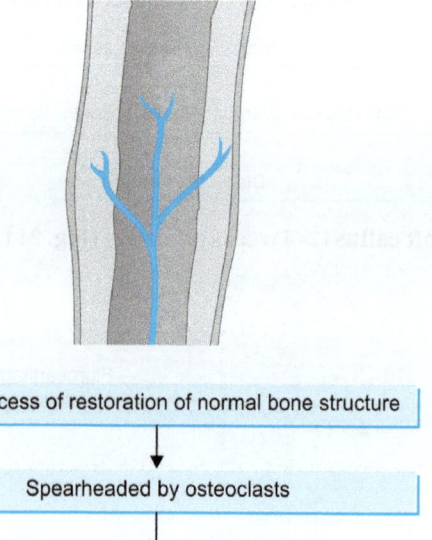

Slow process of restoration of normal bone structure
↓
Spearheaded by osteoclasts
↓
"Cutting cones" in "Howship lacunae"
↓
Osteoblasts lay down new bone

Wolff's law → Functional load and stress pattern on bone

II. DIRECT REPAIR

1. No callus formation
2. Intervening space < 500 μ → cutting cones, cross from one side to other
3. Gap healing → 200-500 μ
4. Contact healing → <200 μ
5. Due to rigid fixation (Compression plating)
6. Intramembranous healing via Haversian remodeling.

III. CREEPING SUBSTITUTION (BY PHEMISTER)

1. Seen in cancellous bone.
2. Typical of articular and periarticular fracture stabilized by rigid fixation.
3. Process of resorption of trabecular network of bone and laying down new bone by appositional ossification on the surface of the scaffold.

Factors Affecting Bone Healing (Expand this in Exam)

1. Patient related: Local/systemic, comorbidities, drugs, smoking.
2. Fracture related: Open/close, soft tissue condition, severity, location
3. Treatment related: Type of fixation.

CARTILAGE

I. INTRODUCTION

1. Specialized connective tissue that serves structural and functional purposes throughout the body.
2. Forms a temporary skeletal model in a growing embryo on which the future bone grows.

II. CLASSIFICATION

Hyaline cartilage	Fibrocartilage	Elastic cartilage
i. Articular cartilage ii. Physis	i. Intervertebral disc Annulus Fibrosus ii. Glenoid iii. Acetabular } labrum iv. Menisci v. Symphysis pubis	i. Epiglottis ii. Pinna

III. HYALINE CARTILAGE

1. Transparent
2. Bluish color
3. Composition → Cells → Chondrocytes
   → Intercellular matrix

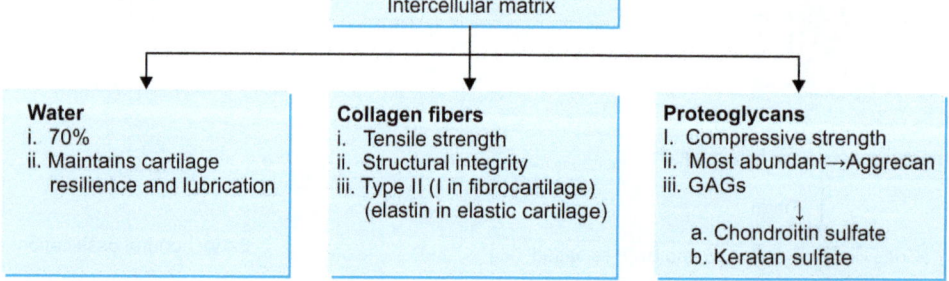

Intercellular matrix
- **Water**
  i. 70%
  ii. Maintains cartilage resilience and lubrication
- **Collagen fibers**
  i. Tensile strength
  ii. Structural integrity
  iii. Type II (I in fibrocartilage) (elastin in elastic cartilage)
- **Proteoglycans**
  I. Compressive strength
  ii. Most abundant → Aggrecan
  iii. GAGs
       ↓
       a. Chondroitin sulfate
       b. Keratan sulfate

IV. ARTICULAR CARTILAGE

1. Highly specialized connective tissue covers the intra-articular ends of long bones.
2. Types of hyaline cartilage → however does not have perichondrium.
3. Function:
   i. Smooth movements of joints → ↓ Friction
   ii. Shock absorbers
   iii. Distributes loads evenly.
4. Relatively acellular.
5. No vascular, neural, lymphatic supply.
6. Gross → Smooth Glistening white surface

7. Microscopy: Four zones (Fig. 24):

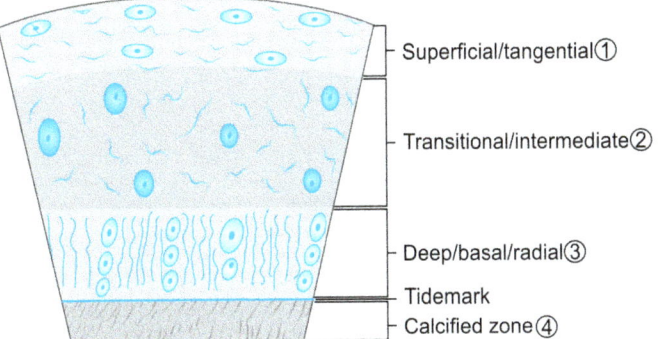

a. Superficial: Parallel collagen fibers.
   Flat chondrocytes
b. Transitional: Random arrangement of collagen fibers
   Round chondrocytes
c. Deep: Perpendicular collagen fibers
   Chondrocytes linearly arranged
d. Calcified zone: Tidemark separates deep and calcified zone.

8. Nutrition → Diffusion: From synovial fluid and subchondral bone.

9.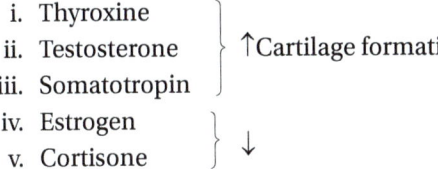

	Aging	OA
i. Water	↓	↑
ii. Elastic	↓	↓
iii. Stiffness	↑collagen crosslinking	Collagen disorganized
iv. GAG	↑ keratin/chondroitin	↑Chondroitin/keratin
v. Proteoglycans	↓ Size	Eventual ↓ in number

10. Hormone effect:
    i. Thyroxine
    ii. Testosterone } ↑Cartilage formation
    iii. Somatotropin
    iv. Estrogen   } ↓
    v. Cortisone

11. Repair/healing
    i. Limited capacity to heal due to:
       ↓
       a. Lack of blood supply
       b. Insufficient fibrin clot formation at site of injury
       c. Low mitotic activity of chondrocytes
       d. Inhibition of synovial cell attachment

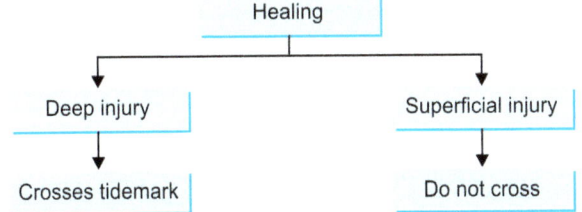

ii. Deep:
    1. Blood vessels from subchondral bone initiate healing process.
       ↓
       Fibrinous arcade scaffold directs the MSCs to form fibrocartilage matrix.
       ↓
       Repaired tissue intermediate between hyaline and fibrocartilage → Poor biochemical properties.
iii. Superficial
    ↓
    Stimulate chondrocyte proliferation but
    ↓
    1. Short-lived
    2. Avascular → No hematoma
                   No fibrin
                   No inflammation
                   No undifferentiated cell supply
    ∴ Never heals.

CARTILAGE INJURIES AND DEFECTS

I. DEFINITION
Spectrum of disease entities from single, focal defects to advanced degenerative disease of articular cartilage.

II. PATHOPHYSIOLOGY
1. Acute trauma
2. Chronic repetitive overload

III. CLASSIFICATION
Outerbridge (Arthroscopic)

Grade:
0: Normal
1: Softening and swelling
2: Small and superficial fissures
3: Deep fissures, crab meat
4: Exposed subchondral bone.

IV. CLINICAL FEATURES
1. Pain
2. Effusion
3. Mechanical symptoms: Locking, catching
4. Background factors predisposing to articular defects:
   i. Joint laxity
   ii. Malalignment
   iii. Compartment overload.

V. RADIOGRAPHS
AP, Lateral, Merchant, Semi-flexed 45° PA view → Most sensitive for early joint space narrowing.
1. Check alignment
2. Rule out bone defects and arthritis
3. Loose bodies
CT: Better evaluation of bone loss
    TT-TG distance
MRI: Most sensitive for evaluating focal defects.

VI. TREATMENT

A. Conservative
First line treatment for mild symptoms and low demand elderly.
1. Rest
2. Pain control → NSAIDs
3. Weight loss
4. Activity modifications
5. PT
6. Orthoses
7. Viscosupplementation and steroid injection

B. Operative
Indications: 1. Failure of non-surgical management
2. Acute osteochondral fracture resulting in full thickness loss of cartilage.
   Based on:

Patient factors	Defect factors
1. Age	1. Size → full / partial
2. Skeletal maturity	2. Location → weight bearing / nonweight bearing
3. Low vs high demand	3. Contained vs uncontained
4. Compliance: Extended rehabilitation	4. Presence of subchondral bone
	5. Traumatic vs degenerative

Management strategies		
Palliative	Reparative	Regenerative
1. Arthroscopic debridement and lavage (chondroplasty)	1. Abrasion chondroplasty 2. Microfracture and Pridie drilling	1. Osteochondral autograft transplantation (OATS)/ Mosaicplasty 2. Allograft implantation 3. Autologous chondrocyte implantation (ACI)

1. **Debridement (Chondroplasty):**
   A. Indications:
      i. Chondral lesions <2 cm²
      ii. Low demand, elderly
   B. Rationale:

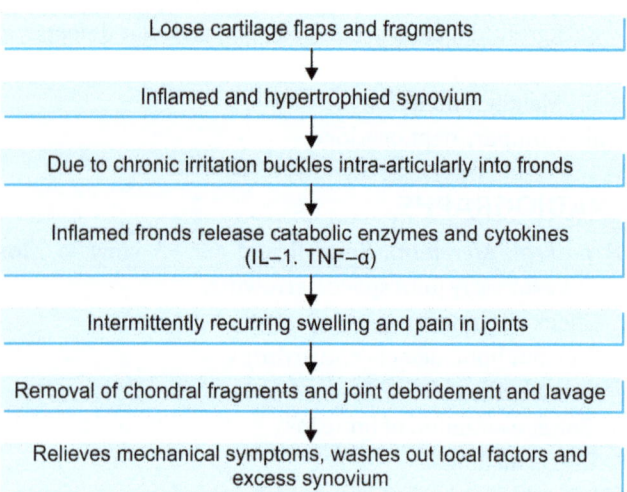

   C. Technique: Arthroscopic **(Fig. 25)**:

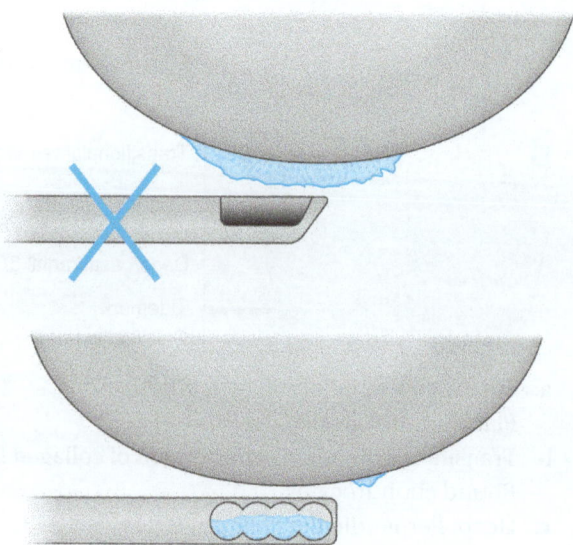

   While debridement cutting edge of arthroscopic blade → kept tangentially to resect articular flap.
   D. Advantages:
      i. Fast and simple procedure
      ii. Faster rehabilitation
   E. Disadvantages:
      i. Exposed layer of articular cartilage and subchondral bone
      ii. Unknown natural history after treatment

2. **Fixation:**
   i. Osteochondral fragment with adequate subchondral bone
   ii. Absorbable or Nonabsorbable screws (head less)

3. **Microfractures:**
   i. Goal: Allow access to marrow elements into the defect → to stimulate the formation of reparative tissue.
   ii. Technique **(Fig. 26)**:

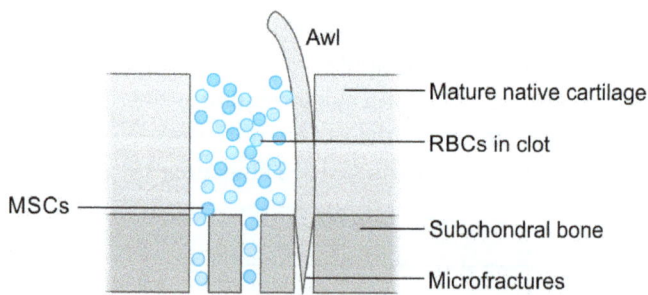

   1. Defect is prepared by debridement to have stable and smooth edges.
      ↓ Calcified layer is removed
   2. Provide a "pool" for the fibrin clot.
      ↓
   3. Awls are used to make multiple perforations in the subchondral bone (3–4 mm) apart.

iii. Indicated for lesions <2–3 cm². Perforations are made 3 mm deep.
iv. Blood clot provides a scaffold for growth factors and MSCs.

↓

Reparative tissue → Fibrous + Hyaline

↓

Weaker biomechanically

v. Advantages:
   a. Minimally invasive
   b. Easy
   c. Minimal surgical morbidities
   d. Cheaper
vi. Postoperative continuous passive movement for healing

4. **Abrasion chondroplasty:**
   i. Marrow stimulation technique
   ii. Exposed subchondral bone beneath cartilage defect at base → abraded using burr
   iii. MOA: Same as microfracture

5. **Osteochondral autograft transplantation (OATS) (Arthrex)/Mosaicplasty (S&N)**
   1. Replace a cartilage defect in a high weight bearing area with normal autologous cartilage and bone plugs from a low weight bearing area **(Fig. 27)**.

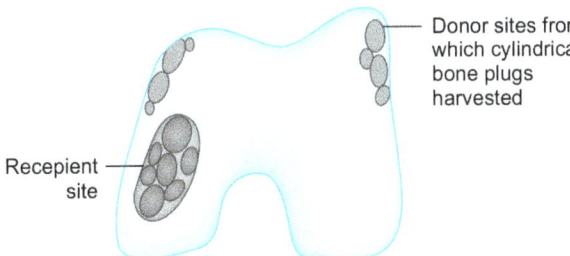

   2. Chondrocytes remain viable
   3. BG is incorporated into subchondral bone and overlying cartilage heals
   4. For full thickness defects = 2–6 cm²
   5. Donor graft slightly > recipient = press fit
   6. Approach → Open Medial parapatellar
                → Arthroscopic
   7. Advantages:
      i. Autologous tissue = No immune, infection
      ii. Single stage
      iii. Cost effectiveness
   8. Contraindications:
      i. Large and deep osteochondral defects
      ii. Arthritic knee
      iii. Degenerative lesions
      iv. Unstable, semidetached surrounding cartilage
      v. Angular deformity
      vi. Untreated instability
      vii. Major meniscal deficiency
   9. Limitations:
      i. Donor site morbidity
      ii. Size constraints
      iii. Matching size and radius of defect – difficult
      iv. Weight bearing – Nil × 3 months
   10. Allograft:
       a. Advantages:
          1. Smaller incision
          2. No donor site morbidity
          3. ↓ Surgical time
          4. Larger graft available
          5. Graft easily matched to contour
       b. Disadvantages:
          1. ↑ Cost, limited availability
          2. Live allograft → infection ↑

AUTOLOGOUS CHONDROCYTE IMPLANTATION (ACI)

I. DEFINITION

Cell-based therapy that involves transplantation of autogenous cells into cartilage defect → to form "hyaline – like" cartilage.

II. TECHNIQUE (FIG. 28)

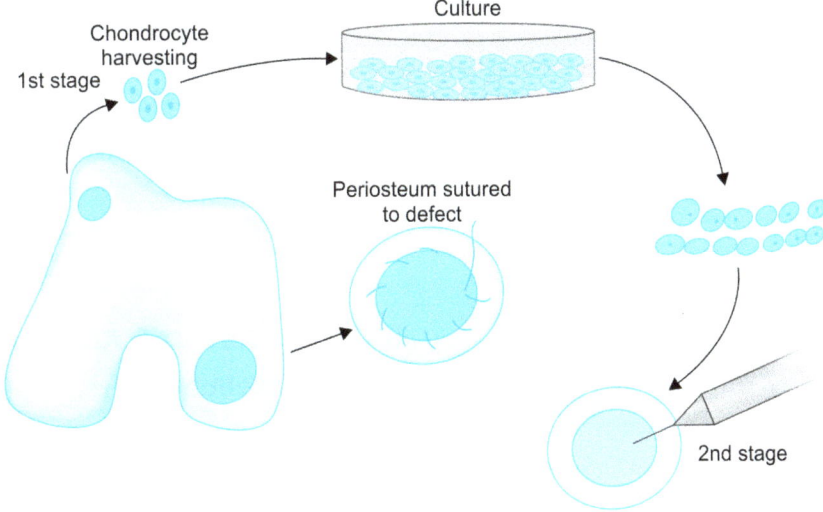

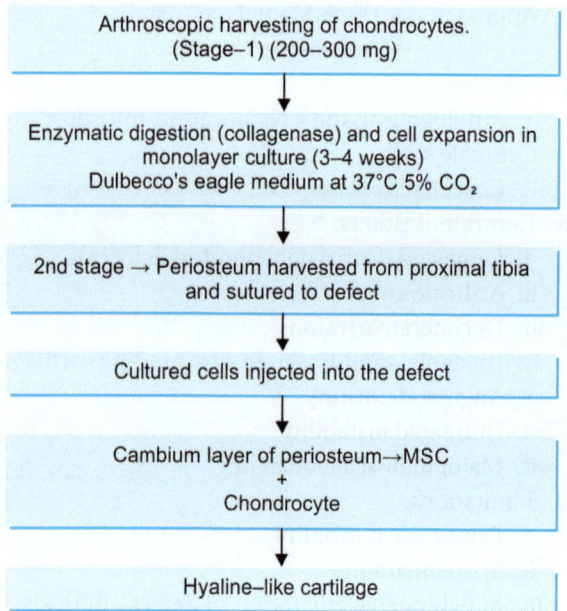

3. Prolonged time interval → ↑ Chondrocyte number
4. High cost
5. Prolonged non-weight-bearing
6. Ectopic calcification
7. Graft hypertrophy.

IX. RECENT ADVANCES

1. Co-culture ACI →
   i. Single-stage
   ii. MSCs + chondrocytes → MSC chondrogenic
   iii. ↓ Need of tedious chondrocyte culture
2. Deep osteochondral defect (>10 mm) → Sandwich technique **(Fig. 29)**

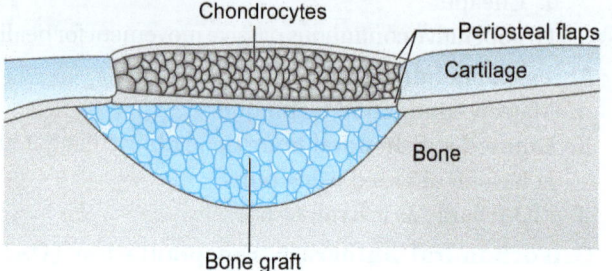

SYNOVIAL FLUID ANALYSIS

I. NORMAL SYNOVIAL FLUID FEATURES

1. Gross appearance: Clear, pale yellow (straw), viscous, does not clot.
2. Amount: 0.5–4 mL (Large joints)
3. Intra-articular pressure: –8 to –12 cmH_2O
4. Sterile
5. Specific Gravity: 1.008–1.005
6. Immune antibodies – Identical with blood serum
7. Cytology – 65/cumm Lymphocytes and Monocytes
8. Protein
   i. 2 g/dL, consisting of mucin, albumin, and globulin.
   ii. Albumin and Globulin → 5-6 times lower than plasma.
   iii. Albumin-to-Globulin ratio → 20:1
9. Synovial fluid contains
   i. Hyaluronic Acid
      a. Nourishes chondrocytes
      b. Reduces friction → lubricates
      c. Provides viscosity
   ii. Lubricin
      a. Glycoprotein
      b. Protects articular surfaces
      c. Controls synovial cell growth

III. INDICATIONS

1. Symptomatic focal chondral/OC defects
2. Defect >2 cm^2 on femur/patella
3. Age: 13–55 years
4. Compliant to postoperative rehab
5. Other modalities failed

IV. PREREQUISITES

1. Appropriate biomechanical alignment
2. Ligamentous stability
3. Range of motion → Normal

V. CONTRAINDICATIONS

1. Joint space narrowing (>50%)
2. Inflammatory joint disease
3. Unresolved septic arthritis
4. Metabolic/Crystal disorder
5. Obesity (>35 kg/m^2)

VI. GENERATIONS

1st = Periosteal flap
2nd = Collagen scaffold
   (Matrix induced chondrocyte implantation)
3rd = Chondrocyte and matrix culture system with growth factors
   ↓
   Biological, phenotypical characteristics

VII. ADVANTAGES

1. Not limited by defect size
2. Can produce hyaline cartilage

VIII. DISADVANTAGES

1. Large open arthrotomy
2. 2-staged

II. SYNOVIAL FLUID ANALYSIS

A. Gross Examination

1. Clarity:
   i. Normally transparent/clear
   ii. Rise in proteins and/or cells → Cloudy.

iii. Flecks can be rice bodies → TB, RA.
iv. In ochronosis, flecks resemble ground pepper or wear particles from prosthesis.
2. Color:
   i. Normally it is clear to a light yellow (straw)
   ii. Xanthochromia is seen in long standing hemorrhage and PVNS.
   iii. Opaque or cloudy white → inflammations and chronic arthritis
   iv. Chylous → Lymphatic obstruction
3. Viscosity:
   i. It is tested by suspending a drop of fluid from a needle tip (syringe drip test) or between two glass slides, a 3–5 cm long "string" is formed.
   ii. Increased water content leads to a shorter string → Inflammation
   iii. Also tested with Hess viscosimeter.
4. Clot formation (rope test):
   i. Glacial acetic acid is used to test for mucin clot formation.
   ii. A tight clump formation is seen when glacial acetic acid is added to synovial fluid due to aggregation of mucin.
   iii. The clump is firm, ropy and does not disintegrate on vigorous shaking.
iv. Inflammation → Mild: Clump is soft and friable.
   → Advanced: Cloudy flocculent precipitate formation.
v. Hemarthrosis → Spontaneous clot formation

B. Cell Counts and Microscopy

1. Normal WBC count → < 100 cumm
2. Differential Count
   i. Neutrophils = 0–20
   ii. Lymphocytes = 0–78
   iii. Monocytes = 0–71
   iv. Histiocytes = 0–26
   v. Synoviocytes = 0–12
3. RBCs → Hemorrhagic effusion
4. Eosinophils (>2%) → Rheumatic, allergic, parasitic diseases
5. Hemosiderin pigment (intra or extracellular) → Intra-articular hemorrhage
6. Iron laden chondrocytes → Hemochromatosis
7. Marrow fragments → Intra-articular fractures
8. Lipid laden macrophages → Traumatic arthritis
9. Ragocytes/Rheumatoid arthritis cells → Neutrophils containing refractile round cytoplasmic inclusions - Seen in RA, SLE.

C. Crystal Examination

TABLE: Characteristics of synovial fluid crystals.

Crystal	Shape		Compensated polarized light	Significance
Monosodium urate	Needles		Negative birefringence	Gout
Calcium pyrophosphate	Rhombic square, rods		Positive birefringence	Pseudogout
Cholesterol	Notched, rhombic plates		Negative birefringence	Extracellular
Corticosteroid	Flat, variable-shaped plates		Positive and negative birefringence	Injections
Calcium oxalate	Envelopes		Negative birefringence	Renal dialysis
Apatite (Ca phosphate)	Small particles require electron microscopy		No birefringence	Osteoarthritis

D. Chemical Examination
1. Glucose
   i. Difference in glucose concentration between plasma and synovial fluid is more important than absolute values.
   ii. Normally, difference is less than 10 mg/dL between serum and joint fluid.
   iii. Infection → Synovial fluid glucose < 20 mg/dL and difference exceeds 50%.
2. Lactate: Synovial fluid lactate rises in infections.
3. Protein:
   i. Limited use, does not differentiate between transudate and exudate.
   ii. Increase in protein concentration > 2.5 g/dL is abnormal and > 4.5 g/dL → inflammation.
   iii. Very low specificity

E. Microbiological and Immunological Examination
1. Gram stain → Rapid test to confirm pathogen.
2. Gene Xpert/TB MGIT → Tuberculosis
3. Latex agglutination → Fungal and bacterial antigens.
4. RA factor → RA

III. SYNOVIAL FLUID ANALYSIS FINDINGS IN VARIOUS DISORDERS

TABLE: Typical synovial fluid results in various disorder.

Gross	Normal fluid composition	Noninflammatory (like traumatic, reactive, degenerative)	Septic arthritis	Inflammatory arthropathies (like rheumatoid)	Crystal arthritis
Appearance	Clear, oil like viscous fluid	Reactive and degenerative effusion—clear, Blood stained—post-traumatic	Turbid	Cloudy	Usually cloudy
Viscosity	High	High	Inconsistent	Low	Inconsistent
Color	Straw	Yellow to red depending on hemorrhage	Cloudy to yellow	Cloudy yellow	Cloudy yellow
WBCs per mm^3	<100, usually monocytes	Up to 2,000 usually monocytes	>80,000, usually poly	2,000–50,000 (poly and mono)	2,000–75,000 (poly and mono)
Neutrophil	<25%	<25%	>75%	≥50	≥50
Crystals	No	No	No	No	Yes
Culture	Sterile	Sterile	±	Sterile	Sterile
Gram stain	–	–	±	–	–
Protein	<2 g/dL	N to (↓-dilutional) with hemorrhage the proteins increase but seldom increase above 5 g/dL	↑↑↑ (both albumin and characteristically globulin rise)	N to ↑↑↑ (complement level reduced in rheumatoid arthritis but N in ankylosing spondylitis). A:G ratio may be reversed in rheumatoid arthritis	↑↑ (globulins increase in proportion to duration of inflammation but unlike rheumatoid arthritis A:G ratio reduces but does not reverse)
Mucin clot	Firm	Firm	Friable, Whole aspirate cloudy	Friable	Friable
Glucose (difference from fasting blood sample)	≈0	≈0	>50 mg%	<50 mg%	>50 mg%

GAIT

I. INTRODUCTION

1. Rhythmic, cyclic movement of the limbs in relation to the trunk resulting in forward propulsion of the body.

   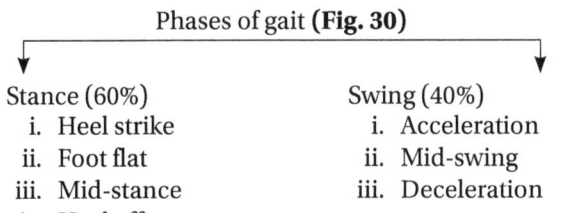
   Phases of gait (Fig. 30)

   Stance (60%)
   i. Heel strike
   ii. Foot flat
   iii. Mid-stance
   iv. Heel off
   v. Toe off (Fig. 30)

   Swing (40%)
   i. Acceleration
   ii. Mid-swing
   iii. Deceleration

2.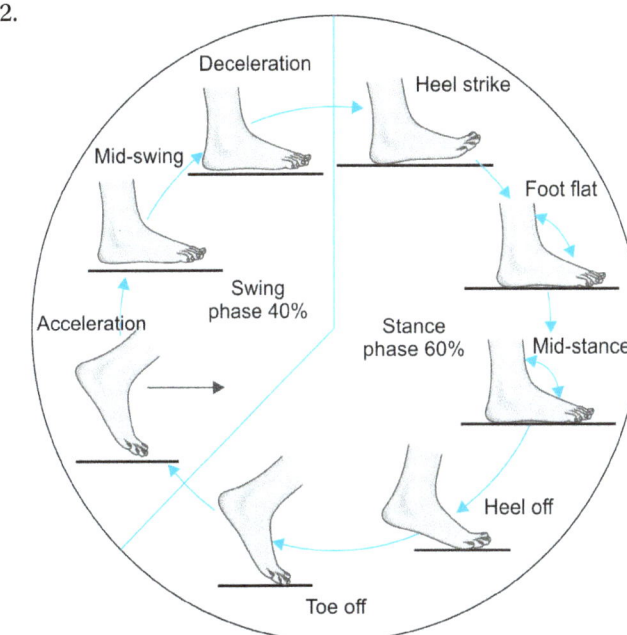

3. *Stride:* (Gait cycle): Distance from heel strike of one limb to heel strike of same limb again. (Stride length) (Fig. 31):

   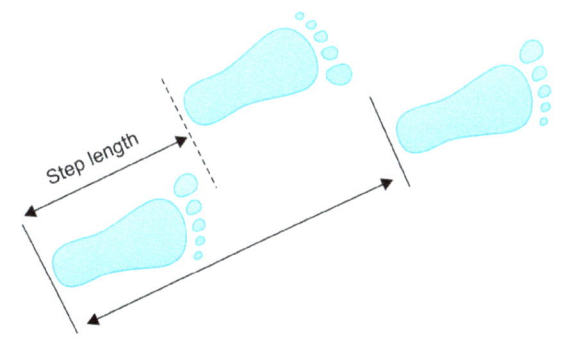

4. *Step length:* Distance from heel strike of one limb to heel strike of the other.
5. *Cadence:* Number of steps/minute. (N) = 70 steps/min.
6. *Double support:* Both limbs on ground
   While running → No double support
   ↓
   Double float

7. *Components of gait:*
   i. *Progression:* Forward fall of the body
   ↓
   Primary force generated by lower limb.
   ii. *Stability:* Controlled fall → maintains upright stability of body.
   ↓
   Body most stable during stance and least → swing.
   iii. *Energy conservation:*
   1. Calculated as O_2 consumed/meter of walking
   2. Efficiency ↑ with ↓ muscular effort to walk
   ↓
   a. Substituting momentum for muscle action
   ↓
   Smooth swinging movements without jerks
   Minimizing displacement of body from line of progression.
   ↓
   b. Ensuring center of gravity shifts only 5 cm up or down and sideways. (Saunders gait determinants)
   COG = 5 cm in front of S_2

II. PHASES

A. Stance

1. **Heel strike**

Ankle	Neutral	D. Flexors (TA, EHL, EDL) prevent foot from slapping
Knee	Extension	Quadriceps concentric contraction
Hip	30° flexion	Gluteus max. and hamstrings prevent flexion beyond 30°

2. **Foot flat**

Ankle	15° PF	PF of ankle control movement of tibia over foot
Knee	15° flexion	Quadriceps concentric contraction
Hip	15° flexion	↓ Flexion by G. maximus

3. **Mid-stance**

Ankle	3° Dorsiflexion	Balancing by plantar flexors
Knee	10° Flexion	Both quadriceps and hamstrings inactive, passive movement
Hip	Neutral	

4. Heel off

Ankle	15° plantar flexion	Active plantar flexor contraction
Knee	Neutral/extension	Active gastrocnemius contraction prevents hyperextension
Hip	7–8° Extension	No activity

5. Toe-off

Ankle	20° Plantarflexion	Plantar flexors become inactive at the end of toe off
Knee	20–30° Flexion	Quadriceps prevents hyperflexion
Hip	10° Extension	Iliopsoas starts getting active at the end

6. Swing phase

1. Ankle	Neutral	Ankle dorsiflexors maintain neutral position of ankle (Foot clearance)
2. Knee	40° flexion ↓ 60° flexion ↓ Extension	Hamstrings first cause further flexion and during late swing quadriceps start contracting
3. Hip	Extension to 20° flexion	Iliopsoas, rectus femoris, Sartorius. Adductors → Bring limb in line of progression

III. GAIT ANALYSIS

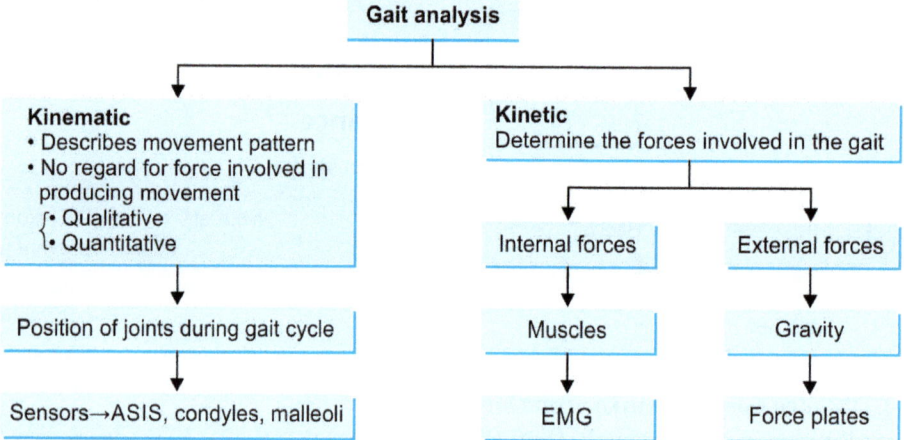

Gait analysis → Observational
　　　　　　→ Instrumental

A. Observational

1. Systemic method of gait assessment for deviations and functional deficits.
　　↓
2. Person walks on smooth surface → 10 feet
　　↓
3. Observed from front, back and sides
4. Three phases:
   i. *Preparation:* Detailed clinical history of gait problem.
   ii. *Observation:* Points 2 and 3
   iii. *Interpretation:* Analysis to identify gait deviations.

B. Instrumental

1. *Movement measurements:* Magnitude and timing of limb – segment motion.
2. *Dynamic electromyography:* Surface electrodes to record → myoelectric potentials
　　↓
　Skeletal muscle activity
3. *Force platform:* Determines stance phase: ground reaction force.
4. *Stride analysis:* Velocity, cadence, step length
　　↓
　By pressure sensors beneath the heel and metatarsal heads

5. *Energetics:* O₂ consumption during gait.
   ↓
   Oxygen spirometry
   ↓
   Energy efficiency of gait.

IV. PATHOLOGICAL GAITS

1. **Hand-to-knee/Quadriceps gait (Fig. 32):**

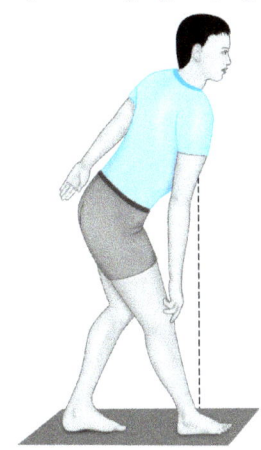

   i. Normally, the knee is locked in extension during foot - flat → mid-stance phase.
      ↓
   ii. Due to contraction of quadriceps
      ↓
   iii. This helps in transmitting weight to the lower limb.
   iv. However, when quadriceps is weak
      ↓
      Buckling of the knee and loss of balance
   v. The patient may be able to prevent buckling if.
      a. Normal hip extensors
      b. Normal ankle plantar flexors
   vi. Compensatory mechanism:
      a. Patient physically pushes the anterior thigh posteriorly to prevent buckling.
      b.

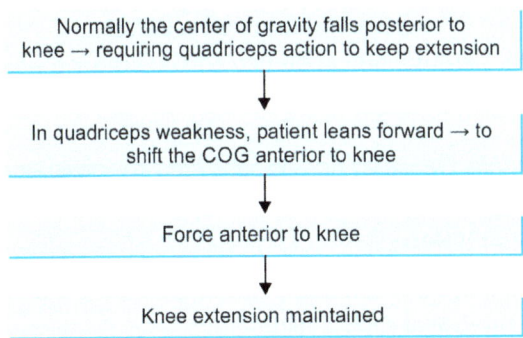

   vii. Etiology:
      1. Poliomyelitis
      2. Stroke
      3. Cerebral palsy
      4. Lyme's disease
      5. Myopathies and muscular dystrophy
      6. Osteoarthritis of knee
      7. Quadriceps tendon rupture → traumatic
      8. PID
   viii. Treatment:
      1. Physiotherapy: Isometric and isotonic quadriceps strengthening exercises
      2. Gait training and balancing
      3. TENS
      4. Orthosis:
         i. Knee ankle foot orthosis (KAFO) **(Fig. 33)**
         ii. Locked knee brace
         iii. Ground reaction AFO

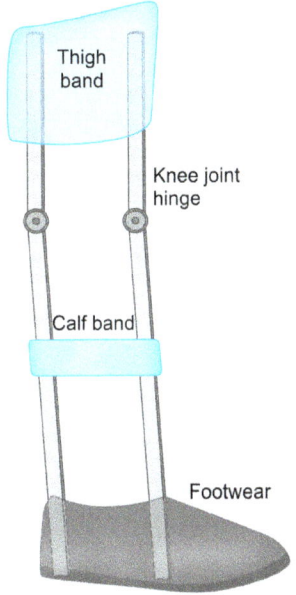

Fig. 33: Knee ankle foot orthosis (KAFO).

2. **Trendelenburg gait (B/L Waddling)**
   i. Abnormal gait resulting from defective hip abductor mechanism
      ↓
      a. Fulcrum: Femur head (hip joint)
      b. Lever arm: Femur neck → GT
      c. Load: Gluteus medius and minimus
   ii. Pathophysiology **(Fig. 34):**

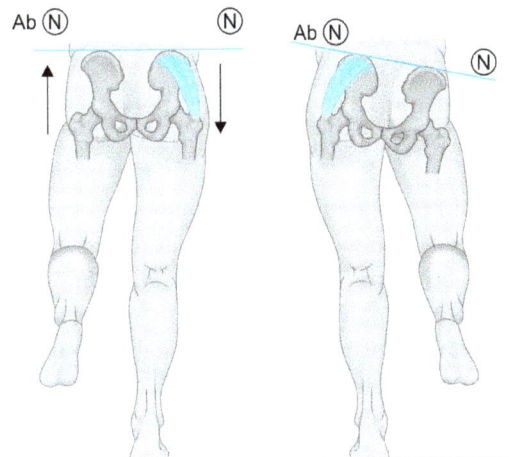

Fig. 34: Trendelenburg gait: "Sound side sags".

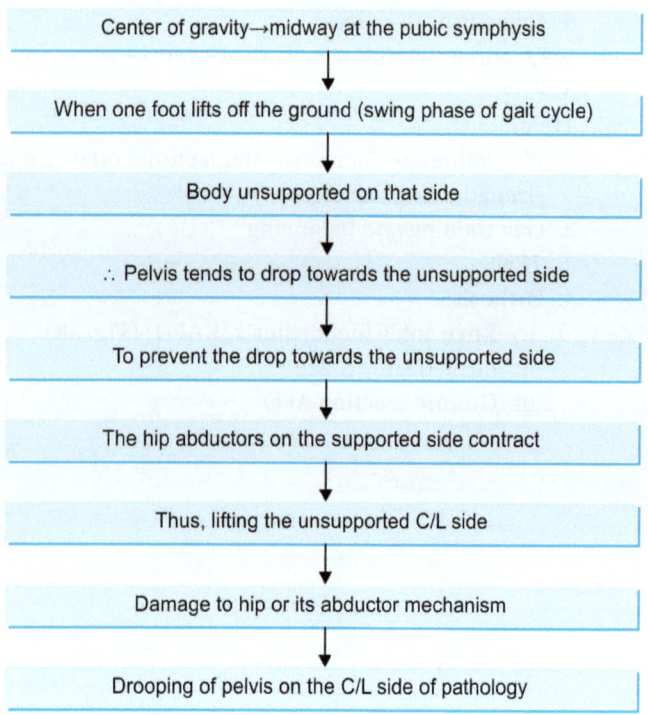

iii. Etiology:
   a. Damage to fulcrum:
      1. ON hip
      2. LCPD
      3. DDH
      4. Chronically dislocated hip
         i. Post-traumatic
         ii. Pathological → TB hip
   b. Failure of lever arm:
      1. Coxa vara
      2. Neck of femur nonunion
      3. GT avulsion
   c. Failure of effort:
      1. Poliomyelitis
      2. L5 radiculopathy
      3. Superior gluteal nerve palsy
      4. Gluteus medius, minimus tendinitis
      5. G. medius abscess
      6. Postoperative THR
      7. Postoperative PFN
iv. Treatment: Treat the cause (elaborate)

3. **Antalgic gait**
   i. Stance phase↓: Pain in the weight bearing limb. OA, fracture, tendinitis
4. **Circumduction gait:** To avoid foot from scrapping the ground → hip and LL rotates outward. Hemiplegia
5. **High stepping gait:** Due to foot drop → the patient flexes the hip and knee extensively to raise the dropped foot.
6. **Sensory/stamping/stomping gait:** Loss of proprioceptive input → slams the foot hard on ground in order to sense it.
   Tabes dorsalis, diabetic neuropathy, Vitamin B_{12} deficiency
7. **Scissoring gait:** One leg crosses directly over the other during each step. CP
8. **Rocking horse gait (Fig. 35):**

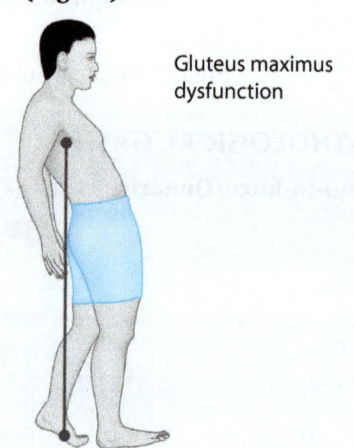

Gluteus maximus dysfunction

Trunk shifts posteriorly to shift the COG posterior to G. Max
↓
Reduces effort required to keep hip in extension in stance phase

9. **Cerebellar (ataxic)** = Reeling gait
   Wide based, clumsy, staggering moves side to side → Titubation
10. **Hamstring/Genu recurvatum gait**
    Knee hyperextension in stance phase
    ↓
    Hamstring ⊗
11. **Short limb gait**: <1.5 cm: Pelvic tilt
    Up to 5 cm: Equinus
    >5 cm: Body dip same side, C/L knee flexion
12. **Shuffling gait:**
    i. Stooped forward, flexion at knee
    ii. Steps → Short, barely clear the ground
    iii. Festination: Difficult to stop once gait is initiated.
13. **Alderman's gait:**
    i. Head and chest thrown backward.
    ii. Protuberant abdomen and legs thrown wide apart
    iii. TB spine → Lower dorsal, upper lumbar.

BLOOD COMPONENTS

I. RATIONALE

1. Separation of blood into components allows optimal survival of each constituent.
2. Transfusion of only specific blood component that patient requires.
3. Avoid use of unnecessary component which maybe C/I to a patient.
4. Multiple patients treated with blood from one donor.
5. Supplements blood supply → Adds to blood inventory.

II. PROCESSING

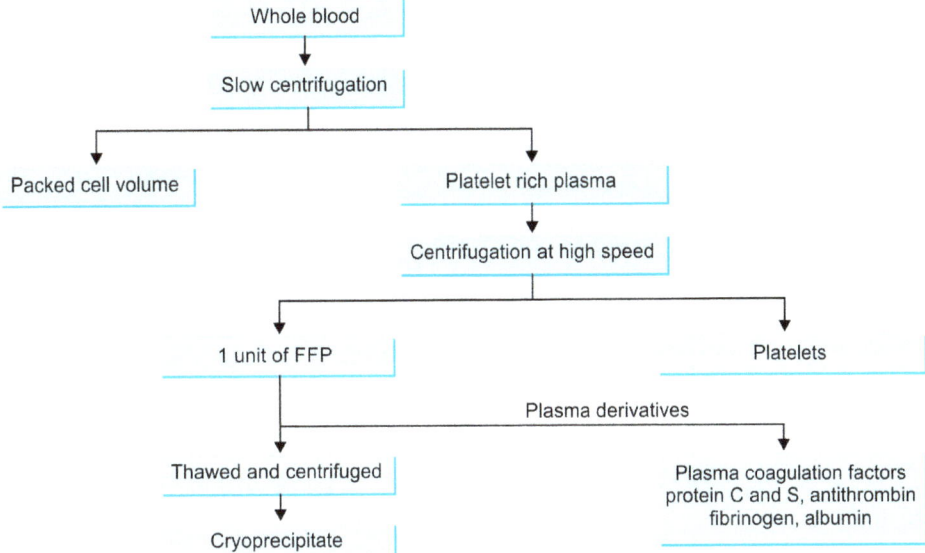

III. COMPONENTS

i. Packed Red Blood Cells

1. Raise oxygen carrying capacity of blood.
2. 1 unit → Raises Hb by 1.2 g/dL
3. For normovolemic patients of chronic anemia without cardiac disease.
4. Acute blood loss → Hemorrhage
   → Surgical blood loss
5. Shelf life: 35–42 days → ↑ by addition of adenosine
6. Storage temp 2–6°C
7. Volume = 250–300 mL
8. Leukocyte reduced - PCV: ↓ Immunological reactions

ii. Platelet Rich Plasma

1. Function:
   i. ↑Extracellular matrix deposition
   ii. ↓ Pro-apoptotic signals
   iii. Minimize joint inflammation
2. Use:
   i. Lateral epicondylitis
   ii. Rotator cuff tears
   iii. Sub acromial impingement
   iv. Patellar tendinosis
   v. Plantar fasciitis
   vi. Nonunion
   vii. Tendoachilles tear
3. PRP: Platelet count 4–5 times than normal.

iii. Platelets

1. Threshold for prophylactic platelet transfusion: 10,000/μL.
   ↓
   Thrombocytopenia with hemorrhage.
2. Levels required for invasive procedure: 50,000 μL
3. Volume = 50–70 mL
4. Storage = 20–24°C
5. If possible ABO specific platelets, but not necessary.

iv. Fresh Frozen Plasma

1. Contains → All coagulation factors.
   → Plasma proteins: Albumin and globulin
2. Volume: 250 mL
3. Shelf life = 1 year
4. Storage temperature = −20°C
5. Uses:
   a. Coagulopathy of massive transfusion
   b. Liver diseases
   c. Disseminated intravascular coagulation
   d. Reversal of warfarin toxicity

v. Cryoprecipitate

1. Fibrinogen, Factor VIII, von Willebrand factor
2. Volume = 10–20 mL
3. Shelf life: Frozen – 1 year
4. Use:
   i. von Willebrand disease
   ii. Hypofibrogenemia
   iii. Hemophilia
   iv. Cryoprecipitate + thrombin = fibrin glue
      ↓
      Sealant

vi. Albumin

1. 5 or 25% solution
2. Use:
   i. Hypovolemia and hypoalbuminemia in surgical setting
   ii. Preoperative and postoperative optimization: Better wound healing, ↓ infection

HAZARDS OF BLOOD TRANSFUSION

Immune mediated: Preformed donor or recipient antibodies	Nonimmune: Chemical and physical properties of stored blood	Infections
1. Acute hemolytic transfusion reactions	1. Hypothermia	**Viral**
2. Delayed extravascular hemolytic reaction	2. Circulatory overload	HIV
3. Febrile non-hemolytic reactions	3. Iron overload	Hepatitis B, C
4. TRALI	4. Electrolyte imbalance	Parvovirus, CMV
5. GVHD		**Bacterial**
6. Septic reaction		Pseudomonas
7. Anaphylaxis		Serratia
		Yersinia
		Parasites
		Plasmodium treponema

Common treatment for immune-mediated reactions:
a. Stop blood transfusion
b. Anti-histaminic
c. Corticosteroids

A. IMMUNE-MEDIATED

1. **Acute hemolytic transfusion reactions:**
   i. Recipients have preformed antibodies to donor RBC antigens (ABO and Rh).
   ii. Hypotension, fever with chills, dyspnea, chest pain.
   iii. Label the post-transfused and untransfused blood → Send to blood bank → Retesting.
   iv. Lysis of RBCs → Renal damage → Diuretics (furosemide)

2. **Delayed extravascular hemolytic reactions:**
   i.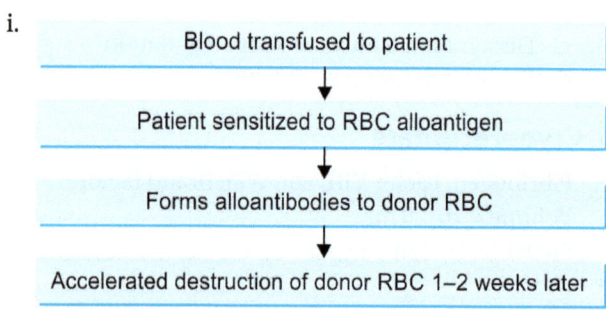
   ii. Rx: Additional transfusion may be required.

3. **Febrile nonhemolytic reactions**
   i. MC transfusion associated reaction
   ii. Antibodies react with donor WBCs and HLA antigen
   iii. Fever with chills and rigor
   iv. Reduced by leukocyte: Reduced PCV

4. **Transfusion-related acute lung injury (TRALI)**
   i. Most common cause of transfusion-related mortality.
   ii. Dyspnea, tachycardia, cyanosis, hypotension.
   iii. Non-cardiogenic pulmonary edema within 6 hours of transfusion.
   iv. Donor plasma has high titer of anti-HLA II Ab
       ↓ bind to
       Recipients WBC → Clumping in pulmonary vessels
       ↓
       ↑ Capillary permeability ← Cytokine storm
       ↓
       Pulmonary edema
   v. Oxygen and ventilator support.

5. **Anaphylactic reactions:**
   i. Severe reaction within minutes of starting BT.
   ii. Coughing, bronchospasm, loss of consciousness, respiratory arrest, shock.
   iii. 1 mL epinephrine (1:1,000) subcutaneously.

6. **Graft-versus-host disease:**
   i. Donor T-lymphocyte → Host HLA antigens.
   ii. Cutaneous eruption, fever, diarrhea, abnormal liver function test.
   iii. Starts 8–10 days after blood transfusion. Death at 3–4 weeks.

7. **Septic reactions:**
   i. Highest with platelet transfusion as they are stored at room temperature.
   ii. *Staphylococcus, Enterobacter, Pseudomonas.*
   iii. Blood culture and sensitivity → Antibiotics, fluid and CVS support.

B. NONIMMUNOLOGIC REACTIONS

1. **Hypothermia:**
   i. Refrigerated blood products transfused soon after removal from refrigerator.
   ii. Cardiac arrhythmia → due to cold fluid → SA node.
   iii. Transfuse at room temperature.
   iv. Rate = 5 mL/minute.

2. **Electrolyte disturbance:**
   i. Massive blood transfusion.
   ii. Concern of pediatrics and neonates
   iii. Hypocalcemia → tingling, numbness, tetany.

3. **Circulatory overload:**
    i. Was seen with whole blood transfusion.
    ii. Patient with compromised cardiac reserve.
    iii. Use diuretics simultaneously.
4. **Iron overload:**
    i. Multiple blood transfusions – Thalassemia, sickle cell anemia
    ii. Iatrogenic hemochromatosis
    iii. Treatment: Deferoxamine and deferasirox. Erythropoietin as alternative.
5. **Infections:**
    i. Compulsory screening: HIV-1, 2, HBV, HCV, Human T-cell lymphotropic virus, Syphilis.
    ii. CMV and Parvovirus B19: Immunocompromised patients.

AUTOLOGOUS TRANSFUSION

Collection and transfusion of patients own blood cells.

I. METHODS

1. **Intraoperative cell salvage (ICS) (Fig. 36)**
    i. Blood collected from suctions and surgical drains.
    ↓
    Washed, filtered → Retransferred.

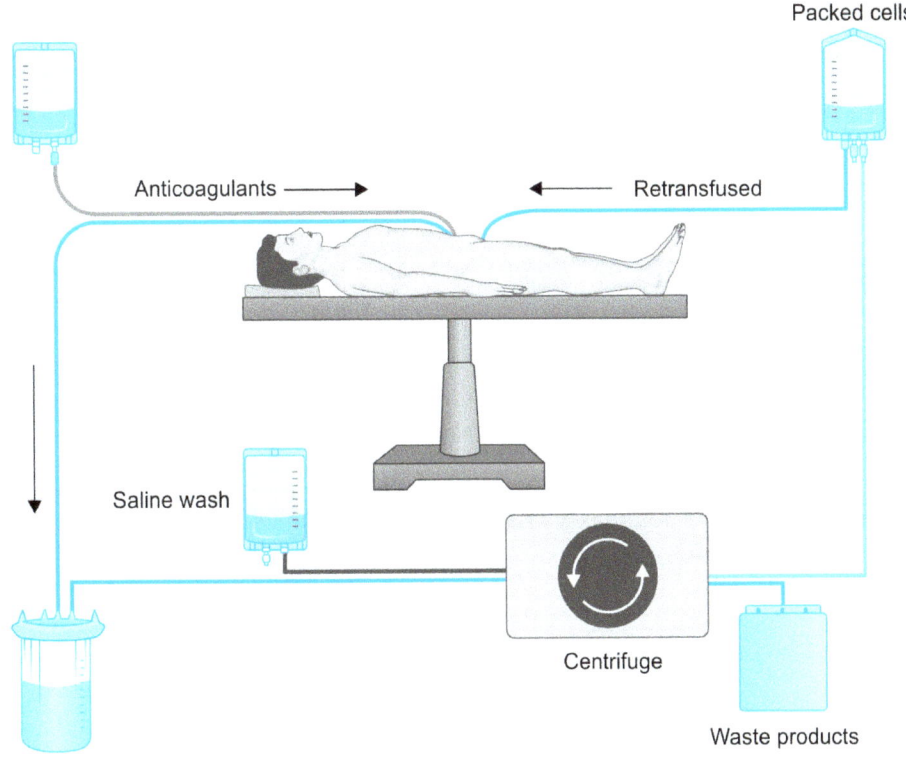

2. **Preoperative autologous transfusion (PAD)**
    i. Blood collected in advance of an elective surgery
    ↓
    Stored in blood bank → Transfused when needed
3. **Acute normovolemic hemodilution (ANH)**
    i. Blood collected immediately prior to surgery
    ↓
    ii. Volume restored by colloid/crystalloid.
    iii. Blood retransfused toward end of surgery
4. **Postoperative cell salvage (not recommended)**
    i. Blood from wound drains of THR and TKR
    ↓
    Filtered and processed → infused

II. INDICATIONS

1. Major elective surgery:
    i. Scoliotic spine surgery
    ii. Revision total hip arthroplasty
    iii. Pelvic tumors
2. Anticipated blood loss >20%
3. Blood collected in abdominal cavity due to organ rupture or during surgery
4. Jehovah's witness → Not willing to accept allogenic blood
5. Rare blood group.

III. ADVANTAGES

1. Reduced allogenic blood transfusion reactions
2. No risk of disease transmission

3. ICS → Fresh RBCs → immediately active, no lag period for oxygen carrying capacity
4. Supplies blood in proportion to losses occurring.

IV. CONTRAINDICATIONS

i. Use of substances in the operative field that are not licensed for using intravenous
   1. Iodine
   2. Topical clotting agents
   3. Non-IV antibiotics
   4. PMMA cement
   5. Irrigation solutions causing damage to blood → Hydrogen peroxide
   6. Extensive bone reaming fragments
ii. Aspiration of body fluids and contaminated fluids into wound site.
   1. Pleural effusions
   2. Fat
   3. Urine
   4. Malignant cells
iii. Sickle cell anemia

DVT AND PULMONARY EMBOLISM

I. INTRODUCTION

1. Venous Thromboembolism = Deep vein thrombosis + pulmonary embolism
2. *Deep vein thrombosis:* Formation of a blood clot (thrombus) in one of the deep veins of the body
3. *Pulmonary embolism:* Occlusion of a pulmonary artery by a thrombus (or fat, air, tumor tissue)

II. ETIOPATHOGENESIS

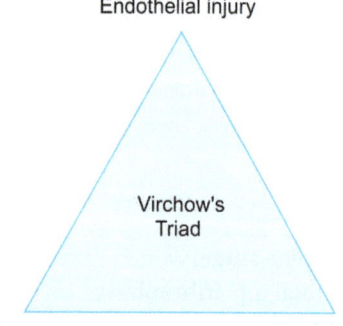

i. *Trauma:*
   1. Polytrauma
   2. Multiple long bone fractures
   3. Severe pelvic fracture
   4. Spine fracture with paralysis
   5. Hip fracture
ii. *Arthroplasty:* Total hip, knee replacement
iii. *Risk factors:*
   1. Previous DVT
   2. Obesity
   3. Age
   4. Pregnancy and OCPs
   5. Immobilization >3 days
   6. Sepsis
   7. Major orthopedic surgery >2 hours.

III. CLINICAL FEATURES

A. DVT:
1. Leg and calf pain
2. Edema: Most specific
3. Phlegmasia alba dolens: Pain, edema and *white blanching skin without cyanosis*
4. Phlegmasia cerulea dolens: Progression from alba dolens with worsening pain and *cyanosis from ischemia*
5. Raised temperature locally
6. Calf tenderness
7. Homan's sign → Pain on DF
8. Erythema

B. PE:
i. *Symptoms*:
   1. Chest pain and tightness
   2. Impending sensation of doom
   3. Cough
   4. Shortness of breath
   5. Palpitations
   6. Hemoptysis
   7. Dizziness
ii. Signs:
   1. Tachypnea
   2. Tachycardia
   3. Hypoxia
   4. Distended neck veins
   5. Hypotension
   6. Diaphoresis → ↑ sweating.

IV. INVESTIGATIONS

A. DVT:
1. Venous Doppler
2. Venography: Gold standard.
3. CT → 90% sensitive, 95% specific

B. PE:
i. Chest X-ray:
   1. Enlarged helium and mediastinum
   2. Atelectasis
   3. Hampton's hump: Pleural based infiltrate
   4. Pulmonary edema
ii. D-Dimer → >500 µg/L
iii. Pulmonary angiography: Gold standard
iv. Helical chest CT
v. Nuclear Medicine: Ventilation perfusion ratio : Dye – sensitive patients
iv. ECG = S1Q3T3

V. TREATMENT

A. PE:
1. Emergency
2. Resuscitation: Basic life support → CAB
3. Management of cardiogenic shock → Fluids
   Inotropes → Dobutamine
4. Anti-coagulant therapy → Heparin

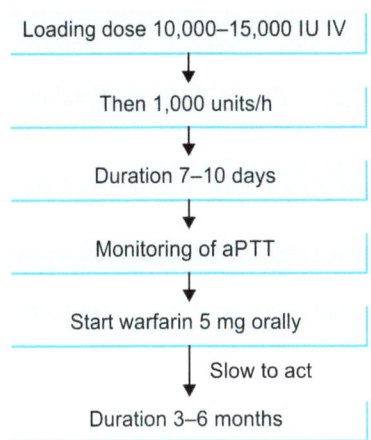

5. Thrombolytic therapy: Fibrinolysis (streptokinase, alteplase)
6. Surgery: Pulmonary embolectomy IVC filters.

B.

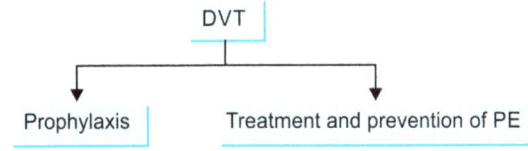

→ Anticoagulant therapy and surgical IVC filters

THROMBOPROPHYLAXIS/NEW ANTICOAGULANTS/LMWH

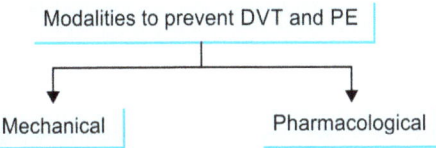

I. MECHANICAL

i. Reduce venous stasis and promote blood flow through external compression.
   1. Graduated compression stockings
   2. Intermittent pneumatic compression devices (IPC)
      ↓
      External pumps → substitute function of calf pumps
      →18 hours compliance
   3. Venous foot pumps
      Foot impulse technology
   4. Mobilization

ii.
Advantages	Disadvantages
1. Lack of bleeding potential	1. Suboptimal compliance
2. No lab monitoring	2. Cannot use in open fracture, PVD, infection, ulceration
3. No clinically significant Side effects	3. Used alone → Not entirely efficacious

II. PHARMACOLOGICAL

i. **Aspirin:**
   1. Acetylsalicylic acid
   2. Inexpensive, oral
   3. Dose (50–100 mg/day)
   4. AAOS → VTE prophylaxis for low-risk patients. (although low efficacy than others)
   MOA → Platelet inhibition

ii. **Unfractionated heparin:**
   1. Anticoagulant + thrombolytic.
   2. Heparin binds to antithrombin (AT)
      ↓
      Heparin – AT complex
      ↓
      Inactivates factor IIa, Xa, XIa, XIIa, IXa
   3. Mode of administration = IV, SC
   4. Bolus of 5,000 units/8 hours: Prophylaxis
   5. *Disadvantages:*
      a. Monitoring aPTT
      b. Heparin-induced thrombocytopenia
      c. Osteoporosis.

iii. **Low molecular weight heparin (LMWH):**
   I. MOA:
      1. Contain active AT III binding site.
         ↓
         Derived from standard heparin
         ↓
         By depolymerization (14–16 KDa → 4–8 KDa)
         Heparin AT III complex → Inactivates IIa, IXa, Xa, XIa, XIIa
      2. Endogenous release of vWF
      3. Reduced platelet aggregation
   II. Dose:
      Enoxaparin – 20 mg BD SC starting 12–14 hours postoperative → Low-to-moderate risk
      High risk → 40 mg SC BD
   III. Use → i. Prophylaxis of DVT: → TKR
         ii. Rx of DVT → THR
         iii. PE → High risk patients undergoing major Sx
         → Polytrauma – immobilized

IV. **Advantages:**
1. More predictable pharmacokinetic and pharmacodynamic properties.
2. No lab monitoring → aPTT or INR
3. Longer $t_{1/2}$
4. Consistent effects → less dose adjustment
5. Low risk of hemorrhagic SE

V. **Complications:**
1. Hypersensitivity reactions
2. Urticaria
3. Rash
4. Anaphylaxis
5. Hemorrhage
6. Hematoma
7. Thrombocytopenia
8. Ulceration
9. Local skin irritation
10. Pain
11. Osteoporosis
12. Reversible alopecia
13. Hyperkalemia.

VI. **Contraindications:**
1. Severely compromised renal and hepatic function
2. Hemophilia
3. Uncontrolled HTN
4. Bacterial endocarditis
5. Active gastric ulcer.

iv. **Warfarin:**
1. Vitamin K antagonist → inhibits carboxylation of coagulation factors.
2. Oral = 5–10 mg
3. Monitor PT INR (2 to 3) (2.5)
4. Takes time to show effect

v. **Fondaparinux:**
1. Direct Xa inhibitor → acts through AT III
2. $t_{1/2}$ = 17 hours
3. Subcutaneous
4. Excreted unchanged in urine
5. More effective than LMWH in prophylaxis of DVT → But major bleeding frequent

vi. **Rivaroxaban, apixaban:**
1. Direct Xa inhibitor
2. Oral, $t_{1/2}$ = 8 hours
3. Dose = 10–20 mg BD
4. Metabolism: Liver
5. Risk → Bleeding

vii. **Dabigatran** (110 mg BD oral)
1. Reversible direct thrombin inhibitor (IIa)
2. Renal, SE = GI upset, bleeding

viii. **Tranexamic acid:** Antifibrinolytic
TXA → ↓ Blood transfusions in THA, TKA
Competitively inhibits activation of plasminogen
IV = 10–20 mg/kg initial bolus dose

Recommendations for thromboprophylaxis
1. Patient classified → Low risk
   → Moderate risk
   → High risk
2. Initiation of TP therapy ≥ 12 pre or postoperative
   ↓
   Not 4 hours.
3. For THA/TKA → Give <u>10–14 days</u> postoperative
4. Combine with mechanical
5. No prophylaxis for arthroscopy
6. Early mobilization

FAT EMBOLISM

I. DEFINITION
Acute respiratory disorder due to inflammatory response to embolized fat globules.

II. ETIOLOGY

Traumatic	Nontraumatic
1. Fracture of long bones.	1. Hemoglobinopathy
2. Major orthopedic surgery: 　i. IMN 　ii. THR 　iii. TKR	2. DM 3. Collagen vascular disease 4. Severe infection 5. Neoplasm
3. Extensive burns	6. Blood transfusion
4. Severe soft tissue injury	7. Osteomyelitis
5. Bone marrow biopsy	

III. PATHOPHYSIOLOGY
1. <u>Mechanical theory</u> → Traumatic injury forces disrupted fat globules into torn venules.
2. <u>Biochemical theory</u> → Triglycerides → Hydrolysis → Free - fatty acids → toxic to lung parenchyma.
3. <u>Metabolic</u> → Hormonal changes due to trauma/infection → systemic release of free fatty acids as chylomicrons

IV. CLASSIFICATION

Sevitt's
1. Subclinical
2. Nonfulminant
3. Fulminant

V. CLINICAL FEATURES
1. Presents 48–72 hours >trauma
2. Triad

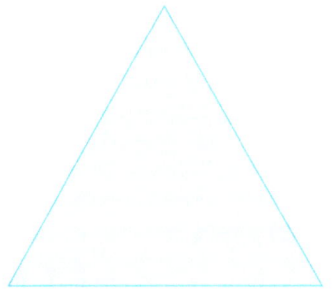

3. Cardiopulmonary:
   i. Early persistent tachycardia
   ii. Tachypnea, dyspnea, hypoxemia
   iii. High grade fever
4. Neurologic:
   i. Acute confusional state
   ii. Aphasia
   iii. Hemiplegia
   iv. Seizures
   v. Retinal hemorrhages (Purtscher's retinopathy)
5. Skin:
   i. Petechial rash → Oral
      → Conjunctival
      → Skin folds (Neck, axilla)

VI. GURD'S CRITERIA

i. Major (At least 1):
   1. Respiratory insufficiency (PaO_2 < 60 mm Hg)
   2. Cerebral dysfunction
   3. Petechial rash
ii. Minor (At least 4):
   1. Tachycardia (>110/min)
   2. Pyrexia (>38.5°C)
   3. Retinal changes
   4. Jaundice
   5. Renal changes = oliguria, lipiduria, hematuria, proteinuria
   6. ↑ ESR
   7. Fat microglobulinemia
   8. Acute ↓ Hb
   9. Sudden thrombocytopenia

VII. RADIOLOGICAL INVESTIGATIONS

1. CXR → Diffuse, patchy pulmonary infiltrate
       ↓
       "Snow storm appearance"
2. CT → Ground glass appearance.
3. MRI brain
4. ECG → Prominent S wave
   Right heart failure pattern

VIII. MANAGEMENT

A. General Measures
1. Maintain airway
2. Maintenance of fluid electrolyte balance
3. Blood transfusion
4. Immobilization of fracture → Slab/splint
5. Antibiotics and analgesics
6. Maintaining → BP, pulse, urine output, PaO_2
7. DVT prophylaxis.

B. Specific
1. Respiratory support: Mechanical ventilation with positive end expiratory pressure (PEEP)
2. Drugs:
   i. *Steroids:* MPS 10 mg/kg/d → 3 divided doses
   ii. *Heparin:* Lipolytic → ↑ Capillary flow
                           → ↓ Plasma flow
   iii. *Dextran:* ↑ Plasma volume
3. Fracture stabilization

C. Prevention
1. Early fracture stabilization (ETC) in a stable patient
2. DCO → Unstable patients
3. Reamer irrigator aspirator.

TOURNIQUET

Constricting or compressing device used to control venous and arterial circulation to an extremity.

I. TYPES

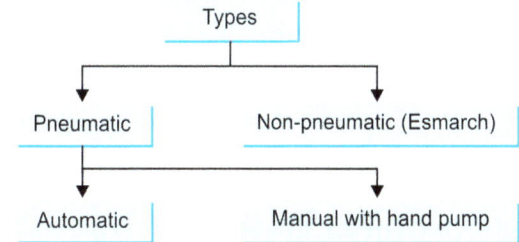

II. PARTS
1. Inflatable cuff → Cylindrical
                  → Conical
2. Gas source
3. Pressure regulator
4. Pressure display
5. Connection tubing.

III. BRUNER'S RULES
1. Size of cuff: Arm = 10 cm
                Thigh = 15 cm or wider in larger

2. Site of application: Upper arm and upper thigh
3. Padding: Two layers of gamgee pad
4. Skin preparation: Prevent soaking of gamgee pad with antiseptic solutions → Chemical burns.
5. Inflation pressure:
   Arm: 50–100 mm Hg > SBP or 200–250 mm Hg
   Leg: Double SBP or 250–300 mm Hg
   Larger limb → Use larger cuffs instead of increasing pressure.
6. Time: Generally must not exceed 2 hours. Absolute maximum – 3 hours
7. Temperature: Keep tissues moist. Avoid heating, cool if possible (NS)
8. Documentation: Duration and pressure
9. Calibration: Weekly → Mercury manometer
10. Maintenance: 3 monthly (Fig. 37)

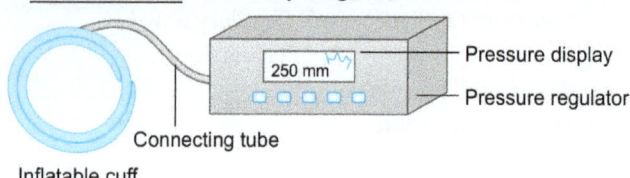

IV. EXSANGUINATION → Before Inflation

1. Improves quality of bloodless field and ↓ Pain
2. Methods → Elevation only
   → Elevation + mechanical compression (Esmarch)
3. No exsanguinations or simple elevation

   Done in cases of malignancy, infection

V. CONTRAINDICATIONS

1. Peripheral arterial disease
2. Severe crush injury
3. Deep vein thrombosis
4. Sickle cell anemia
5. Arteriovenous fistula

VI. PHYSIOLOGICAL EFFECTS

A. Local

1. Muscles: Increased lactic acid, ↓ pH
   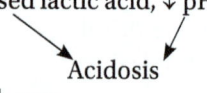
   Acidosis
   ↓ PO_2, ↑ PCO_2, ↓ ATP
2. Nerves: Reversible physiological conduction block.

B. Systemic

1. Hemodynamic: Compromised cardiovascular function (inflation)
   ↓
   Circulatory overload → Cardiac arrest.
   Deflation → ↓BP, CVP → Arrhythmia

2. CNS → ↑CBF
3. RS → End tidal PO_2 concentration ↑
4. Hematological: Inflation → Hypercoagulable
   Deflation → ↑ Fibrinolytic activity
5. Temperature: ↑ Core body temperature → Inflation
   ↓ Core body temperature → Deflation

VII. COMPLICATIONS

1. Tourniquet paralysis → Mechanical effect of tourniquet pressure → Insufficient oxygenation
2. Post-Tourniquet Syndrome
   i. Edema, joint stiffness, pallor, motor weakness
   ii. Ischemic effect
   iii. Recovers in 1 week
3. Reperfusion syndrome
4. Pulmonary embolism → Symptomatic
   → Asymptomatic
5. Chemical burns
6. Superficial abrasions
7. Rhabdomyolysis: Rare
8. Compartment syndrome
9. Vascular complications

COMPARTMENT SYNDROME

I. INTRODUCTION

1. *Compartment*: Closed area of muscle groups, nerves and blood vessels surrounded by fascia. Normal = 5–15 mm Hg
2. *Compartment syndrome*: An elevation of interstitial pressure in closed osteofascial compartment that results in microvascular compromise and affects tissue viability.
3. True orthopedic emergency.

II. ETIOLOGY

i. ↑*Compartment content*:
   1. Fractures (open and closed) (most common cause) → Tibia, forearm
   2. Blunt trauma → Soft tissue injury
   3. Coagulation abnormality
   4. Fluid infusion (arthroscopy)
   5. Major vascular disruption
   6. Snake bite.
ii. ↓ *Compartment size*:
   1. Tight casts, dressings, splints
   2. Tourniquet
   3. Entrapment under collapsed weights
   4. Burns
   5. Tight closure of fascial defects.

III. PATHOPHYSIOLOGY

1. **Eaton and green vicious circle (Edema-ischemia cycle)**

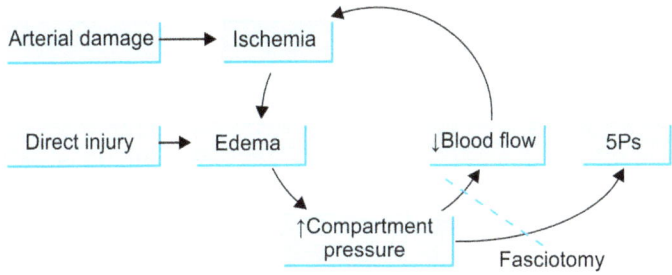

   Normal pressure = 0-10 mm Hg
2. Absolute pressure theory - 30 mm Hg (Mubarak)
3. Arteriovenous pressure gradient theory
   Local blood flow = Pa-Pv/VR
   Pa = arterial pressure
   Pv = venous pressure
   VR = vascular resistance.
4. Whiteside's: ΔP = Diastolic BP - Intracompartmental pressure
   Difference < 30 = Compartment syndrome

IV. CLASSIFICATION

→ Acute → Medical emergency
→ Chronic: Exertional compartment syndrome
↓
Athletes, pain and cramping during exercise
↓
Subsides on stopping activity.

V. TISSUE SURVIVAL

Muscles: 3-4 hours - Reversible changes
6 hours - Variable
8 hours - IRREVERSIBLE
Nerves: 2 hours - Reversible → loses nerve conduction
4 hours - Neuropraxia
8 hours - Irreversible

VI. CLINICAL PRESENTATION

i. *The P'*:
   1. Pain - out of proportion
   2. Palpably tense compartment } Most reliable
   3. Pain with passive stretch
   4. Paresthesia
   5. Paralysis
   6. Pallor } missed the bus
   7. Pulselessness

ii. *Pediatric compartment syndrome—3A's*:
   ↑ Analgesia requirement
   Anxiety
   Agitation

VII. INVESTIGATIONS → Clinical Diagnosis

1. X-ray → Fractures
2. Lab → CPK - MM, myoglobin
3. Compartment pressure monitoring:
   i. Ventilator
   ii. Obtunded
   iii. Alcoholic
   iv. Regional anesthesia
      a. Whitesides technique (**Fig. 38**)
      b. Slit catheter method
      c. Solid state transducer (STIC)
      d. Wick catheter method
      e. Near-infrared spectroscopy (NIRS)

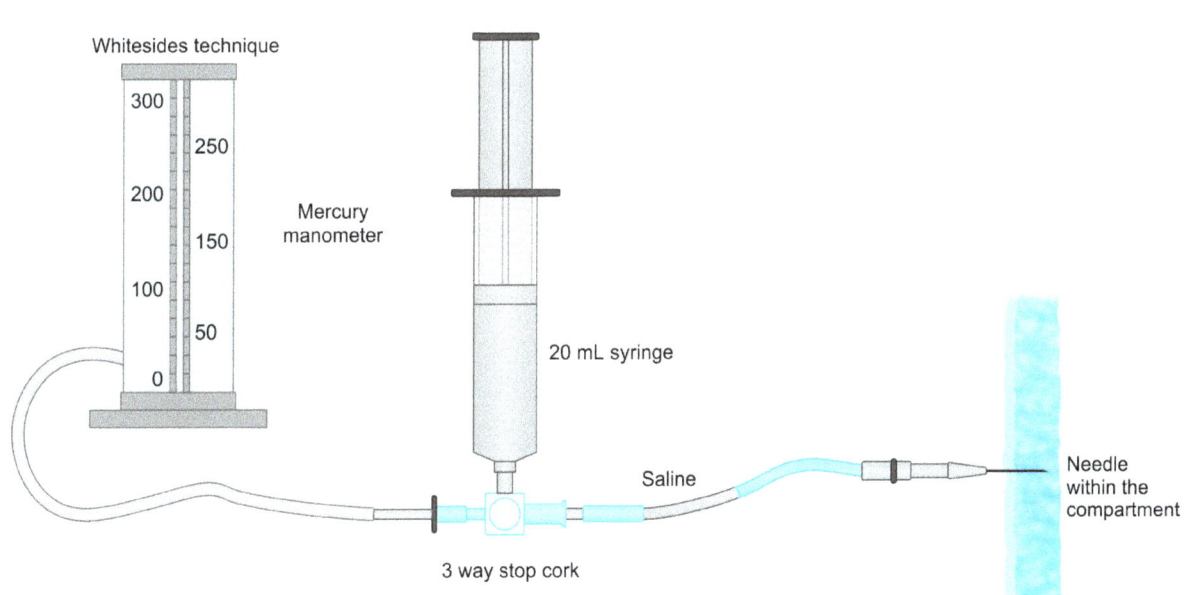

VIII. TREATMENT

1. High index of clinical suspicion → Compartment syndrome unless proven otherwise
2. Ensure hemodynamic stability (normotensive) Hypotensive → ↓ Perfusion pressure
3. Maintain limb at level of heart → elevation reduces arterial inflow
4. Supplemental O_2 administration.
5. *Remove circumferential casts:*
   i. Split on one side → Falls by 30%
   ii. Split and spread → by 65%
   iii. Splitting the padding → further 10%
   iv. Complete removal → another 15%
6. Treatment is surgical → Fasciotomy
7. *Principles:*
   i. Make early diagnosis
   ii. Long extensile incisions
   iii. Release all fascial compartments
   iv. Preserve neurovascular structures
   v. Debride necrotic tissue
   vi. Coverage in 7–10 days
8. Leg: Single incision (Matsens): Just posterior to fibula
9. Double incision (Mubarak): Two vertical incisions separated by at least 8 cm.
   i. Anterolateral compartment
   ii. 1 cm behind posteromedial border of tibia
10. Forearm: Three compartments **(Fig. 39)**:
    i. Volar
    ii. Dorsal
    iii. Mobile wad

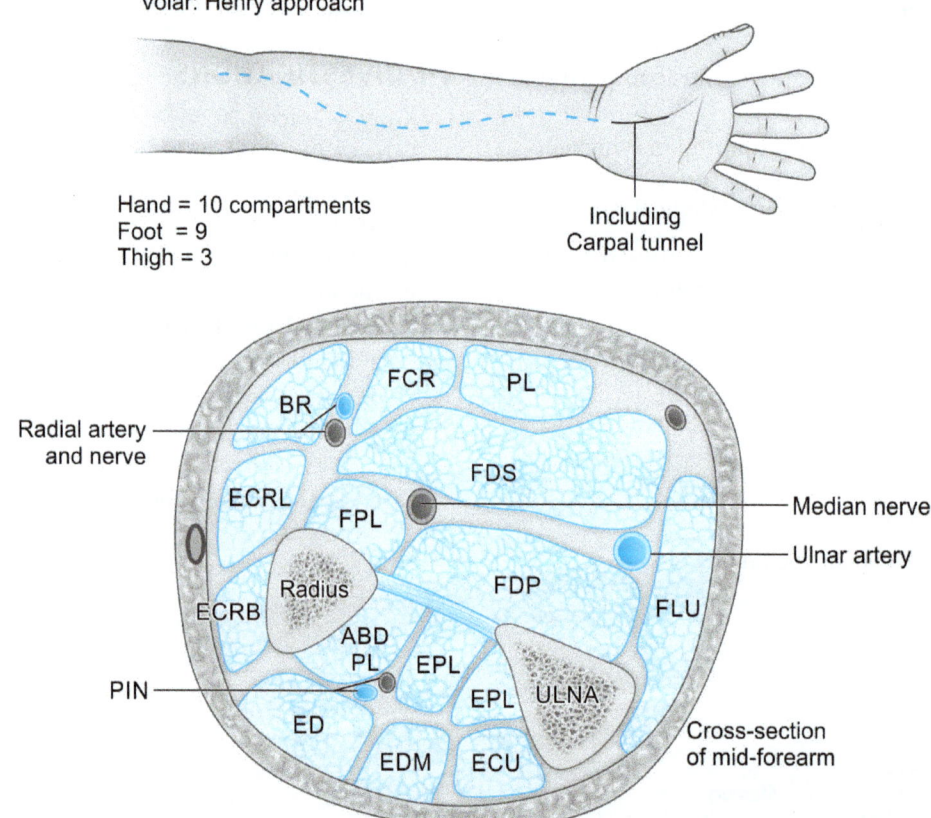

11. Interim coverage:
    i. VAC
    ii. Vessel loop "Bootlace"
    iii. Simple absorbent dressing
12. Second look = 48-72 hours
13. Definitive coverage:
    i. Skin graft
    ii. Flap - exposed bone
    iii. Delayed primary with relaxing incisions

IX. COMPLICATIONS
1. Volkmann's ischemic contracture
2. Equinus
3. Claw toes
4. Sensory loss
5. Chronic pain
6. Amputation.

STRESS AND STRAIN

I. STRESS
1. Force acting on a surface divided by the area over which it acts.
2. *Example*: When an equal force (hammer blow) is applied to both a sharp and a dull osteotome, the sharp osteotome will concentrate the same force over a smaller surface area than a dull osteotome because of the sharp edge. Therefore, the sharp osteotome will create a greater stress at the osteotome-bone interface, resulting in cutting of the bone.

II. STRAIN
1. Change in the height or length of the object (displacement) under load divided by its original height or length.
2. *Example*: If two plates of different lengths are both subjected to loads that lengthen the plate by 1 cm, the shorter of the two plates will be subjected to more strain as change in length is spread over a shorter distance than it is for the longer plate.

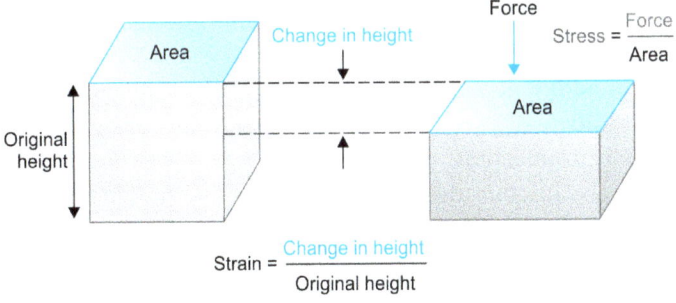

III. YOUNG'S MODULUS OF ELASTICITY
i. Mechanical property of solid materials which measures its resistance to elastic deformation under stress.
ii. It is defined as the ratio of the stress (force per unit area) applied to the object and the resulting axial strain (displacement or deformation) in the linear elastic region of the material.

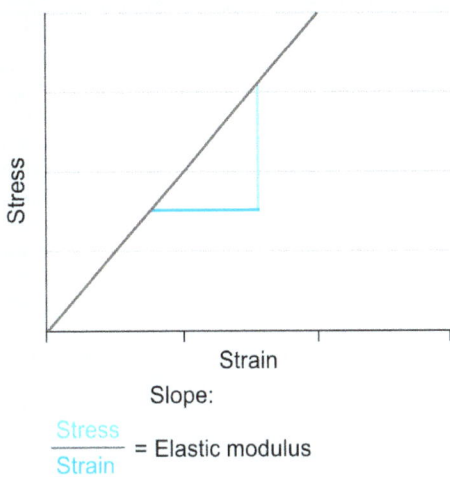

IV. TESTING OF MATERIALS
1. Mechanical testing is used extensively to analyse the properties of different constructs as well as new implant designs.
2. The testing usually consists of a fractured bone fixed with a certain implant in different configurations.
3. This construct is then loaded into an apparatus that applies a specific load in either a constant or cyclic manner.
4. Sensors can measure the forces applied to the bone as well as any deformity or eventual failure.
5. Depending on the purpose of the experiment the data can be collected measuring the structural properties of the bone-fixation construct; i.e., the properties of the fixation device and the bone combined.
6. Alternatively, the data can measure the material properties which relate to the properties of the substances that make up each component (bone, stainless steel, titanium).
7. The graph represents the data measured in this experiment plotted on a stress-strain graph.
8. The force and displacement are measured and normalized to stress and strain.

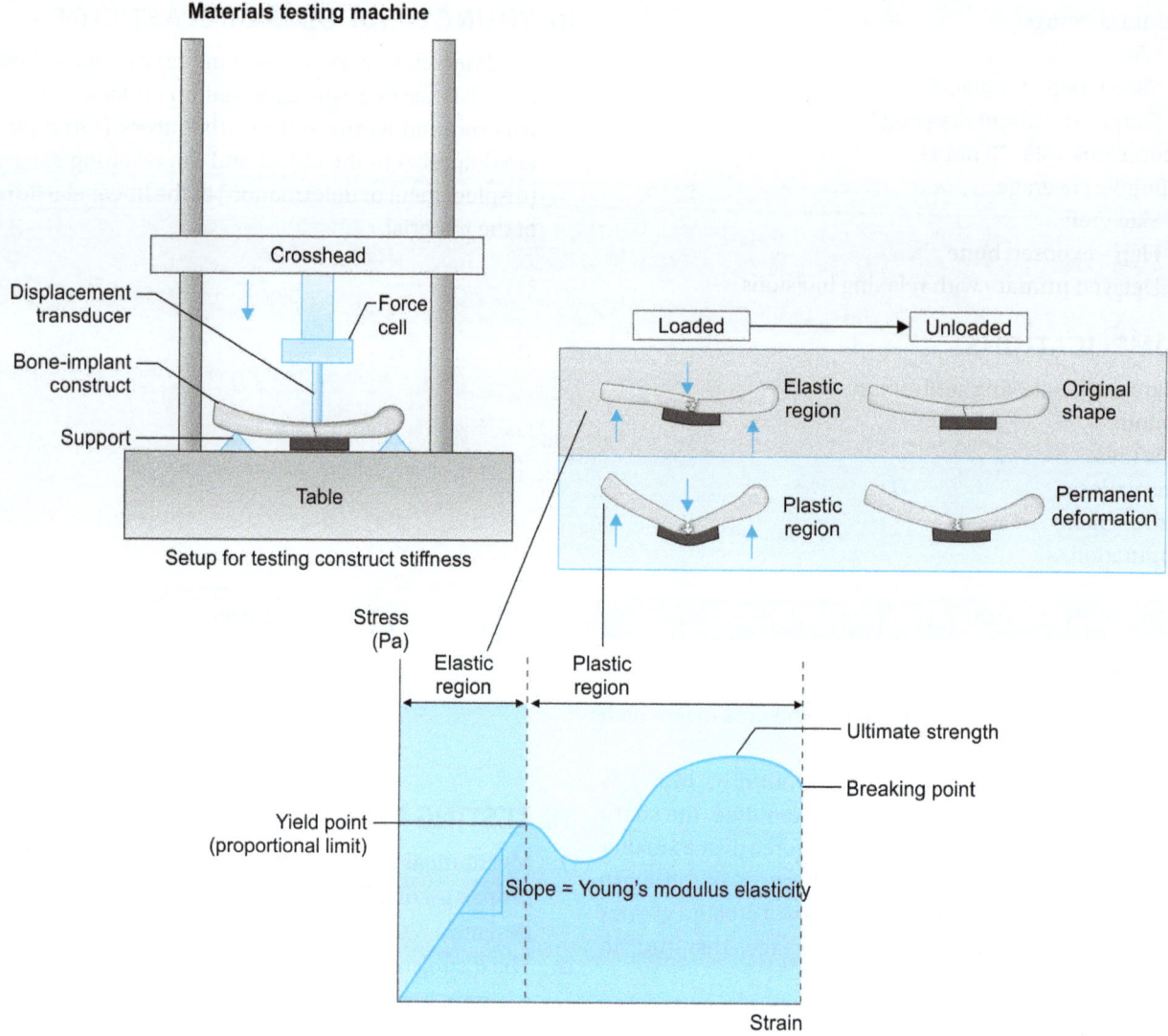

9. The initial deformation is termed elastic because when the load is removed, the plate will return to its original shape.
10. This is represented by the linear portion of the graph, termed the elastic region.
11. At some load, however, the construct becomes overloaded, entering the plastic range.
12. If the load is released after loading in the plastic range but before failure, some permanent deformation remains in the construct.
13. The point at which elastic behaviour changes to plastic is termed the yield point.
14. As previously mentioned, the slope of the stress–strain curve is the elastic (Young's) modulus.

Material	Elastic Modulus (MPa)
Cortical Bone	15,000
Cancellous Bone	1,000
Titanium (Al 4V) (Alloy F 136)	100,000
Stainless Steel (316L)	200,000

15. Stainless steel is twice as stiff as Titanium material → Higher modulus of elasticity.
16. Titanium more closely matches the elasticity of the bone.

V. STAINLESS STEEL (SS) VERSUS TITANIUM

1. SS alloys are significantly stiffer than bone and have traditionally proven to be durable enough to allow healing.
2. In addition, stainless steel is relatively inexpensive and biologically well tolerated, → smooth surface from electropolishing.
3. It also has the advantage of being ductile enough to allow contouring of the plate without fracture.
4. Electro-polished stainless steel overall has an excellent clinical track record in most fracture types and anatomic locations; however, questions have arisen regarding whether it may be too stiff to allow for fracture healing in some anatomic locations or fracture types, such as the distal femur.

5. Titanium, on the other hand, more closely matches the modulus of elasticity of bone.
6. This flexibility may be more conducive to fracture healing in areas where more strain is required for a healing response to develop.
7. Additionally, titanium alloy is more resistant to cyclic load and notch sensitivity.
8. Titanium has a good clinical track record when used in internal fixation devices for fractures.
9. Previous issues of "cold-welding" of screws to plates when commercially pure titanium was used have been essentially eliminated with the introduction of titanium alloys.
10. The use of titanium has been limited by regional surgeon preference and increased cost compared with electro-polished stainless steel, although these barriers are decreasing.
11. Comparing the advantages and disadvantages of the mechanical properties of each metal does not lead to an obvious conclusion about which is better for fracture fixation.
12. It may be that neither metal is universally superior to the other, but that each has properties that may make it superior to the other in specific anatomic locations.
13. In addition, the strength and durability of the construct also depends significantly on the number, type (i.e., locking vs. nonlocking, uni- vs. bi-cortical), and composition/position of the screws used.

SECTION 2

Pediatric Orthopedics

PROXIMAL FEMORAL FOCAL DEFICIENCY (PFFD)

I. INTRODUCTION

1. Deficient development of the proximal femur (PF) leading to abnormal iliofemoral articulation, malrotation of the femur and limb length discrepancy.
2. *Broad spectrum:*
   i. Congenital short femur
   ii. Femoral neck pseudoarthrosis
   iii. Complete agenesis of femur
   iv. Absent hip joint
3. *Most commonly:* Partial skeletal defect in the PF with a variably unstable hip joint and shortening.
4. *Associated anomalies:*
   i. Fibular hemimelia (50%)
   ii. Knee cruciate ligaments deficiency
   iii. Coxa vara
   iv. Knee contractures
   v. Club foot
   vi. Spinal dysplasia
5. *B/L:* 15%
6. Pathophysiology: Defect in the 1° ossification center (Cartilage anlage) ⊗ → Sonic *hedgehog* gene
7. *Risk factors:*
   i. Maternal diabetes
   ii. Thalidomide

II. CLASSIFICATIONS

1. Aitken
2. Pappas
3. Gillespie and Torode
4. Hamanishi

A. Aitken (Fig. 1)

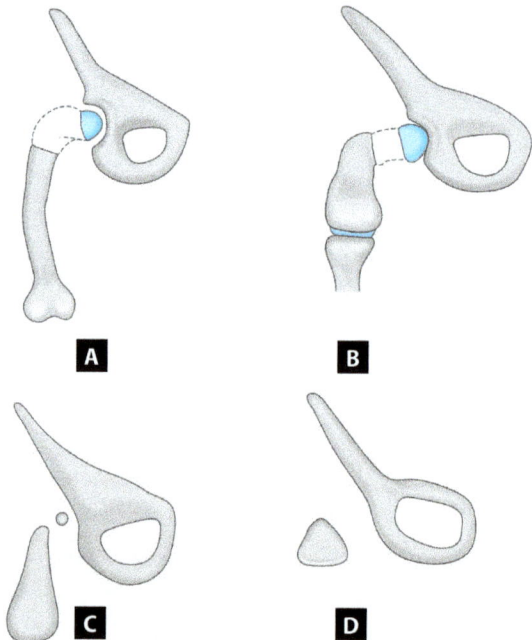

Type	Femur head	Acetabulum normal	Femoral segment	Relationship
A	Present	Moderately dysplastic	Short	• Between femoral parts = Bony connection • Femoral head in acetabulum • Subtrochanteric varus angulation • ± Pseudoarthrosis
B	Present	Severe dysplasia	Short, proximal bony tuft	• No osseous connection between head and shaft • Femoral head in acetabulum
C	Absent/ossicle	Absent obturator foramen	Short, proximal Tapered	No articular relation between femur and acetabulum
D	Absent	Enlarged	Short, deformed	None

B. Pappas

1. Complete absence of femur.
2. PF absent, acetabulum not developed (Aitken D)
3. PF deficient, no bony continuity between femur shaft and head.
4. PF deficiency, fibro-osseous connection between shaft and head (Aitken A).
5. Mid-femoral deficiency with hypoplastic proximal or distal femur (Aitken A).
6. Distal femoral deficiency.
7. Short femur with coxa vara and sclerosis of diaphysis.
8. Short femur with coxa valgum
9. Congenital short femur

C. Gillespie and Torode

Group A (Congenital Short Femur)
1. Affected femur up to 50% shorter than normal
2. Foot → Mid-tibia of normal side
3. Limb lengthening possible

Group B
1. >50% shorter than normal
2. Foot → Above mid-tibia
3. Rotationplasty, prosthetic management and amputation

Group C
Subtotal absence of femur (Aitken D)

D. Hamanishi (Fig. 2)

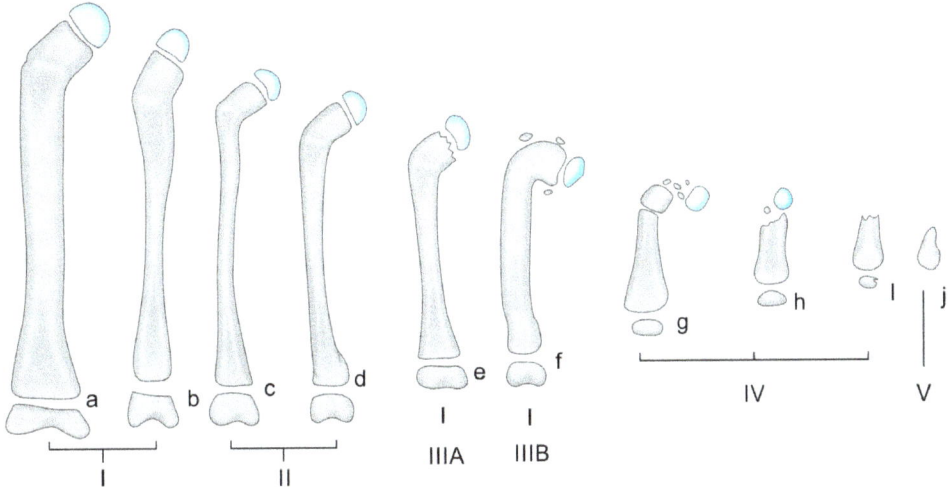

Consider limb deficiency a continuous spectrum representing varying degrees of response to an insult.

III. CLINICAL FEATURES

1. Femoral segment → Short, flexed, abducted, externally rotated.
2. Hip and knee → Flexion contractures
3. Fibular hemimelia (50%)
4. Proximal thigh is bullous and rapidly tapers to knee joint (inverted conical shape).
5. LLD → short limb gait
6. Assisted gait → Unipedal, equinus
7. Galeazzi test → [+]
8. Telescopy maybe [+]
9. High riding greater trochanter
10. Exaggerated lumbar lordosis

IV. RADIOLOGY

1. Proximal femur ossification delayed
2. Arthrography or fluoroscopy: To detect mobility across pseudoarthrosis
3. Subtrochanteric bow
4. Absence of both tibial spines, absence of notch in tunnel view → anterior cruciate ligament deficiency
5. MRI:
   i. Acetabulum → Posterior wall deficient, retroverted
   ii. Cartilaginous femoral head
   iii. Ligament abnormalities of knee

V. TREATMENT

A. Goals

1. Individualized treatment
2. Restore hip function
3. Correct length discrepancy of limb
4. Flexion and ER deformity of femur, flexion and instability of knee and fibular deficiency also needs Rx

B. Conservative

1. Up to 5 cm → Shoe raise
2. B/L PFFD → Extension prosthesis maybe provided

C. Operative

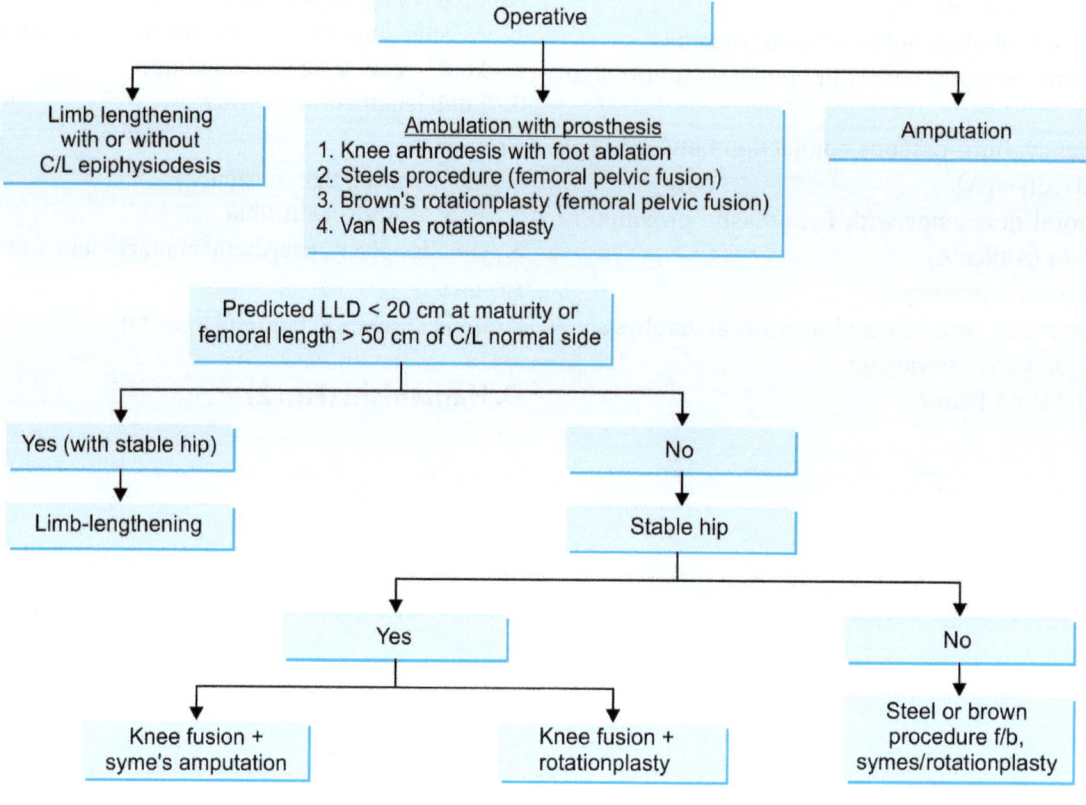

A. Stable Hip with Minimal Shortening

1. Surgical limb lengthening with or without C/L shortening
2. Aitken A and B (FH present)
3. Normal adult femur ≈ 40–45 cm.
4. Maximum amount of lengthening in single long bone → 10–12 cm.
5. Combined C/L shortening → 17–20 cm
6. Therefore, limb lengthening only for patients with predicted shortening < 20 cm/>50% femur length

B. Stable Hip with Severe Shortening

1. Knee arthrodesis + Syme's amputation
   ↓
   Creates a single bone segment from the tibia and shortened femur
   ↓
   Functions as AK amputation > foot amputation
2. Van Nes rotationplasty:
   i. Limb is rotated by 180° and ankle substitutes the knee. Knee is fused.
   ii. Ankle ROM must be sufficient (more than 60%)
   iii. Aitken C and D
   iv. Ankle DF becomes knee flexion
   v. Allows use of below knee prosthesis → improves gait and efficiency **(Fig. 3)**.

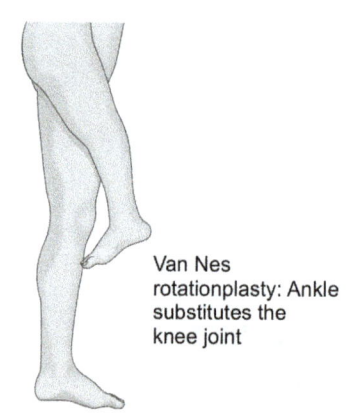

Van Nes rotationplasty: Ankle substitutes the knee joint

C. Unstable Hip

1. Steel's procedure = Iliofemoral fusion + Chiari osteotomy
2. Chiari osteotomy creates a suitable bony bed to receive the small femoral remnant.
3. Knee functions as hip joint → Knee extension is hip flexion because femoral fragment fused at 90° flexion relative to pelvis
4. Brown modification of steel
   ↓
   Distal femur rotated 180° before fusion to ilium.
   ↓
   Knee flexion → Hip flexion allows additional hip flexion for sitting **(Fig. 4)**.

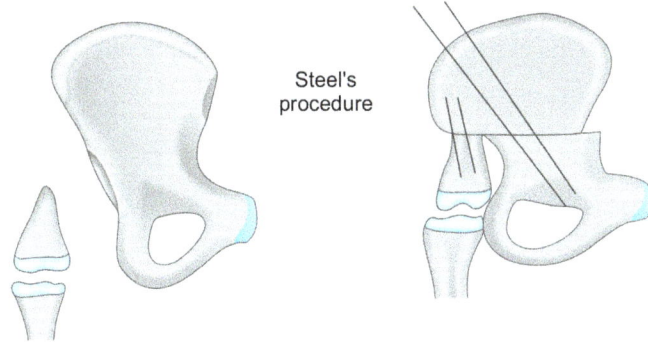

Reduction of thigh: To aid prosthesis fitting → liposuction or Sx reduction.

PERTHES DISEASE

I. DEFINITION

Avascular necrosis of femoral head epiphysis in a child.

II. EMBRYOLOGY

1. Ossification of femur: 7th week IU life
2. At birth, single physis at PF
3. Femoral head epiphysis: 4 months
4. Trochanteric epiphysis: 4 years
5. Fusion of these with PF: 14–16 years **(Fig. 5)**

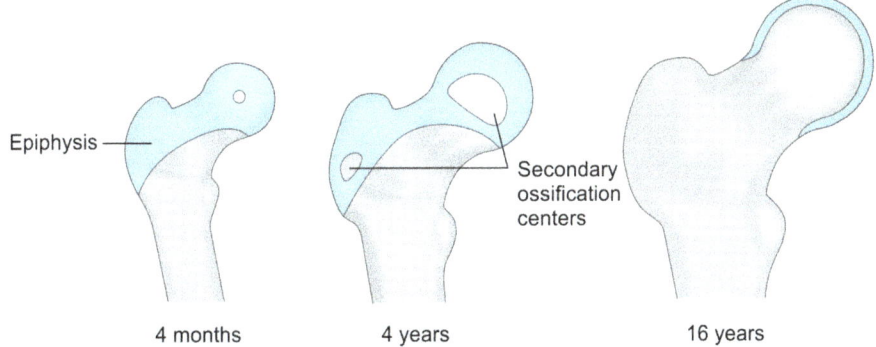

III. BLOOD SUPPLY (FIG. 6)

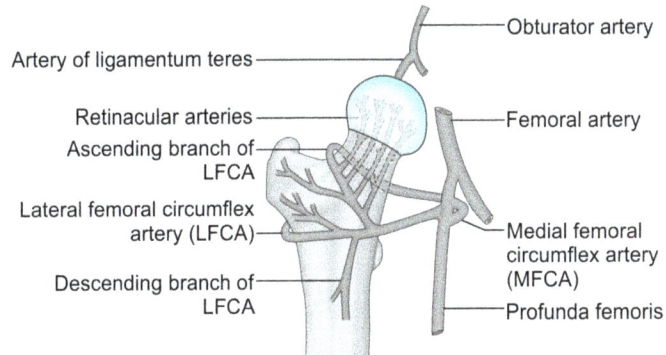

Most important: Lateral ascending cervical artery – Branch of medial circumflex artery.

IV. ETIOLOGY

1. Trauma
2. Coagulopathy: Protein C or S deficiency, Factor V Leiden mutation, hypofibrinolysis. (**Caffey's Hypothesis**)
3. Hereditary: *COL2A1* gene
4. Hyperactive child (ADHD)
5. Passive smoking
   Prothrombotic effect by inhibiting tissue plasminogen activator
   ↓
   Venous occlusion of femoral vessels

V. PATHOPHYSIOLOGY

1. Disruption of capital femoral epiphysis blood supply → Epiphyseal osteonecrosis → Growth of ossific nucleus hampered.
2. **Trueta's hypothesis:**
   i. <4 years: Metaphyseal and retinacular arteries
   ii. **4–8 years: Only retinacular**
   iii. >8 years: Retinacular + artery of ligamentum teres
3. Vascular occlusion → Bone necrosis → Synovitis, cartilage and ligamentum teres hypertrophy → Muscle spasm → Femur head extrudes out laterally of the acetabulum → Weight bearing stress on extruded avascular bone.
   ↓
   Femoral head deformation → If extruded >20%.

VI. CLINICAL FEATURES

1. Age: 4–8 years
2. Sex: Boy : Girl – 4 : 1
3. Bilateral: 1 in 10 cases
4. Painless limp: Most common
5. Pain in hip, knee: Referred to knee
6. Small, often thin, extremely active, constantly running and jumping
7. Limited range of motion (Abduction and internal rotation)

8. Muscle wasting: Gluteus, hamstring, quadriceps atrophy.
9. Antalgic + Trendelenburg gait (Body leans over the affected hip)
10. Trendelenburg test: Positive

VII. RADIOGRAPHIC STAGING: MODIFIED WALDENSTROM (FIG. 7)

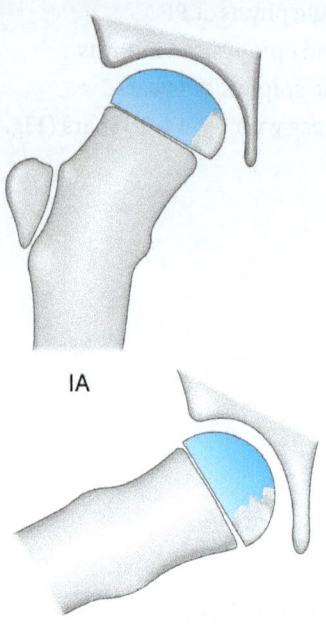

IA

I. Initial (Avascular necrosis):
   IA. Sclerosis of the epiphysis without any loss of epiphyseal height **(Fig. 8)**

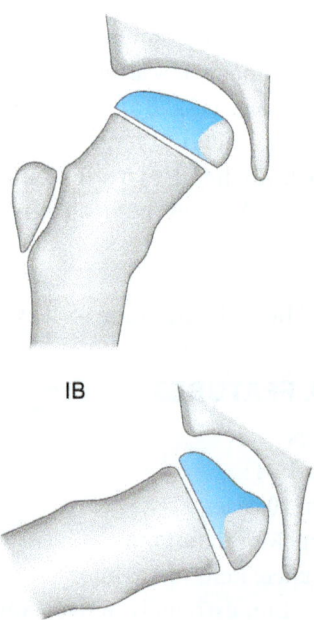

IB

   IB. Sclerosis of the epiphysis with some loss of epiphyseal height.

II. Fragmentation:
   IIA. One or two vertical fissures in the epiphysis **(Fig. 9)**

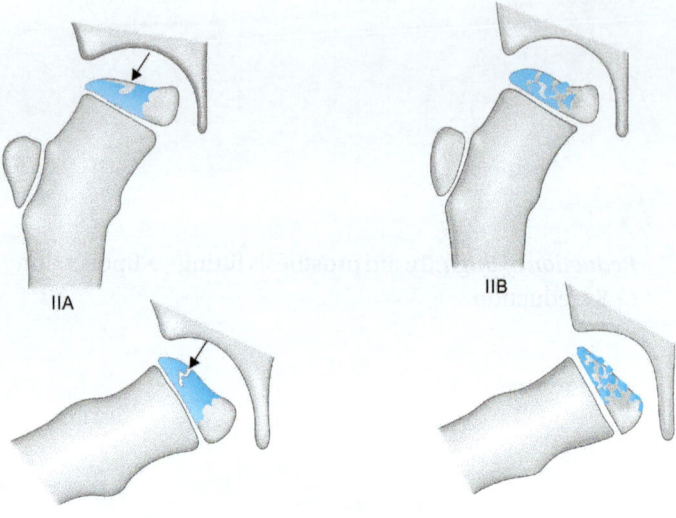

IIA   IIB

   IIB. Advanced fragmentation without evidence of new bone formation lateral to the fragmented epiphysis

III. Reconstitution **(Fig. 10)**

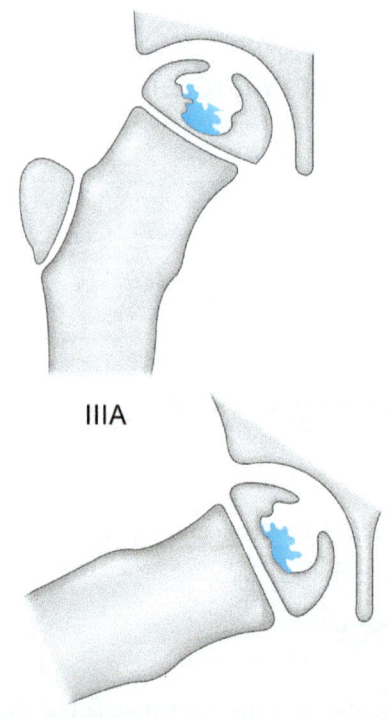

IIIA

   IIIA. New bone formation at the periphery of the necrotic fragment.
   <1/3rd of the circumference of the epiphysis.
   IIIB. New bone formation at the periphery of the necrotic fragment.
   >1/3rd of the circumference of the epiphysis.
IV. Complete healing

VIII. CLASSIFICATIONS

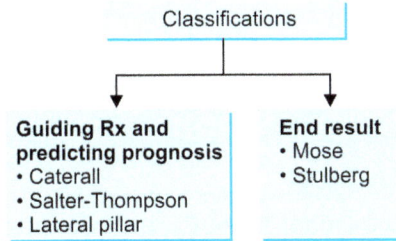

A. Caterall

Extent of Epiphyseal Involvement

Group 1:
1. Only anterior portion of epiphysis affected
2. No collapse

Group 2:
1. More anterior portion involved
2. Central sequestrum present
3. May collapse, but epiphyseal height preserved.

Group 3: Most of the epiphysis is sequestered barring a medial or lateral segment.

Group 4: Entire epiphysis is sequestered.

Head at risk signs:
1. Lateral subluxation of femur head
2. Gage's sign: V-shaped lucent defect at the lateral portion of the epiphysis and/or adjacent metaphysis.
3. Horizontal physis
4. Calcification lateral to epiphysis
5. Metaphyseal cysts

B. Salter–Thompson

Subchondral Fracture – Crescent Sign

Group A: <50% of head involved
Group B: >50% of head involved

C. Lateral Pillar (Herring)

1. Extent of epiphyseal collapse and extrusion
2. Herring divided the capital epiphysis into lateral, middle and medial pillars.
3. Lateral pillar is the principal load bearing part of the head. Decides prognosis **(Fig. 11)**.

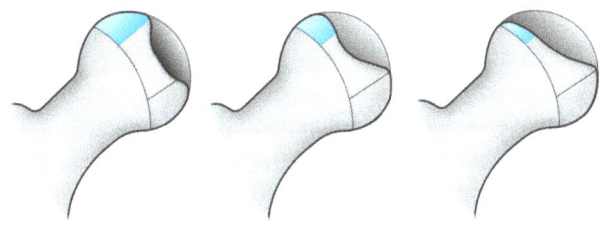

A: NO loss of height of lateral pillar. Minimal density change
B: Loss of height less than 50%. Radiolucency present.
C: Loss of height more than 50%.
B/C: Lateral pillar narrow (2–3 mm), poorly ossified with height around 50%.

D. Stulberg

Stulberg grading		Congruence
I	Normal spherical femoral head	Spherical congruence
II	Spherical head: Coxa magna or coxa breva	
III	Nonspherical head (mushroom), acetabulum matches head	Congruous incongruity
IV	Flattened head, acetabulum also flattened	
V	Head collapsed, acetabulum not flattened	Incongruous Incongruity

IX. MANAGEMENT

Based on modified Waldenstrom staging by Dr Benjamin Joseph.
1. Onset: IIA → Early part of the disease → Preventive intervention
2. IIB: IIIB → Late part of the disease → Remedial intervention
3. Stage IV → Healed disease → Salvage for residual deformity

A. Early (Onset – IIA)

Containment

1. Any intervention that places the anterolateral part of femoral epiphysis well into the acetabulum.
   ↓
2. Protects the vulnerable part from being subjected to deforming forces

Variable	Contain	Not to contain
Age	>7 or <7 with extrusion	<7 (no extrusion)
Stage of evolution	Ia, Ib, IIa	IIb, IIIa, IIIb, IV
Extrusion	Present	Absent (<7 years)
Range of hip motion	Normal	Restricted

3. Containment → Conservative (Cast, bracing) or surgical
4. Conservative
5. Petri cast: Broomstick cast
6. Toronto brace
7. Atlanta Scottish rite brace

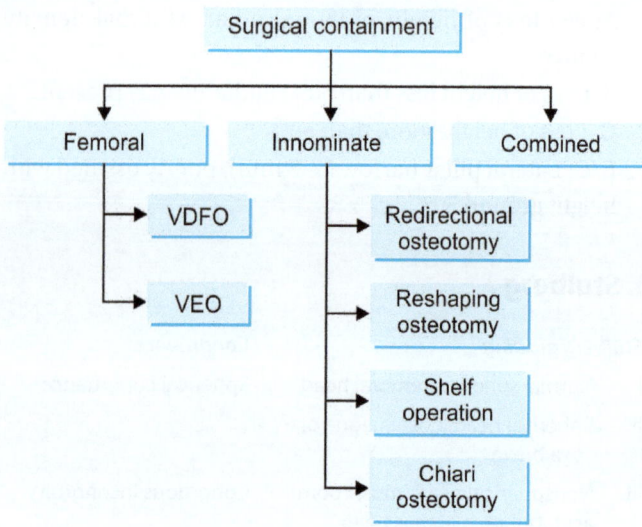

1. *Varus derotational femoral osteotomy:*
   i. Level: Intertrochanteric or subtrochanteric
   ii. Proximal fragment: Abduction and internal rotated
   iii. Distal fragment: Adducted and externally rotated
   iv. Sufficient: 20° varus
      20–30° of derotation
   v. Restoration of Hip ROM a **MUST** before containment surgery
2. *Varus extension osteotomy*:
   i. Indication: Passive internal rotation restricted even after traction and trial of broomstick cast.
   ii. Distal fragment: Adducted and Ex. Rotated 20°

B. Late (IIB–IIIB) – Remedial

1. *Valgus osteotomy*:
   i. Indication: Hinged abduction
   ii. Femur head hinges on acetabular margin causing pain and restriction of motion.
2. *Arthrodiastasis*:
   i. Joint distraction with external fixation
   ii. Unloads the hip joint
   iii. Maintains synovial fluid circulation
3. *Epiphyseal drilling*

C. Salvage for Sequelae

1. *Aims of treatment*:
   i. Relieve pain
   ii. Correct Trendelenburg gait
   iii. Minimize the risk of development of degenerative arthritis
2. *Options*:
   i. Valgus osteotomy, joint distraction
   ii. Improving acetabular coverage
   iii. Arthrodesis
   iv. Cheilectomy
   v. Greater trochanteric advancement

3. Recent advances in management:
   i. Bisphosphonates
   ii. Bone morphogenic proteins
   iii. Biological treatment

DDH

I. INTRODUCTION

1. Structural relationship of PF and acetabulum is intermittently or continuously abnormal.
2. ~~Congenital dislocation of hip (CDH)~~ → Developmental dysplasia of hip (DDH):
   i. Congenital → Developmental
   ii. Dislocation → Dysplasia
3. Spectrum:
   i. Dislocatable hip
   ii. Acetabular dysplasia
   iii. Subluxation
   iv. Dislocated hip

II. ETIOLOGY

1. Ligamentous laxity → Single most important factor
   i. Familial → Wynne-Davies criteria
   ii. Hormonal → Relaxin: Crosses placenta induces laxity in baby.
2. Breech position:
   i. Complete breech
   ii. Footling breech 2%
   iii. Frank breech 20%
3. Postnatal positioning → Swaddling
4. Primary acetabular dysplasia
5. Crowding effect:
   i. First born child
   ii. Oligohydramnios
6. Left side > Right side (MC fetal position: Left Occipito-anterior)
7. Packaging disorders:
   i. Congenital muscular torticollis (20%)
   ii. Metatarsus adductus (10%)
   iii. Congenital dislocation of knee
8. Gradually progressive disorder → Malformation of anatomic structures → Developed normally during embryonic period → due to gentle forces, but persistent and is initially reversible.

III. OBSTACLES TO REDUCTION

1. Pulvinar hypertrophy
2. Elongation and thickening of Ligamentum teres
3. Transverse acetabular ligament pulled upward
4. Iliopsoas tendon → Hourglass narrowing
5. Narrowing of capsule → "Chinese Finger-trap" mechanism

IV. CLINICAL PRESENTATION

A. Neonate
1. **Ortolani test**: The examiner grasps the child's thigh between the thumb and the index finger and, with the fourth and fifth fingers, lifts the greater trochanter while simultaneously abducting the hip. → Reduces the hip joint.
2. **Barlow's test**: Dislocation of hip joint by adduction.

B. Infant
1. Limitation of abduction: Most reliable sign of a dislocated hip.
2. Galeazzi/Allis sign: Shortening of thigh
   Both hips 90° flexion and compare knee height.
3. Asymmetric thigh folds
4. Klisic test:
   i. Middle finger → Greater trochanter
   ii. Index finger → ASIS
   iii. Normal → Line points to umbilicus
   iv. Dislocated → Between umbilicus and pubis (Fig. 12).

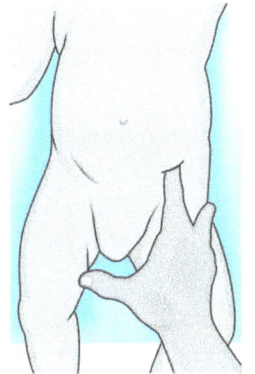 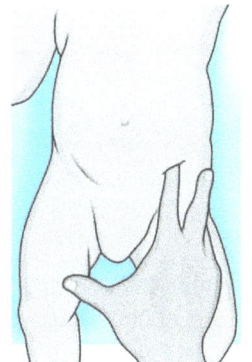

C. Walking Child
(Apart from findings of infant)
1. Trendelenburg gait/Abductor lurch
   Body leans over the affected hip (sound side sags)
2. Excessive lumbar lordosis
3. Short limb

V. RADIOLOGICAL INVESTIGATIONS

A. USG
1. Why ultrasonography in neonate?
   Because femur head primarily composed of cartilage. And USG → Soft tissue anatomy (Fig. 13)
2. "Baseline" → Line of ilium intersecting the acetabulum
3. "Inclination line" → Along the margin of the cartilaginous acetabulum
4. "Acetabular roofline" → Along the bony roof
5. α → Baseline + Roofline
6. β → Baseline + Inclination line (Fig. 14)

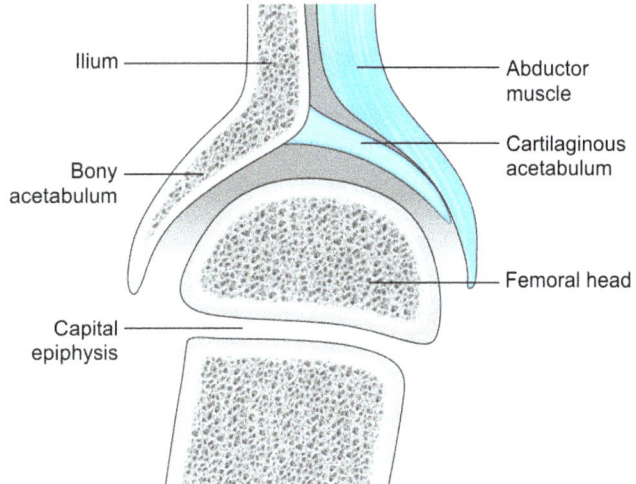

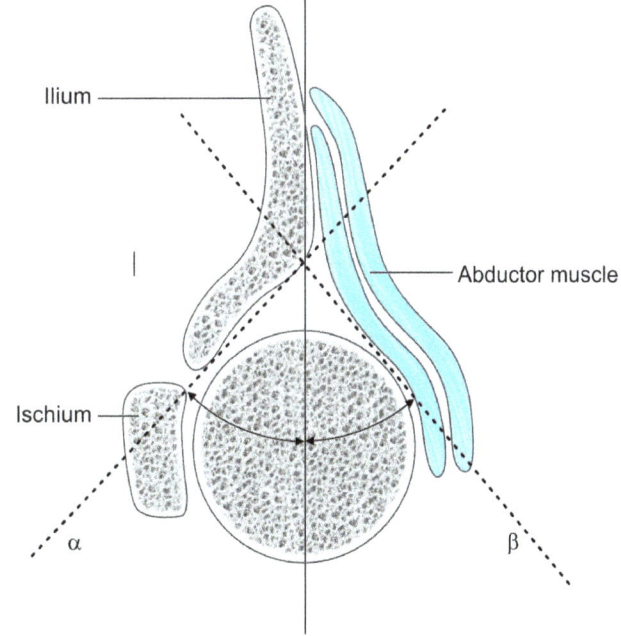

Class	Alpha angle	Beta angle	Description	Treatment
I	>60°	<55°	Normal	None
II	43–60°	55–77°	Delayed ossification	Variable
III	<43°	>77°	Lateralization	Pavlik harness
IV	Unmeasurable	Unmeasurable	Dislocated	Pavlik harness/ closed vs open reduction

B. X-ray
1. After the age of 3 months.
2. Lines assessed on PBH
   i. Hilgenreiner line: A horizontal line through the triradiate cartilages.

ii. Perkins line: Drawn at the lateral margin of the acetabulum, is perpendicular to the Hilgenreiner line (Fig. 15).

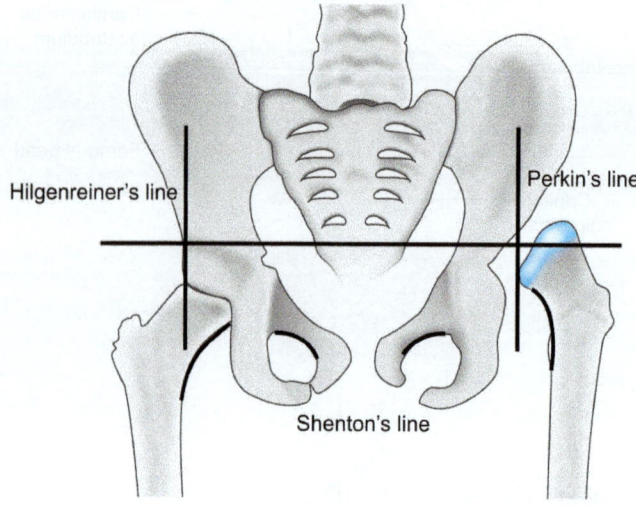

iii. Shenton's line: Begins at the lesser trochanter, goes up the femoral neck, and connects with a line along the inner margin of the pubis.
3. Acetabular index:
   i. Hilgenreiner line + Line along the acetabular surface.
   ii. Newborns → 27.5°, 6 months → 23.5°, 2 years → 20°
   iii. 30° upper limit of normal (Fig. 16).

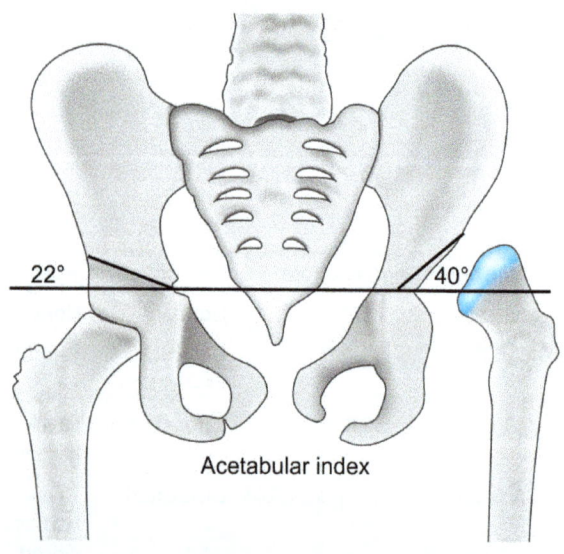

Acetabular index

4. Lateral center edge angle of Wiberg (Fig. 17):
   i. Vertical line along the center of femur head
   ii. Line drawn from center of femur head to lateral margin of acetabulum
   iii. Reliable after 5 years
   iv. 6–13 year → >19° (6 + 13 = 19)
   v. 14 years → >25°

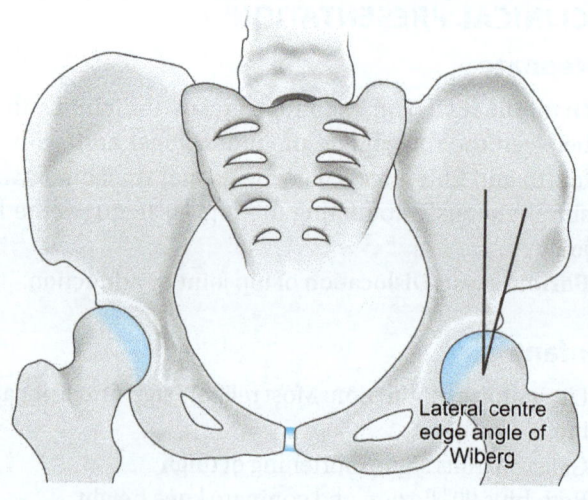

5. Von Rosen view:
   i. Abducted, internally rotated and extended hip
   ii. Normal → line extending from femur shaft intersects acetabulum
   iii. DDH → Line crosses above acetabulum (Fig. 18)

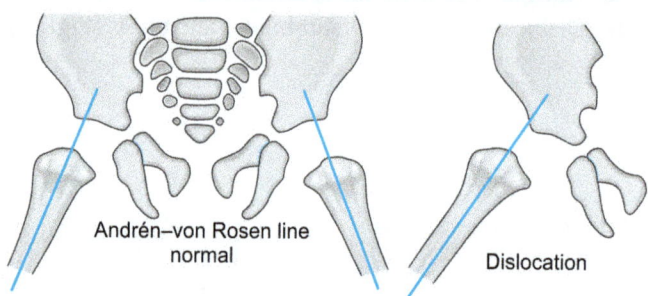

6. Acetabular tear drop:
   i. Normally, appears by 6–24 months
   ii. DDH → Fails to appear or tear drop loses convexity. Becomes wider.

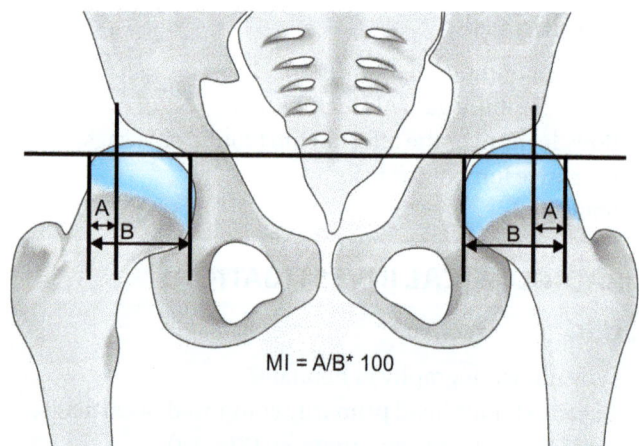

MI = A/B* 100

7. Reimer's migration index (Fig. 19):
   i. Percentage of femoral head uncovered by the acetabulum
   ii. Normal → 17–27%
   iii. Acetabular dysplasia → >27%

8.

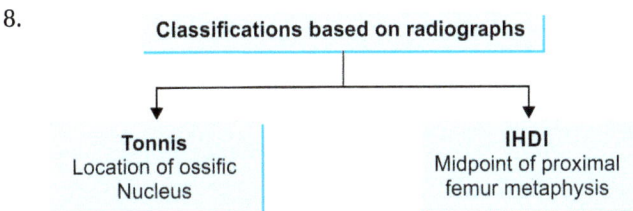

C. Arthrogram

1. *Purpose:*
   i. Assessment of reduction
   ii. Depth of acetabulum
   iii. Stability of reduction
2. Normal hip → **"Rose-thorn" appearance**: Free border of labrum sharp and overlying femur head.
3. Dislocated hip: Capsule enlarged with increased dye in medial gap.
   i. Adequate reduction → 5-6 mm
   ii. Poor reduction → >6 mm

VI. MANAGEMENT

1. Management is age wise:
   A. Newborn → Birth-6 months
   B. Infant → 6-18 months
   C. Toddler → 18-24 months
   D. Child → 3-8 years
   E. Adolescents → >8 years

A. Newborn → Birth to 6 Months

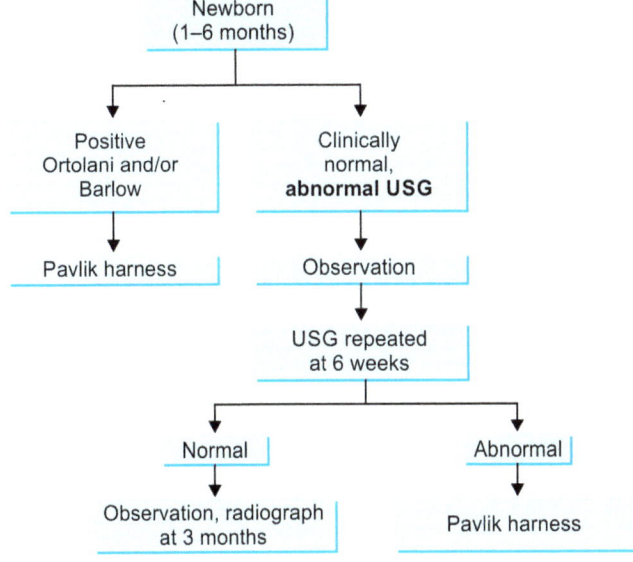

2. **Pavlik harness:**
   i. It is a dynamic flexion-abduction orthosis (95% successful treatment)
   ii. Chest strap: Level of nipples
   iii. Shoulder strap
   iv. Feet in stirrup
   v. Flexion strap: Anteromedial – 110-120°
   vi. Abduction strap: Posteromedial. Must be gravitational. Forceful abduction can lead to AVN.
   vii. To be worn full-time
   viii. Weekly follow-up
   ix. Look for active knee flexion at each F/U: Femoral nerve palsy
   x. Infants outgrow in 3-4 weeks
   xi. Repeat USG at 3 weeks (**Fig. 20**)

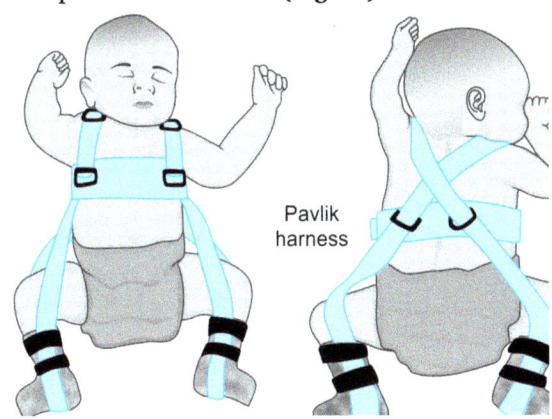

3.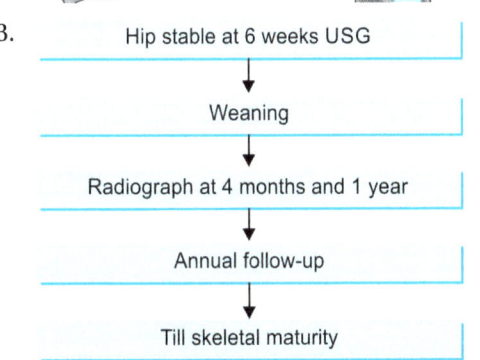

4.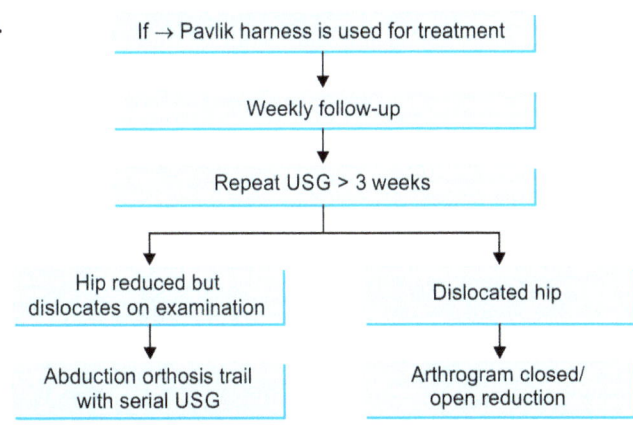

5. *Pavlik disease:*
   i. Erosion of the pelvis superior to acetabulum.
   ii. Prevention of development of posterior wall of acetabulum due to prolonged hip flexion and abduction
   iii. Therefore, discontinue harness if hip is not reduced by 3-4 weeks.
6. Other orthosis → von Rosen splint, Ilfeld/Craig splint.
7. Not to be used → Frejka pillow, triple diaper (Never forcefully abduct the child hip → leads to AVN).

B. Infants 6–18 Months (Fig. 21)

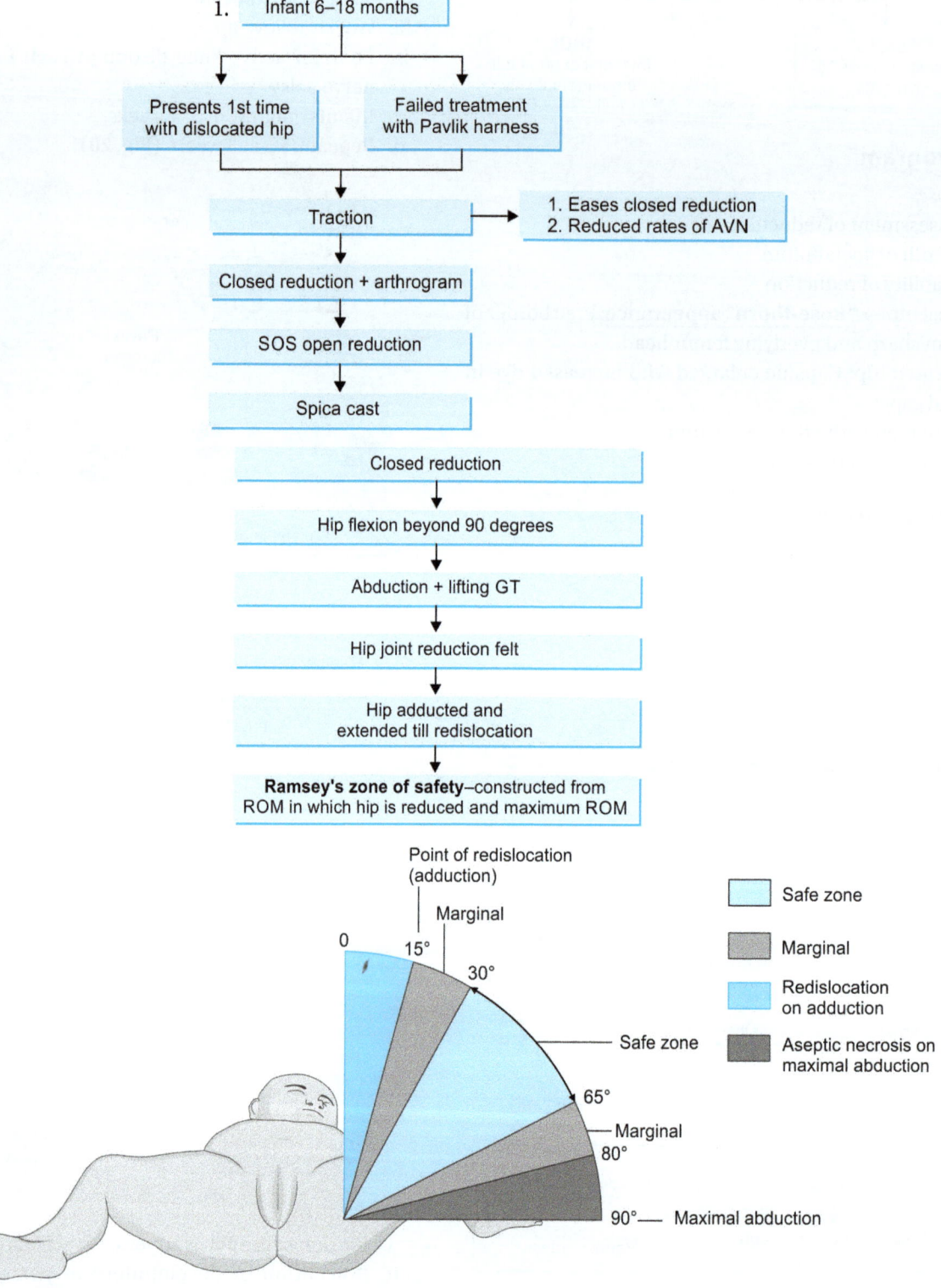

3. *Spica cast: In "Human position":*
   i. Hip flexion 90–100°
   ii. Abduction 45°
   iii. Immobilization for 4 months
4. *Arthrogram:*
   i. Assessment of reduction
   ii. Depth of acetabulum
   iii. Stability of reduction
   iv. Normal hip: "Rose-thorn" appearance
      a. Free border of labrum sharp and overlying femur head.

v. Dislocated hip: Capsule enlarged with increased dye in medial gap.
   a. Adequate reduction → 5-6 mm
   b. Poor reduction → >6 mm
5. Open reduction → When CR fails

Medial approach	Anterior approach
<12 months	>12 months
Directly addresses block to reduction	MC used → decreased risk of injury to MCFA
Unable to perform capsulorrhaphy	Capsulorrhaphy
Higher risk of AVN	
Separate incision for pelvic osteotomy	

C. Toddler (18–24 Months)

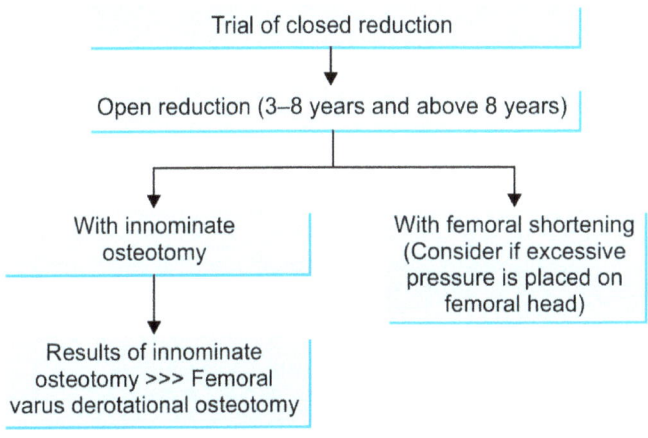

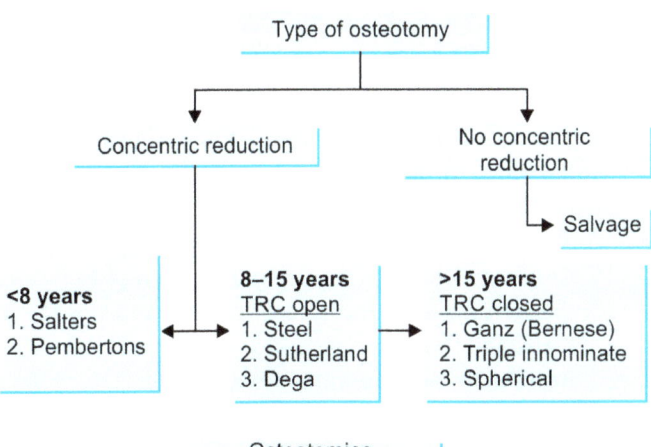

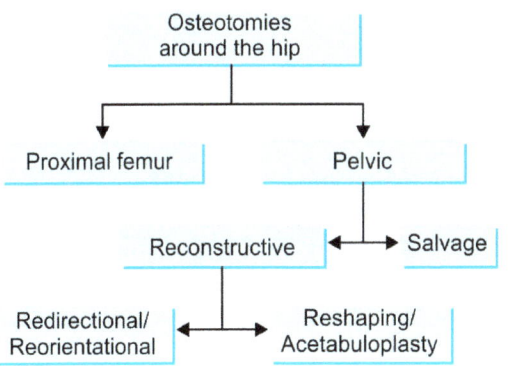

Pelvic osteotomies		
Reconstructive		Salvage
Redirectional	Reshaping	
Salters (Single Innominate)	Pemberton	Shelf
Sutherland (Double Innominate)	Dega	Chiari
Tonnis and Steel (Triple Innominate)	San Diego	
Ganz		
Spherical osteotomies		

1. **Salter's osteotomy:**
   i. Age: 1.5-9 years
   ii. Improves Anterolateral coverage → 10°
   iii. Limb length increases by 1 cm
   iv. Single transverse cut
   v. AIIS → Sciatic notch
   vi. Kalamchi modification
      a. Prevents medial and posterior displacement.
      b. Added limb length eliminated
      c. Decreased pressure on femoral head, increased stability (**Fig. 22**)

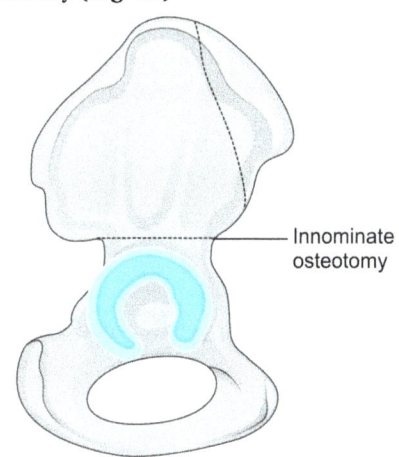

2. **Pemberton's osteotomy:**
   i. Pericapsular osteotomy of ilium
   ii. 18 months-10 years
   iii. Correction better than Salters
   iv. Acetabulum hinges on pubic symphysis Anteriorly and TRC posteriorly (**Fig. 23**).

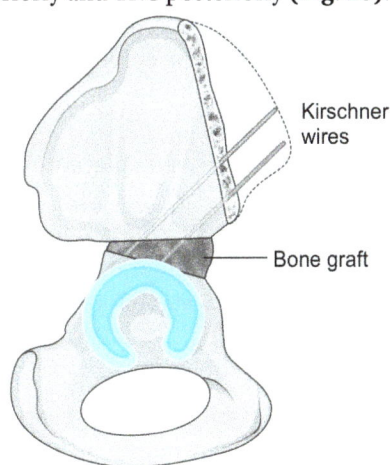

3. **Salvage osteotomies: For incongruous hips:**
   i. Chiari (**Fig. 24**)

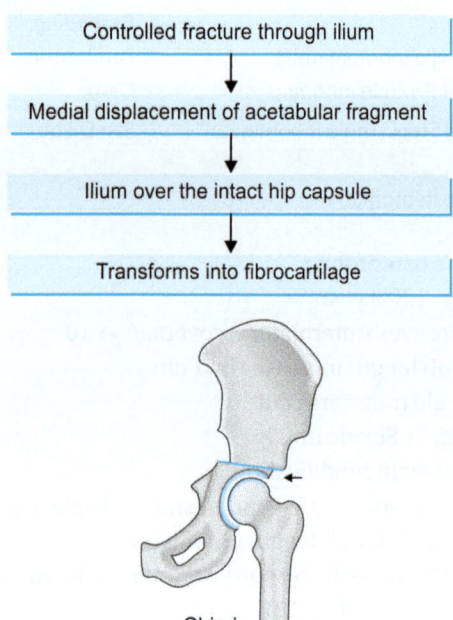

Chiari

ii. Staheli's shelf osteotomy: Shelf is constructed over femur head using local shavings of iliac wing (**Fig. 25**).

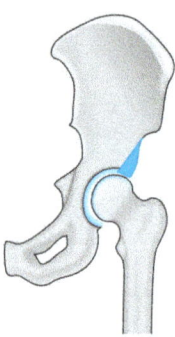

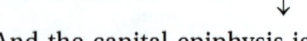

Shelf arthroplasty

SLIPPED CAPITAL FEMORAL EPIPHYSIS

I. INTRODUCTION

1. SCFE (Adolescent coxa vara) occurs during the adolescent rapid growth period when the epiphyseal growth plate is weakened
   ↓
2. And the capital epiphysis is displaced downward and backward.
3. "SCFE" → misnomer: Actually the femoral neck and shaft are displaced upward and anteriorly while the femoral epiphysis remains in the acetabulum.

II. ETIOLOGY

1. *Age:* Rapid growth between 10 and 17 years.
   ∴ SCFE occurs in this age group.
2. *Sex:* Males > females (2:1.4)
3. *Body type and obesity:*
   i. Single greatest risk factor
   ii. Frolic type obesity with underdeveloped genitalia
4. *Location:*
   i. L > R
   ii. B/L in 25%
5. *Trauma:*
   i. Trivial trauma history maybe present
   ii. The pressure of weight-bearing or muscular contraction superimposed on the weakened epiphyseal growth plate is sufficient to cause displacement.
   iii. Rarely, severe trauma causes acute separation through the growth plate (acute slip)
6. *Hormone theory:*

   1. Separation occurs through the hypertrophied layer of physis
   ↓
   2. At this level, the chondrocytes are large and the intercellular matrix, on which the tissue strength depends is thin
   ↓
   3. Growth hormone ↑ rate of proliferation of chondrocytes and further ↑ area of hypertrophied cells
      This further lessens resistance to pressure
   ↓
   4. Sex hormone (especially estrogen)
      Decreases secretion of GH and rate of skeletal growth
   ↓
   5. Estrogen also stimulates enchondral bone formation
      → Newly formed trabeculae are thick and strong
   ↓
   6. ∴ During growth, the structure of epiphyseal plate depends on relative levels of GH and sex hormone

7. *Mechanical theory:*
   i. The periosteum spanning the epiphyseal plate becomes progressively thinner from childhood, through adolescence as adulthood reaches.
      ↓
   ii. Consequently, during the period of rapid growth, the periosteal covering is stretched and unable to withstand the shearing forces.
   iii. Acetabular and femoral retroversion.

III. PATHOLOGY

1. The epiphysis slowly displaces posteriorly and inferiorly, with the femur neck shifting upward and rotating anteriorly.
2. Varus, adduction and ER deformity.
3. The interval produced by separation becomes filled with fibrous tissue, embryonic cartilage and callus.
4. The head remains attached to posterior periosteum (retinaculum) through which the major vessels reach the epiphysis.

5. After several months, the epiphyseal junction heals and the exposed portion of the neck superiorly and anteriorly becomes covered with fibrocartilage.
6. If displacement persists over the years → degenerative changes supervene.
7. Chondrolysis → Pathological degeneration and erosion of articular cartilage, chronic inflammation and fibrosis of capsule and synovium. Fibrous ankylosis may develop.
8. AVN results when the posterior epiphyseal attachment and it is combined vessels are torn by forcible manipulation and surgical trauma.
9. Abduction and internal rotation restricted due to:
    i. Large "**herndon hump**" formed by fibrous cartilage overgrowth on the anterior exposed portion of the neck → impinges against the anterior and superior margins of the acetabulum.
    ii. The capital epiphysis is fixed posterior and inferior
    ↓
    Further outward movement is limited by its impingement against the posterior capsule.

IV. CLASSIFICATION
A. Loder
(Prognostic value): Based on ability to bear weight.
1. Stable: Able to bear weight with or without crutches (90%)
2. Unstable: Unable to ambulate (not even with crutches). ↑ risk of ON.

B. Temporal
Based on duration of symptoms:
1. Pre-slip: Prodromal
2. Acute: Symptoms for <3 weeks
3. Chronic: >3 weeks
4. Acute on chronic: Acute exacerbation of long standing symptoms.

C. Southwick Slip Angle
1. Based on femoral epiphyseal-diaphyseal angle difference.
2. Difference between normal and affected site (**Fig. 26**).

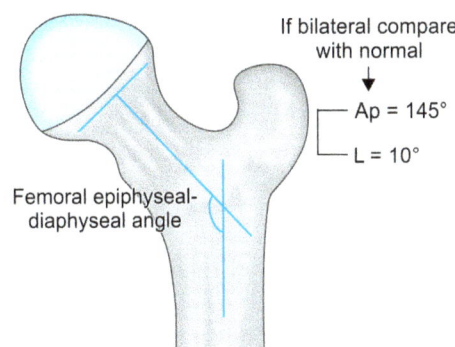

Femoral epiphyseal-diaphyseal angle

If bilateral compare with normal
- Ap = 145°
- L = 10°

   i. Mild: <30°
   ii. Moderate: 30–50°
   iii. Severe: >50°

V. CLINICAL PRESENTATION
A. Symptoms
1. **Pain**:
    i. Groin or thigh pain → MC presentation
    ii. Knee pain → medial obturator nerve.
2. **Limp**:
    i. Antalgic gait
    ii. Externally rotated foot progression angle
3. Patient prefer to sit in a chair with affected leg crossed over the other
4. Symptoms are usually present for weeks and months before Dx is made.

B. Physical Examination
1. *Abnormal gait:*
    i. Antalgic
    ii. Waddling → B/L involvement
    iii. Externally rotated gait
    iv. Trendelenburg gait
2. ↓ *Hip ROM:*
    i. **Drehmann sign** → Obligatory external rotation during passive flexion of hip due to
    ↓
      a. Synovitis +
      b. Impingement of the displaced anterior - lateral femoral metaphysis on the acetabular rim
    ii. Loss of hip abduction, IR and flexion
    iii. Thigh muscle atrophy.

VI. INVESTIGATIONS
1. Views: AP ⎫
        Frog leg lateral ⎬ both hips
                        ⎭
   ↓
   Hips in 90° flexion and 45° IR
2. Lateral better than AP X-ray for diagnosing subtle slips.
3. Earliest findings in the preslipping stage
    i. Globular swelling of joint capsule
    ii. Irregular widening of epiphyseal line
    iii. Decalcification of the epiphyseal border of the metaphysis
4. Continuity of Shenton's line broken
5. **Blanch sign of steel**: Area of ↓ bone density in the proximal femoral neck.
6. **Trethowan's sign**: Failure of Klien's line to intersect femur head (**Fig. 27**).

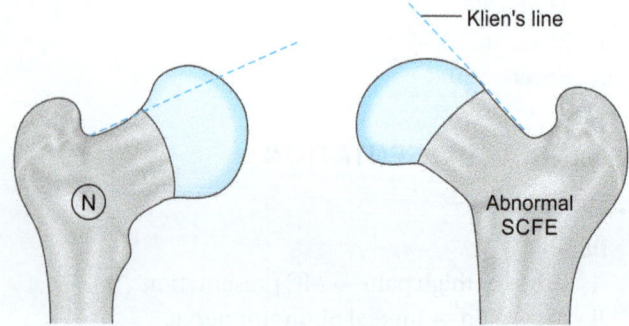

7. Chronic SCFE:
   i. Rounding of superior portion of FN
   ii. Reduced height of epiphysis
   iii. Callus at epiphysio metaphyseal junction
8. X-ray used to grade severity of slip.
   i. Linear displacement → Wilson's method
   ii. Angular displacement → Southwick
9. CT scan
   i. To evaluate penetration of head of femur by fixation device.
   ii. To confirm closure of PF physis
10. Technetium 99 → ↑ uptake B/L → Chondrolysis
11. USG → Joint effusion, step between femoral neck and epiphysis.
12. MRI → May help in diagnosis of pre-slip when X-ray negative.
13. Blood investigation → Endocrine profile.

VII. TREATMENT
A. General
1. Strictly nonweight-bearing as soon as diagnosis is made.
2. Bed rest, ↑ traction crutches, brace → to prevent further displacement
3. There is no role of conservative management in SCFE, surgery is the only option.

B. Operative
1. *Principles:*
   i. Prevent further slippage
   ii. Stimulate early physeal closure
   iii. Reduction of epiphyseal displacement
   iv. Avoid complications like ON, chondrolysis and OA
2. *Three broad treatment methods available:*
   i. To prevent further slippage → in situ fixation
   ii. To reduce degree of slippage → corrective osteotomies
   iii. Salvage procedure
3. Prophylactic treatment of C/L hip → Controversial. Maybe considered in patients at high risk (Endocrine abnormalities)
4. Gentle manipulative reduction may only be attempted in acute and acute on chronic slips.
5. Contraindicated in chronic slips → ↑ ON
6. *In situ pins or screw fixation:*
   i. Percutaneous in situ pinning is currently the most often Rx for mild and moderate slips
   ii. Open pinning may be indicated for more severe acute or acute on chronic slips
   iii. Single large diameter central pin/screw should be passed perpendicular to physis
   iv. Persistent pin penetration → Complication
7. *Bone peg epiphysiodesis* (Fig. 28):

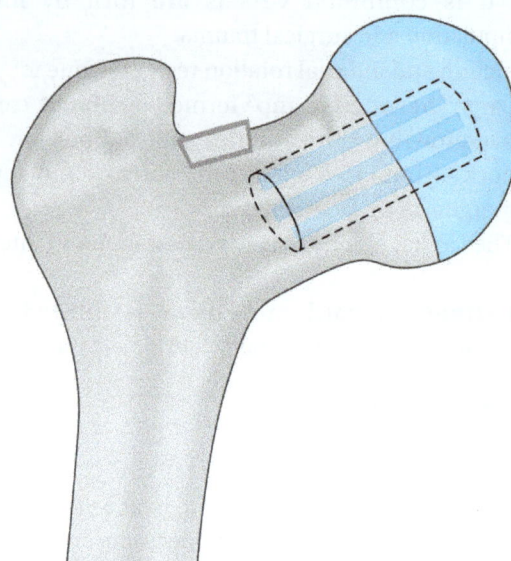

   i. Rapid closure of physis and ↓ chondrolysis
   ii. Bone grafts cross the physeal plate and are deeply embedded in the FH
8. *Osteotomies* (Fig. 29):

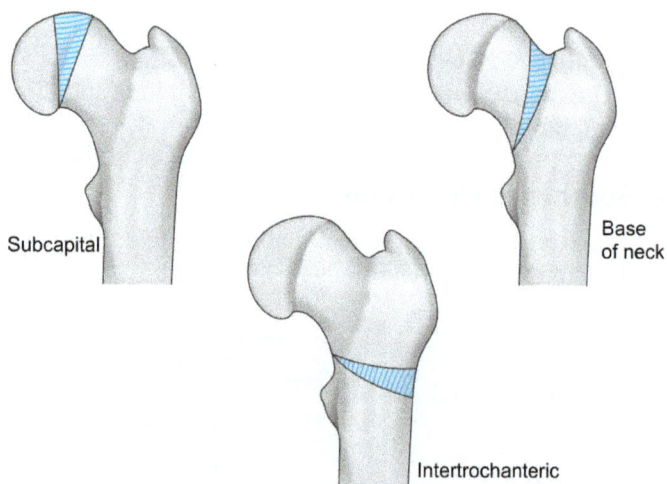

   i. Goals:
      a. Restore the normal relationship of the FH and neck
      b. Delay the onset of degenerative joint disease

ii.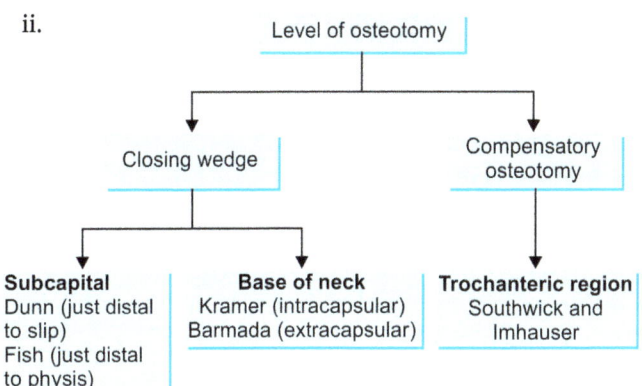
iii. The advantage of subcapital osteotomy is that deformity itself is corrected.
iv. Disadvantage → High incidence of ON and chondrolysis
v. The osteotomy at the base of the neck avoids disruption of the neck avoids disruption of the bloody supply to FH
vi. *Trochanteric osteotomy:*
   a. Ball and socket osteotomy (Campbell)
   b. High subtrochanteric osteotomy (Tachdjian)
   c. Biplane intertrochanteric osteotomy (Southwick)
vii. Trochanteric osteotomy is far away from FH blood supply but,
   ↓
   Substitutes one deformity for another. Does not accurately restore mechanisms.
viii. Osteoplasty of femoral neck (Heyman–Herndon) (Cheilectomy) → Simple resection.
   Large bony prominence on the anterosuperior aspect of FN → blocks IR and abduction by impinging against acetabulum
ix. Reconstruction → Hip arthroplasty
x. Salvage: Hip arthrodesis

COXA VARA

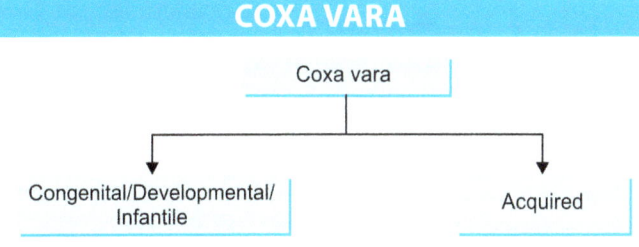

I. INTRODUCTION
Developmental coxa vara is a primary ossification defect in the inferomedial part of the neck leading to decreased neck–shaft angle.

II. CLASSIFICATION–ETIOLOGY
1. *Developmental:* → Isolated
   → Associated with dysplasia (Cleidocranial dysostosis)
2. *Acquired:*
   i. SCFE
   ii. LCPD
   iii. Septic arthritis
   iv. DDH reduction
   v. Post-traumatic → FN fracture
   vi. Associated with pathologic bone disorders:
      a. OI
      b. Fibrous dysplasia
      c. Renal osteodystrophy
      d. Osteoporosis
3. *Congenital:* Associated with congenital femoral deficiency (PFFD).

III. PATHOPHYSIOLOGY
1. Proximal femoral cartilaginous physis defect.
   ↓
   ↓ Proximal femur neck–shaft angle.
2. Vertical position of PF physis + Varus
   ↓
   Inferomedial neck compressive forces
   Physeal sheering forces

IV. CLINICAL PRESENTATION
A. History
1. Family
2. Trauma } Rule out 2° causes.
3. Skeletal abnormalities

B. Symptoms
1. Incidence: Boys = Girls
2. Present at walking age (18 months–3 years)
3. Painless limp → Trendelenburg
   → Waddling (if B/L)

C. Examination
1. LLD: Shortening
2. Decreased abduction and IR: Nontender
3. High riding trochanter
4. Excessive lumbar lordosis
5. Galeazzi test: Femoral shortening.

V. INVESTIGATIONS
1. Radiograph → AP with hip IR
   → Lateral hip
   i. Varus neck shaft angle = <120°
   ii. Short femoral neck: Coxa breva
   iii. Vertical physis
   iv. Increased Hilgenreiner's epiphyseal angle (Normal < 25°)

Pediatric Orthopedics

v. Triangular metaphyseal fragment in the inferomedial femoral neck: Inverted Y-lucency (Fairbanks triangle) **(Fig. 30)**

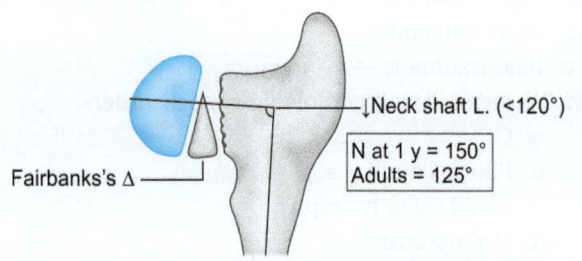

vi. ↓ Femoral anteversion

2. *CT scan*:
   i. Surgical planning
   ii. Delineates PF defects
   iii. Orientation of deformity

VI. TREATMENT
A. Based on HEA (Fig. 31)

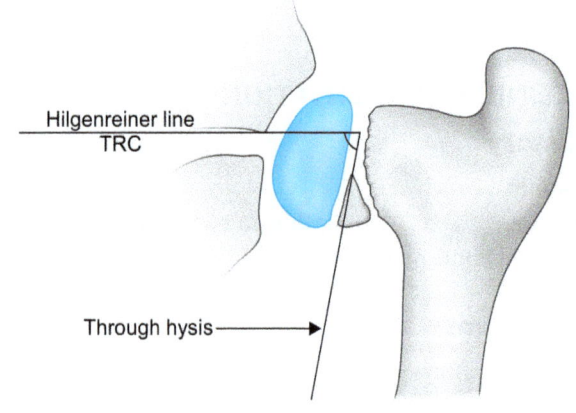

1. <45° → Observation alone
2. 45–60° → May progress
   Close follow-up → if nonsymptomatic
3. >60 or 45–60° (symptomatic) → Operative
   NS angle = <110°

B. Corrective Valgus Derotational Osteotomy (VDRO)

1. *Goals*:
   i. Overcorrect NS angle. HEA < 38°
   ii. Correct LLD
   iii. Correct hip anteversion
   iv. Re-establish abductor muscle tensioning.
2. Approach: Direct lateral
3. Procedure: Valgus trochanteric osteotomy
   Fixation → Blade plate
4. Others → GT transfer
            → GT epiphysiodesis

VII. COMPLICATIONS
1. Premature close of physis
2. Loss of correction
3. Overgrowth of PF
4. Acetabular dysplasia

ANGULAR DEFORMITIES OF LL IN CHILDREN

Physis → "nature" (greek)
↓
Injury → Abnormal longitudinal growth
       → Angular deformity

I. GROWTH AT PHYSIS (% OF BONE) (FIG. 32)

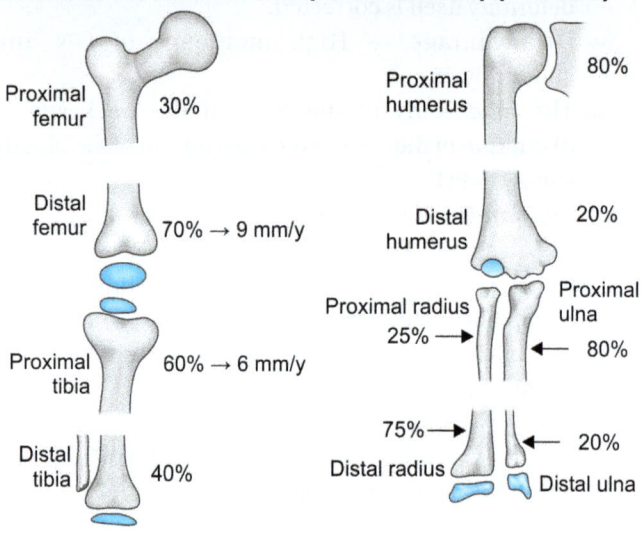

II. BLOOD SUPPLY (FIG. 33)

Epiphyseal blood vessels → danger zone
↓
No other blood supply in epiphysis

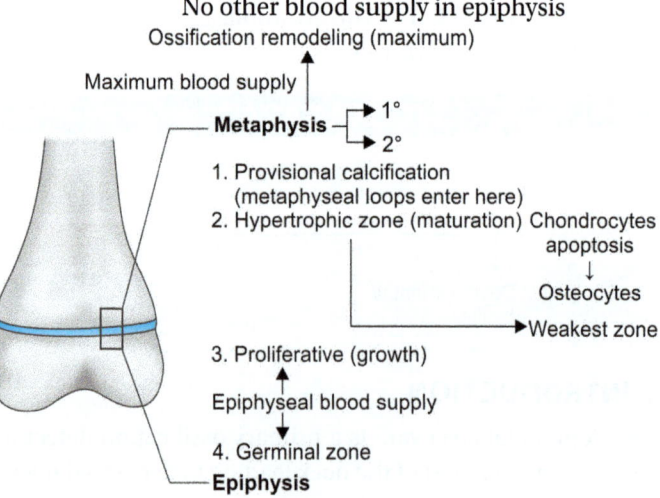

III. HUETER-VOLKMANN LAW

Mechanical forces → (influence) → Longitudinal growth
Compressive forces → Inhibit growth
Tension forces + + Cortical bone

Physeal arrest classification (Fig. 34):

↓

Peterson

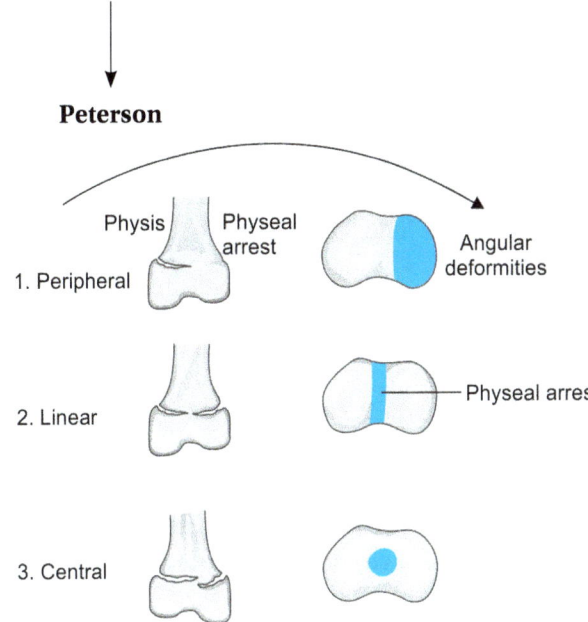

1. Peripheral — Physis, Physeal arrest → Angular deformities
2. Linear — Physeal arrest
3. Central

Children → Tibiofemoral angle:

0–18 months	18–30 months	3–4 years	8–18 years
Varus	Straight	Excessive valgus	Normal adult valgus
10–15°	0°	10–15°	6–8°

("Selenius and Venka" 1975 JBJS)

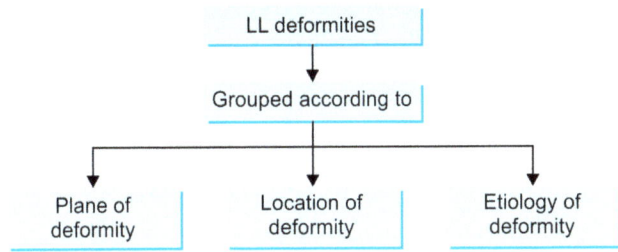

LL deformities → Grouped according to:
- Plane of deformity
- Location of deformity
- Etiology of deformity

IV. PLANE

Varus / Valgus } Frontal/Coronal

Procurvatum / Recurvatum } Sagittal

Intorsion / Extorsion } Axial

Oblique → Combination

V. ETIOLOGY

1. Physiological: Normal variant
2. Traumatic
3. Infective
4. Metabolic: Rickets, renal osteodystrophy
5. Congenital: Syndromes, dysplasias
6. Developmental: Blount's, tibia vara
7. Neoplastic: HME
8. Neuromuscular: CP
9. Idiopathic
10. Iatrogenic

Children → 10% fractures involve physis
4% of these are associated with bar formation.

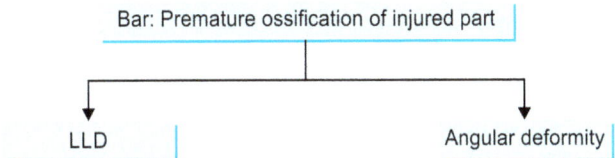

Bar: Premature ossification of injured part
→ LLD
→ Angular deformity

Distal femur physis → "undulating and irregular" → Predisposed to bar formation
SH 2: Usually no bar formation
SH 3 and 4: Most common cause of bar formation.
Because involvement of epiphysis (Poor blood supply)

VI. HISTORY

1. Age of onset (remember normal development of Genu)
2. Progression or regression of deformity
3. History suggestive of etiology:
   i. Family (hypophosphatemic rickets, etc.)
   ii. Dietary (milk allergy)
   iii. Past history of trauma/infection

VII. SYMPTOMS

1. Parental concern → Appearance
2. Gait disturbance → Circumduction, waddling
3. Function → Frequent falls, unable to run
4. Anterior knee pain

VIII. GENERAL EXAMINATION

1. Height: Short stature → Achondroplasia? Rickets?
2. Weight: Obese → Blounts?
3. Ligamentous laxity: Exaggerated deformity on weight bearing.
4. Multiple swellings: Enchondromatosis, HME.

IX. LOCAL EXAMINATION

1. U/L or B/L
2. Symmetrical or asymmetrical
   U/L or asymmetrical
   ↓
   look for pathological cause
3. Intercondylar distance } In standing position
4. Intermalleolar distance
5. Tibiofemoral angle (Goniometer)

6. Knee flexion test
   ↓
   Deformity disappears completely on flexion knee joint
   ↓
   Source: Distal femur → posterior condyles do not contribute to axial plane deformity
7. *Cover-up test:*
   i. Screening test
   ii. To assess alignment of upper part of leg
   iii. In children with bow legs of age 1–3 years
   iv. Positive: Bowing in upper tibia
   v. Negative: Slight valgus at upper tibia (physiological bowing)
8. *Torsional profile:*
   i. Femoral torsion
      In prone position
      Check for hip external and internal rotation
      ↑ IR → Excessive femoral anteversion
      Tibial torsion
      ↓
      Thigh-foot angle → (N) 15–30° external tibial torsion
      Prone position
      Assessment of instability:
      a. Genu valgum: Patellofemoral maltracking/subluxation
      b. Genu varum: LCL laxity
9. *Gait*:
   i. Waddling/Circumduction
   ii. Lateral thrust: Tibia vara

X. RADIOGRAPH

Full length standing AP view
↓
Iliac crest to ankle
1. Both feet flat on floor (use blocks to level iliac crest if LLD)
2. Both knees max extension
3. Both patellae facing forward.
4. If severe deformity/obesity → Each limb separate
5. Distance between X-ray tube and patient → 10 feet (focus on knee)
6. Lateral view → 10° externally rotated for femoral condyles overlap.

MRI

Fat suppressed images: Bony Barr.

XI. BIOCHEMICAL INVESTIGATIONS

1. Sr. calcium
2. Sr. alkaline phosphatase
3. Vitamin D
4. PTH
5. Urine calcium
6. Renal profile

XII. LOWER LIMB ALIGNMENT

1. Alignment: Collinearity of the hip, knee, ankle
2. Joint orientation: Position of the articular surface relative to the axis of the limb ligament.

Malalignment Test
1. Is there a deformity?
2. Which bone/area?
3. Exactly where in the bone? (CORA)

A. Mechanical Axis of the Limb

Line between center of femoral head → center of ankle.
Normally passes through center of knee (±8 mm)
Passes → Laterally → Valgus
       → Medially → Varus

B. Mechanical Axis of Bone

1. Center of joint above to center of joint below
2. Femur → Center of FH → Center of knee
3. Tibia → Center of proximal tibia → Center of ankle
4. Normal MA of femur and tibia → colinear
5. Angle between distal femur joint line and proximal tibia joint → JLCA
6. Joint line convergence angle (JLCA) → N = 0–2°
7. *Source of deformity* (**Fig. 35**):

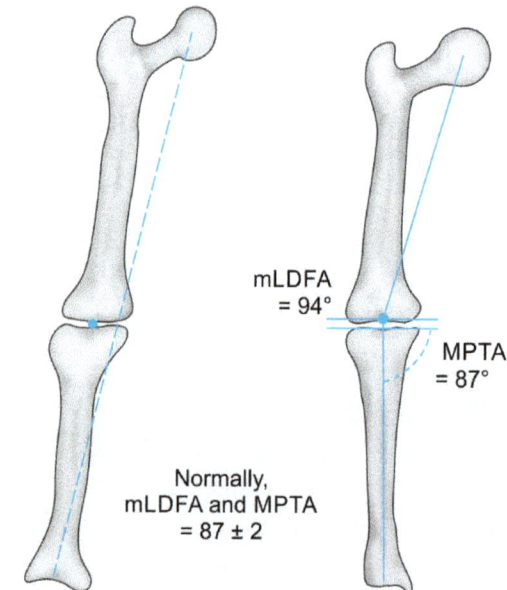

mLDFA = 94°
MPTA = 87°
Normally, mLDFA and MPTA = 87 ± 2

1. Draw MA of LL → If passing medial to knee joint → Varus. Where but?
   Distal femur or proximal tibia?
2. Draw MA of LL → Medially ∴ VARUS
3. Draw MA of femur and tibia

mLDFA	MPTA	Source
94	87	Femur
87	82	Tibia
94	82	Both

3. Exactly where in the bone is the deformity??

MA   vs   Anatomic axis
↓
Mostly we use MA → Because goal of surgery is to restore this.
In tibia, MA = AA

Femur
AA: Piriformis fossa to slightly medial to deepest point of IC notch.
Angle between MA and AA of femur: **6°**

So, where in bone?
CORA = Center of rotation of angulation
Draw proximal axis and distal axis **(Fig. 36)**

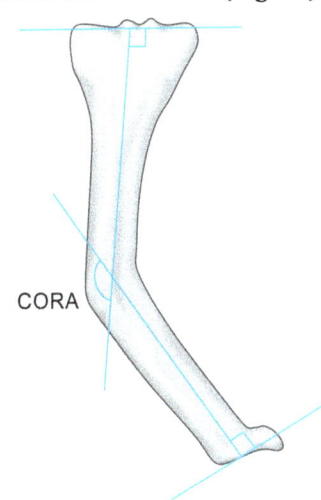

But most CORAs in children will come around physis **(Fig. 37)**.

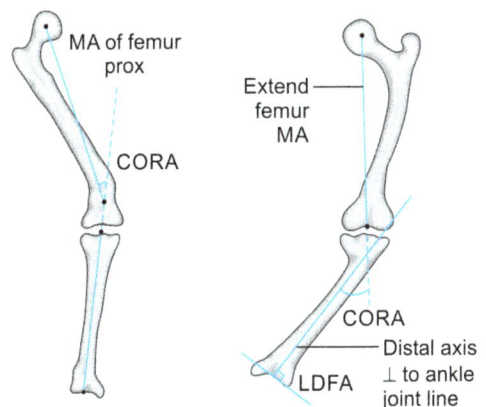

XIII. GROWTH MODULATION FOR ANGULAR DEFORMITIES OF LL

1. Cessation of deceleration of the natural growth across a growing point to correct deformities of the axial/appendicular skeleton
2. Stop growth on convex side
3. Continue of concave side ∴ correct deformity.
4. **GROWTH MODULATION**
   ↓   ↓
   Temporary   Permanent
   ↓   ↓
   8 - plates   Physeal ablation
                        Transphyseal screws
5. *Implant placement:*
   i. Extraperiosteal
   ii. Epiphyseal → centered in frontal plane
   iii. Equicortical → centered between anterior and posterior cortex in sagittal plane
6. *Indication of growth modulation:*
   i. Skeletally immature with at least 2-3 years of growth remaining
   ii. 1.5 degree of correction/month = Idiopathic
   iii. 0.5° in dysplastic.
7. *Phases of growth*:

   Prenatal   -Exponential
      ↓
   Birth-5 years   -Fast growth
      ↓
   5 years-puberty -Stable growth
      ↓
   Puberty   -2nd spurt
      ↓

   Important here, as majority of angular deformities present during this phase.

8. Growth modulation   v/s   Osteotomy **(Fig. 38)**
        ↓   ↓
   1-2 years growth remaining   <1-2 years remaining

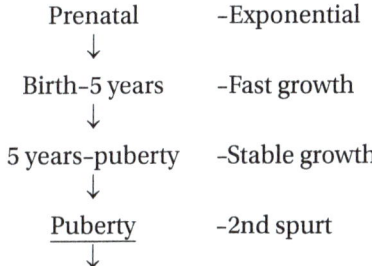

9. Chronological age dose not correlate with stage of growth
   Skeletal age strongly correlates to stage of growth.
   ↓
   Indicator of biological maturity of child
10. Appearance of sesamoid bone at base of thumb.
    ↓
    Onset of puberty (G11, B13)
    Closure of TRC (G12, B14)

11. *Dimeglio = Olecranon*
Five stages:
i. Two ossification nuclei: At onset of puberty
ii. Half moon

iii. Rectangular stage
iv. Beginning of fusion
v. Completion of fusion → at PHV
12. *Risser = iliac apophysis*
13. Sauvegrain method = elbow
Matching of charts
25 = PHV
If >25 → not much growth remaining.

XIV. PRINCIPLES OF DEFORMITY CORRECTION

1. Identify CORA by midalignment test
2. Femur/tibia/ankle joint
3. Resolve to single CORA if deformity <10°
4. Multiapical deformity: multilevel osteotomy
5. Recognize coexisting torsional component
6. Closed-wedge/open wedge/dome osteotomy
7. As close to CORA as possible
8. Accommodate ligament laxity especially in dysplasias
   i. When measuring IC distance in genu varum
   ↓
   Keep patella facing forward

XV. DEFORMITY CORRECTION INDICATIONS

1. Skeletally mature
2. Complex/multiapical deformities
3. Severe deformities ≥30°
4. Dysplasias or syndromes where growth modulation is less reliable
5. Attempt bar excision if:
   i. >2 years growth remaining
   ii. <30% bar compared to total physis

CONGENITAL PSEUDOARTHROSIS OF TIBIA (CPT)

Tibial bowing
- Anterolateral → CPT
- Posteromedial → Physiological
- Anteromedial → Fibular hemimelia

1. A congenital bowing of tibial diaphysis (anterolateral apex), associated with diaphyseal pseudoarthrosis.
2. Pseudoarthrosis is usually not congenital, and develops postnatally due to fracture nonunion.
3. Continuum of disease: Anterolateral bowing of tibia = CPT.
4. Associated condition → **NF1** is found in 55% of patients with AL bowing. 15% associated with fibrous dysplasia.
5. Rare, 1: 200,000

I. PATHOLOGY

Upper and lower end of tibia have a normal structural appearance
↓
Diaphysis becomes progressively tapered near the defect
↓
Medullary canal obliterated and bone ends sclerotic
↓
Gap occupied by hypercellular fibrous tissue, continuous with thickened periosteum

Congenital ALB → Fracture → CPT
1. AL bowing   ⎫
2. Congenital CPT   ⎬ Precursors of CPT
                     ⎭

II. INVESTIGATIONS

A. Radiograph

1. Absence of bone formation of tibia at junction of **middle 2/3rd and distal 1/3rd**.
2. Varying degrees of:
   i Diaphyseal tapering
   ii Sclerosis
   iii. Obliteration of medullary canal
3. Usually fibula unaffected, but may display pseudoarthrosis at same level.
4. The distal tibial segment is angulated backward = equinus of foot.

III. CLASSIFICATION

Boyd, Crawford, Anderson: Do not guide management or outcome.

Paley's classification (2019): Guides treatment.

Type 1: No fractures
Type 2: No fracture tibia, fracture fibula with fibula (a) at station (b) proximal migration
Type 3: Fracture tibia, no fracture fibula
Type 4: Fracture tibia and fibula with fibula (a) at station (b) proximal migration (c) bone defect tibia with proximal migration fibula.

Crawford (Fig. 39)

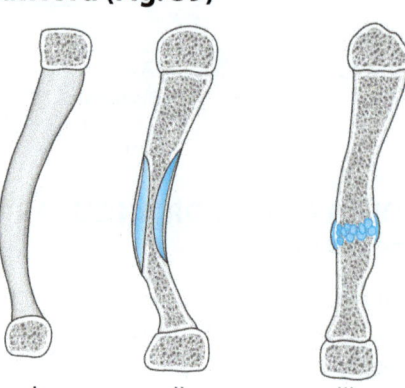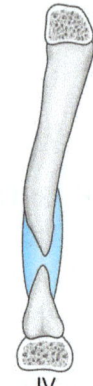

I II III IV

1. *Nondysplastic:*
    i. Anterolateral bowing
    ii. Increased cortical density (medullary sclerosis)
2. *Dysplastic:*
    i. Failure of tabulation
    ii. Narrow medullary canal
3. *Cystic*
4. *Atrophic/frank pseudoarthrosis*

IV. CLINICAL FEATURES
1. Majority present in 1st year with bowing
2. Deformity
3. NF = café au lait spots, neurofibromas, Scoliosis, Lisch nodules

V. TREATMENT
A. Conservative
1. Bracing in clamshell orthosis or patellar tendon bearing (PTB) orthosis.
   Indications:
     i. Ambulatory age
     ii. Bowing without PA/Fracture
   Goal:
     i. Prevent further Bowing or fracture
     ii Maintained unit skeletal maturity
     iii Osteotomy for bowing alone is a contraindication.
2. BMP: 2 and 7 = Promising results [postoperative IV pamidronate (Bisphosphonates)]
3. Electrical stimulation

B. Operative
1. Goals:
    i. Achieve union: Excision of pseudoarthrosis
    ii. Refracture prevention: Splinting till skeletal maturity
    iii. Limb length discrepancy correction
        ↓
        Early intervention for union and limb equalization procedures
    iv. Correction of growth abnormalities
    v. Ankle deformity correction: Retain intramedullary nail that crosses the ankle joint (until skeletal maturity) or ilizarov technique.
2. Options:
    i. Intramedullay nailing and cortical bone graft. (1st procedure of choice)
    ii. Operative frame fixation with ilizarov lengthening or bone transport
        ↓
        (<5 years = poor result)
        (>5 years = good result)
    iii. Microsvasculature free fibular grafting (Farmer's procedure)
    iv. *Amputation*:
        Indications:
         a. Multiple failed surgical attempts at union
         b. Severe LLD
         c. Dysfunctional angular deformity
            Syme's or Boyd amputation
            ↓
            Prosthesis

C. Complications
1. Recurrent fractures (50%)
2. Valgus deformity
3. LLD at skeletal maturity (average 5 cm)

TIBIA VARA

I. INTRODUCTION
Developmental disorder characterized by growth retardation at the posteromedial aspect of the proximal tibial epiphysis and physis resulting in a persistent or progressive low leg.

II. TYPES

Infantile	Adolescent
2–5 years	>10 years
B/L : 50%	U/L
More common	Less
More severe	Less
Early stages can resolve spontaneously	Progressive
Bracing and surgery	Surgery only

III. ETIOPATHOGENESIS
1. *Risk factors*:
    i. Overweight/obese
    ii. Early walkers
    iii. African–American
    iv. Hereditary
2. Mechanical overload in a genetically susceptible individual
   ↓
   Excessive medial pressure
   ↓
   Osteochondrosis of the medial proximal tibial physis and epiphysis
   ↓
   May progress to physeal bar formation

IV. CLINICAL FEATURES
1. Genu varum
2. Flexion deformity ±
3. Internal tibial torsion: Thigh foot angle
4. LLD
5. Positive "cover-up" test.
6. Usually NO → tenderness, ROM restriction, effusion.
7. Lateral thrust on walking.

V. RADIOLOGY

A. Langenskiold

1. Classification (Fig. 40):

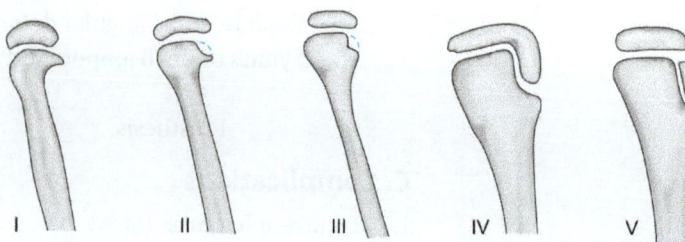

Stage:
   I: Medial metaphyseal beaking
   II: Saucer-shaped defect of medial metaphysis
   III: Saucer deepens into step
   IV: Sloping of epiphysis into metaphysis
   V: Double epiphysis
   VI: Medial physeal bone bar

2. Measurements:
   i. Metaphyseal: Diaphyseal angle (Drennan) (Fig. 41)

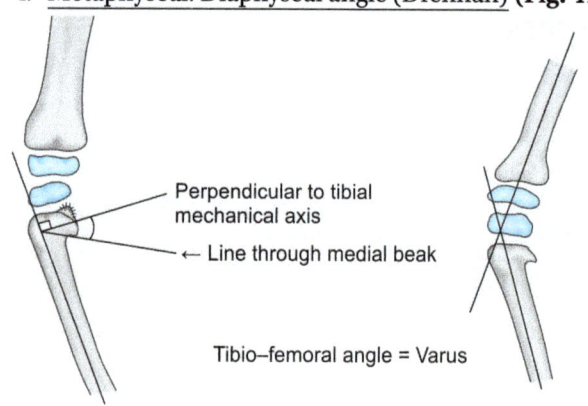

   a. >16° → 95% progress = Tibia vara
   b. <10° → 95% resolve
   c. 11–16° → Observe
   ii. Tibiofemoral angle = Varus

VI. TREATMENT

Depends upon:
1. Age
2. Severity of disease

A. Conservative

1. Brace → Knee ankle foot orthosis (KAFO)
2. For stage I and II <3 years
3. Worn for 2 years
4. Good prognosis → U/L,
5. Bad prognosis → B/L, obese

B. Operative

1. *Indications*:
   i. Stage I and II >3 years
   ii. III, IV, V, VI stages <3 years
   iii. Any stage ≥4 years
   iv. Failure of brace Rx → Progression
   v. MD Angle: >20°
2. Proximal tibia and fibula osteotomy: Overcorrect to 10–15 valgus.
   Technique:
   i. Osteotomy below TT
   ii. Staged → IV, V, VI
   iii. Epiphysiolysis → V, VI
   iv. Medial opening wedge → For LLD
3.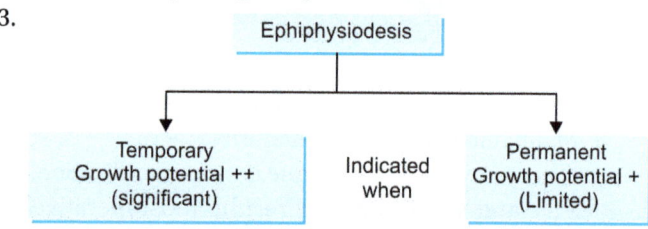

4. Hemiplateau elevation → Intraepiphyseal osteotomy. Restore joint stability (Fig. 42).

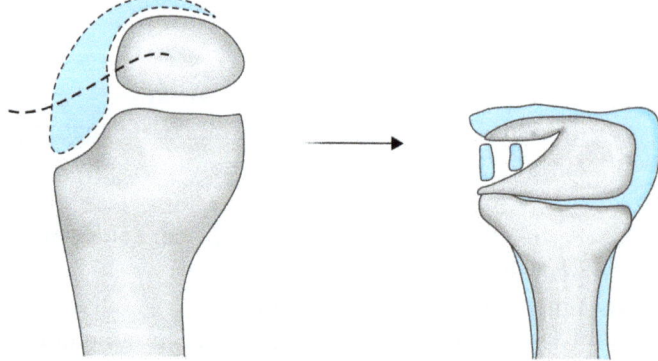

Immobilization after osteotomy = Cast, pins
Ex. Fix plate, screws

5. Immobilization after osteotomy = Cast, Pins
   Ex. Fix
   Plate, screws

VII. COMPLICATIONS

1. Compartment syndrome
2. Recurrence
3. Chronic joint pain
4. CPN palsy
5. Vascular injury

CTEV

I. DEFINITION
Congenital anomaly of the foot characterized by a typical and fixed pattern of cavus, adductus, varus and equines deformities.

II. EPIDEMIOLOGY
1. Most common musculoskeletal birth defect
2. 1:1000, M:F = 2:1
3. B/L = 50%
4. Isolated deformity → 80%

III. ETIOLOGY AND CLASSIFICATION

Idiopathic	Associated with syndromes	Neurogenic
↓	1. Arthrogryposis multiplex congenita 2. Down's syndrome 3. Streeters dysplasia 4. Mobius syndrome 5. Fetal alcohol syndrome	1. CP 2. Polio 3. Postburn VIC of calf muscles 4. Leprosy

Idiopathic:
1. Genetic defect
2. Intrauterine pressure therapy (Packaging defect)
3. Germ-plasm defect → talus.
4. Myogenic: Defective innervations of peroneal muscles
5. Defect in cartilaginous anlage of talus.
6. Retracting fibrosis: "Crimp" collagen - Ponseti
7. Infecting pathogen: Enterovirus
8. Amniocentesis
9. Absent anterior tibial artery (vascular)

IV. PATHOPHYSIOLOGY AND DEFORMITIES
1. Rotatory subluxation of talocalcaneonavicular joint complex
2. Talus in plantar flexion
3. Subtalar complex in medial rotation and inversion

Tight muscle - contractures:
4. Cavus → Midfoot → Intrinsics, FHL, FDL
5. Adductus → Forefoot → Tibialis posterior
6. Varus → Hindfoot → Tendoachilles, tibialis posterior and anterior
7. Equinus → Ankle → Tendon achilles
8. Calcaneum → Varus → rotated medially around talus
9. Navicular and cuboid displaced medially.

V. CLINICAL EXAMINATION
1. Most commonly evaluated by Pirani score **(Fig. 43)**

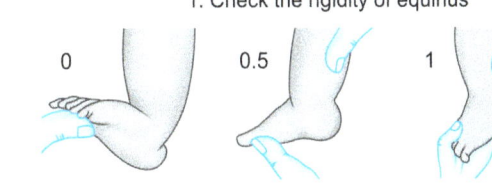

MOVE — 1. Check the rigidity of equinus
- 0
- 0.5
- 1

FEEL
2. The heel
- 0 Tuberosity palpable
- 0.5 Tuberosity partially palpable
- 1 Tuberosity nonpalpable

3. Lateral part of the head of talus
- 0 Complete reduction
- 0.5 Partial reduction
- 1 Fixed subluxed

EVALUTE
- 0 Normal
- 0.5 Moderate
- 1 Severe

4. Curvature of lateral border
5. Medial crease
6. Posterior crease

2. Small foot and calf
3. Shortened tibia

VI. RADIOLOGY

Diagnosis is clinical, usually not required.
Indication → Recurrent, relapse, resistant.
1. Dorsiflexion lateral: Turco's view
   ↓
   Hindfoot parallelism between talus and calcaneum (angle < 25°). Normally convergent.
2. AP:
   i. Talocalcaneal angle = Kite's view
      Normal = 20–40° CTEV < 20°
   ii. Talus–1st MT angle → Negative = Adductus
       Normal = 10–20°

VII. MANAGEMENT

Goal → to obtain pain free, supple, plantigrade foot with good function with cosmesis with no special footwear required.

Correct deformity early → entirely → develop muscle power of limb to maintain.

1. Ponseti Method of Serial Manipulation and Casting

i. Gold standard
ii. Rationale (Fig. 44):

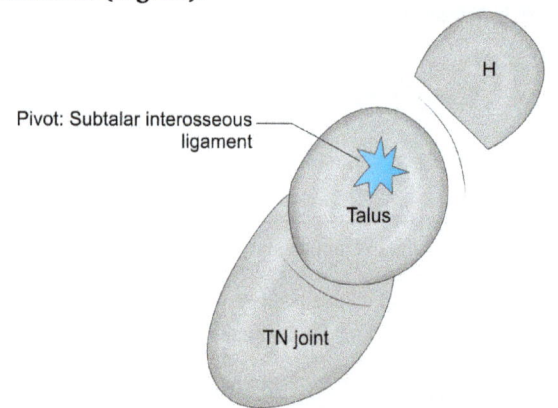

a. Kinematic coupling of foot
b. Relaxation of collagen and atraumatic remodeling of joints.

iii. Two phases → Correction
                 → Maintenance

iv.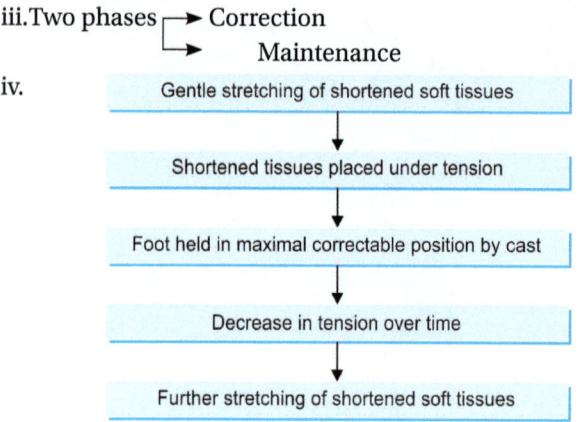

A. Correction

1. Basics:
   i. Child in mother's lap
   ii. Gentle manipulation
   iii. No tincture
   iv. Appropriate cast padding
   v. Long leg cast up to upper thigh
   vi. Knees in 90° flexion
   vii. Toes covered on plantar surface, free dorsally
2. Simultaneous correction achieved at TN, CC, Talocalcaneal joints
3. *Manipulation*:
   i. "Pronation twist" (Cavus) → Corrected by lifting the 1st MT head
      a. Apparent ↑ in deformity.
      b. Forefoot in supinated to bring in line with mid and hindfoot supination.
   ii. Varus and adductus = Tarsal bones distal to talus abducted in supinated foot.
       ↓
       a. Navicular comes in front of talus.
       b. Cuboid in front of calcaneum
       c. Calcaneus glides below talus in corrected position (kinematic coupling)
   iii. Equinus
        a. Only >70° of abduction
        b. Avoid DF before correction of hindfoot varus
           ↓
           Rocker-bottom foot
        c. Dorsiflex = 5–10° before tenotomy
        d. 15–30° DF > tenotomy held in cast for 3 weeks.

B. Maintenance

1. Started immediately > casting
2. 23 hours/day for 3 months → followed by night time → 2–4 years
3. Dennis–Brown splint
   Steenbeek splint (Fig. 45)

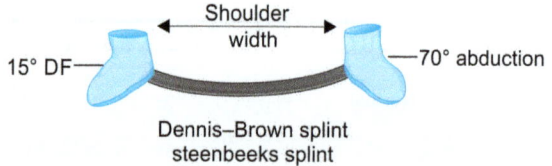

Dennis–Brown splint
steenbeeks splint

4. Casts changed every 7 days → 5–7 sessions
5. Cost-effective, reproducible, Consistent results (>90%)

2. Modified French technique (DiMeglio)

Daily PT and adhesive tapes.

3. Operative → Soft tissue procedures
                → Bony procedures

i. Indications:
   1. Resistant

Pediatric Orthopedics

2. Recurrent
3. Relapse
4. Neglected

ii. "A la carte": Personalized for every case
↓
iii. Extensive dissection → Rigid, painful feet

A. PMSTR of McKay

1. Approach

TURCO	CINCINATI	CARROL
↓	↓	↓
Hockey stick, posteromedial incision	Circumferential	Two incisions: 1. PM 2. Small lateral over subtalar joint

2. Timing → 9-10 months } Structures are larger
   or } Therefore, it is easier,
   8 cm size of foot } As ossification present.
3. TN joint with ST joint fixed with K wires.

B. Tendon Transfers

Dynamic supination of midfoot ↓ Split anterior tibialis tendon transfer → to lateral cuneiform ↓ As there is evertor deformity	For calcaneus gait (Triceps insufficiency) ↓ Peroneus brevis split and rerouted to calcaneal tuberosity

C. Bony Procedures

1. Metatarsus adductus: MT osteotomy. Age > 5 years
2. Hindfoot varus
   <2-3 years: Modified McKay PMSTR (Posteromedial soft tissue release)
   3-10 years:
   i. **Dwyer osteotomy** = Lateral closing wedge calcaneal osteotomy
   ii. **Dilwyn–Evans** → Partial excision of calcaneocuboid joint and fusion.
   iii. **Lichblau's** → Calcaneocuboid excisional arthroplasty.
   >10 years: Triple arthrodesis
3. Equinus
   Severe deformity
   Lambrinudi procedure: Excision of portion of talus
4. Cavus > 6 years → Japas V osteotomy
   → Dome osteotomy
5. All deformities > 10 years → Triple arthrodesis
   → Wedge tarsectomy
   ↓
   Remove dorsolateral wedge.

6. External fixation → JESS
   → Ilizarov
   → Taylors spatial frame.

CONGENITAL VERTICAL TALUS (CVT)

I. INTRODUCTION

1. Rare congenital foot deformity that presents as rocker bottom foot.
2. A.k.a. Convex pes valgus
3. M:F – 2:1
4. It is a rare foot deformity consisting of an irreducible dorsal dislocation of the navicular on the talus, producing a rigid flat foot
5. *Congenital oblique talus:* Patients with reducible navicular dislocation that realigns on stretched plantar flexion lateral films.
6. 1/5th cases are familial (genetic)
7. Associated with:
   i. Spina bifida
   ii. Sacral agenesis
   iii. Arthrogryposis
   iv. Diastematomyelia
   v. Genetic and chromosomal abnormalities

II. ETIOPATHOLOGY

1.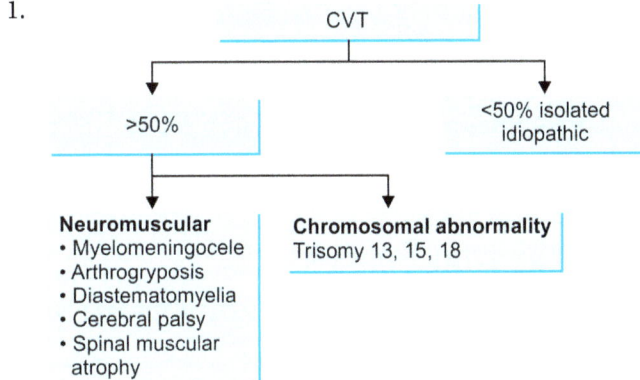

2. Hallmark → Irreducible dorsal dislocation of navicular.
3. Vertically oriented Talus
4. Coleman et al. classified CVT based on calcaneocuboid joint:
   i. Type 1: Normal calcaneocuboid joint
   ii. Type 2: Dislocated calcaneocuboid joint → Resistant to treatment

III. CLINICAL FEATURES

1. Presentation: 1st year of life
2. Bilateral: 50%
3. Fixed hindfoot equinovalgus → due to contracture of TA and peroneal tendons.
4. Rigid mid foot dorsiflexion → due to dislocated navicular
5. Forefoot abducted and dorsiflexed → due to contractures of EDL, EHL and tibialis anterior tendons.

6. Prominent talar head: Medial border of foot and sole is convex.
7. Convexity of foot persists on weightbearing unlike flexible flatfoot.
8. "Peg-leg"/Calcaneal gait
9. Neurological examination mandatory.

IV. RADIOLOGY
1. Plantar flexion lateral view → Diagnostic
    i. Persistent dorsal dislocation of the talonavicular joint.
    ii. Meary's angle > 20° [between line of longitudinal axis of talus and longitudinal axis of 1st metatarsal **(Fig. 46)**].
    iii. Vertically oriented talus

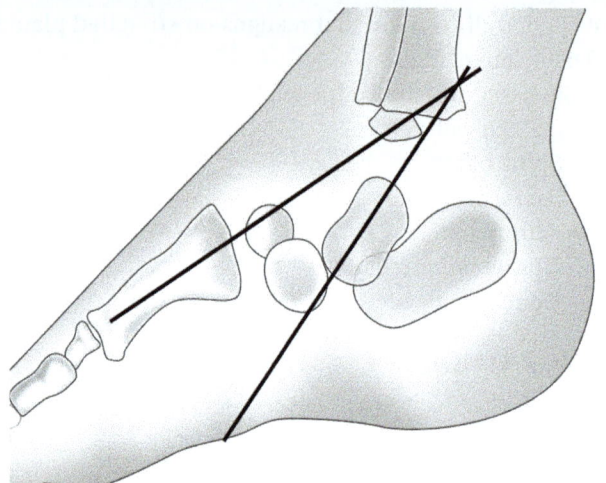

2. AP view: Kite's angle (Talocalcaneal angle) >40° (Normal 20–40°)
3. MRI: Neuraxial imaging

V. DIFFERENTIAL DIAGNOSIS
1. Congenital oblique talus → Reduced on forced plantar flexion
2. Tarsal coalition
3. Pes valgus deformity

VI. TREATMENT
1. Goal: Plantigrade, pain-free, and normal appearing foot.
2. Serial manipulation and cast: Reverse Ponseti method (Dobbs et al.)
    i. Pressure applied to the medial part of talus while the forefoot is adducted and plantarflexed to reduce the joint and held by cast.
    ii. Combined with operative management.
3. Talonavicular reduction and pinning:
    i. Required in most cases
    ii. Age: 6–12 months
    iii. A la carte lengthening of soft tissues → TA, Peronei, EDL, tibialis anterior
    iv. Surgical pantalar release, capsulotomy of TN joint
4. Talectomy: Resistant cases
5. Coleman's subtalar arthrodesis ⎫ Salvage surgery
6. Triple arthrodesis ⎭
7. Postoperatively: Ankle foot orthosis for 2 years along with medial arch support.

CALCANEOVALGUS FOOT

I. INTRODUCTION
1. Postural deformity of infancy characterized by dramatic hyperdorsiflexion of the foot that appears to be plastered up against the anterior surface of the tibia.
2. Plantar flexion of foot is frequently limited as a result of contracture of anterior ankle and foot structures.

II. ETIOLOGY
1. Abnormal in utero positioning of the foot described as a "packaging' defect"
2. Associated conditions:
    i. DDH
    ii. Metatarsus adductus
    iii. Congenital muscular torticollis

III. CLINICAL FEATURES
1. Higher in 1st born child
2. Girls > Boys
3. Ankle is in hyperdorsiflexion → Passively correctable
4. Heel is in valgus.
5. Forefoot abduction
6. Calcaneus is palpable in the heel pad and is noted to be in "dorsiflex position"

IV. DIFFERENTIAL DIAGNOSIS
1. Posteromedial bowing of tibia → Apex is distal tibia (Calcaneovalgus foot → Ankle)
2. CVT → Rigid deformity, hindfoot in equinus whereas Calcaneovalgus foot is flexible and hindfoot is in dorsiflexion.
3. Paralytic foot deformity

V. TREATMENT
1. Prognosis is excellent
2. Gentle stretching exercises by parents in cases of severe deformity with marked reduction in plantarflexion
   ↓
3. Foot position normalizes within 3–6 months
4. Corrective casting or splinting → if foot cannot be plantarflexed beyond neutral.
   ↓
Ankle foot orthosis splint (AFO)

TORTICOLLIS

I. DEFINITION

Torticollis (Wryneck) is the deformity of tilting of the head toward one side and rotation towards the opposite side.

II. CLASSIFICATION

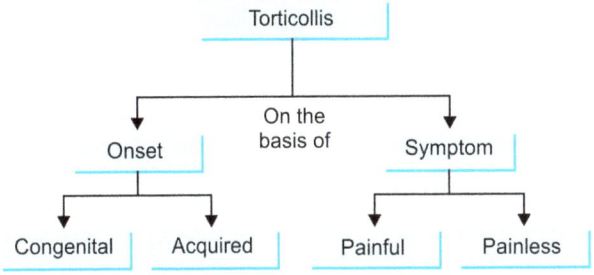

1. *Congenital – painless:*
   i. Congenital muscular torticollis (CMT) (MCC of infantile torticollis)
   ii. Vertebral anomalies
      a. Klippel–Feil syndrome
      b. Occipitalization of C_1
      c. Congenital hemiatlas
      d. Ocular torticollis
2. *Acquired – painful:*
   i. Traumatic
      a. Atlantoaxial rotatory displacement
      b. Os odontoideum
      c. C_1 fracture
   ii. Inflammatory and infective
      a. Atlantoaxial rotator displacement (Grisel syndrome)
      b. Juvenile RA
      c. Osteomyelitis
   iii. Tumors
      a. Eosinophilic granuloma
      b. Osteoid osteoma
   iv. Sandifer syndrome
3. *Acquired, nonpainful (but maybe painful too):*
   i. Paroxysmal torticollis of infancy
   ii. CNS tumors → Posterior fossa
      → Acoustic neuroma
   iii. Syringomyelia
   iv. Hysterical torticollis
   v. Oculogyric crisis
   vi. Associated with ligamentous laxity:
      a. Down's syndrome
      b. Mucopolysaccharides

III. ETIOPATHOGENESIS

1. *Risk factors*:
   i. Oligohydramnios
   ii. Primigravida
   iii. Traumatic delivery
   iv. Breech delivery
2. Associated conditions → "Packaging disorders"
   i. DDH
   ii. Metatarsus adductus
   iii. Calcaneovalgus feet
3. Intrauterine malposition
   ↓
   Venous outflow obstruction
   ↓
   ↓ Blood supply → compartment syndrome (Intrauterine/perinatal)
   ↓
   Ischemia and fibrosis of the SCM

IV. CLINICAL FEATURES

1. M > F = 3:2
2. Head tilted toward affected side
3. Chin rotated away
4. Painless passive motion (restricted)
5. Palpable neck mass:
   i. Newborn/within 4 weeks
   ii. Elongated, indurated nontender SCM
   iii. Rigid, nonelastic
6. Ruling out other abnormal → Hip, spine, foot
7. Older children:
   i. Restricted rotation and lateral flexion of neck
   ii. Plagiocephaly
   iii. Facial asymmetry
   iv. Fixed scoliosis in cervical spine
   v. Diplopia

V. INVESTIGATIONS

1. USG → Hyperechoic fibrotic lesion → SCM
   Differentiates CMT from others
2. X-ray → Rule out bony causes (Failure of segmentation)
3. MRI = Central causes
4. CT scan (dynamic): Rule out C_1-C_2 rotatory subluxation

VI. TREATMENT

1. Conservative (90-95% success rate): Child <1year
   i. Passive stretching: Gentle, by parent
   ii. Strategic positioning of toys and crib. Child forced to look on opposite side
   iii. Orthotics
   iv. Excessive program
   v. Traction.
2. Operative: CMT does not resolve spontaneously beyond 1 year of age.
   i. Indications:
      a. Failure of conservative management
      b. Progressive or recurrence
      c. Significant restricted ROM

ii. Options:
   a. Tenotomy → Open
                → SC
   b. Bipolar release of SCM
   c. Z-lengthening of SCM
   d. Radical resection of SCM (contracted)
iii. Complications → Spinal XI injured
iv. Postoperative torticollis brace

CONGENITAL RADIO-ULNAR SYNOSTOSIS

I. INTRODUCTION

Congenital disorder characterized by failure of differentiation that leads to the presence of a bony bridge between the proximal radius and ulna.

II. ETIOPATHOPHYSIOLOGY

1. Development of forearm begins as a single cartilaginous anlage → then in the 7th week in utero → divides from distal to proximal into the radius and ulna.
   ↓
   Failure of differentiation → Radioulnar synostosis.
2. Bilateral in 60% and at the upper 1/3rd of the forearm, although the junction can occur anywhere.
3. Marrow cavity of the synostosis maybe continuous with that of both bones.
4. Upper end of the radius may/may not be completely formed.
   ↓
   Anterior/Posterior dislocation of elbow
5. Supinator muscle is absent.
6. Pronator teres/Quadratus imperfectly formed/absent.
7. Shaft of radius crosses over the ulna in a close relationship so that fixed pronation of forearm and tightened, narrow interosseous membrane results.

III. CLASSIFICATION

Based on tissue type at synostosis site and +/– radial head dislocation.

A. Cleary Classification

1. Fibrous synostosis
2. Bony synostosis
3. Associated with posterior dislocation of elbow
4. Associated with anterior dislocation of elbow

IV. CLINICAL FEATURES

1. M > F: 3:2
2. 5–6 years of age
3. Symptoms:
   i. Asymptomatic (most common) → noted by parents
   ii. Painless

4. Examination:
   i. Inability to supinate forearm
   ii. Flexion, extension of elbow normal
   iii. Fixed pronating deformity of forearm
   iv. Increased compensatory movement of elbow joint (shoulder)
   v. Associated with DDH, CTEV **(Fig. 47)**

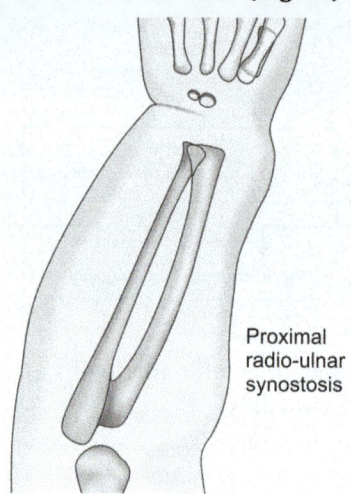

Proximal radio-ulnar synostosis

V. RADIOLOGY

1. Radius is wide and bowed.
2. Ulna is narrow and straight
3. Proximal synostosis
4. Radial head malformed

VI. TREATMENT

1. Observation → Asymptomatic and unilateral cases
2. Surgical:
   i. Indications:
      a. Activities of daily living affected (sports, hygiene, eating)
      b. Severe pronation deformity >60°
      c. Bilateral deformities
   ii. Excision of synostosis with soft tissue interposition:
      a. Restores active forearm rotation
      b. Excise synostosis and interpose vascularized fascio-fat graft
      c. Vascularized fat better than free fat graft
      d. Excision alone without graft interposition → nearly 100% recurrence of synostosis
   iii. Forearm derotational osteotomy:
      a. Places the forearm in more functional resting position
      b. Candidate age group → 3–6 years of age
      c. Osteotomy location →
         1. Distal to synostosis
         2. Through synostosis → Then rotation of forearm
         3. Bifocal osteotomy → Distal osteotomy of ulna + proximal osteotomy of radius

iv. Position:
   a. Unilateral: Forearm in 0–30° pronation
   b. Bilateral: Dominant forearm in 0–15° pronation and nondominant forearm in neutral
v. Stabilization:
   a. Casting alone (no fixation)
   b. Circular external fixator frame (Ilizarov)
   c. Percutaneous pins

VII. COMPLICATIONS
1. Recurrence of synostosis
2. Recurrence of malrotation
3. Compartment syndrome
4. Neurological deficit

POLYDACTYLY

I. INTRODUCTION
Congenital malformation of the hand characterized by an extra digit in the hand.

II. TYPES
1. Preaxial → first digit (thumb)
2. Central → 2nd, 3rd, 4th digit
3. Postaxial → 5th digit (little finger)

III. PREAXIAL (RADIAL, THUMB POLYDACTYLY OR THUMB DUPLICATION)
1. 1 in 1000–10,000 live births
2. M > F
3. Sporadic occurrence

A. Wassel Classification
Based on number of bifid or duplicated phalanges or metacarpals, from distal to proximal.
1. Type 1 → Bifid distal phalanx
2. Type 2 → Duplicated distal phalanx (2nd most common)
3. Type 3 → Type 2 + bifid proximal phalanx.
4. Type 4 → Duplicated proximal and distal phalanx (most common)
5. Type 5 → Type 4 + bifid metacarpals
6. Type 6 → Duplication of all phalanges and metacarpal
7. Type 7 → Any duplication with a triphalangeal thumb (associated with syndromes → Holt-Oram, Fanconi's anemia, cleft palate, Blackfan-Diamond anemia) (**Fig. 48**)

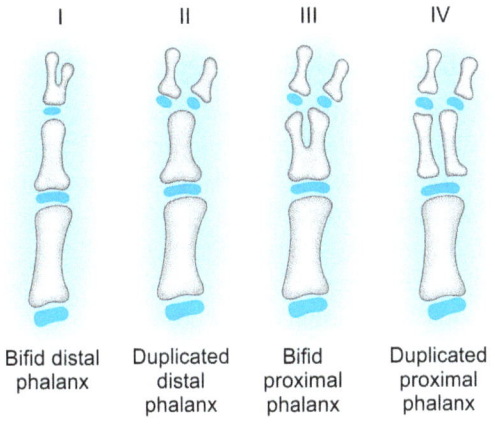
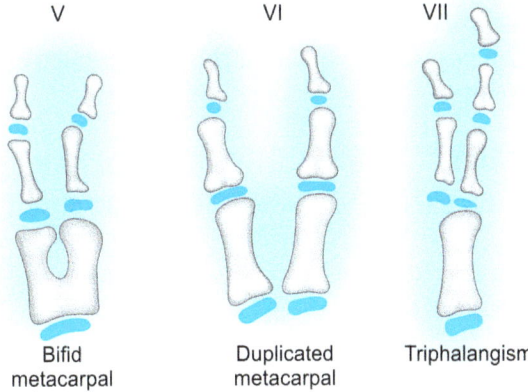

B. Treatment
1. Principles:
   i. Reconstruction of a thumb → 80% of the size of the contralateral thumb
   ii. Resect smaller thumb (usually radial component)
   iii. Preserve medial collateral structures in order to preserve pinch function
   iv. Reconstruction of all components typically done in one procedure
   v. Chondroplasties or corrective osteotomies of the metacarpals or phalanges.
   vi. Deepening of 1st web space by Z-plasties.
   vii. Thus, providing a single, stable, mobile, functional thumb.
2. Bilhaut-Cloquet: Type 1 combination:
   i. Indicated in type I, II and III.
   ii. Both digits are combined into one and central tissue is removed.
3. Type 2 combination: For type III and IV:
   i. Skeleton and nail of one digit is preserved, soft tissue augmentation from the other and ablation of the lesser digit.
4. Type 3 combination: For V, VI and VII:
   i. Superior proximal part in one digit and distal part in the other
   ii. On-top plasty: Segmental distal transfer is done.

IV. POSTAXIAL
1. Type A:
   i. Fully developed digit
   ii. Rx.: Reconstruction by type 2 combination

2. Type B:
   i. Rudimentary and pedunculated digit
   ii. Rx.: Amputate before the age of 1 year.

CONGENITAL TRIGGER THUMB

Pediatric disorder of the thumb in which there is abnormal flexion at the interphalangeal joint.

I. ETIOPATHOLOGY
1. Three infants per 1,000 live births
2. A palpable mass, a nodule called **Notta nodule** → represents the FPL constriction at the A1 pulley.
3. Abnormal collagen degeneration and synovial proliferation
4. Caused by size mismatch or a differential growth of a tendon and its pulley leading to progressive constriction → Abnormal tendon gliding
5. No inflammatory component involved.

II. CLINICAL EVALUATION
1. M = F
2. Bilateral → 30%
3. Painless
4. Palpable nodule of the FPL tendon at the A1 pulley with:
   i. Triggering or
   ii. Fixed flexion contracture of the IP joint
5. In long-standing cases, compensatory hyperextension of the MCP joint.

III. TREATMENT
1. Spontaneously resolved by 9 months of age in 30–50% of patients
2. Intermittent extension splint
3. Surgical release of A_1 pulley:
   i. Indications:
      a. For patients >1 year
      b. Fail to resolve spontaneously
      c. Patients presenting after 1 year of age with fixed PIP
   ii. Care should be taken to preserve neurovascular bundle and the oblique pulley.
   iii. Transverse incision → cosmetic.

IV. COMPLICATIONS
1. Digital nerve injury
2. Wound complications
3. Interphalangeal joint movement restriction
4. Bow-stringing of flexor tendon → iatrogenic release of oblique pulley

LIMPING CHILD

I. TODDLER/PRESCHOOL (1–4 YEARS)
1. Infection (septic arthritis, osteomyelitis in the hip/spine)
2. Mechanical (trauma and nonaccidental injury)
3. Congenital/developmental problems (developmental dysplasia of the hip, talipes, leg length discrepancy)
4. Reactive arthritis/transient synovitis (toxic synovitis, irritable hip)
5. Legg-Calve-Perthes disease
6. Neurologic disease (cerebral palsy, hereditary syndromes)
7. Inflammatory arthritis (most commonly juvenile idiopathic arthritis)
8. Metabolic (e.g., osteomalacia)
9. Hematologic (hemophilia)
10. Malignant disease (e.g., leukemia, neuroblastoma)

II. CHILDREN (5–10 YEARS)
1. Mechanical (trauma, overuse injuries, sport injuries)
2. Reactive arthritis/transient synovitis (toxic synovitis, irritable hip)
3. Legg-Calve-Perthes disease
4. Inflammatory arthritis (juvenile idiopathic arthritis most common)
5. Infection (septic arthritis, osteomyelitis)
6. Metabolic (e.g., osteomalacia)
7. Tarsal coalition
8. Complex regional pain syndromes
9. Malignant disease (e.g., leukemia, neuroblastoma, lymphoma).

III. ADOLESCENTS (OLDER THAN 10 YEARS)
1. Mechanical (trauma, overuse injuries, sport injuries)
2. Slipped capital femoral epiphysis
3. Inflammatory arthritis (most commonly juvenile idiopathic arthritis)
4. Infection (septic arthritis, osteomyelitis)
5. Tarsal coalition
6. Complex regional pain syndromes.

SPINA BIFIDA

I. INTRODUCTION

Myelodysplasia is a common group of congenital disorders caused by various chromosomal abnormalities that lead to the failure of closure of the fetal spinal cord and present with anatomic anomalies and neurological impairment of varying degree.

II. ETIOLOGY
1. *Risk factors:*
   i. Folate deficiency: Supplementation can decrease risk by 70%
   ii. Maternal hyperthermia
   iii. Maternal diabetes
   iv. Valproic acid
2. *Chromosomal abnormalities*:
   i. Trisomy 13
   ii. Trisomy 18

iii. Triploidy
iv. Single-gene mutations

III. PATHOPHYSIOLOGY

Local failure of primordia of the two laminae to unite leaves vertebral canal open dorsally.

IV. TYPES

1. Spinal bifida oculta → defect in vertebral arch with confined cord and meninges within skin
2. Spina bifida aperta:
   i. Meningocele → protruding sac without neural elements
   ii. Myelomeningocele → Protruding sac with neural elements
   iii. Rachischisis → Neural elements exposed with no covering **(Fig. 49)**

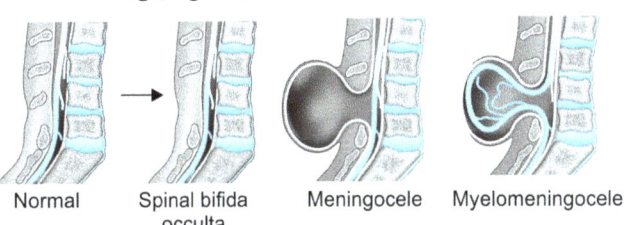

Normal | Spinal bifida occulta | Meningocele | Myelomeningocele

Level	Function level (described by lowest functioning level)	
	Function	Primary motion
L2	Nonambulatory	
L3	• Marginal household ambulator • High risk of hip dislocation	• Hip flexion • Hip adduction
L4	• Household ambulator plus • Key level because quadriceps can function	• Knee extension • Ankle dorsiflexion and inversion
L5	Community ambulator	• Toe dorsiflexion • Hip extension • Hip abduction
S1	Normal ambulator	Foot planter flexion
S2	Normal ambulator	Toe planter flexion
S3, 4	Normal ambulator	Bowel and bladder function

Lab → Raised alpha fetoprotein

V. ASSOCIATED ORTHOPEDIC CONDITIONS AND TREATMENT

A. Pathologic Fractures

1. Long bones fractures → common due to osteopenia
2. ↑ Frequency → higher the level of the defect
3. Fractures are often confused with:
   i. Infection
   ii. Osteomyelitis
   iii. Cellulitis
4. Treatment → Short period of immobilization in a well-padded splint

B. Scoliosis → Defined as Curve >20°

1. Muscle imbalance (neurogenic)
2. Congenital malformation (e.g., hemivertebrae)
3. Rapidly progressing deformities → Cord tethering
4. Treatment → Bracing not effective
5. Anterior and posterior spinal fusion with pelvic fixation for progressive curve
6. Complications:
   a. High pseudoarthrosis rate
   b. High incidence of infection → Poor soft tissue coverage of posterior spine

C. Congenital Kyphosis

Kyphectomy with fusion and posterior instrumentation: Indication → Progressive deformity.

D. Hip Disorders

1. **Dislocation** → L3 → unopposed hip flexion and adduction → Pathological dislocation Rx → Open reduction and San Diego osteotomy
2. Abduction contracture → Ober-Yount procedure → proximal division of fascia lata and distal iliotibial band release.
3. Flexion contracture → >40°: Anterior hip release with tenotomy of the iliopsoas, sartorius, rectus femoris, and tensor fascia lata.

E. Knee Disorders

1. Weak quadriceps → Knee ankle foot orthosis (KAFO)
2. Flexion contracture → hamstring lengthening +/- posterior capsulotomy → greater than 20° of knee flexion contracture
3. Supracondylar extension osteotomy → Older patients, failed soft tissue procedures.
4. Tibial rotational deformities (torsion):
   a. Observation and orthotics → <5 years old
   b. Distal tibial derotational osteotomy → >5 years

F. Foot Deformities

90% incidence. **CTEV** → Serial casting → if not resolved → Posteromedial soft tissue release (PMSTR)

TRASH LESIONS (THE RADIOGRAPHIC APPEARANCE SEEMED HARMLESS)

I. INTRODUCTION

1. A group of special injuries around the elbow resulting from high energy trauma that are routinely missed at initial presentation because of seemingly normal X-rays.
2. Described by Waters et al. in 2010, these are a group of osteochondral injuries having a high propensity for surgical intervention and usually have poor outcomes if not treated adequately.

3. Prompt diagnosis warrants a high index of suspicion even when a radiograph appears to be normal with a disproportionately swollen elbow in a child.

II. TRASH LESIONS

1. Radial head osteochondral fractures
2. Medial condylar fractures in unossified elbow
3. Transphyseal separations of the distal humerus
4. Monteggia lesions
5. Entrapped incarcerated medial epicondylar fractures
6. Capitellar shear fractures
7. Lateral condylar fractures extending to the cartilage

III. APPLIED ANATOMY

(Mnemonic for the ossification centers - Age mentioned is more close to boys, for girls subtract by 1 year for most centers.)

Age	Appearance of ossification centers
1	**C**apitellum
3	**R**adial head
5	**I**nternal epicondyle
7	**T**rochlea
9	**O**lecrenon
11	**E**xternal epicondyle
	Fusion of ossification centers
13	**C + T + E** to each other
15	**CTE** with distal humerus
17	**I** with distal humerus

IV. CLINICAL FEATURES

1. H/O → Significant trauma, fall from height
2. Significant swelling which does not match the benign radiographic appearance.
3. Tenderness around the elbow
4. Restricted painful range of motion
5. Muffled crepitus (cartilage moving against cartilage/bone)

V. INVESTIGATIONS

A. Radiograph
   1. Might appear normal on screening look in a busy emergency.
   2. Closer look might reveal bony fragment and joint malalignment.
   3. Must be investigated further keeping high degree of suspicion.
B. USG: Might identify cartilage injuries
C. MRI
   1. Diagnostic
   2. Sedation for young child.
D. Intraoperative arthrogram: Definitive

VI. TREATMENT

1. Most injuries are unstable → Require operative fixation
2. Displaced injuries → Anatomic articular reduction
3. Instrumentation is based on age of the patient and size of fragment.
4. Options include:
   i. K-wires (1–2.5 mm): Removed after 3–4 weeks.
   ii. Osseous screws (PTCC, Herbert)
   iii. Suture anchors
   iv. Plates: 1.5–3.5 mm (if near skeletal maturity)

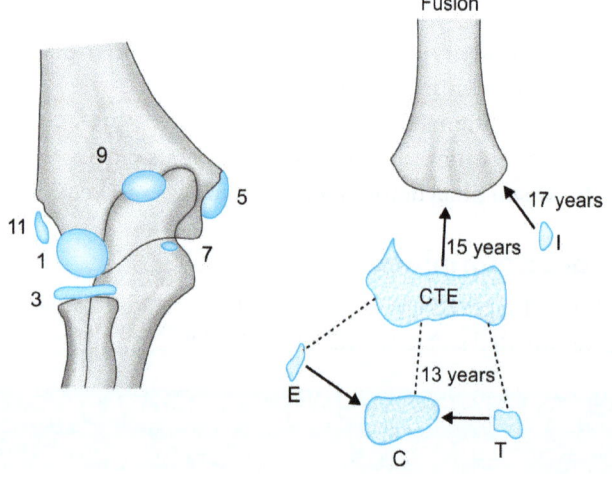

SECTION 3

Hip

HIP BIOMECHANICS

I. BIOMECHANICS

1. Biomechanics is the study of forces (internal and external) acting on a living body.
2. Hip acts as a class I lever **(Fig. 1)**.

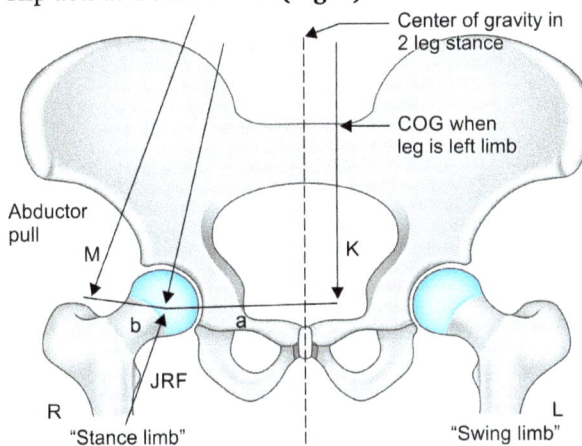

3. When both legs are on the floor → each hip carries 1/3rd body weight equally.
   (weight of the trunk and upper limb = $\frac{4/6}{2}$ = 1/3rd).
4. They do not have to carry contralateral limb weight.
5. The center of gravity is centered between both hips.
6. Moment (torque) = Product of force and the distance from which it acts.
7. Joint reduction force (JRF) → Force generated within a joint in response to the forces acting on a joint.

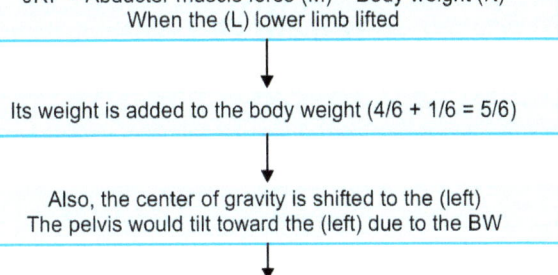

- The abductors exert a counterbalancing force to maintain equilibrium
- Body weight (K) × moment arm (a) = Abductor force (M) × moment arm (b)
- [N] lever arm → a = 2.5b to 3b
- Therefore, the abductor pull must be three times that of BW

↓

Longer the abductor lever arm

↓

Less abduction force required to maintain balance

↓

Less pressure force on femoral head

II. APPLICATIONS

1. In Trendelenburg gait → Patient tilts toward the affected hip
   ↓
   Shifting the center of gravity toward it → ↓ BW lever arm
   ↓
   Less abductor pull needed → ↓ force on FH
2. Use of cane in C/L limb **(Fig. 2)**

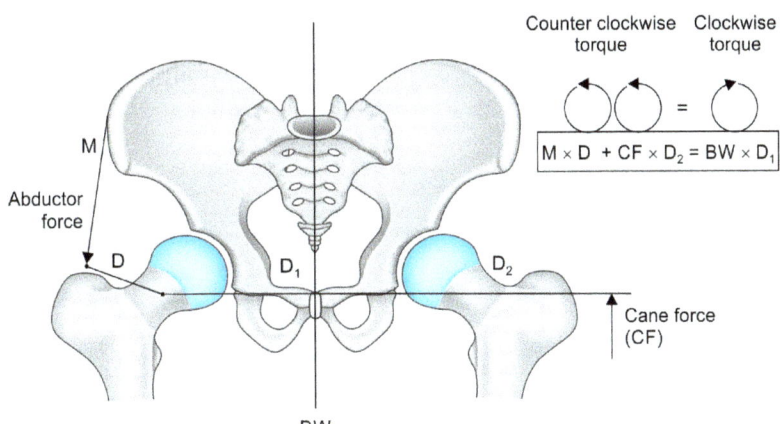

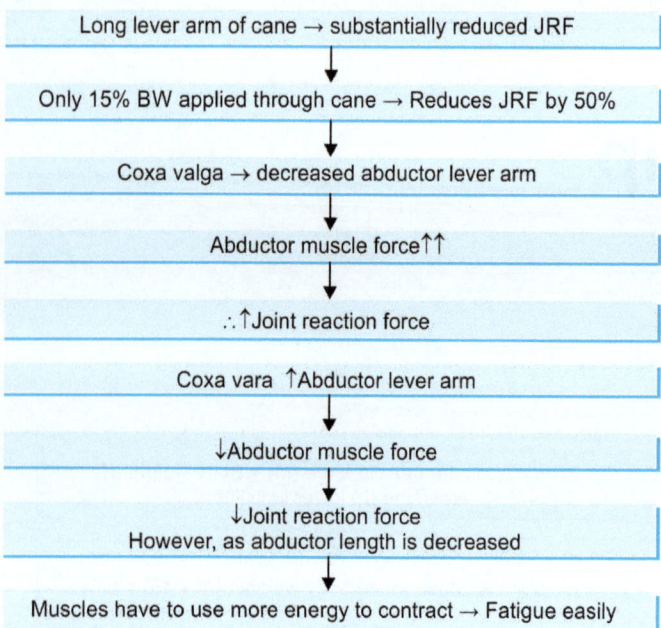

Other biomechanical aspects (Elaborate on these headings in the exam).
1. Mechanical aspects of LL
2. Anatomical axis of femur
3. Femoral anteversion
4. Femoral neck – shaft angle
5. Center of gravity → In front of S_2

III. APPLICATIONS IN THR

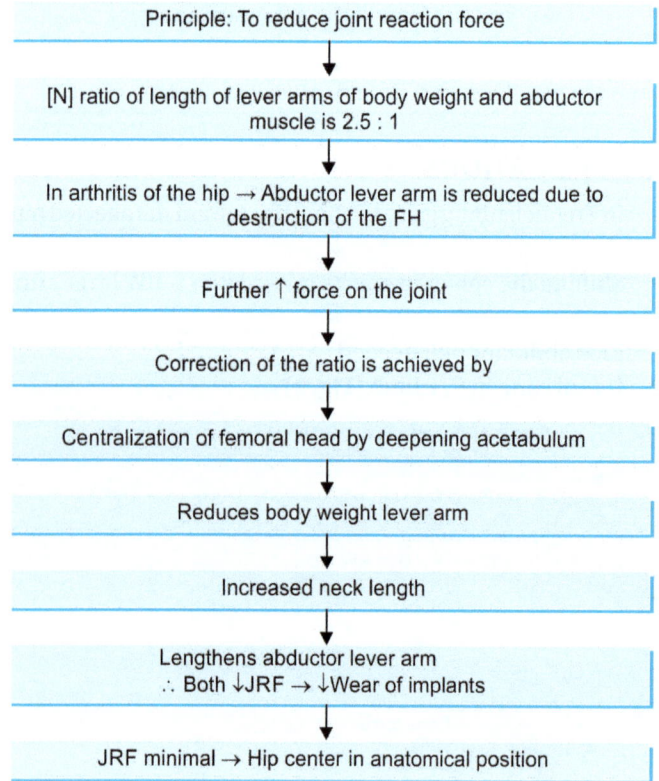

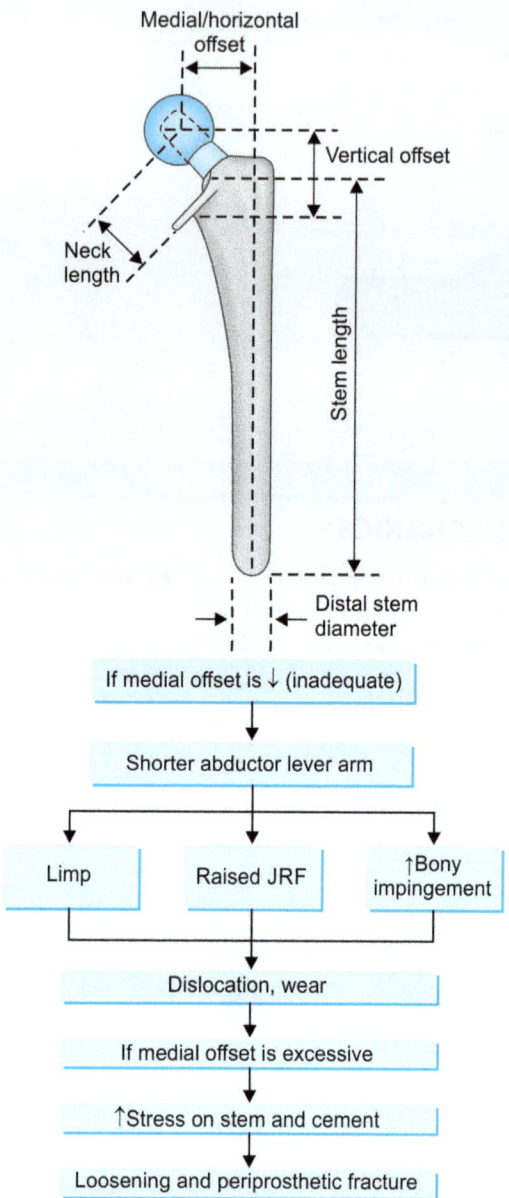

1. Neck length is very important as it affects both vertical and horizontal offset **(Fig. 3)**.
2. Principle of medialization has given way to → preserving subchondral bone.
   ↓
3. Deeper acetabulum only as much necessary → to obtain bony coverage.
4. THRs are done without GT osteotomy → Abductor lever arm altered only relative to the offset of head and stem.
5. ROM → influenced by prosthesis design **(Fig. 4)**.

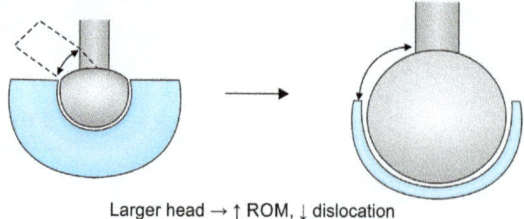

Larger head → ↑ ROM, ↓ dislocation

6. **Component orientation**
   1. *Acetabular position*: (Lewinnek safe zone)
      1. Anteversion: 15–20°
      2. Abduction: 45–50°
   2. *Femoral stem position*:
      Anteversion → 15°
      ↑ → Anterior dislocation
      ↓ → Posterior dislocation.
   3. Further reading: Spinopelvic alignment and its effect on acetabular shell positioning. (Recent hot topic)

APPROACHES TO HIP JOINT

I. CLASSIFICATION
A. Based on Direction

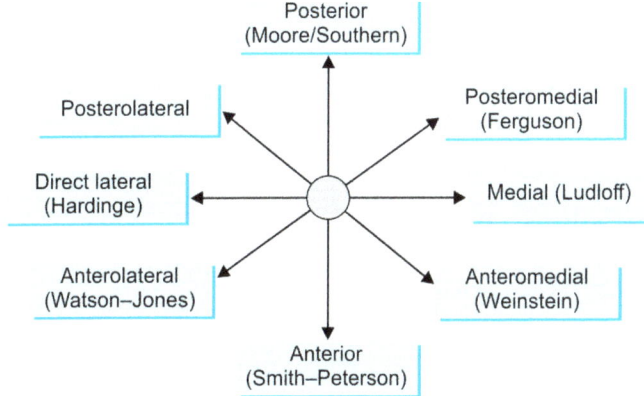

B. Based on Incision and Invasiveness
1. Standard incision (e.g., posterior)
2. Mini incision (MIS)

C. Based on Type of Surgery
1. Open
2. Arthroscopic

a. **Anterior approaches:**
   Indications:
   i. Arthrotomy (Infections)
   ii. Synovial biopsies
   iii. Pelvic osteotomies
   iv. Excision of tumors, myositis ossificans
   v. Anterior column fractures of acetabulum
   vi. Open reduction of developmental dysplasia of the hip (DDH) when dislocated femoral head lies anterior superior to the true acetabulum.
   vii. Intra-articular fusions.
   viii. Arthroplasty ⎯→ Total
                        ⎯→ Hemi

1. **Smith-Peterson: Iliofemoral (Fig. 5)**

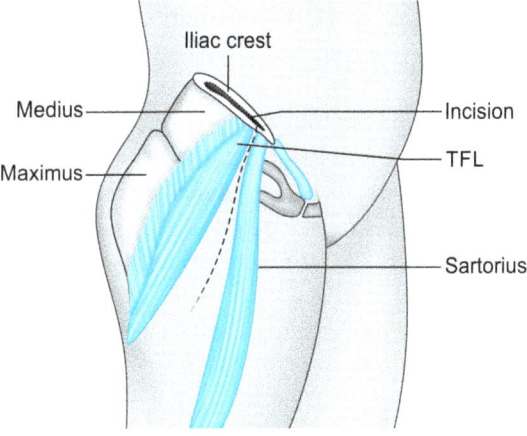

   i. *Position:* Supine with sandbag under the pelvis on the operating side.
   ii. *Incision:* Longitudinal incision between anterior iliac crest toward upper thigh curving over the anterior superior iliac spine.
   iii. *Soft-tissue dissection:*
       1. Superficial: Sartorius and TFL
       2. Deep: Rectus femoris and gluteus medius
   iv. *Internervous plane:* Femoral nerve (sartorius) and superior gluteal nerve (TFL)
   v. *Arthrotomy:* Adduct and externally rotate
       ↓
       Excision capsule longitudinally or F – shaped
   vi. *Dislocation:* By ER
   vii. *Closure:* In layers, capsule rarely closed. Fascial planes closed and skin.
   viii. *Advantages:*
       1. Preservation of vascularity.
       2. Limits chances of dislocation
          ↓
       3. Limits muscle cutting and separation.
       4. No abductor disruption→No postoperative limping.
   ix. *Disadvantages:* Limited access → technically demanding to place components in arthroplasty.
   x. *Specific complications:*
       1. Lateral cutaneous femoral nerve
2. **Somerville-Transverse bikini incision**
3. **Anterolateral: Watson-Jones (Fig. 6)**

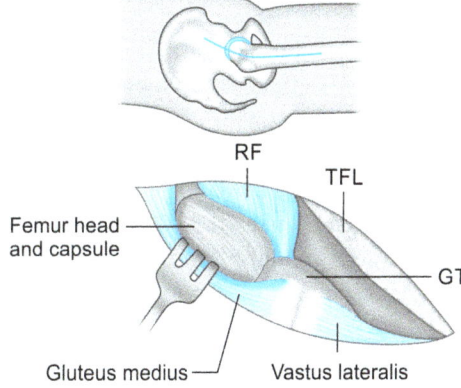

i. *Position:* Supine or lateral.
ii. *Incision:* 10-15 cm longitudinal incision centered over tip of greater trochanter.
↓
Incision crosses the posterior third of the GT before running down the shaft.
iii. *Soft-tissue dissection:* Plane between tensor fascia lata and gluteus medius ↓
No internervous planes →–Both muscles supplied by SGN.
iv. *Extending:* Incising the fascia lata anteriorly or posteriorly.
↓
Extending down the lateral aspect of thigh → splitting the vastus lateralis to gain access to the lateral aspect of femur.
Trochanteric osteotomy may be needed.
v. *Arthrotomy:* Capsule is divided longitudinally over the anterior superior femoral neck.
vi. *Dislocation:* ER, traction and adduction.
vii. *Closure*:
1. Wound closed in layers starting with the capsule.
2. If a trochanteric osteotomy was done, it has to be reattached.
viii. *Advantages*:
1. Better stability.
2. ↓ Chances of dislocation → posterior
3. ↓ Sciatic nerve damage.
ix. *Disadvantages:*
1. Injury to SGN → Weakness of abductors
2. Damage to LCFA
x. *Modifications*:
1. Mueller's anterolateral minimally invasive approach
2. Ganz-trochanteric flip osteotomy
b. **Lateral:**
1. McFarland and Osborne
2. Hardinge
3. McLaughlin and Hay
4. Harris
1. **Hardinge**
Transgluteal approach:
i. *Position:* Lateral or supine position.
ii. *Incision:* Posteriorly directed lazy J incision central over the GT, and in line with the femur shaft.
iii. *Soft-tissue dissection:* Gluteal fascia and ITB divided → Plane between tensor fascia and gluteus maximus identified.
↓
Gluteus medius tendon and muscle fibers and vastus lateralis split

→ ∴ No true internervous plane.
↓
G. medius split → Not >5 cm from tip of GT → to prevent injury to SGN **(Fig. 7)**.
iv. *Dislocation:* ER and abduction.
v. *Closure:* G. medius tendon repaired → non-absorbable suture. ITB required.
vi. *Advantages*:
Avoids need for trochanteric osteotomy → Early mobilization
↓ Sciatic nerve ⊗ compared to posterior approaches
vii. Complications:

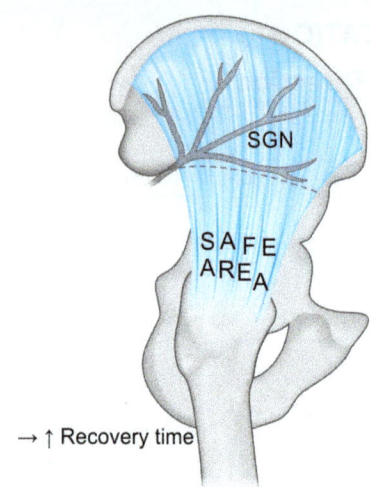

→ ↑ Recovery time

viii. Damage to G. medius → ↑ Recovery time.
ix. Heterotopic ossification.
c. **Posterior:**
1. Gibson–Posterolateral
2. Moore (Southern)
3. Osborne
Modified Gibsons:
1. *Position:* Lateral
2. *Incision:* Begin 6-8 cm anterior to posterior superior iliac spine (PSIS), just distal to iliac crest.
↓
Extend it distally to the anterior border of G. max.
↓
Distally along the line of the femur
3. *Soft-tissue dissection:*
i. ITB incised in line of its fibers.
ii. Extend incision along anterior border of G. maximus.
↓
iii. Separate posterior border of G. medius and piriformis.
↓
iv. Divide G. medius and minimus at their insertions → but leave enough for reattachment.

4. *Dislocation:* Flex and IR hip.
5. *Advantage:*
   i. Excellent exposure to acetabulum and femoral neck.
   ii. Easy insertion of THR prosthesis.
6. *Disadvantage:* ↑ Posterior dislocation
   ↑ Sciatic nerve injury.

Posterior–Moore (Fig. 8):

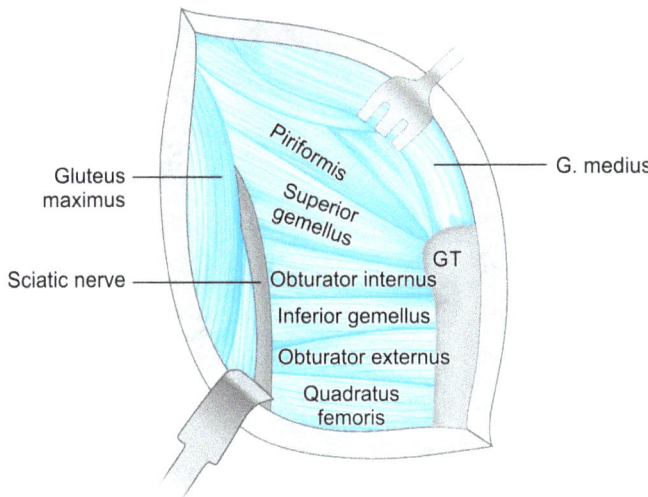

1. *Incision:* 10 cm distal to PSIS
   ↓
   Extending distally and laterally with the fibers of G. max.
   ↓
   To the posterior margin of GT.
   ↓
   Continued 10–15 cm distally parallel to the femoral shaft.
2. *Soft-tissue dissection:* Separate the fibers of G. max through blunt dissection → Not >7 cm → prevent IGN ⊗
   ↓
   G. medius retracted anteriorly
   ↓
   Short external rotators identified and cut > stay sutures.
   ↓
   Retracted posteriorly and prevent sciatic nerve injury.
3. *Arthrotomy:* T-shaped incision
4. *Dislocation, advantages, disadvantages:* Same as modified Gibsons.

II. MEDIAL APPROACH

1. *Indications:*
   i. Mainly in children → Protects blood supply and soft tissue.
   ii. Open reduction of DDH
   iii. Psoas release
   iv. Obturator neurectomy
   v. Adductor release
2. *Disadvantages:*
   i. Close to perineum
   ii. Limited exposure.
   iii. Deep incision → vascular injury
3. *Position:* Supine with flexion, Abduction, and external rotation, sole of foot lies along medial side of opposite knee.
4. *Incision:* Longitudinal incision on medial side of thigh → 3 cm below pubic tubercle.
5. *Ludloff:* Between pectineus and adductor longus and brevis.
6. *Weinstein:* Pectineus and neurovascular bundle.
7. *Ferguson:* (Superficially) A. Longus and Gracilis, (Deep) A. Brevis and Magnus **(Fig. 9)**.

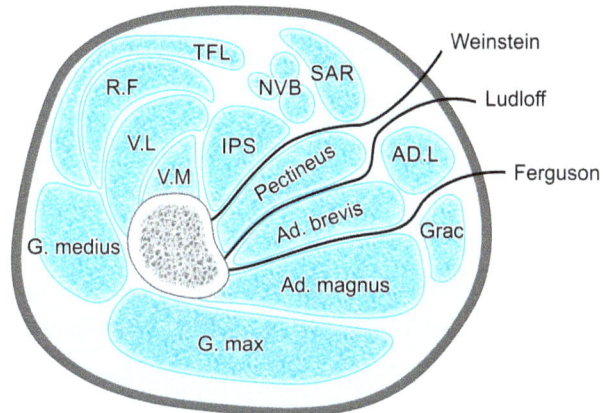

OSTEONECROSIS (HIP)/AVN/ CHANDLER'S DISEASE

Progressive destruction and alteration of bony architecture because of compromised vascularity.

I. ETIOLOGY AND CLASSIFICATION

ON ⎡ 1°: Idiopathic
   ⎣ 2°: Underlying cause present

ON ⎡ Post-traumatic → Fracture of femur head, acetabulum, neck or hip dislocation
   ⎣ Nontraumatic
   1. Idiopathic
   2. Drug induced
      1. Steroids (>20 mg/d for 3 months)
      2. Chemotherapy
      3. Smoking (>20 pack years)
      4. Alcohol (400 mL/week)
      5. Antiretroviral therapy
   3. Irradiation
   4. Hematological ⎡ Sickle cell
                    ⎣ Thalassemia
   5. Infection and autoimmune ⎡ HIV → SLE
                                ⎣ RA → Septic arthritis

6. Endocrine:
   1. Cushing's syndrome
   2. Hyperparathyroidism
   3. Pregnancy
7. Dysbarism-Caisson's disease
8. Metabolic → Gaucher's disease
   CRF
   Hepatic failure
   Hyperlipidemia

II. PATHOPHYSIOLOGY

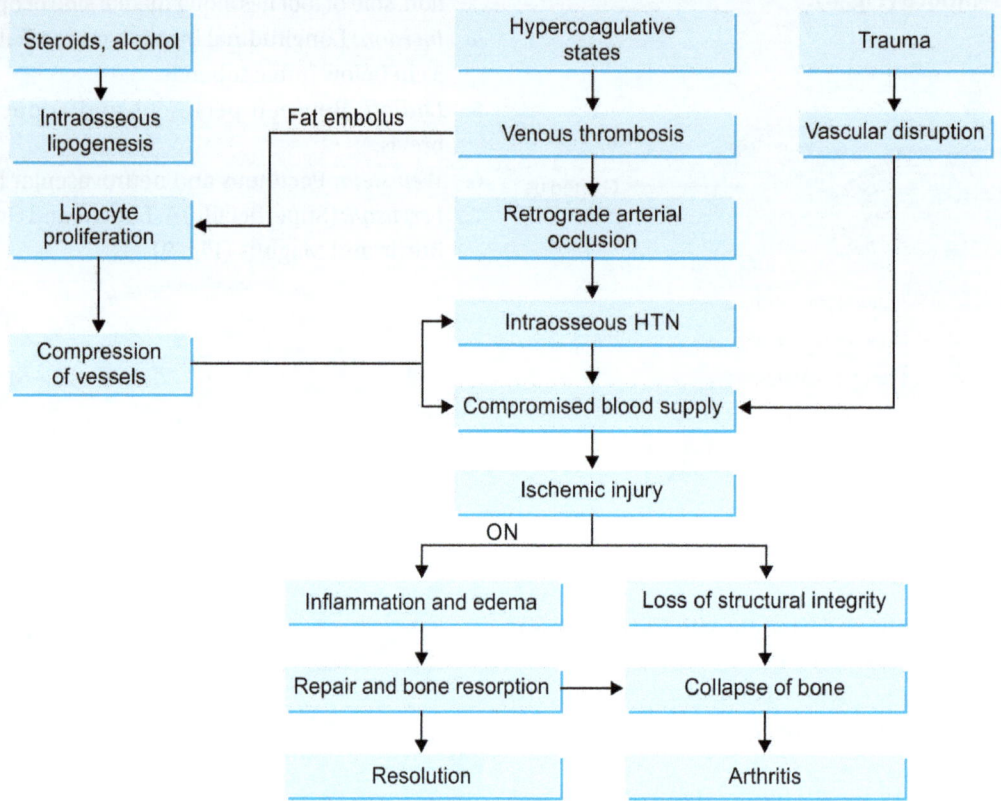

"Starlings resistor" → Femoral head (Fig. 10)

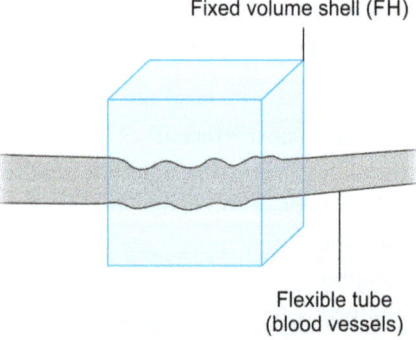

Fig. 10: "Starlings resistor" → Femoral head. Pressure within the shell determines the flow within the tube.

III. CLINICAL PRESENTATION

1. Males > Females
2. *Age:* 35–50 years
3. *B/L:* 50%, steroid: 80%
4. *Pain:*
   i. Most common presenting symptom
   ii. Groin
   iii. Insidious onset
   iv. Progressive
5. *Limp:*
   i. Antalgic gait
   ii. Trendelenburg gait
6. *Restricted ROM:* Earliest IR
   ↓
   Knee to axilla sign
7. Thomas test → Flexion deformity
8. Sectoral sign – Differential rotation
9. Limb length discrepancy

IV. RADIOLOGICAL INVESTIGATIONS

1. *Classification:*

   | Modified Ficat and Arlet |
   | Steinberg – University of Pennsylvania |
   | ARCO: Association of Research Circulation Osseous |

2. Modified Ficat and Arlet (Fig. 11)

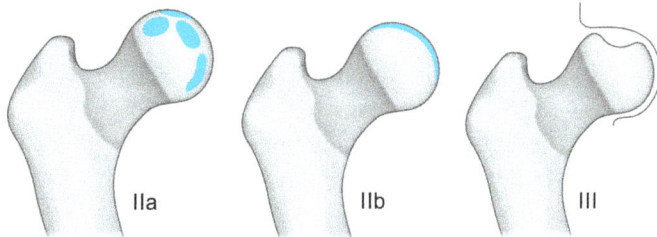

0: Normal/Silent hip
I: Cold spot on FH → Bone scan
II: Density changes in FH
IIA: Sclerosis, subchondral cysts
IIB: Crescent sign
III: Collapse of FH, JL—normal
IV: Joint space narrowing, acetabular changes (arthritis)
3. *MRI*:
   1. Highest sensitivity (99%) and specificity (99%)
   2. Double density sign
4. Bone scan → Doughnut sign
5. Modified Kerboul's angle → Midcoronal and midaxial sections
   Collapse risk **(Fig. 12)**
   >240° = High
   190–240° = Moderate
   <190° = Low

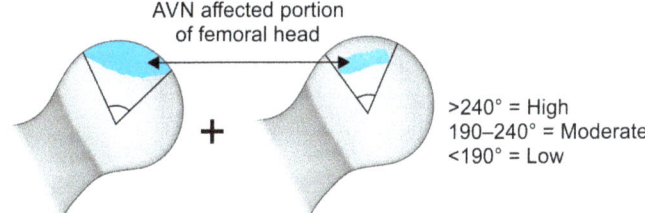

V. MANAGEMENT

A. Conservative

1. *Bisphosphonates:*
   i. Indicated in Ficat 0–II → Precollapse
   ii. Alendronate 70 mg/week × 3 years (Oral)
   iii. Zoledronic acid IV yearly 5 mg + alendronate 70 mg/week × years
2. *Other drugs (questionable efficacy):*
   i. Lipid lowering agents → Statins
   ii. Teriparatide
   iii. LMW heparin - Coagulopathy pts
3. *Adjuvant modalities:*
   i. Pulsed electromagnetic field (PEMF)
   ii. Extracorporeal shockwaves
   iii. Hyperbaric O_2 therapy

B. Operative

Hip preserving	Hip sacrificing
Aimed to relieve pain and prevent progression: 1. Core decompression 2. Vascularized and nonvascularized bone grafting 3. Revascularization procedures 4. Proximal femur osteotomies 5. Osteochondral reconstruction	1. Hip arthroplasty 2. Arthrodesis 3. Excisional arthroplasty 4. Hip resurfacing

a. **Hip preserving:**
   1. **Core decompression (Fig. 13):**
      Described by Ficat and Arlet in 1960s
      ↓
      Incidentally when they were trying to find cause of pain in ON
      i. *Indications*:
         1. Stage I and II → Relieves pain significantly.
         2. Age < 50 years
      ii. *Contraindications:* After FH collapse
      iii. *Technique*:
         1. *Traditional:* Drill an 8-10 mm hole through subchondral necrosis.
         2. *Alternative:* Multiple 3.2 mm channels drilled in different direction.
      iv. *Mechanism*:
         Decompression of starling's resistor → Compartment syndrome resolved
         ↓
         A. Relieves intraosseous pressure → relieves pain
         B. Stimulates healing response via angiogenesis
      v. *Additional modifications*:
         a. Fibula grafting:
            1. Most commonly used in India
            2. Mechanical support → prevents collapse
               ↓
            3. Predominantly cortical → Slow resorption
            4. Less regenerative tissue required to fill the defect
            5. ┌►Nonvascularized
            6. └►Vascularized
               i. Better channel for revascularization and regeneration.
               ii. Technically, demanding

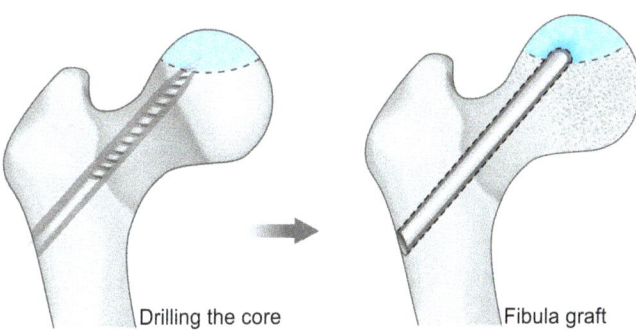

Fig. 13: Core decompression and fibula grafting.

b. Bone marrow aspirate:
   1. Technique:
      i. Aspirated from iliac crest.
      ii. Pooled aspirate → 150 mL
      iii. Filtered to removed fat and clotted blood
      iv. Concentration done at 400 g for 5 minutes
      v. Leukocytes removed → Aspirate = 30 mL
      vi. Concentrate injected through core decompression hole under pressure.
   2. Rationale:
      Core decompression alone fails due to
      ↓
      Insufficient creeping substitution from small number of progenitor cells in the necrotic and surrounding bone
      ↓
      Bone marrow → Hematopoietic component
      ↓
      Stromal component → Osteoprogenitor cells
   vi. *Postoperative management:* Protected weight bearing for 6 weeks
   vii. *Pearls*:
      1. Avoid window below LT → Pathological fracture
      2. Avoid entry in anterior half of femur
         ↓
         Lesion anterolateral
      3. Avoid FH perforation
   viii. *Prognosis*:
      a. Poor:
         1. More 15% area of acetabular surface
         2. Combined necrotic angle >240°
      b. Good → Young patient
2. **Curettage and bone grafting techniques:**
   i. Merle d'Aubigne light bulb: Through cortex of FH - Neck junction **(Fig. 14A)**
   ii. Trapdoor (Mont): Through articular surface **(Fig. 14B)**.

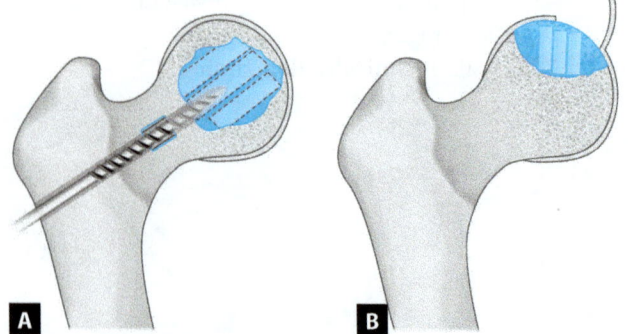

Figs. 14A and B: (A) Merle d'Aubigne light bulb; (B) Trapdoor (Mont).

   iii. Local pedicle vascular bone graft
      a. Meyer's quadratus femoris
      b. TFL

   c. Gluteus medius
   d. Sartorius
3. **Osteotomies:**
   i. Damaged painful region → out of weight bearing axis → relieves pain.
   ii. Gives damaged region time to heal
   iii. Indications and prerequisites:
      1. Young (<50 years)
      2. Stages 2–3 (ARCO)
      3. Small Kerboul necrotic angle (<200)
      4. <30% FH involvement
      5. Minimal acetabular involvement
      6. No ongoing RF (steroids, alcohol)
   iv.

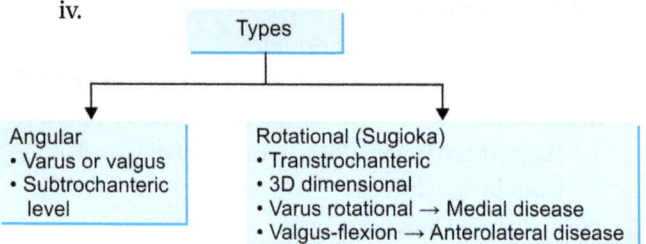

   Angular
   • Varus or valgus
   • Subtrochanteric level

   Rotational (Sugioka)
   • Transtrochanteric
   • 3D dimensional
   • Varus rotational → Medial disease
   • Valgus-flexion → Anterolateral disease

b. **Hip-sacrificing:**
   1. **Total hip arthroplasty:**
      i. Current gold standard for advanced disease
         ↓
      ii. Most reliable → Pain relief, immediate return of function
      iii. Pain relief, immediate return of function
      iv. Young patients:
         a. Uncemented > Cemented
         b. COC > Metal–on poly
            ↓
         c. High rate of linear wear and osteolysis.
      v. Indications:
         a. Advanced arthritis
         b. Age >50
         c. Kerboul >240
         d. All failed previous surgery
   2. Arthrodesis: Stable hip → at cost of ROM. Manual laborer.
   3. Hip resurfacing: Advanced DJD → Small focus, C/I in ongoing etiology (steroid use).

FEMOROACETABULAR IMPINGEMENT

I. INTRODUCTION
1. Early abnormal contact between the bony prominences of the acetabulum and femur
   ↓
2. Mechanically limits the physiological movements of hip
   ↓
3. Producing pain at terminal hip ROM

II. CLASSIFICATION

1. Cam
2. Pincer
3. Combined

A. Cam (Fig. 15)

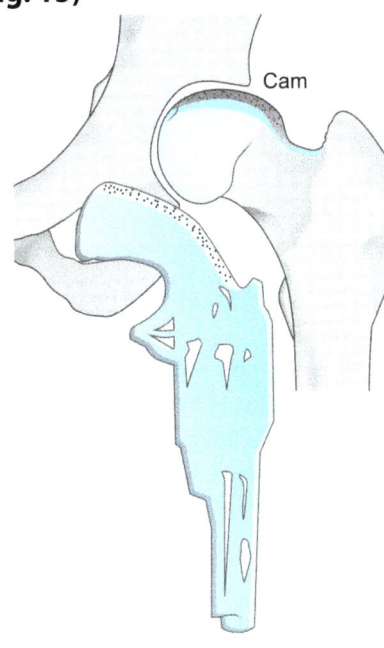

Fig. 15: Cam lesion: Pistol grip deformity.

1. Femoral cause → due to aspherical portion of the femoral head-neck junction.
2. Two morphological features of femoral head in cam.
   i. "Pistol grip" deformity – ↓ Femoral head-neck offset on the superior/anterolateral region.
   ii. "Bump" or exuberant bone in the anterosuperior region of the femoral neck. ↓
       Classic anterior impingement.
3. Sphericity mismatch
   ↓
   Shearing at chondrolabral junction.
   ↓
   Cartilage delamination and labral separation.

B. Pincer (Fig. 16)

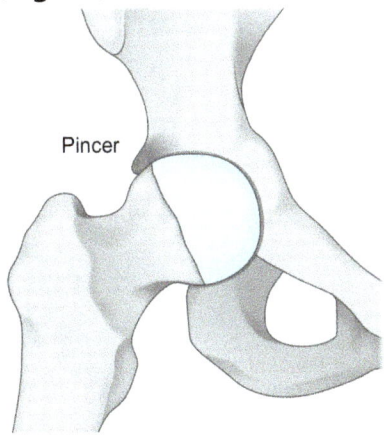

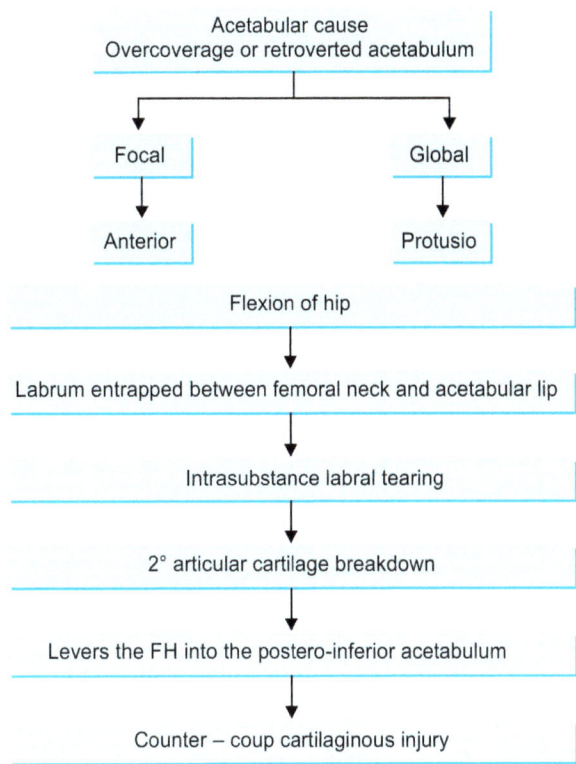

III. CLINICAL FEATURES

1. M: F ┬→ Cam → 14:1
        └→ Pincer → 1:3
2. Age ┬→ Cam → Early middle age (21–51 years)
        └→ Pincer → Late middle age (40–57 years)
3. Pain → i. Activity related
         ii. Groin (deep) or anterior thigh
         iii. Increases on hip flexion and IR
4. Mechanical symptoms → Clicking/Popping
5. ROM hip flexion
   | Adduction
   ▼ IR
6. Pincer → Sudden stop in ROM
   Cam → Gentle stop
7. FADIR test +ve
8. Drehmann's sign +ve → Passive ER of hip while performing hip flexion. (Gearstick sign)

IV. INVESTIGATIONS

A. X-ray

1. True AP (hip in 15° IR)
2. Modified Dunn view
3. False profile view.

B. Cam

1. *Pistol grip deformity:* Asphericity and abnormal contour of femoral head and neck
2. Break in the reverse Shenton's line
3. α angle >50° = Cam **(Fig. 17)**

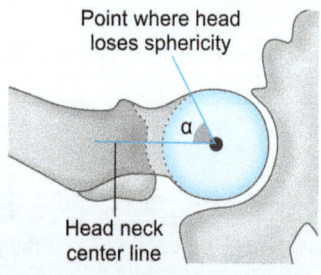

Lateral view

4. Anterior offset:
   i. Anterior offset = Anterior femoral head radius – Anterior femoral neck radius
   ii. Normal >10 mm, Cam: < 8 mm
5. Head-neck offset ratio (Cam: <0.17) $= \dfrac{\text{Anterior offset}}{\text{FH diameter}}$

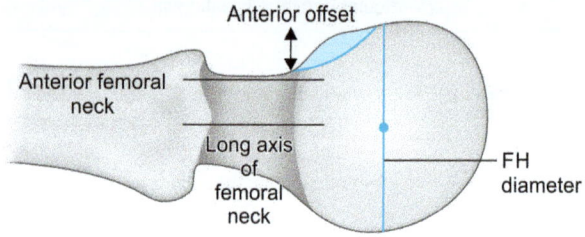

6. Horizontal growth plate
7. Femoral retroversion
8. Cam + Pincer = Kissing lesions

C. Pincer

1. Coxa profunda, protrusio acetabuli
2. Crossover sign/Figure of 8 sign: Acetabular retroversion, anterior overcoverage
3. Posterior wall sign:
   i. Normal → Very close to FH center
   ii. Retroversion → Medial to FH center
4. Lateral center-Edge angle of Wiberg **(Fig. 19)**
   Normal = 25–39°
   ≥40° = Pincer

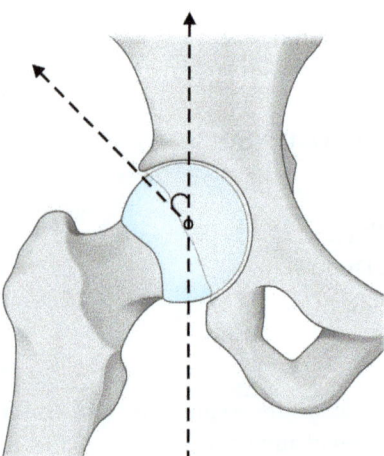

Fig. 19: Lateral center-edge angle of Wiberg > 40° in pincer FAI.

5. Tonnis roof angle → <0° Pincer **(Fig. 20)**

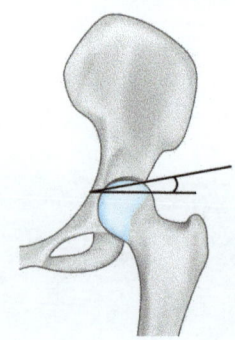

Fig. 20: Angle between a line along the superior acetabulum and the horizontal (normal hip shown in the figure).

6. Extrusion index → Normally 25% head is not covered by the acetabulum.
   In Pincer: <15° is not covered.
7. *Acetabular index:* Normal = 33–38°, <15° = pincer
   (Inter- teardrop line to lateral acetabular roof)
   MRI → Articular cartilage, labral tear.

V. MANAGEMENT

A. Conservative

1. *Modality*:
   i. Activity modification
   ii. PT
   iii. NSAIDs
2. *Indications*:
   i. Minimal symptoms
   ii. No mechanical symptoms
3. Structural abnormality does not improve with conservative management, hence many patients → Surgery.

B. Operative

1. *Benefits*:
   i. Pain relief due to removal of structural abnormality
   ii. Early recognition and management prevents OA
2. *Goals of surgery*:
   i. Precise deformity correction: Intra- and extra-articular
   ii. Treatment of soft tissue abnormality (labrum, articular cartilage, etc.) **(Fig. 21)**

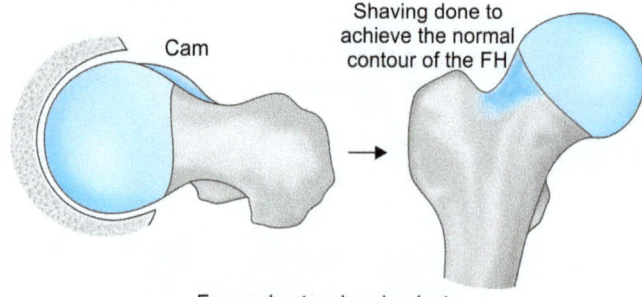

Fig. 21: Shaving off of the cam lesion.

3.
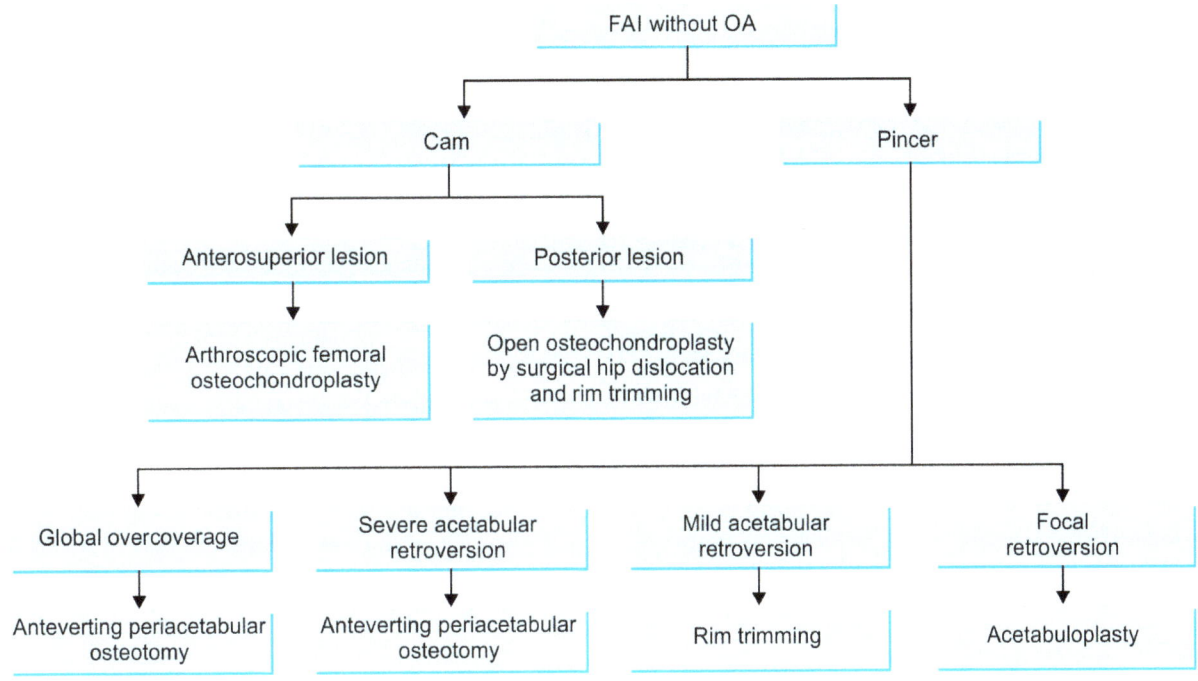

4. Osteochondroplasty **(Figs. 21 and 22)**:

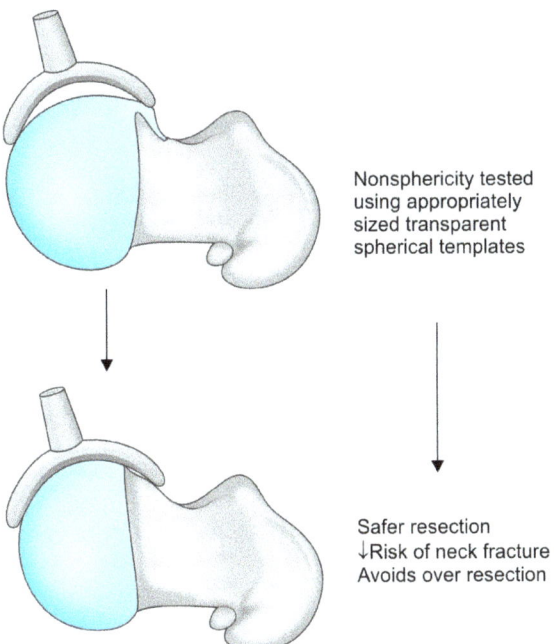

i. Nonsphericity tested using appropriately sized transparent spherical templates
   ↓
   a. Safer resection
   b. ↓ Risk of neck fracture
   c. Avoids over resection
ii. Presence of cyst near the peripheral border of the nonspherical segment is sometimes noted, which indicates point of maximum impingement.
iii. Perfusion confirmed by bleeding from raw cancellous bony surface following neck debridement.
iv. Bone wax applied to debrided surface prior to relocation
v. Postoperative → NWB Gait training → 6 weeks
   a. Avoid flexion >70° and abduction to allow healing of osteotomy site.
   b. Radiological healing >6 weeks → Weight bearing.
5. FAI with OA → Arthroplasty.

VI. COMPLICATIONS
1. Femoral neck fracture
2. Heterotopic ossification
3. Residual deformity following arthroscopic treatment.

HIP ARTHROSCOPY

I. INTRODUCTION
1. Hip arthroscopy is a minimally invasive surgical procedure that uses an arthroscope to diagnose and treat hip disorders.
2. It provides excellent visualization of the articular surface of the joint, peritrochanteric and extra-articular region around the hip.
3. It is technically demanding because of the sphericity of the femoral head and the dense capsule and musculature that surround the joint.
4. In arthroscopic anatomy, hip is divided into central, peripheral and peritrochanteric regions.
5. Image intensifier is required.

II. INDICATIONS

Intra-articular	Periarticular
1. Femoroacetabular impingement (FAI; cam and pincer type) 2. Labral pathology 3. Chondral lesions 4. Ligamentum teres injuries 5. Loose bodies 6. Synovial chondromatosis 7. Septic arthritis 8. Synovial-based diseases 9. Adhesive capsulitis 10. Capsular laxity and instability 11. Isolated femoral head fractures	1. Greater trochanteric pain syndrome 2. Snapping hip syndromes 3. Proximal hamstring repair 4. Sciatic nerve entrapment 5. FAI [ischiofemoral and anterior inferior iliac spine (AIIS) subspine type] 6. Gluteal tears 7. Iliopsoas tendon pathologies 8. Piriformis release

III. CONTRAINDICATIONS

Absolute	Relative
1. Advanced osteoarthritis 2. Severe proximal femoral deformity (Legg–Calvé–Perthes disease, slipped capital femoral epiphysis) 3. Ankylosis 4. Dysplasia with femoral head migration 5. Severe acetabular retroversion 6. Joint contracture 7. Protrusio acetabuli	1. Moderate osteoarthritis 2. Mild dysplasia 3. Obesity

IV. COMPARTMENTS

1. Central compartment → Requires traction for access. Consists of,
    i. Acetabular fossa and femoral head articular surfaces
    ii. Acetabular rim and labrum
    iii. Ligamentum teres
    iv. AIIS and capsule
2. Peripheral compartment
    i. After completion of the central compartment procedure, the leg is removed from traction and the hip is flexed to 45°.
        ↓
    ii. Relaxation of the capsule
        ↓
    iii. Better access to the peripheral compartment.
    iv. Consists of,
        a. Femur head-neck junction
        b. Iliopsoas tendon
        c. Medial synovial fold
3. Peritrochanteric and extra-articular compartment → No traction needed
    i. Iliotibial band and bursa
    ii. Hip abductor tendons
    iii. Piriformis muscle
    iv. Sciatic nerve
    v. Hamstring origin at ischial tuberosity

V. SETUP

1. Instrumentation
    i. 70° arthroscope
    ii. Long cannula and guides
    iii. Flexible instruments
2. Fluoroscopy is needed for hip arthroscopy.
3. Positioning
    i. Supine →
        a. Utilizes fracture table
        b. Patient position becomes easy
        c. Surgeon familiarity
    ii. Lateral →
        a. Easier in obese patients
        b. Requires distractor devices
4. 10–12 mm distraction needed to cannula placement.
5. Traction time must be < 2 hours to ↓ neuropraxia chances.

VI. PORTALS

Portal	Function	Site	Risk
Anterolateral	1. Primary viewing portal 2. Instrumentation → anterolateral	1. 1 cm superior and anterior to the anterior border of GT 2. Made first under fluoroscopy	Superior gluteal nerve
Anterior	Central compartment access and instrumentation	1. Intersection of a line drawn from tip of GT and line drawn inferiorly from ASIS 2. Second portal to be made	1. Lateral femoral cutaneous nerve 2. Ascending branches of lateral femoral circumflex artery 3. Femoral neurovascular bundle
Distal anterolateral	Access to peripheral compartment near femoral neck	1. Starting point 3–4 cm distal to the anterolateral portal 2. Traction is removed and the hip is placed in either neutral flexion and extension or in 45° of flexion to relax the anterior capsule	Ascending branch of lateral femoral circumflex artery

Portal	Function	Site	Risk
		3. Fluoroscopy and direct arthroscopic visualization is used to guide portal placement	
Mid-anterior	Like anterior portal	Between anterior and anterolateral portals	Same as anterior
Posterolateral	Access and instrumentation of posterior hip	1 cm posterior proximal to the posterosuperior tip of the greater trochanter	Sciatic nerve

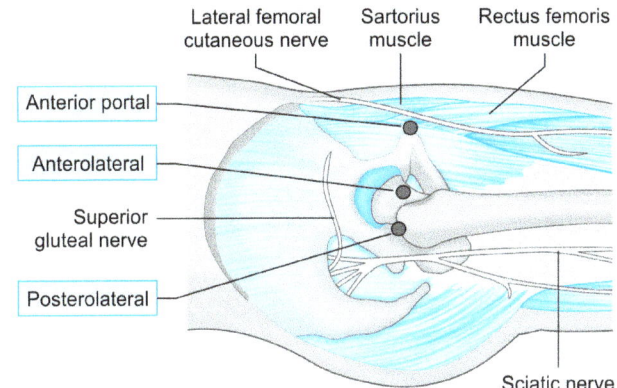

VII. COMPLICATIONS

1. Traction neuropraxia of femoral, sciatic, pudendal or lateral femoral cutaneous nerves
2. Damage to articular surface and labrum
3. Hip instability
4. Bony over-resection and under-resection in impingement procedures
5. Heterotopic ossification
6. Abdominal compartment syndrome
7. Heterotopic ossification

HIP RESURFACING ARTHROPLASTY (HRA)

A conservative surgical procedure of arthroplasty of hip.

I. PRINCIPLES AND BENEFITS

1. **Femoral bone reservation:**
   i. Enhanced implant stability → due to additional bone support.
   ii. Larger femoral head used
       ↓
       ↓ Rates of dislocation
   iii. More bone available at the time of revision surgery
2. **Near normal bone loading:**
   i. HRA transmits load through the preserved bone in FH and neck.
       ↓
   ii. ↑ Density postoperative compared to THR.
   iii. No stress shielding effect that is seen in THR.
3. **Higher activity level → ↑ROM:**
   i. Larger FH → ↑ Stability → ↓ Dislocation
   ii. Return to sports, sitting on the floor, use of Indian commode possible.
4. **Improved biomechanics:**
   i. Does not disrupt the normal biomechanics of hip joint.
   ii. Native offset maintained.
   iii. No LLD.
5. Decreased morbidity at the time of revision surgery.
6. Improved outcome in the event of infection.
7. Does not violate femoral canal.
8. Reduced prevalence of thromboembolic phenomena
9. ↑ Natural feel
10. Rapid recovery

II. INDICATIONS

1. Primary osteoarthritis
2. Secondary osteoarthritis:
   i. Post-childhood hip disorders: Perthes, SCFE
   ii. Dysplasia
   iii. AVN (<25% of FH inv.) } results not very favorable
   iv. Post-traumatic
3. Young patient (< 65 years)
4. Male → Larger bone stock
5. Active and motivated
6. Preserved proximal femoral bone stock.

III. CONTRAINDICATIONS

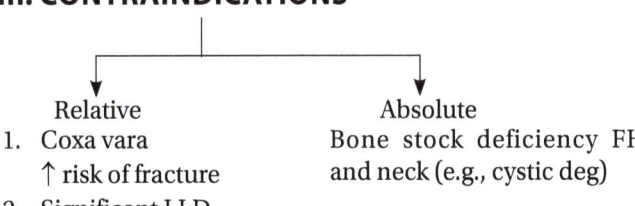

1. Coxa vara
   ↑ risk of fracture
2. Significant LLD
   HRA cannot correct LLD
3. Female sex of child bearing age
   Risk of metal ions crossing placenta.
4. Renal failure
5. >65 years age
6. Severe osteoporosis

Absolute: Bone stock deficiency FH and neck (e.g., cystic deg)

IV. DISADVANTAGES

1. Femoral neck fractures
   ↓   ↓
   i. Vertical fractures.
   ii. MC mechanism of failure in less than 3 years and in acute postoperative period

iii. Risk factor → Femoral neck notching → ↓sed by placing the component in slight valgus (10°)
2. Femoral vascularity ⊗ → loosening and ON
3. Metal ion dispersal
4. Metal sensitivity
5. Difficulty in inserting acetabular component with intact FH and N
6. Heterotopic ossification >THR
7. Require larger exposure than THA
8. No long-term safety data compared to THA
9. More technically demanding.

V. BEARING

1. Metal-on-metal (currently)
2. First generation → Metal-on poly
   ↓
   Large femoral head on polyethylene
   ↓
   ↑ Volumetric wear
   ↓
   ↑ Osteolysis rate → Abandoned
3. Latest C-O-C trials

VI. COMPONENTS

1. Acetabular → Uncemented cup → cobalt, chromium, titanium
2. Fixation by circumferential pins
3. HA coating **(Fig. 23)**

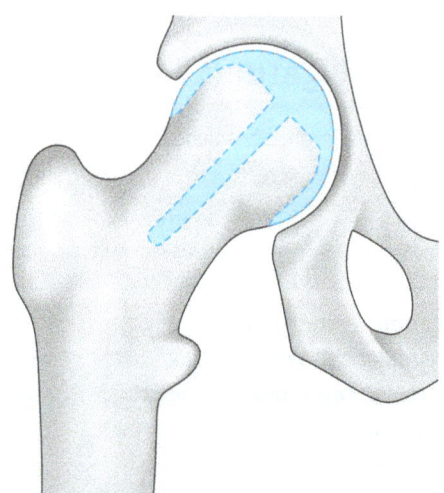

VII. RECENT ADVANCES

1. Robot assisted
2. Navigation
3. Minimally invasive HRA.

FEMORAL NECK FRACTURE NONUNION

I. INTRODUCTION

1. Fracture shows no signs of visible healing till **3 months** after injury
2. Other fractures → 9 months (US FDA)

II. BLOOD SUPPLY OF PROXIMAL FEMUR (FIG. 24)

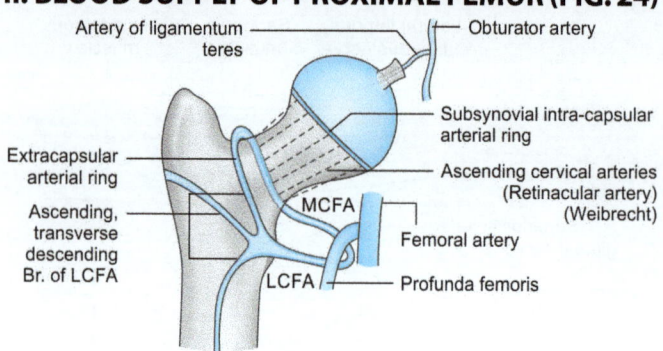

MCFA: medial circumflex femoral artery
LCFA: lateral circumflex femoral artery

III. PATHOGENESIS

A. Compromised Biology (1° Factors)

1. Cambium layer absent → No osteoprogenitor cells.
2. Poor callus formation due to continuous bathing of fracture in synovial fluid.
3. Poor vascularity → Atrophic non-union.
4. Tamponade effect.

B. Fracture Configuration

1. Displaced fracture (Garden III or IV).
2. Posterior comminution leads to retroversion and varus.
3. High Pauwels angle → ↑ Shear forces.

C. Treatment Related

1. No treatment
2. Poor reduction
3. Poor fixation
4. Delay of fracture fixation (>24 hours)

D. Neglected Presentation

1. Osteopenia
2. Neck resorption
3. Osteonecrosis.

IV. CLASSIFICATION

A. Sandhu et al. (CORR 2005)

I. Irregular fracture surfaces (fresh)
   i. Proximal fragment (PF) size > 2.5 cm
   ii. Gap between fracture fragments <1 cm.

II. Smooth fracture surfaces:
   i. PF > 2.5 cm
   ii. Gap = 1–2.5 cm
III. i. PF < 2.5 cm
   ii. Gap >2.5 cm
   I, II, III → With or without osteonecrosis.

B. Leighton
1. Inadequate fixation or nonanatomic reduction.
2. Loss of fixation with fracture displacement.
3. Fibrous nonunion with no displacement and intact fixation.

V. CLINICAL PRESENTATION
Neck of femur fracture (NOF)
<48 hours—Acute NOF
48–3 weeks—Delayed presentation
>3 weeks—Neglected
>3 months—NU

A. History
1. Trauma to hip.
2. Prior surgery.

B. Symptoms
1. Pain in hip → Groin, buttock.
2. Unable to bear weight.
3. Difficulty in walking and carrying ADL.

C. Examination
1. Surgical scar.
2. Antalgic gait.
3. LLD
4. Atrophy of thigh gluteal muscles.
5. Tenderness at hip joint.
6. Painful and decreased ROM
7. Unable to carry out active SLR
8. Telescopy [+]
9. Log roll pain [+]

VI. INVESTIGATIONS
1. Radiograph (AP, cross table lateral, traction IR):
   i. Persistent fracture line
   ii. Resorption of fracture surfaces
   iii. Hardware failure
   iv. Calcar comminution
   v. Varus malalignment
   vi. ON
2. MRI: ON femur head
3. CT:
   i. Most definitive way to diagnose N-U
   ii. Surgical planning
4. Tc^{99} Bone scan:
5. Lab: ESR, CRP, WBC → Rule out infection
6. Hip joint aspiration.

VII. MANAGEMENT
Depends upon:
1. Age at presentation
2. Presence of ON
3. Functional demands of patient

A. Valgus Intertrochanteric Osteotomy (Fig. 25)

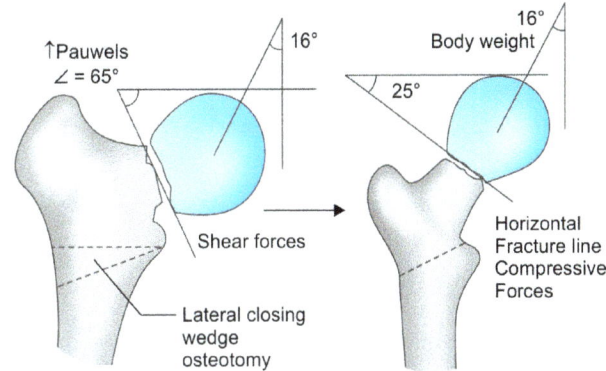

1. *Indications:*
   i. Failure of fracture fixation
   ii. NU > 3 months postoperative
   iii. Varus collapse
   iv. Young patient, active
2. *Contraindications:*
   i. Significant bone loss
   ii. Joint incongruity
   iii. Age > 65 (relative)
3. MC salvage procedure
4. Reorients vertical → horizontal fracture line.
5. Improves abductor function.

   Restores femoral length and abductor lever arm.

B. Bone Grafting
Indications:
1. Well aligned nonunion with loss of posterior bone stock
2. Quadrants femoris vascularized pedicle graft → Meyers
3. Free vascularized fibula graft

C. Total Hip Arthroplasty
1. *Indications:*
   i. Femoral bone defect
   ii. Poor acetabular bone quality
   iii. Older patients with active lifestyle
   iv. Presence of ON
2. *Technique:*
   i. Cemented or uncemented
   ii. Metal-on-poly or C-O-C
   iii. Dual mobility THR → ↓ Dislocation
3. *Complications:*
   i. Dislocation
   ii. Loosening
   iii. Infection
   iv. Need for revision

D. Hip Hemiarthroplasty
1. Elderly patients with comorbidities.
2. Not active, low physical demand.

E. Hip Arthrodesis
1. Young patient with nonviable femoral heads.
2. Heavy manual labors.

EVOLUTION OF THR

There has been a significant evolution of hip arthroplasty over the past 200 years

↓

1820—Anthony White performed excision arthroplasty

↓

1830–1900—Leopold and Ollier performed interpositional arthroplasties using fat (1912 Sir Robert Jones used gold foil as an interpositional material)

↓

1890—Professor Themistocles Glück used and ivory ball and socket, fixed with nickel plated screws, plaster of Paris, Pumice and resin was used to provide fixation to bone

↓

1917—William Baer used a chromicized pig bladder as an interpositional material

↓

1919—Delbert used a rubber femoral prosthesis

↓

1923—Smith Peterson used a glass mold over freshened articular surfaces with the Idea of guiding the natural repair processes to form a smooth articulating surface
Advantage—Biocompatible
Disadvantage—Could not withstand pressures and failed

↓

1937—Smith Peterson used a vitallium prosthesis (an alloy of chrome, cobalt and molybdenum)

↓

1930—Philip Wiles-first metal on metal prosthesis using preciously fitting stainless steel components with nuts and bolts

↓

1944—Judet Brothers - Acrylic prosthesis

↓

1950—Thompson prosthesis
1952—Moore — Metallic chrome cobalt alloy proximal femoral

↓

Mid 1950s—Kenneth McKee-modified metal on metal prosthesis (modified Thompson style prosthesis with a cemented acetabular component)

↓

1963—Sir John Charnley (father of total hip arthroplasty) – Charnley's low friction arthroplasty
– metallic femoral stem, small head (22 mm), cemented polyethylene (PTFE-polytetrafluoroethylene-high wear rate-0.5 mm/month and severe foreign body reaction) acetabular component, acrylic bone cement
Charnley's assistant: Despite Charnley's reluctance tested HDPE (High density polyethylene)
Much better wear characteristics and lesser foreign body reaction

↓

Evolution of bearing surfaces
HDPE–High density polyethylene
UHMWPE–Ultra high molecular weight polyethylene
XLPE–Highly cross-linked polyethylene
Ceramic–Alumina and zirconia
Metal on metal–Discarded
Metalized ceramic–Oxinium
Dual mobility

Evolution of fixation methods
Osteolysis attributed to cement–biologic fixation with bone ingrowth
Late 80s–early 90s–Uncemented femoral stems
• Grit blasting
• Plasma spraying
• Porous coating
• HA coating
Cementless acetabular components
• Porous coated
• Trabecular metal
• Screws

BEARING SURFACES IN TOTAL HIP ARTHROPLASTY

I. INTRODUCTION
1. Several options are available to the surgeon when choosing the bearing surface in THA [ceramic-on-ceramic (CoC), ceramic-on-polyethylene (CoPE), metal on polyethylene (MoPE)], each with advantages and drawbacks.
2. The most common material for acetabular liners is polyethylene (PE), either ultra-high molecular weight polyethylene (UHMWPE) ("standard" or "conventional" PE) or highly cross-linked poly (XLPE), or ceramics or metal (nowadays abandoned and withdrawn from the market for THA).
3. Heads can be made of ceramics or metal alloys, usually CoCr (Cobalt-Chromium).

II. IMPORTANT DEFINITIONS
1. *Wear:* The surface damage with progressive loss of material (debris) due to friction between moving surfaces.
2. *Debris:* Particles of different material and size shed from the surface of the various parts of the implant due to wear.
3. *Fretting:* Relative low amplitude movement (oscillation and sliding) between two mechanically joined parts, under load conditions (between 1 and 100 μm). All modular junctions are susceptible.
4. *Corrosion:* Surface degradation due to electrochemical interactions producing metallic ions and salts which applies only to metals.

III. BEARING SURFACES FOR ACETABULAR CUP

A. Polyethylene
1. Ultra-high molecular weight polyethylene:
   i. Introduced in the early 1960s by Charnley
   ii. Until 1990s Sterilization by Gamma radiation: 2.5 Mrad (25 kGy)
2. XLPE: Highly cross linked polyethylene:
   i. UHMWPE exposed to higher doses of radiation 5–10 Mrad (50–100 kGy) of gamma/electron beam radiation
   ii. Radiation-increases cross linking in poly, but forms free radicals, which cause oxidation, make poly brittle and more susceptible to wear
   iii. The cross-linking process, while increasing the wear properties of PE decreases the mechanical ones, making the liners more at risk of fatigue fracture.
   iv. Methods to reduce oxygen free radicals:
      a. **Remelting:**
         1. Heating the material above its melting point (approximately 135°C).
         2. Free radicals are virtually eliminated, but the crystallinity of the is also reduced, reducing the physical properties.

3. Show good oxidation resistance but less fatigue resistance (decreased fracture toughness and ultimate tensile strength)
   b. **Annealing:** Process of heating the material just below the melting point.
      1. This avoids the reduction in crystallinity and consequent reduction in mechanical properties
      2. Less effective than remelting in extinguishing residual free radicals.
      3. Show good wear and fatigue performances but poor oxidation resistance
   c. **Vitamin E Doping:**
      1. Vitamin E, strong anti-oxidant added in PE powder/by diffusion after machining, scavenges free radicals, avoids need for annealing
      2. Final sterilization by ethylene oxide/gas plasma with oxygen-free packaging.

B. Ceramic

Most commonly alumina (silica and aluminum).
1. *Advantages*:
   i. Wear particles are inert
   ii. Extremely hard-lower wear rate
   iii. For a same sized acetabular cup, thinner shell acceptable-larger size femoral head can be used
2. *Drawbacks*:
   i. Edge loading can cause fracture, chipping
   ii. Squeaking
   iii. Higher cost

IV. BEARING SURFACES FOR FEMORAL HEAD

A. Metal

1. Conventional choice CoCr alloy. Mated to UHMWPE/XLPE
   1. *Advantages*:
      i. Cheap
      ii. Less risk of fracture
   2. *Disadvantage*:
      i. More wear than ceramic
      ii. Risk of trunnionosis/fretting/head neck junction corrosion.

B. Ceramic

1. *Advantage*:
   i. Surface finish smoother than metal implants
   ii. Harder than metal
   iii. More resistant to scratching from third-body wear particles.
   iv. Higher wettability
   v. Surface finish with only negative peaks
   vi. No trunnionosis
2. *Disadvantage*:
   i. High cost
   ii. Risk of fracture, chipping, flaking

C. Ceramicized Metal

1. *Oxidized zirconium*:
   i. Zirconium metal alloy that is placed through an oxidation process
   ii. Yields an implant with a zirconia ceramic surface of approximately 5 µm in thickness.
   iii. The enhanced surface is integral to the metal substrate and not a surface coating.
2. *Advantage*: Same surface hardness, smoothness, and wettability of typical ceramics, but are not susceptible to chipping, flaking, or fracture.
3. *Disadvantage*: Available only with a polyethylene liner, not as a ceramic on ceramic configuration.

Various combinations of bearing surfaces available with main disadvantages.

Couplings	Main disadvantage
Metal-on-polyethylene	Wear and osteolysis
Ceramic-on-polyethylene	Wear and osteolysis
Metal-on-XLPE	Decreased mechanical properties
Ceramic-on-XLPE	Decreased mechanical properties
Ceramic-on-ceramic	Breakage and squeaking
Metal-on-metal	ARMD (ALVAL, high ion levels, osteolysis, pseudotumors)

TRIBOLOGY

"TRIBOS" → RUBBING

Branch of science and technology which deals with the study of friction, wear, and lubrication.

A. Friction

Resistance to relative motion between two bodies in contact.
1. *Types*:
   a. Static: Prevent surfaces from moving altogether.
   b. Dynamic/sliding: Hinder the continued motion of already moving surfaces.
2. Components of friction **(Fig. 26)**
   (F: Friction force; N: Perpendicular force across surfaces; µ: Coefficient of friction)

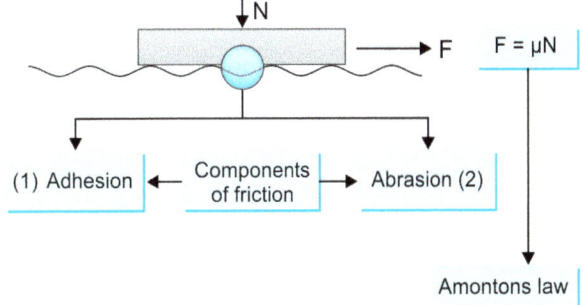

1. Adhesion:
   Force between surface atoms and molecules of two adjacent surfaces.
   ↓
   Electrostatic, metallic bonds.

ii. Abrasions:
Cyclic elastic or plastic deformation of contact spots (asperities)
↓
Generation of particles.

B. Wear

Removal or displacement of material from one body when subjected to contact or relative motion with another body.

I. **Types:**
  1. *Adhesive (fretting) 20-30%* **(Fig. 27)**

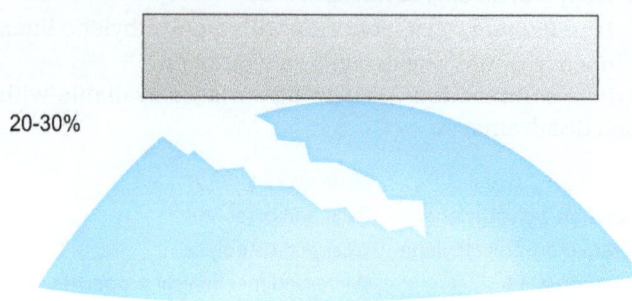

20-30%

Strength of adhesion during contact of two bearing surfaces is greater than strength of material.
  2. *Abrasive (erosive) (30-50%)* **(Fig. 28)**

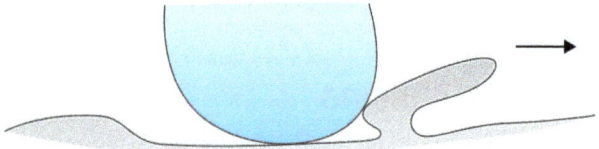

Hard projection of one surface cuts through the opposing soft surface.
  3. *Third-body wear* **(Fig. 29)**

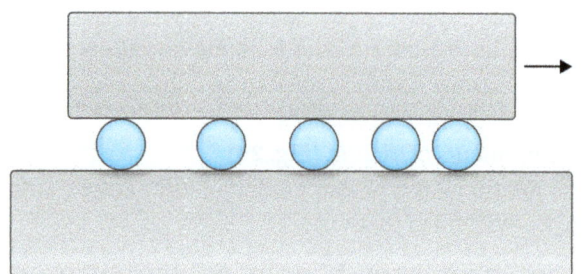

Hard particles such as bone or PMMA trapped between bearing surfaces → abrasive damage.
  4. *Fatigue wear* **(Fig. 30)**

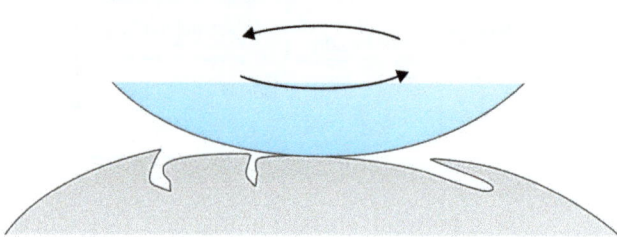

Repeated loading and unloading of bearing surfaces during articulation.

  5. *Corrosive wear* **(Fig. 31)**

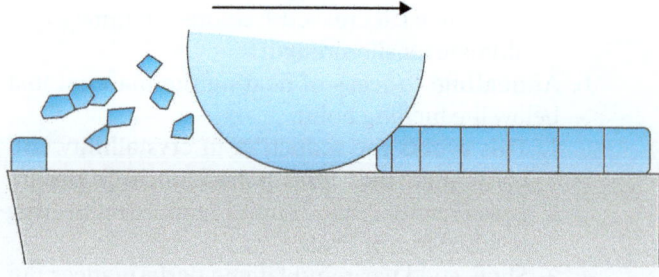

Mechanical wear + chemical reaction
↓
Material released
↓
Third-body wear

II. **Wear modes**
↓
Condition under which prosthesis was functioning when wear occurred.

Mode 1: Motion of two primary bearing surfaces against each other.

Mode 2: Primary bearing surface moving against a secondary surface that was not intended to come in contact with the first (subluxating hip).

Mode 3: Contaminant particles directly abrade one or both of 1° bearing surfaces (third-body wear).

Mode 4: Two secondary surfaces rub against each other (backside wear).

Osteolysis → Causes aseptic loosening of the implanted prosthesis.

Largest cause of revision surgery and failure of arthroplasty. Results from resorption of bone as a result of biological reaction to wear particles (acetabular comp > femoral).

Lubrication

Interposes a material between two contacting solids to minimize usual interaction between them.

COMPLICATIONS OF THR AND PERIPROSTHETIC HIP FRACTURES

1. Early / Late 2. Local / Systemic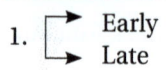

A. EARLY

1. *Wound complications:*
   i. Superficial infection
   ii. Wound necrosis
   iii. Instability and dislocation
   iv. Neurovascular injury
2. *Cardiopulmonary:*
   i. Chest pain
   ii. Palpitations
   iii. Dyspnea
   iv. Pulmonary complications
   v. Congestive heart failure
   vi. Blood loss.

3. *Neuropsychiatric*:
    i. Altered sensorium
    ii. Post-surgery psychosis
    iii. Hyponatremia
    iv. Delirium
4. *Renal*:
    i. Oliguria
    ii. Urinary retention
    iii. UTI
    iv. Chronic renal failure
5. *Nonspecific*:
    i. Fever
    ii. Nausea
    iii. Abdominal pain
    iv. Pain → Groin/buttock → Acetabulum
       Thigh → Femoral stem
    v. Stress shielding → Proximal femur bone loss in a setting of well-fixed stem.

B. LATE
1. Aseptic loosening
2. Heterotrophic ossification
3. Late instability prosthetic fractures
4. Prosthetic joint infection
5. Stress fractures
6. Periprosthetic fractures
7. Metal hypersensitivity
8. Malignancy.

I. DEEP INFECTION
A. Etiology
1. *S. aureus* and *S. epidermidis* >50% infections
2. Patients skin → Most frequent source of infection
3. Gram -ve → P. aeruginosa
    Klebsiella
    E. coli
4. Other Gram +ve → Streptococci
    Enterococcus

B. Risk Factors
1. Patient
    i. Advanced vascular disease
    ii. Rheumatoid arthritis
    iii. Renal disease
    iv. Immunosuppressive medications
    v. Diabetes
    vi. Hemophilia
    vii. Obesity
    viii. Malnutrition
    ix. Smoking
2. Local
3. Operative
    i. History of multiple surgeries
    ii. Revision surgery
    iii. ↑ OT time
    iv. Hematoma formation.

C. Classification
Tsukayama and treatment:
1. *Positive intraoperative cultures*:
    i. S. epidermidis (coagulase negative) during a revision THR for a presumed aseptic failure.
    ii. 6 weeks IV antibiotics, no additional Sx intervention
2. *Early postoperative infections*:
    i. Within 1st month = <4 weeks
    ii. Wound colonization, infected hematomas, superficial infections spreading to periprosthetic space.
       Rx → wound wash → debridement → attempt prothesis salvage.
3. *Acute hematogenous infections*:
    i. Sudden deterioration in previously well-functioning THA
    ii. History of pyogenic infection elsewhere in the body.
4. *Late chronic infections*:
    i. >1 month, insidious onset >4 weeks
    ii. Prosthesis removal and staged revision
    iii. 1st stage → Implant removal and spacer
       Spacer can be → Static or articulating
    iv. Serves 2 functions → Structural support and local antibiotic delivery.
    v. 2nd stage → Usually after 6 weeks, revision arthroplasty.
    vi. Final option → Arthrodesis.
    vii. Debilitated patient → Long-term antibiotic suppressive therapy.

D. 2018 Diagnostic Criteria for Prosthetic Joint Infection

Major criteria (at least one of the following)	Decision
Two positive cultures of the same organism	Infected
Sinus tract with evidence of communication to the joint or visualization of the prosthesis	

		Minor criteria	Score	Decision
Preoperative diagnosis	Serum	Elevated CRP *or* D-dimer	2	≥6 infected
		Elevated ESR	1	
	Synovial	Elevated synovial *WBC count or LE*	3	2–5 possibly infected[a]
		Positive alpha-defensin	3	
		Elevated synovial PMN (%)	2	0–1 not infected
		Elevated synovial CRP	1	

	Inconclusive preoperative score or dry tap[a]	Score	Decision
Intraoperative diagnosis	Preoperative score	–	≥6 infected
	Positive histology	3	4–5 inconclusive[b]
	Positive purulence	3	
	Single positive culture	2	
			≤3 not infected

E. Prevention
1. Chlorhexidine skin bath
2. Controlled blood sugar
3. Albumin > 3, Hb >10
4. Systemic antimicrobial prophylaxis 30-60 minutes before skin incision (cefazolin)
5. Correction of modifiable risk factors
6. Surgical technique and operating room environment
7. Laminar air flow
8. Reduction of traffic flow
9. Dental prophylaxis

II. ASEPTIC LOOSENING
1. Implant loosening as a result of
   ↓
2. Noninfective osteolysis
3. Main cause → Ultra high molecular weight polyethylene
4. Polyethylene wear debris → Phagocytosed by macrophages
   ↓
5. Chronic granulomatous inflammation
   ↓
   Bone resorption
6. Loosening-types
   1. Definite → Migration of stem
      Fracture of stem
      Fracture in cement mantle
   2. Probable → Continuous radiolucent line at the cement bone interface.
   3. Possible: Radiolucent line between 50 and 100% of cement bone interface (**Fig. 32**)

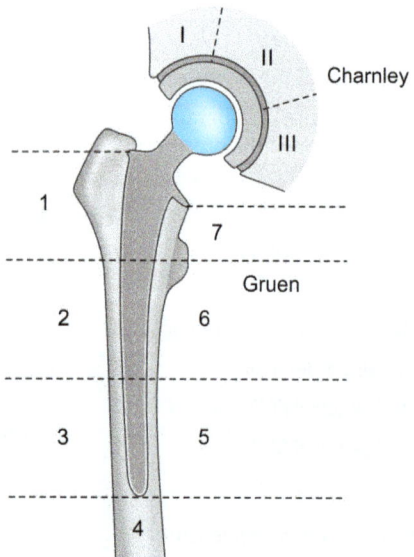

Fig. 32: Zones of cementing.

III. NEUROVASCULAR INJURY
1. MC nerve injury → Sciatic (peroneal > tibial division)
2. Others → Femoral (anterior approach), obturator, gluteal.
3. *Cause*:
   1. Direct trauma → Retractors, dissection
   2. Traction
   3. Constriction by wire or sutures
   4. Thermal injury from cement
   5. Ischemia after hematoma formation
   6. Dislocation of components
4. *Prevention and management*:
   1. Knee immobilizer to prevent knee from buckling → Femoral nerve.
   2. Foot splint → Prevents equinus deformity. Sciatic nerve injury.
   3. Intraoperative assistance of vascular surgery.
   4. Preoperative angiography → Complex cases.

IV. INSTABILITY
A. Risk Factors
1. Disease conditions:
   i. Prior sepsis
   ii. DDH
   iii. RA
   iv. Nonhealed fracture
   v. Infection
2. Surgical factors:
   i. Posterior approach
   ii. Retroverted acetabular cup
   iii. Excessively anteverted → Anterior dislocation
   iv. Vertical orientation (>55%) acetabular cup
   v. Small femoral head and reinforcements at base (skirted head)
   vi. Less experience
   vii. Reduced femoral offset
   viii. Trochanteric fracture
   Greatest risk ≤ 3 months
3. Patient factors:
   i. F > M
   ii. Frail elderly
   iii. Alcohol abuse
   iv. Neuromuscular disease
   v. Obese
   vi. Emotionally unstable

B. Classification–Dorr
1. Malposition of extremity
2. Soft tissue imbalance
3. Component malposition

C. Prevention and Rx
1. Good surgical planning → Reproduce normal offsets
2. Immediate treatment → Closed reduction in OT
3. Postreduction immobilization
   ↓
   Long knee brace
4. Identify underlying cause → Rx
5. Dual mobility THR and large femur heads

V. HETEROTOPIC OSSIFICATION

1. Aberrant bone formation in places where bone does not form normally.
2. ↑ rates → Anterior approaches.
3. Brooker classification of HO **(Fig. 33)**:

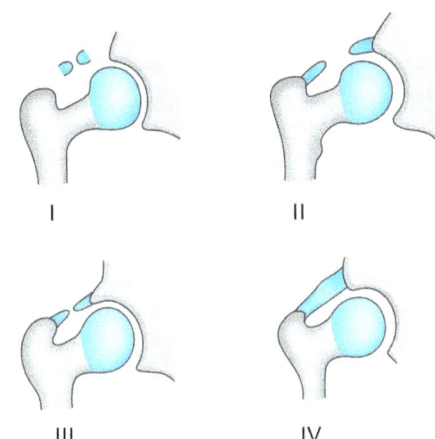

   i. Islands of bone with soft tissue of hip
   ii. Bony spurs at pelvis and femur >1 cm intervening space
   iii. <1 cm intervening space
   iv. Bony ankylosis

4. **Risk factors**
   a. *Patient factors*:
      i. Previous heterotopic ossification
      ii. History of trauma to hip
      iii. Hypertrophic OA
      iv. DISH
      v. Males
      vi. AS
   b. *Surgical factors*:
      i. Approach → Anterior or trochanteric
      ii. Surgical trauma → G. medius
      iii. Postoperative hematoma
      iv. Dislocation
      v. Fracture
      vi. Infections
5. **Prevention**
   i. Minimize soft tissue trauma
   ii. Irradiation – 800 cGY dose
   iii. NSAIDs → Indomethacin 25 mg TDS for 3 months
   iv. Bisphosphonates
6. **Treatment:** Only when HO → Mature → No signs of active disease → Excision (if interferes).

VI. LEG LENGTH DISCREPANCY

1. Preoperative templating – Prevention
2. Up to 2 cm → Body compensates
3. Up to 5 cm → Shoe raise

VII. VENOUS THROMBOEMBOLISM

A. Virchow's Triad

Venous stasis → Positioning, limb swelling
↓Mobility preoperative and postoperative

Endothelial injury
Limb manipulation, intraoperative

Hypercoagulability
Perioperative → B. loss

Prophylaxis

Pharmacological
1. LMWH
2. Dabigatran
3. Warfarin
4. Aspirin
5. Fondaparinux
6. Rivaroxaban

Mechanical
1. DVT Stockings
2. Venous foot pump
3. Pneumatic compression devices

VIII. PERIPROSTHETIC FRACTURES

1. Intraoperative
   Postoperative
2. ↑ Incidence → Prolonged survival time
   → Increased number of 1° and revision THRs
3. Etiology and RF
   i. Low energy fall
   ii. Main risk factor → Osteolysis → Implant loosening
   iii. Osteoporosis
   iv. F > M
   v. RA
   vi. Revision surgery
   vii. Paget's disease
   viii. Tumors
   ix. Trauma
   x. Polyneuropathies
   xi. Stress risers
   xii. Varus stem.
4. **Classification**
   a. **Callaghan:** Intraoperative acetabular fracture:
      1. Anterior wall
      2. Transverse
      3. Inferior hip
      4. Posterior wall
   b. **Peterson:** Postoperative acetabular fracture:
      1. Clinically and radiologically stable
      2. Unstable
   c. **Vancouver:** Most commonly used

Three factors considered:
  i. Site of fracture
  ii. Stability of implant
  iii. Quality of bone

Types (Fig. 34)

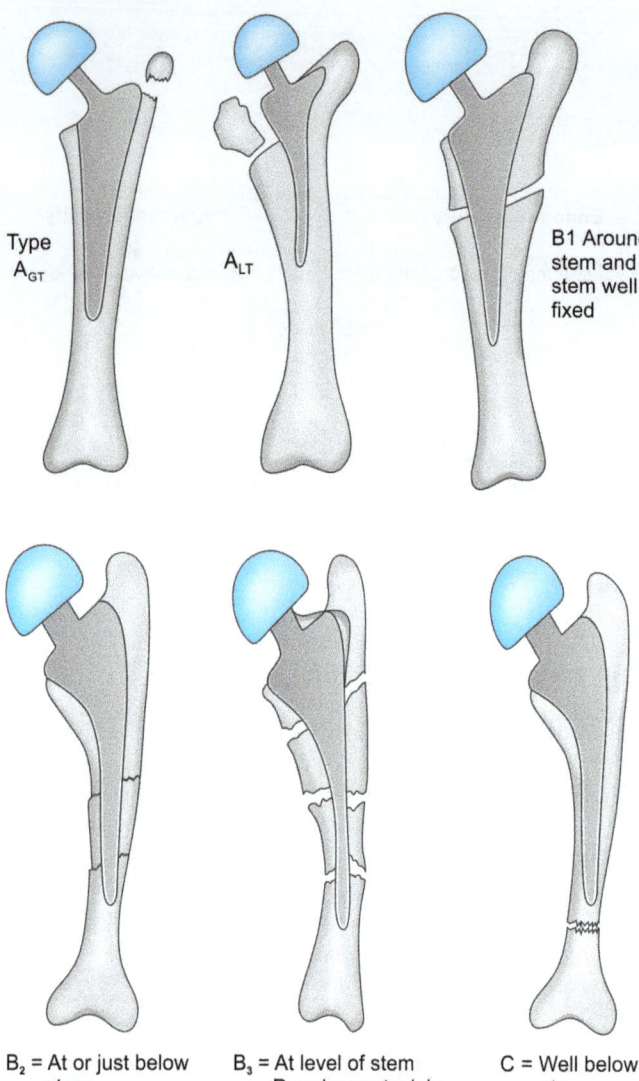

A_{GT}, A_{LT}
B_1 = Fracture around stem and stem well fixed
B_2 = At or just below stem, stem loose
B_3 = At level of stem, poor bone stock in proximal femur
C = Well below stem

5. **Management**
   i. *Acetabular fracture:*
      1. Stable (intra- or postoperative) → Conservatively
      2. Unstable → Require fixation and weight-bearing restrictions
      3. Late postoperative acetabular fracture + Osteolysis
         ↓
         Operative intervention → Revision
   ii. *Femoral fracture:*
      1. A_{GT} → Stable undisplaced
         ↓
         a. Conservatively
         b. Protected weight bearing
         c. Avoid abduction for 6–12 weeks.
            Unstable → >2.5 cm displaced
               → Pain, instability, abductor weakness.
            Treatment → Bone grafting + Trochanteric fixation
      2. A_{LT} → Nonoperative usually
         If large portion of calcar compromised
            ↓
         Cerclage wiring
      3. B → MC fracture
         a. B_1 → ORIF with or without BG (cortical strut)
            Locking trochanteric plate with
               +
            Proximal unicortical screws with cables
               +
            Distal bicortical screws
         b. B_2 →
            i. Revision → Long femoral stem preferably uncemented
               ↓
            ii. Bypassing the fracture by a minimum distance of two femoral diameters + at least 5 cm of diaphyseal fit.
               +
            iii. Fracture fixation with cerclage wires ± cortical strut.
            iv. Cemented stem → osteoporosis and wide canals, irradiated bones
            v. Cement-in cement → When cement mantle is reasonably fixed to bone. Adv. → Faster, technically less demanding
            vi. Extensively porous - coated stems with distal interlocking screws.
            vii. Tumor prosthesis
         c. B_3 →
            i. Revision arthroplasty but high rate of complications due to loss of bone stock.
            ii. Essential for implant to obtain adequate distal fixation to gain axial and rotational stability.
            iii. Young → allograft + prosthesis

iv. Old → low functional demand → Proximal femur replacement or mega prosthesis. Immediate weight bearing.
4. **C** → ORIF locking plate, unicortical and bicortical screws hybrid cable construct. May use IMN too
↓
↓ Stress risers

OSTEOARTHRITIS HIP

Degenerative disease of the hip joint that causes progressive loss of articular cartilage of FH and acetabulum.

I. CLASSIFICATION

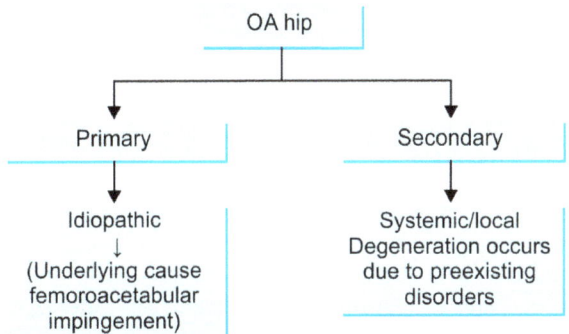

II. ETIOLOGY AND RISK FACTORS

1. Age: >60 years → 1°
2. Gender: Males > Females
3. Occupation: Manual heavy lifting laborers
4. Sports: High impact sport activities
5. Genetics
6. Race: ↓1° in Indians, ↑ Europeans
7. BMI: ↑ → Faster progression
8. LLD
9. Previous trauma to hip
10. Muscular dysfunction
11. Developmental disorders:
    i. DDH
    ii. LCPD
    iii. SCFE
    iv. Dysplasia:
        a. Coxa magna
        b. Coxa vara
        c. Coxa valga
        d. Coxa profunda
    v. Acetabular — Retroversion
                    — Anteversion
    vi. Femoral — Retroversion
                 — Anteversion.
12. FAI → MC underlying cause of 1°
13. Paget's disease

III. PATHOPHYSIOLOGY

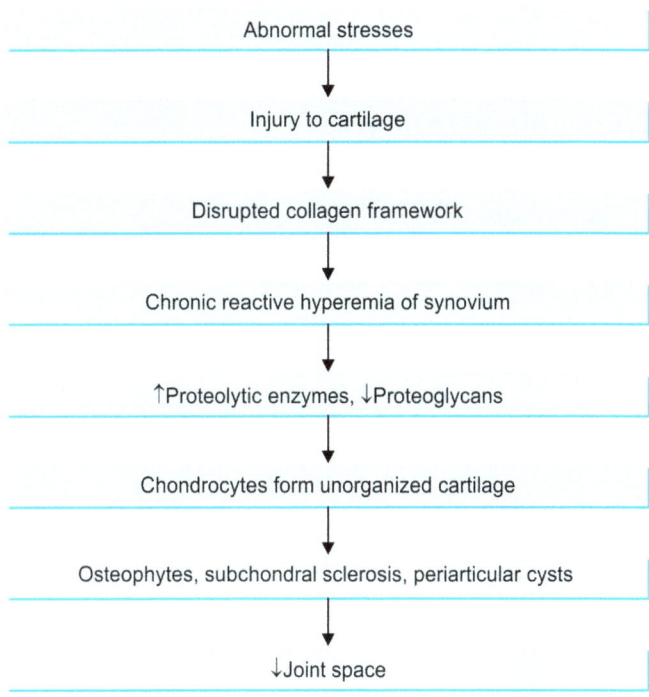

IV. CLINICAL FEATURES

A. Symptoms

1. Pain (Groin)
   i. Function limiting
   ii. Activity related
   iii. Decreased with rest
   iv. Night pain ±
2. Stiffness
3. Locking catching sensations
4. Limp.

B. Physical Examination

1. Trendelenburg gait
2. Limb in external rotation and adduction
3. Thomas test → Flexion deformity
4. Muscle wasting
5. LLD

V. DIAGNOSIS

American College of Rheumatology

A. Clinical Criteria A

1. Hip pain
2. IR < 15°
3. ESR ≤ 45 mm/h or flexion ≤15°

OR

B. Clinical Criteria B

1. Hip pain
2. Pain on IR

3. Morning stiffness ≤60 minutes
4. Age > 50 years
              OR

C. Clinical + Radiological

Hip pain + 2/3 of the following:
1. Osteophytes → Femoral
                → Acetabular
2. Joint space narrowing
3. ESR < 20 mm/h

VI. RADIOLOGIC

1. Joint space narrowing → Best, most important indicator of severity.
   Normal = 3–5 mm, Moderate <2.5 mm, Severe: <1.5 mm
2. **Tonnis classification**
   Grade:
   0: Normal
   1: Mild
   2: Moderate
   3: Severe

VII. MANAGEMENT

A. Conservative

1. Analgesia →
   i. NSAIDs
   ii. Opioids → Tramadol
   iii. Duloxetine
   iv. Steroid injections
2. Walking stick – C/L limb, ↓ JRF
3. Weight loss, activity modification, physiotherapy.

B. Operative

1. THA → End-stage, severe arthritis, Age > 50 years
2. Arthroscopic debridement: Degenerative labral tears
3. Arthrodesis
4. Periacetabular osteotomy ± Femoral osteotomy → symptomatic dysplasia in young adult
5. Hip resurfacing
6. Femoral head resection.

SAFE SURGICAL DISLOCATION OF HIP/GANZ SURGICAL DISLOCATION OF HIP

I. INTRODUCTION

1. It is a surgical technique described by Ganz which provides full access to the femoral head and acetabulum without the risk of avascular necrosis.
2. It involves anterior dislocation of hip from posterior approach with trochanteric flip osteotomy.

II. VASCULAR ANATOMY

Given in chapter of Perthes disease.

III. INDICATION

1. Osteochondral lesions of femoral head and acetabulum
2. Femoral-acetabular impingement
   i. Repair of acetabular labrum
   ii. Reshaping of acetabular margin (acetabuloplasty)
   iii. Removing bony bumps from femoral head (femoral osteoplasty)
3. Femoral head fractures
4. Acetabular fractures (to aid in reduction)
5. Removal of loose bodies in fracture dislocations of hip
6. SCFE
7. Perthes disease
8. Hip arthrodesis
9. Other condition:
   i. Rheumatoid arthritis (for synovectomy)
   ii. Synovial chondromatosis

IV. TECHNIQUE

1. Positioning: Lateral decubitus position with pillow between the legs.
2. Incision (**Fig. 35**)
   i. Greater trochanter (GT) and ASIS are marked with a sterile surgical marker
   ii. Incision starts proximal to the level of ASIS and continues in a straight line along the axis of the femur on the anterior aspect of GT.

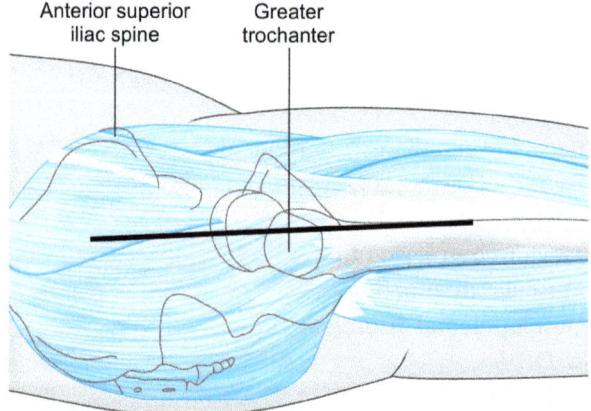

3. Superficial dissection
   i. Dissection continues to the fascia lata distally and to the fascia over the gluteus maximus proximally.
   ii. The fascia lata is incised longitudinally and proximally from the most distal extent of the wound up to the greater trochanter.
   iii. The approach is continued along the anterior border of the gluteus maximus (Gibson interval).
   iv. The gluteus medius is visible proximal to the greater trochanter.

v. Interval between gluteus maximus and gluteus medius is identified. Extension of hip—relaxes gluteus maximus and improves exposure of gluteus medius

vi. Once the fascia is completely opened, the following landmarks are readily identifiable:
   i. Greater trochanter
   ii. Vastus lateralis
   iii. Gluteus medius
   iv. Anterior border of gluteus maximus

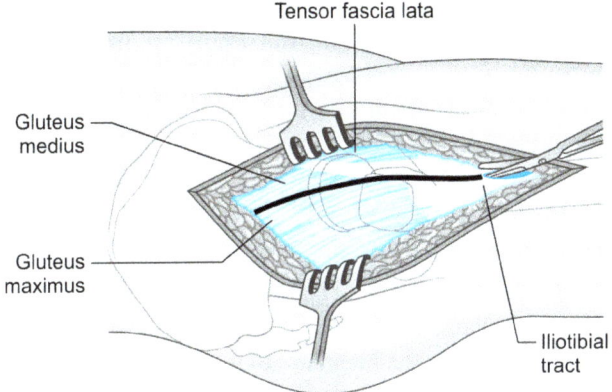

4. Deep dissection
   i. Trochanteric bursa flap is created by an anterior incision, to expose the short external rotators (flap is repositioned and repaired when wound is closed—prevents development of adhesions between GT and fascia lata)
   ii. Gluteus medius is retracted anteriorly, piriformis is then identified (overlapped by gluteus medius)
   iii. The posterior border of gluteus minimus is identified and interval between gluteus minimus and piriformis is sharply dissected over distance of 1–2 cm.

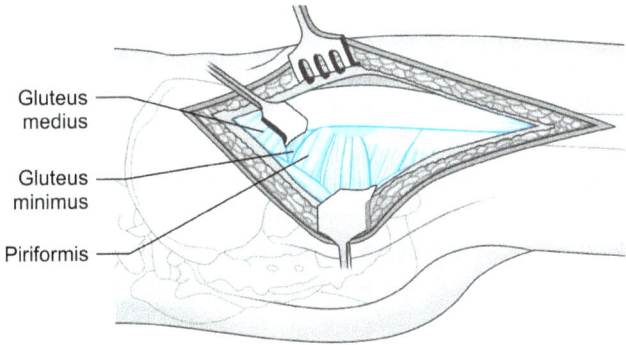

5. Trochanteric flip osteotomy
   i. To identify the distal starting point of the trochanteric flip osteotomy, the vastus lateralis is elevated from the proximal femur up to its insertion at the greater trochanter → Vastus ridge
   ii. Trochanteric fragment should be around 15 mm thick.
   iii. 5 mm of cuff of posterior border of gluteus medius is left behind—will remain attached to position of trochanter attached to shaft, thereby decreasing the risk of injury to vessels.
   iv. Using cautery, the osteotomy line is marked.
   v. Hip is internally rotated to facilitate the osteotomy.
   vi. Osteotome is used to lift the fragment initially and remaining periosteum and gluteus medius are cut.
   vii. This fragment of GT along with the tissues is retracted anteriorly with Hohmann retractor placed anteriorly to the femur.

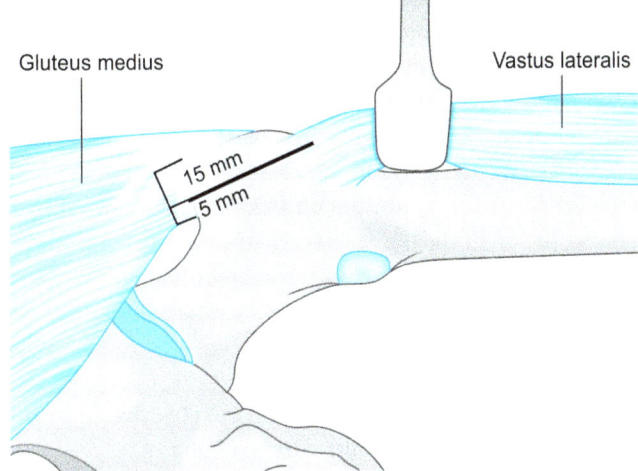

   viii. An alternative technique is step cut osteotomy of greater trochanter—facilitates more stable attachment of greater trochanter.
   ix. Retractor holds the gluteus minimus in a posterior direction.

6. Z-shaped capsular incision
   i. Taken in three steps:
      a. Starting from the trochanteric physis at the anterior edge of the trochanteric osteotomy, a longitudinal incision is made toward the acetabulum (1).
      b. The second cut runs along the distal anterior insertion of the capsule around the calcar (2).
      c. The third cut runs parallel to the edge of the acetabulum in a posterior direction (3).

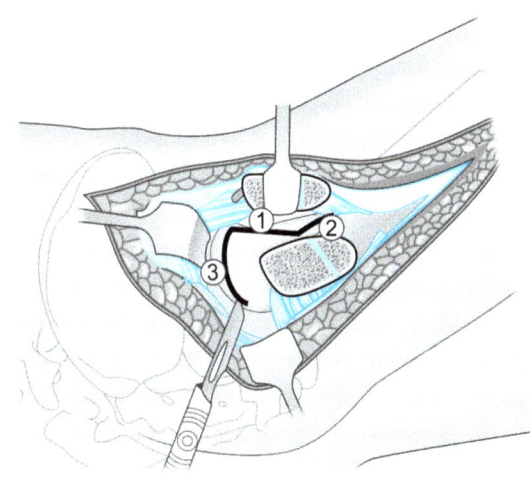

ii. On opening the capsule following structures are visible:
   a. Anterior and lateral aspect of femoral head
   b. Acetabular labrum
   c. Distal attachment of capsule
7. Dislocation
   i. Femoral head can be subluxated with progressive flexion and external rotation at hip.
   ii. Initial inspection of hip joint and associated pathology is made
   iii. If fragment/pathology can be seen and managed without complete dislocation, then dislocation is not done
   iv. If dislocation is necessary, then obstetric scissor is used to cut ligamentum teres.
   v. Dislocation is done with flexion and external rotation of limb, leg is placed in a sterile bag, allows visualization of most of the acetabulum.
8. Reduction: Achieved with traction, internal rotation and extension of the limb.
9. Closure of capsule
   i. Capsule is loosely closed with 2-0 absorbable suture, sutures should remain extra-articular
   ii. Loose closure is preferred, decreases chances of hemarthrosis
10. Reduction and fixation of osteotomy
    i. Trochanteric fragment is held with sharp bone clamp. The assistant brings the extended leg to 20–30° of abduction—relaxes gluteal muscles and facilitates reduction
    ii. Trochanteric fragment is held with K-wires, can be fixed with 2 × 3.5 mm cortical screws.
    iii. Screws are to be inserted perpendicular to the plane of osteotomy and should reach the contralateral cortex. This is followed by removal of K-wires.
11. Closure of fascia
    i. Trochanteric bursa is closed first—prevent development of adhesions between trochanter and fascia
    ii. Fascia lata and fascia over gluteus maximus are closed with continuous running interlocking sutures.
12. Skin and subcutaneous tissue are closed as per surgeon's preference

V. COMPLICATIONS

1. Fracture of greater trochanter
2. Damage to vascularity of femoral head leading to AVN
3. Injury to sciatic nerve
4. Injury to intra-articular structures
5. Nonunion of trochanteric osteotomy
6. Migration of trochanteric osteotomy
7. Lateral hip pain
8. Heterotopic ossification
9. Osteonecrosis of femoral head

SECTION 4

Knee

KNEE ARTHROSCOPY

Minimally invasive video-assisted surgical intervention for intra-articular pathologies of the knee.

I. INDICATIONS → Diagnostic
↳ Therapeutic

1. Meniscal tears
2. ACL tear
3. PCL tear
4. Removal of loose bodies
5. *Synovectomy:*
    i. PVNS
    ii. Infections → Pyogenic
    ↳ TB
    iii. Synovial chondromatosis (loose bodies)
    iv. Rheumatoid arthritis
6. Articular cartilage → Defects
    ↳ Injuries
    i. Abrasion arthroplasty
    ii. Mosaicplasty
    iii. Autologous cartilage implantation (ACI)
7. Lateral retinacular release → Patellar maltracking
8. Patellar clunk syndrome
9. Evaluation of knee joint before UKR, HTO
10. Arthroscopic fixation of tibial plateau fracture.
11. Joint debridement → OA (Controversial)
12. Synovial biopsy.

II. PORTALS (FIG. 1)

Primary (1°)	Secondary (2°)
i. Anterolateral	i. Posteromedial
ii. Anteromedial	ii. Posterolateral
iii. Superomedial (SM)	iii. Transpatellar
iv. Superolateral (SL)	iv. Proximal superomedial
	v. Far medial and far lateral

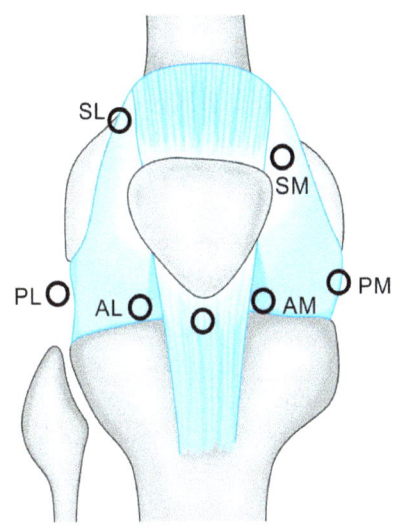

A. 1°

1. Anterolateral:
    i. Primary viewing portal
    ii. Incision 1 cm lateral to patellar tendon, and below the patella, over the "soft spot" of the joint line
2. Anteromedial:
    i. Primary working portal
    ii. Just medial to patellar tendon, slightly inferior to AL portal on the Joint line
3. SM/SL:
    i. Accessory portal
    ii. MC used for water inflow or outflow
    iii. Used for suprapatellar pouch procedures:
        a. Loose body removed
        b. Medial retinaculum plication
        c. Synovectomy

B. 2°

1. Posteromedial:
    i. 1 cm above joint line, behind MCL
    ii. Visualizes → Posterior horn and PCL

2. Posterolateral:
    i. 1 cm above JL between LCL and biceps tendon
    ii. Posterior horn and PCL
3. Transpatellar:
    i. 1 cm distal to patella splits the tendon
    ii. Access to intercondylar notch
4. FM and FL:
    i. 2 cm lateral/medial to their respective anterior portals
    ii. Accessory instrument placement → Posterior to femoral condyles
    iii. Loose body removal

III. DIAGNOSTIC ARTHROSCOPY – METHODICAL SEQUENCE

1. Knee fully extended → <u>suprapatellar pouch</u>
   ↓
   Adhesions, loose bodies
2. Patellofemoral joint → Cartilage
                        → Maltracking
3. Trochlear grove → trochlea and anterior aspects of medial and lateral FC
   Cartilage → Softening, fissures, unstable flaps
4. Lateral gutter:
    i. Between lateral femoral condyle and lateral capsule of knee
    ii. Insertion of popliteus
    iii. 3 lateral popliteomeniscal fascicles
5. Lateral compartment:
    i. Anterior horn of lateral meniscus
    ii. LM attachment to capsule
6. Medial gutter:
    i. Loose bodies
    ii. Medial meniscal cysts
    iii. Displaced flap tears
7. Medial compartment – Flexing knee to 90°:
    i. Medial meniscus
    ii. Articular cartilage → Femoral condyle and tibial plateau
8. Intercondylar notch → ACL
                       → PCL
                       → <u>Posteromedial corner</u>
   Best seen → 70° scope through notch: Modified Gillquist view **(Fig. 2)**
9. Knee in figure of 4 finish lateral compartment
    i. Lateral meniscus
    ii. Popliteal hiatus
    iii. Articular cartilage → Femoral condyle and tibial plateau

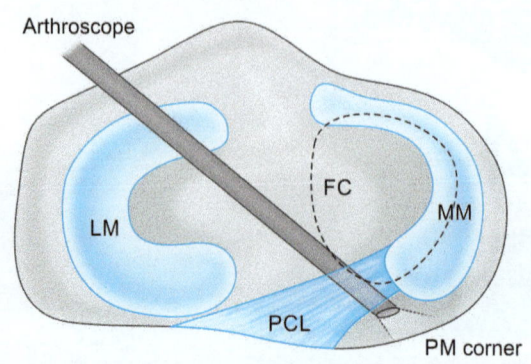

Fig. 2: Modified Gillquist view: Posteromedial corner of knee.

IV. COMPLICATIONS

1. Iatrogenic cartilage damage – MC complication
2. Hemarthrosis
3. Neurovascular injury, popliteal artery → posterior intercondylar attachment of meniscus
   PM → Saphenous nerve
   PL → CPN
4. Compartment syndrome
5. Injury to ACL, PCL, Menisci.

V. RECENT ADVANCES

1. *ACL repair:* Resurgence of interest, despite initial failures
    i. Refixation with suture anchors
    ii. Internal brace ligament stabilization
    iii. Dynamic intraligamentous stabilization (DIS)
    iv. Bridge enhanced ACL repair (BEAR)
2. *Individualized ACL reconstruction:*
   Appreciate native anatomy, individualized surgery as per patient needs, graft choices, tibial slope (↑ posterior slope: ACL tear ⊗, Failure of ACL reconstruction)
3. Double bundle → AM and PL separate grafts
4. Anterolateral ligament (ALL) reconstruction along with ACL for rotator instability
5. *Lateral extra-articular tenodesis:* Central band of ITB rerouted under LCL and attached to tibia.
6. *Remnant sparing ACL reconstruction:*
   Spare viable ACL remnants during recon
   ↓
   ↑Vascularity, Proprioception
7. *Orthobiologics:*
    i. Mesenchymal stem BMAC cells (MSC) from BM
    ii. Platelet rich plasma (PRP)
    iii. BMP: 2 and 7
   ↓
   Cartilage repair and regeneration
   Meniscal repair
8. *ACL reconstruction in skeletally immature:*
    i. Delay surgery >12 weeks: ↑↑↑ Meniscal injuries
    ii. Early surgery better than nonoperative Mx
    iii. Techniques:
        a. Transphyseal

b. Physeal sparing
   c. Hybrid
9. *Hormonal role and programs*:
   i. Women → ↑ ACL tear in ovulatory phase
   ii. OCP → ↓ 20% ACL tears
   iii. Athlete training programs
10. *Meniscal repair augmentation*:
    Trephination, rasping, abrasion of synovium
11. Meniscal allografts
12. Meniscal scaffolds: Allows for native cells and tissues to grow in, biodegrades over time
13. 3D printed scaffolds impregnated with autologous meniscal or stem cells
14. Gene therapy → Meniscal regeneration
15. Cartilage Rx

Palliative	Repair	Restorative
↓	↓	5. Autologous chondrocyte implantation (ACI)
Chondroplasty and debridement	Drilling and micro fracture	6. Osteochondral autograft transfer (OATS)
		7. Osteochondral allograft

16. MPFL repair
17. Computer-assisted navigation in knee arthroscopic surgery (CANS): Accuracy of tunnel placement
18. Robotic knee arthroscopy: Steerable robot tools, leg manipulators
19. OPD diagnostic arthroscopy

ANTERIOR CRUCIATE LIGAMENT TEAR

INTRODUCTION
Anterior cruciate ligament (ACL) tear leads to disruption of its fibers causing anterior and lateral knee rotatory instability.

I. PATHOANATOMY
1. Intra-articular, extrasynovial
2. Length = 33 mm, width = 7–11 mm diameter
3. *Tibial insertion*:
   i. Broad, irregular, diamond shaped.
   ii. Immediately anterior and adjacent to the medial tibial eminence,
4. *Femoral attachment:* Semicircular area on posteromedial aspect of lateral femoral condyle.
5.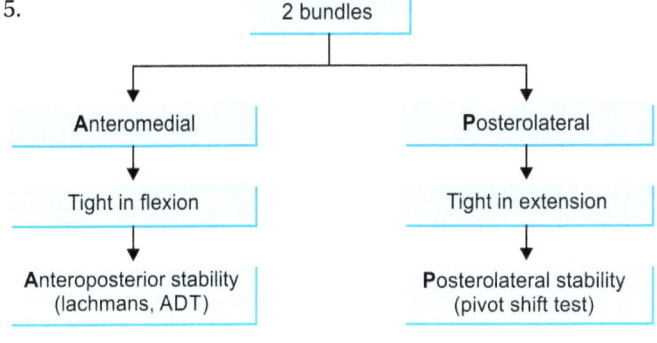

6. Collagen: Type I – 90%
              Type III – 10%
7. Blood supply: Middle geniculate artery.
8. Mechanoreceptor nerve endings within ACL → Proprioceptive role

II. PATHOPHYSIOLOGY
1. Noncontact pivoting injury (70%)
   ↓
2. Internally rotated tibia translates anteriorly while knee is in slight flexion and valgus.
3. Common in soccer, basketball, skiing.
4. Direct blow to knee (30%)
5. Continued valgus stress on IR tibia → MCL rupture
   ACL + MCL+ Medial meniscus → **Unhappy triad of "O – Donoghue"**
   ↓
   Although originally described MM, lateral meniscus injury is more common in acute ACL tears, MM injury → Chronic ACL tears.
6.
```
                    Tear
                   /    \
           Partial (20%)  Complete (80%)
                          More common
                          Middle third MC location (90%)
    Few fibers to near complete
    Either AM or PL bundle
```

III. RISK FACTORS
A. Extrinsic
1. Uneven playing field
2. Level of conditioning
3. Higher intensity of play → Championship > training
4. Skill acquisition
5. Rainy weather
6. Aggressive playing attitude

B. Intrinsic
1. Female (4.5:1) – hormonal fluctuations
   ↑ in ovulatory and postovulatory phase
2. ↑ Ligament laxity, ↓ muscle strength, poor reaction time
3. ↑ Q-angle, valgus knee, ↑ Pelvic width
4. Narrow IC notch of femur
5. ↑ Recurvatum
6. Small ACL size
7. Neuromuscular factors – muscle activation latencies

IV. NATURAL HISTORY
1. Patients with a high level of participation in jumping or cutting sports and significant side-to-side differences (>5 mm on KT-1000 arthrometer)
   ↓
   High risk of recurrent injury without ACL construction. Accelerated progression of arthritis.

2. However, ACL reconstruction has failed to prevent arthritis
3. Infact, in some researchers have demonstrated increased incidence of arthritis in ACL reconstructed knees.
4. Incidence of meniscal tears and chondral injuries reduces after ACL reconstruction.
5. It is hypothesized that double - bundle ACL - reconstruction might decrease incidence of arthritis.

V. CLINICAL PRESENTATION

A. History
1. Patient may describe a non-contact pivoting injury, involving change of direction/deceleration.
2. Hearing or feeling a "pop".
3. Immediate swelling of knee (70%) (Hemarthrosis)
4. Was not able to return to play.

B. Symptoms
1. Generalized knee pain
2. Instability preventing return to sport.
3. Difficulty weight - bearing
4. Knee instability → Feeling of giving away while getting down the stairs.

C. Physical Examination
1. Effusion
2. *ROM:* Loss of extension → due to displaced bucket - handle tear or arthrofibrosis (stiff knee)
   Loss of flexion → knee effusion
3. Quadriceps avoidance gait
4. **Lachman's test** → Most sensitive test. PCL tear may give false +ve Lachman due to posterior subluxation.
5. **Pivot shift test**: Knee is flexed from an extended position in a valgus and IR state
   [Pivot shift from ACL → MCL (Pre-requisite - Intact MCL)]
   → Anterior subluxated tibia reduces at around 20-30° of flexion due to IT band tension.
6. ADT → Not very sensitive, but helpful to rule out PCL injury
7. A complete evaluation of the knee to rule out other injuries is a must.
   i. Meniscal tears:
      a. Joint line tenderness.
      b. Mcmurray test
      c. Apley's compression test
      d. Childress, Eges test
   ii. MCL and LCL → Valgus and Varus stress tests
   iii. PCL → PDT, Godfrey sign
   iv. PLC injury → Injury to popliteus, popliteofibular ligament, biceps, ITB or posterior capsule → Dial test with ER asymmetry.
   v. Patellar instability → Apprehension test.

VI. INVESTIGATIONS

A. Radiograph (Fig. 3)
1. *Segond fracture:*

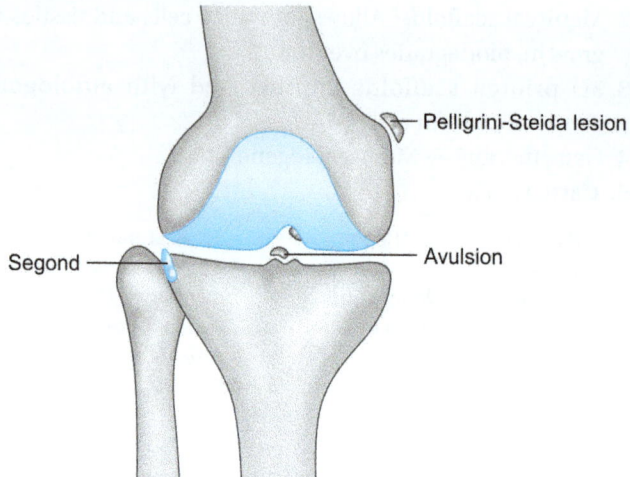

   i. Cortical avulsion fracture of proximal lateral tibia (just below plateau)
      ↓
   ii. Pathognomonic of ACL tear
   iii. Represents bony avulsion of ALL.
   iv. Associated with ACL tear 75–100% of the time
2. *Deep sulcus (terminalis) sign (lateral knee X-ray):*
   i. Depression on lateral femoral condyle at the terminal sulcus.
   ii. At the junction between the weight-bearing surface (tibial) and the patellar articular surface of the femoral condyle.
3. *Pellegrini-Stieda lesion:* Calcification at the femoral origin of the MCL.
4. ACL avulsion injury in young patients
5. *Arcuate sign:* Avulsion fracture of head of fibula.

B. MRI
1. "Empty-notch" sign: Fluid signal at the expected ACL attachment site on the intercondylar notch.
2. Primary sign is
   i. Discontinuity of fibers visible on oblique sagittal plane
   ii. Absence
   iii. Too flat in orientation to Blumensaat
       Grade I: Sprain→ hyperintense signal but continuous
       Grade II: Partial
       Grade III: Complete

C. CT Scan

To evaluate for bone loss in revision setting.

VII. MANAGEMENT

Individualized treatment based on:
1. Age
2. Activity level
3. Functional demands
4. Concomitant pathology

A. Nonoperative

1. *Indications:*
   i. Low demands with decreased laxity
   ii. No giving away episodes
   iii. Near normal range of motion on extension
   iv. Minimal or no meniscal damage on MRI
   v. Unwilling for surgery
2. Early symptomatic treatment → Knee extension brace for 3 weeks, ice fomentation, NSAIDS
3. This is followed by supervised PT
   ↓
   → Balance training
   → Hamstring strengthening
   → Hip abductor and core strengthening

B. Operative

1. *Indications:*
   i. Overt knee instability
   ii. High demand athletes, dancers
   iii. Concomitant operative meniscal injury
   iv. Pre-requisite = Restoration of full ROM post-injury. (unless mechanical block by meniscal tear)
2. Gold standard → Intra-articular ACL reconstruction
3. Acute reconstruction within 3 weeks is avoided → Fear of arthrofibrosis
4. *Goals:*
   i. Anatomical reconstruction of ACL to restore anterior and rotational stability
   ii. Maintain normal knee motion
   iii. Minimal donor site complications
   iv. Return of patient to desired level of activity
5. If violent pivot shift thrust > consider simultaneous <u>anterolateral ligament (ALL) reconstruction.</u>
6.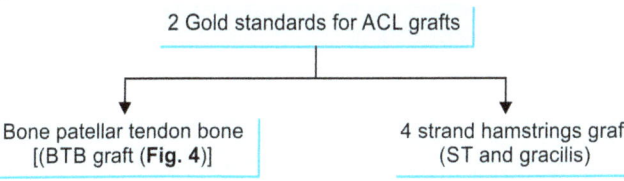

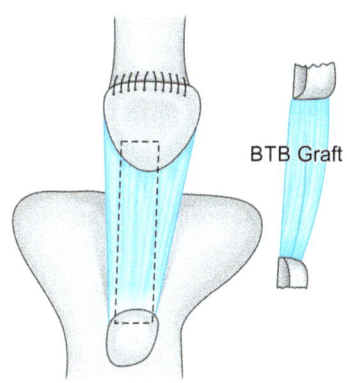

7. *Hamstring tendon graft harvesting:*
   i. 2–3 cm paramedian incision centered at the level of tibial tubercle → 6 cm below medial joint line
   ii. Sartorial fascia exposed; tendons palpated
   iii. Gracilis tendon insertion superior to ST
   iv. Reflect overlying sartorial fascia
   v. Whipstitch taken in the tendons near their insertion for mobilization
   vi. All tendinous slips/bands must be freed
   ↓
   vii. Harvest using tendon stripper
   viii. Muscle fibers removed using curette
8. *Arthroscopic portals made:*
   i. Anterolateral → Video, Viewing portal
   ii. Anteromedial → Working portal
9. Diagnostic arthroscopy performed; all pathology identified.
10. Meniscal tears repaired if indicated
11. Articular cartilage lesions addressed
12. Loose bodies are identified and removed
13. Torn ACL → Debrided with shaver
14. Small amount of femoral footprint left behind → to assist in identifying proper tunnel location.
15. The tibial footprint → cleared of all tissue
16. *Tibial tunnel placement* (**Fig. 5**):

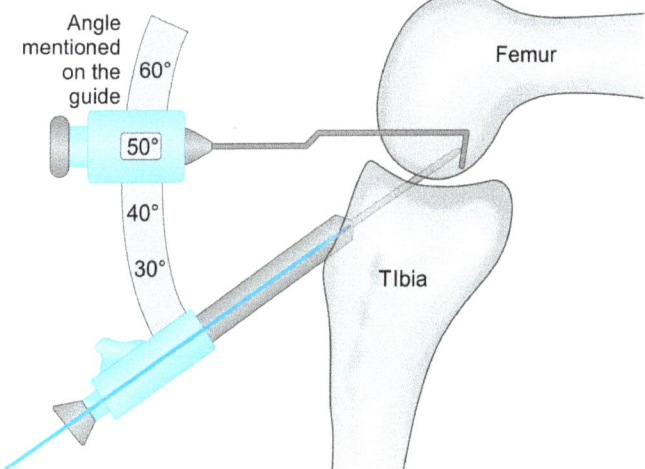

i. Commercially available guide is used
   ii. Intra-articular landmarks:
      a. Posteromedial aspect of ACL footprint
      b. Just anterior to medial eminence
      c. Along a line extended from the posterior border of anterior horn of LM
      d. Extra-articular portion of the guide
         ↓
         Positioned midway between the tibial tubercle and the posteromedial tibia
      e. Guide set at angle of 45–50° for hamstring graft.
      f. Once guide wire is inserted and confirmed.
         ↓
      g. Cannulated drill bit to complete tunnel (tibial drill must be of same diameter as hamstring drill)
17. *Femoral tunnel placement* (**Fig. 6**):

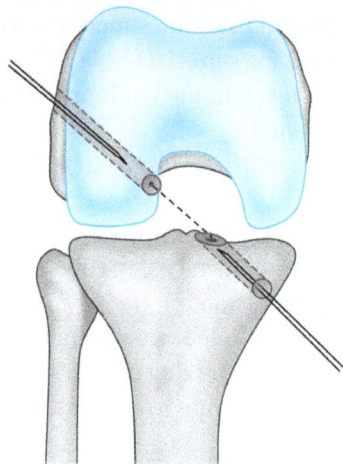

   i. Transtibial tunnel drilling
   ii. Knee in 90° flexion, pass a beath pin through the femur and then out through the anterolateral thigh.
   iii. Position of femoral tunnel: 10:30 o' clock right knee
        : 1:30 o' clock left knee
         ↓
         Creates a more horizontal graft
         ↓
         Reduces rotational laxity.
18. Pass the graft through the final tunnel
19. *Graft fixation:*
   i. Femoral side → Endobutton (**Fig. 7**)

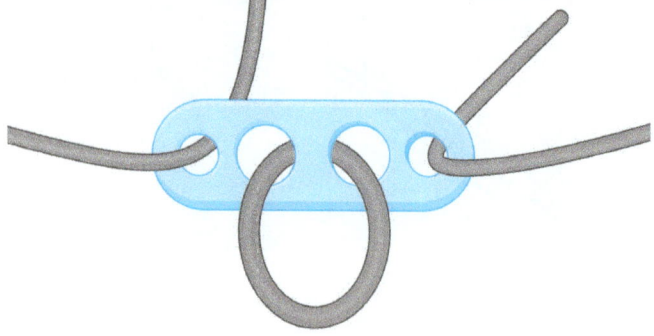

   ii. Tibial side:
      a. Interference screw – 1 mm larger than the diameter of the tunnel and graft
      b. Metallic (titanium) or bioabsorbable

VIII. COMPLICATIONS

1. *Arthrofibrosis:* Loss of knee ROM due to extensive fibrous tissue growth postsurgically (intra-articular, extraarticular, globally)
   i. Risk factors:
      a. Acute ACL reconstruction
      b. CRPS
      c. Prolonged immobilization
      d. Open ACL reconstruction
   ii. Management:
      a. Progressive active and passive rehabilitation
      b. Pain management
      c. Intra-articular steroids
      d. Arthroscopic lysis of adhesions
2. *Graft malpositioning:*
   i. Leads to postoperative loss of motion
   ii. Femoral malposition: Due to resident's ridge → Raised bony landmark just anterior to the femoral attachment of ACL
   iii. Cyclops lesion: Anterior tibial placement of graft → development of fibrotic tissue between the notch and reconstructed ligament
   iv. Patellar fracture → BTB graft
   v. Infection
   vi. Early graft failure: Due to poorly tensioned and lax fixation

IX. CONTRAINDICATIONS

1. Established arthritis
2. Local infection in joint
3. Noncomplaint patient about postoperative protocol
4. Restricted ROM

X. RECENT ADVANCES

BEAR = Bridge enhanced anterior cruciate ligament repair.

XI. POSTOPERATIVE REHABILITATION

1. *0–2 weeks:*
   i. Continuous passive motion (CPM) started next day after surgery. 5 h/day
   ii. Cold therapy with ice
   iii. Knee immobilization after surgery → Prevents flexion contracture
   iv. 90° knee flexion → by 1 week
   v. Full knee ROM → 2–3 weeks
   vi. Exercises are closed chain

2. *2–6 weeks:*
    i. Bracing continued to protect knee, but ROM to be completely regained by 3 weeks
    ii. If meniscus repair is done simultaneously knee brace locked in full extension for 6 weeks
    iii. Stationary bicycle program started
    iv. Strengthening exercises → Quadriceps training and hamstring rehabilitation
    v. Exercises remain closed chain
3. *6–12 weeks:*
    i. Braces discontinued
    ii. Hip and core strengthening exercises
    iii. Wall slides and chair squats, lunges
    iv. Open chain exercises started
4. *12–16 weeks:*
    i. Begin cardiovascular conditioning
    ii. Jump and plyometric training
    iii. Begin jogging when quadriceps strength >65%
    iv. Progressive knee strengthening program
5. *5–6 months:*
    i. Agility training
    ii. Sport specific drills (45° cutting, figure of 4)
6. *6 months:* Return to sports if:
    i. Motion > 130°
    ii. Hamstrings > 90°
    iii. Quadriceps > 85°
    iv. Sports specific agility training completed
    v. Maintenance exercises 2–3 times/week

POSTERIOR CRUCIATE LIGAMENT INJURIES

I. PATHOANATOMY

1. Intra-articular, but extrasynovial, static stabilizer of the knee.
2. *Origin:* Posterior tibial sulcus below the articular surface (1.5 cm)
3. *Insertion:* Anterolateral medial femoral condyle → Broad, crescent-shaped footprint
4. *Dimensions:*
    i. 38 mm in length × 13 mm in diameter
    ii. 30% larger than the ACL
5. *Two bundles* **(Figs. 8 and 9)**:
    i. Anterolateral bundle
        a. Tight in flexion
        b. Strongest and most important for posterior stability at 90° of flexion
    ii. Posteromedial bundle—tight in extension
        a. Lies between the meniscofemoral ligaments
6. Ligament of Humphrey (anterior) and ligament of Wrisberg (posterior) → originate from the posterior horn of the lateral meniscus and insert into PCL substance.

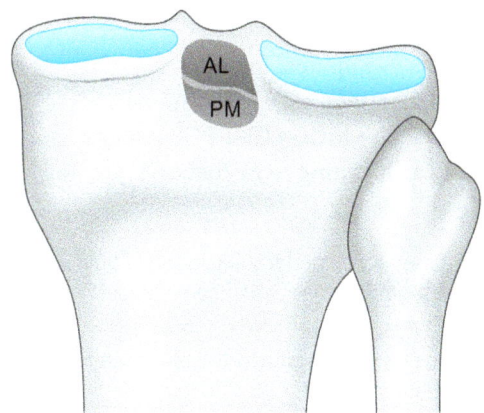

II. FUNCTION

1. Primary restraint to posterior tibial translation
2. Prevents hyperflexion
3. Isolated injuries cause the greatest instability at 90° of flexion
4. Tibial external rotation and varus/valgus stress in the extended knee → secondary restraint

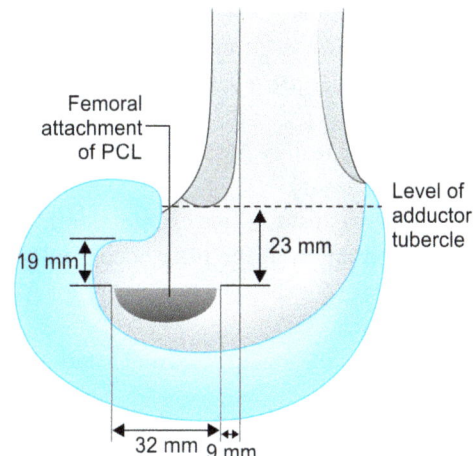

III. PATHOPHYSIOLOGY

1. *Mechanism:*
    i. Direct blow to proximal tibia with a flexed knee → Dashboard injury
    ii. Noncontact hyperflexion with a plantar-flexed foot
    iii. Hyperextension injury
2. *Associated conditions:*
    i. Combined PCL and posterolateral corner (PLC) injuries
    ii. Multiligamentous knee injuries
    iii. Knee dislocation

IV. CLINICAL FEATURES

A. Symptoms

1. Pain → back of knee
2. Instability

B. Examination
1. Tenderness → Popliteal fossa
2. Varus/valgus stress test
   i. Laxity at 0 → MCL/LCL + PCL injury
   ii. Laxity at 30° alone → MCL/LCL injury only

PCL injury classification	
Based on posterior subluxation of tibia relative to femoral condyles with knee in 90° of flexion	
Grade I	1. A partial tear 2. Examination shows 1–5 mm posterior tibial translation 3. Tibia remains anterior to the femoral condyles
Grade II	1. A complete isolate tear 2. Examination shows 6–10 mm posterior tibial translation 3. Complete injury in which the anterior tibia is flush with the femoral condyles
Grade III	1. A combined PCL + capsuloligamentous injury 2. Examination shows >10 mm posterior tibial translation 3. Tibia is posterior to the femoral condyles and often indicates an associated ACL and/or PLC injury

3. Posterior sag sign (Godfrey's sign): Hip and knee in 90° in supine position → Posteriorly-directed tibial step-off
4. Posterior drawer test → Most accurate manoeuvre for diagnosing PCL injury
5. Quadriceps active test → Knee extended from 90° flexion → anterior reduction of the tibia occurs relative to the femur
6. Positive dial test:
   i. PLC + PCL injury → >10° external rotation difference at 30° and 90°
   ii. Isolated PLC injury → >10° external rotation difference at 30° only

V. RADIOLOGY
1. Radiographs:
   i. Avulsion fractures
   ii. Posterior tibiofemoral subluxation
   iii. Medial and patellofemoral compartment arthrosis → chronic injuries
   iv. Lateral stress view
      a. Application of stress to anterior tibia with the knee flexed to 70°
      b. Asymmetric posterior tibial displacement indicates PCL injury
      c. Becoming the gold standard in diagnosing and quantifying PCL injuries
2. MRI → Confirmatory study for the diagnosis of PCL injury

VI. MANAGEMENT
1. Acute injury: RICE
2. Protected weight bearing and rehabilitation
   i. Indicated in → Isolated Grade I (partial) and II (complete) injuries
   ii. Quadriceps rehabilitation
3. Immobilization → long knee brace in extension for 4 weeks
   i. Indicated in → isolated Grade III injuries
   ii. Immobilization is followed by quadriceps strengthening
4. PCL repair of bony avulsion fractures → ORIF: Screw/suture anchor fixation
   Isolated Grade II or III injuries with bony avulsion
5. PCL reconstruction
   i. Indications
      a. Combined ligamentous injuries
         1. PCL + ACL or PLC injuries
         2. PCL + Grade III MCL or LCL injuries
      b. Isolated chronic PCL injuries with a functionally unstable knee
   ii. Allograft → Hamstring, bone-patellar tendon-bone, achilles, and anterior tibialis
   iii. **Arthroscopic transtibial technique**
      a. Standard arthroscopic portals with an accessory posteromedial portal
         1. Posteromedial portal → 1 cm proximal to the joint line posterior to the MCL
         2. Branches of the saphenous nerve are at risk during placement
      b. Posteromedial corner of the knee is best visualized with a 70° arthroscope either through the notch (modified Gillquist view) or using a posteromedial portal
      c. Technique
         1. Transtibial drilling anterior to posterior
         2. Fix graft in 90° flexion with an anterior drawer
6. High tibial osteotomy - Chronic PCL deficiency
   Medial opening wedge osteotomy to treat both varus malalignment and PCL deficiency → Increases tibial slope → Prevents posterior tibial translation

VII. COMPLICATIONS
1. Popliteal artery injury
2. Patellofemoral arthrosis
3. Medial sided arthritis

POSTEROLATERAL CORNER (PLC) INJURY

INTRODUCTION
Traumatic knee injuries that present with lateral knee instability and are usually associated with concomitant cruciate ligament injuries.

I. PATHOANATOMY

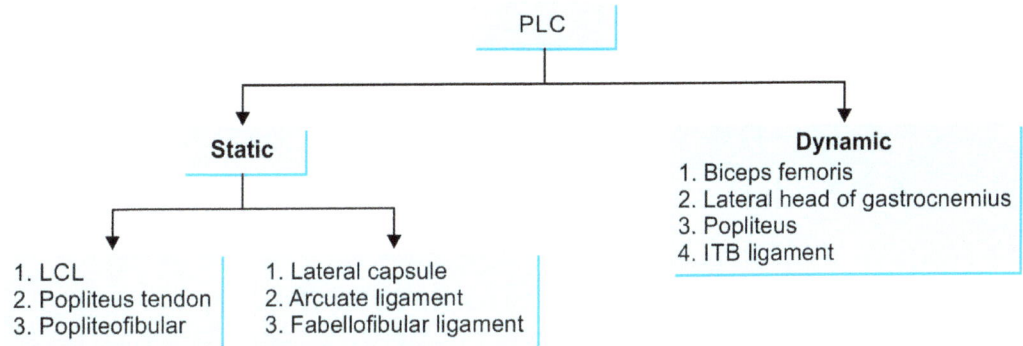

II. FUNCTIONS

1. Resists posterolateral rotation of the tibia on the femur
2. Resists varus angulation and posterior displacement of the tibia on the femur

III. ETIOLOGY

1. Blow to anteromedial knee
2. Varus blow to flexed knee
3. Contact and noncontact hyperextension injuries
4. External rotation twisting injury
5. Knee dislocation

IV. CLASSIFICATION

Modified Hughston classification		
	Examination	Findings
Grade I	0–5 mm of lateral opening on varus stress 0°–5° rotational instability on dial test	Sprain, no tensile failure of capsuloligamentous structures
Grade II	6–10 mm of lateral opening on varus stress 6°–10° rotational instability on dial test	Partial injuries with moderate ligament disruption
Grade III	>10 mm of lateral opening on varus stress, no endpoint >10° rotational instability on dial test, no endpoint	Complete ligament disruption

V. CLINICAL FEATURES

A. Symptoms

1. Pain → outer aspect of knee
2. Instability
3. Difficulty climbing stairs, playing sports

B. Examination

1. Tenderness → Posterolateral aspect of knee
2. Varus/valgus stress test
   i. Laxity at 0° → MCL/LCL + PCL injury
   ii. Laxity at 30° alone → MCL/LCL injury only
3. Positive dial test
   i. PLC + PCL injury → > 10° external rotation difference at 30° and 90°
   ii. Isolated PLC injury → > 10° external rotation difference at 30° only
4. Posterolateral Drawer test
5. Reverse shift test
6. External rotation recurvatum test
7. Gait → Varus thrust
8. Neurological symptoms → CPN injury: Altered sensation to dorsum of foot and weak ankle dorsiflexion

VI. RADIOLOGY

A. Radiographs

1. Arcuate sign – Avulsion fracture at the arcuate ligament complex insertion on the proximal fibula. Tell-tale sign of associated cruciate ligament injury (90%)
2. Stress X-rays
3. X-rays Scanograms – Lower limb alignment → Varus

B. MRI

1. Bony bruising and edema → Medial femoral condyle and tibial plateau
2. Hyperintense signal → LCL, popliteus and biceps tendon

VII. MANAGEMENT

1. Long knee brace immobilization in extension for 4 weeks
   i. PLC grade I injury
   ii. Isolated midsubstance grade II injury
2. PLC avulsion fractures → Screw/suture anchor fixation
3. PLC reconstruction
   i. **Larson → Fibula-based reconstruction (Fig. 10)**

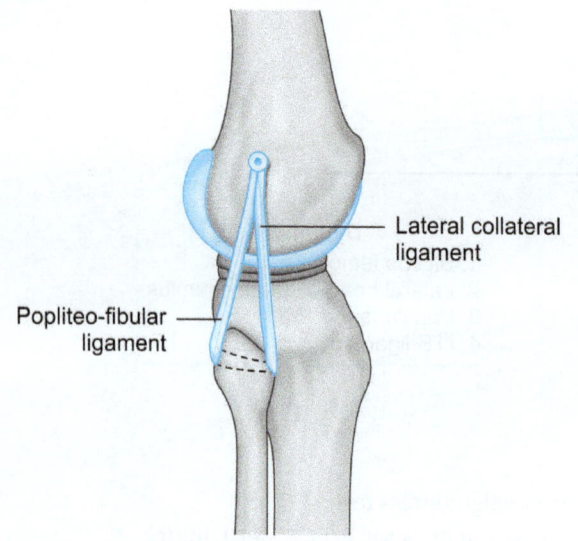

Fig. 10: Larson: PLC reconstruction.

   ii. **LaPrade anatomic reconstruction (Fig. 11)**
      a. LCL and popliteofibular ligament reconstruction +
      b. Popliteus tendon reconstruction

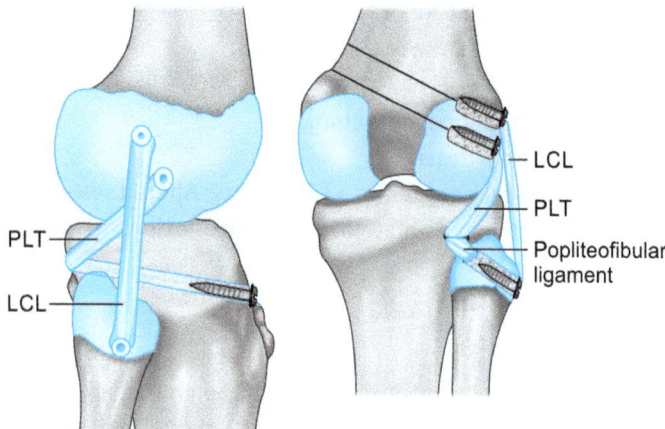

4. ACL/PCL reconstruction   } Combined with PLC
5. Valgus high tibial osteotomy ±   management

VIII. COMPLICATIONS
1. Arthrofibrosis
2. Missed PLC injury → Failure of ACL reconstruction
3. Peroneal nerve injury (25%)
4. Residual Laxity
5. Persistent knee pain
6. Early onset knee arthritis
7. CRPS

MENISCUS

INTRODUCTION
These are semilunar cartilages, 2 crescentic plates of fibrocartilage on the tibial condyles.

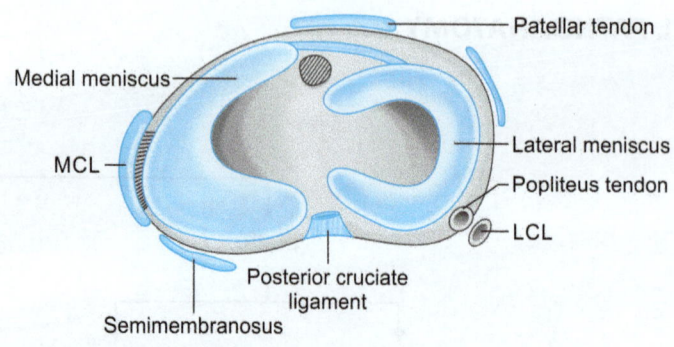

I. ANATOMY (FIG. 12)
1. Triangular in cross-section, wide base facing externally, apex internally.
2. Horns: Two fibrous extremities attached about the intercondylar area on tibia.
3. Superior surface: Concave, Inferior – flat.
4. Made of fibroelastic cartilage
5. 60–75% = Water
   Collagen → 90% type I
       ↓
   Arrangement → 1. Radial
                  2. Circumferential
                      → Helps dissipate hoop stresses
                      → Vertical mattress captures
6. *Lateral meniscus:*
   i. Circular: Covers larger portion of articular surface
   ii. Meniscofemoral ligaments → Connect the posterior horn of lateral meniscus to intercondylar wall of the medial femoral condyle
           ↓
   Ligament of Humphrey (anterior to PCL)
           Wrisberg (posterior to PCL)
7. *Medial meniscus:*
   i. C – shaped → Semicircular
   ii. Outer aspect of medial meniscus → attached to posterior deep fibers of the tibial collateral ligament and capsule
         ↓
   Less mobile → prone to injury
8. Transverse (Intermeniscal ligaments) – connect medial and lateral meniscus anteriorly.
9. Coronary ligaments – Connects the menisci peripherally to the rim of tibia.
10. Vascular anatomy (Miller Warner classification) **(Fig. 13)**

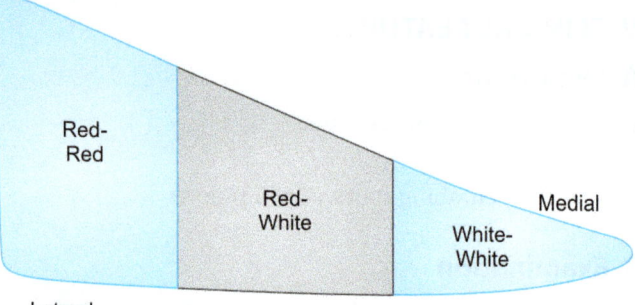

i. Red–Red: Largest amount of vascular channels → best prognosis
ii. Red–White: Intermediate vascular channels → Rx techniques: synovial abrasion, fibrin clot → Improve results.
iii. White–White: Poor prognosis.

II. FUNCTION

1. *Joint filler:* Compensates for gross incongruity between femoral and tibial articulating surfaces.
2. *Force transmission* (**Fig. 14**):
    i. Shock – absorption – More elastic than articular cartilage.
    ii. ↑ Congruency - ↑ contact area, ↓ point loading
    iii. Transmits 50% weight bearing in extension and 85% in flexion

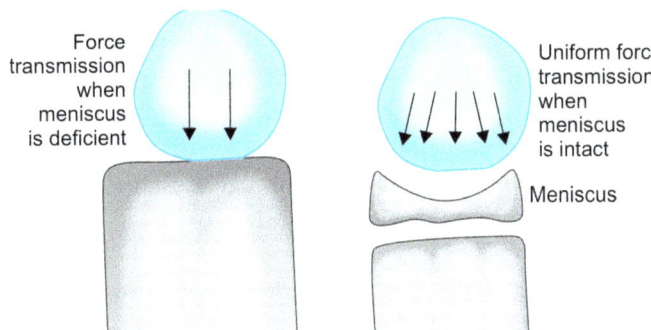

3. Stability – in all planes:
    i. Rotatory stabilizers – smooth transition from pure hinge to gliding motion from flexion to extension
    ii. Posterior horn of medial meniscus → main secondary stabilizer to anterior translation.
        ↓
    iii. Primary stabilizer in ACL deficient knee
4. Proprioception – joint position sense

III. MECHANISM OF TEAR

In extreme flexion → Posterior half of meniscus compressed between tibia and femoral condyles
    ↓
Sudden extension of knee (twisting injury) → Posterior horn trapped → tear
Risk factor = ACL deficient knee.

IV. CLASSIFICATION OF TEARS
O' CONNOR (Fig. 15)

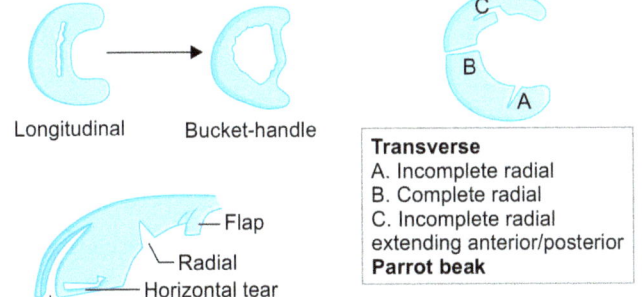

1. *Longitudinal:*
    i. Due to trauma to normal meniscus
    ii. Vertically oriented
    iii. Bucket – handle tear – inner fragment displaces over into the intercondylar notch.
    iv. Most frequently associated with ACL injuries
2. *Horizontal:* shear injury – superior, inferior tear surfaces.
3. *Radial:* vertical, from inner edge of meniscus toward its periphery.
4. *Flap tears:* Horizontal cleavage element.
5. *Complex:* Combination, usually degenerative.

V. CLINICAL PRESENTATION

1. *History:* Twisting injury to flexed knee
2. *Symptoms:*
    i. Pain localizing to medial or lateral side
    ii. Mechanical symptoms – locking, clicking
    iii. Giving – away or buckling when walking on uneven ground
    iv. Swelling
3. *Physical examination:*
    i. Joint line tenderness – Most sensitive
    ii. Quadriceps atrophy
    iii. Effusion
    iv. McMurrays test
    v. Apleys grinding test
    vi. Thessalys test
    vii. Ege's test
    viii. Childress test
    ix. Bounce home test

VI. INVESTIGATIONS

1. X-ray:
    i. For bony pathology associated with tear
    ii. Patellofemoral arthrosis – skyline view
    iii. Long standing cases – degenerative joint pathology, ↓ joint space
2. *MRI*: Tears and cysts (**Fig. 16**)

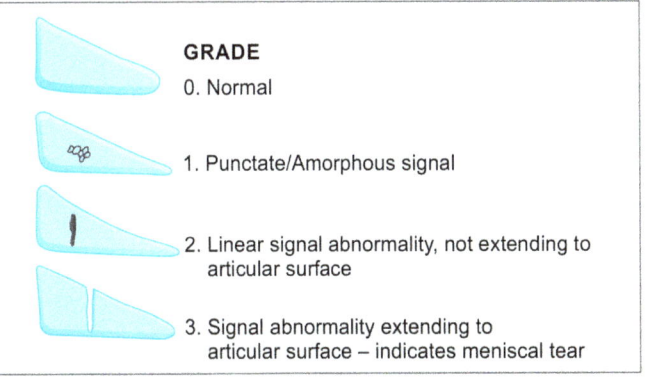

    i. Tears
    ii. Meniscal cysts
3. *Arthroscopy*: Diagnostic, gold standard

VII. TREATMENT

A. Conservative
1. Rest, pain control drugs, no weight bearing (acute)
2. Physiotherapy – rehabilitation
3. Hinge knee brace
4. *Indications*:
    i. Degenerative tears
    ii. Incomplete or small (<3 mm)
    iii. Stable peripheral tear with no associated pathology.

B. Meniscal Repair
1. *Criteria for best results*:
    i. Location: Red–Red zone – within 3 mm of periphery (lower rim width)
    ii. Stability: Partial thickness
    iii. Tear pattern: Longitudinal, vertical, peripheral and root tear
       (Flap, degenerative, complex, radial and bucket – handle → excision preferred)
    iv. Age < 45 years
    v. Chronicity: Acute tears < 8 weeks heal better.
    vi. Ligament stability: ACL deficiency must be corrected simultaneously to prevent instability.
2. *Repair techniques*:
    i. **Inside-out: Gold standard (Fig. 17)**:
       a. Posterior horn tears
       b. Peripheral capsular tears
       c. Meniscal allografts
       d. Displaced bucket – handle tears
       e. Mid-third tears

Double armed sutures with long flexible needles
↓
Medial or lateral incision to retrieve suture needles as they exit joint capsule
Vertical mattress → superior, ability to repair almost all tear patterns
Disadvantage: Neurovascular injury → Medially → Saphenous nerve and vein
Laterally → Peroneal nerve

    ii. **Outside-in (Fig. 18)**
       a. Anterior horn tears
       b. Radial tears
       c. Complex tears
       d. Mid-third tears
          Developed to avoid risk to NV structures.

18 - gauge spinal needle is inserted across the tear from outside the inside the joint.
↓
O polydioxanone suture inserted through the needle into the joint → knot tied in the suture.
↓
Knot pulled back into the joint against the meniscus to hold it in a reduced position.
↓
Free ends of adjacent sutures tied over joint capsules.

    iii. **All inside** (suture devices with plastic or bioabsorbable anchors) **(Fig. 19)**

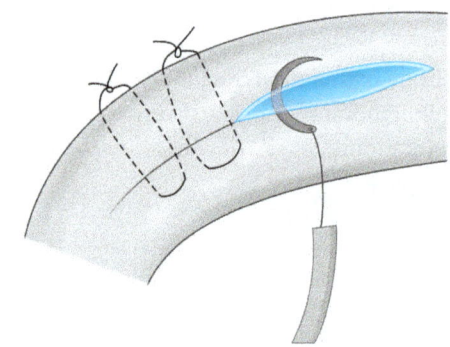

Fig. 17: Inside-out.

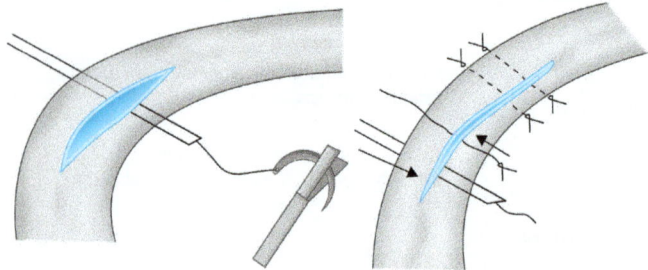

Fig. 18: Outside-in.

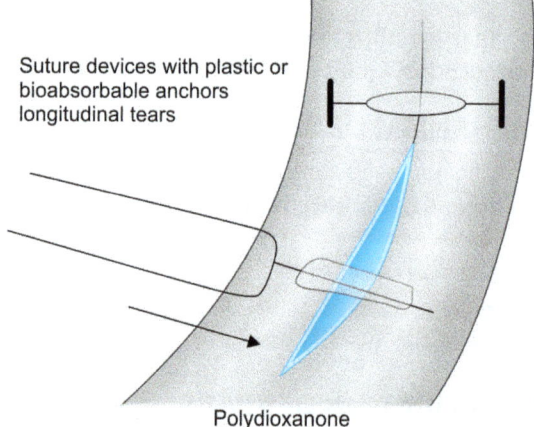

Fig. 19: All–inside.

       a. Unstable vertical longitudinal tears. Posterior (peripheral) horns of menisci
       b. Use curved cannulated suture passing hooks

C. Meniscectomy
1. *O'Connor classification*:
    i. Partial: Only loose, unstable fragments excised, stable and balanced peripheral rim preserved.
    ii. Subtotal: Requires excision of portion of peripheral rim of meniscus.

iii. Total meniscectomy – rarely indicated
   a. Meniscus is detached from its peripheral meniscosynovial attachment.
   b. When intrameniscal damage and tears are extensive.
2. *Principles*:
   i. All mobile fragments that can be pulled past the inner margin of the meniscus into the center of the joint → Remove
   ii. Remaining meniscal rim → smoothened to remove any sudden changes
       ↓
       Leads to further tears
   iii. Meniscocapsular junction and peripheral meniscal rim protected
       ↓
       Maintains meniscal stability, vital in preserving load transmission of meniscus.

D. Nonfixation Healing
1. Synovial abrasion on femoral and tibial surfaces of meniscus
2. Meniscus trephination
3. Fibrin clot

E. Meniscal Transplantation
1. Allograft meniscus
2. Autograft fascial material
3. Biologic scaffold

DISCOID MENISCUS

INTRODUCTION
Abnormal development of the meniscus leading to a hypertrophic and discoid shaped meniscus.

I. ETIOPATHOGENESIS (FIG. 20)

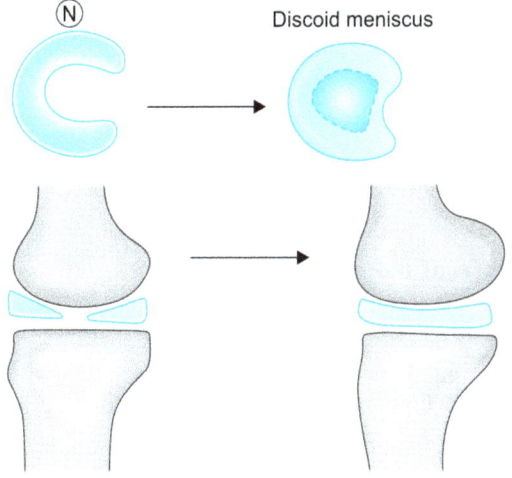

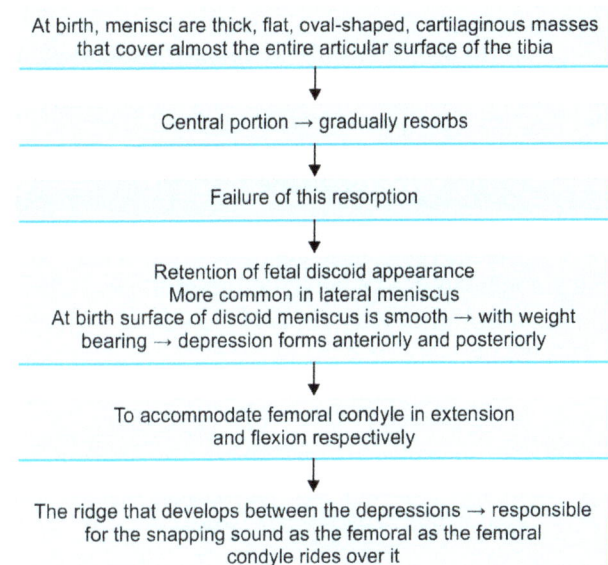

II. CLASSIFICATION
Watanabe
1. Complete
2. Incomplete
3. Wrisberg (lack of posterior meniscotibial attachment to tibia)

III. CLINICAL FEATURES
1. *Age:* young, athlete, 20–30 years
2. Pain
3. Clicking, mechanical locking → More in extension
4. Signs and symptoms of meniscus tear

IV. INVESTIGATIONS
1. Radiographs
   i. Widened joint pace
   ii. Squaring of lateral condyle
   iii. Cupping of lateral tibial plateau
   iv. Hypoplastic lateral intercondylar spine.
2. MRI-Investigation of choice
   i. ≥3–5 mm sagittal images with meniscal continuity (bowtie sign)
   ii. Thick and flat meniscus

V. TREATMENT
A. Conservative
Observation – asymptomatic

B. Operative
1. Partial meniscectomy and saucerization
2. *Indications*:
   i. Pain and mechanical symptoms
   ii. Meniscal tear or meniscal detachment

3. *Technique:*
    i. Obtain anatomic looking meniscus with debridement
    ii. Repair meniscus if detached (Wrisberg variant)
    iii. Repair for peripheral tears

MENISCAL CYSTS

INTRODUCTION

Localized collection of synovial fluid within or adjacent to the meniscus most commonly as a result of a meniscal tear **(Fig. 21)**.

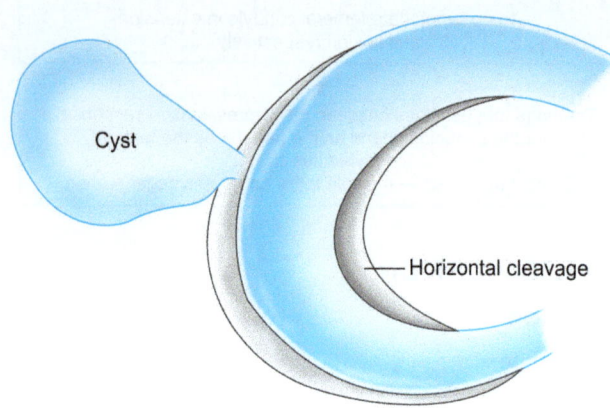

I. TYPES

1. Perimeniscal

1. Small lesions of fluid within the meniscus.
2. Medial > Lateral = 2:1
3. Medial cysts: Posterior horn
4. Lateral cysts: Anterior horn

2. Parameniscal (e.g., Bakers Cyst)

1. External fluid outside the meniscus (MC)
2. Between semimembranosus and medial head of gastrocnemius

II. PATHOPHYSIOLOGY

1. Meniscal tear → One way valve ↓
2. Synovial fluid extrudes and then concentrates to form gel like material
3. Horizontal and complex tears - parameniscal cysts
4. Radial or vertical tears - perimeniscal cysts
5. *Associated condition*:
    i. Articular cartilage injury
    ii. ACL tear

III. CLINICAL PRESENTATION

1. History → Trauma
2. *Symptoms*:
    i. Asymptomatic
    ii. Pain: Localized to medial/lateral or posterior
    iii. Mechanical symptoms
        → Clicking
        → Locking
    iv. Delayed or intermittent knee swelling
    v. Weakness or claudication (Neurovascular impingement)
3. *Examination*:
    i. Popliteal mass: Best visualized with knee in extension
    ii. Crepitus
    iii. Joint line tenderness

IV. INVESTIGATIONS

1. *X-ray:* Normal in acute setting
2. *MRI:* Most sensitive diagnostic test
    Cyst → Bright T_2 signal

V. TREATMENT

A. Conservative

1. Rest
2. Pain control
3. Physiotherapy → Rehabilitation
4. Indication → Small cysts

B. Operative

1. *Aspiration and steroid injection:* Isolated bakers cyst in young patient
2. Arthroscopic debridement, cyst decompression and meniscal resection
    Indication: Perimeniscal cyst associated with tear not amenable to repair (complex, degenerative)
3. Cyst excision: Posterior approach
    Indication: Symptomatic parameniscal – not amenable to conservative Rx

SYNOVIAL PLICAE/PLICA SYNDROME

PLICAE = "Fold"

I. INTRODUCTION

1. Membranous infolds that are part of the synovial lining of knee capsule.
2. Remnants of embryonic development.
3. Plica syndrome → Painful impairment of knee function resulting from thickened and inflamed synovial folds.

II. PATHOANATOMY

A. Origin

Persistence of membranes of mesenchymal tissue that separates the 3 synovial compartments (medial, lateral, suprapatellar).

B. Plica Types (Fig. 22)

1. *Ligamentum mucosum:* Most common located in intercondylar notch.

2. *Suprapatellar:* 2nd MC. Divides quadriceps bursa into 2 parts.
3. *Medial:* Rare, but most symptomatic. Medial aspect of knee from superior pole of patella to medial tibial fat pad.

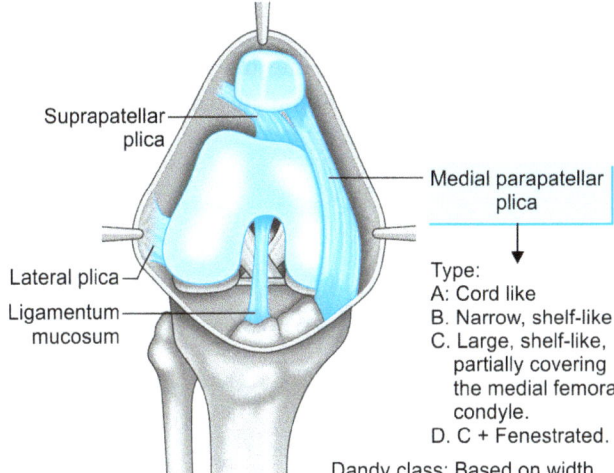

III. ETIOPATHOGENESIS

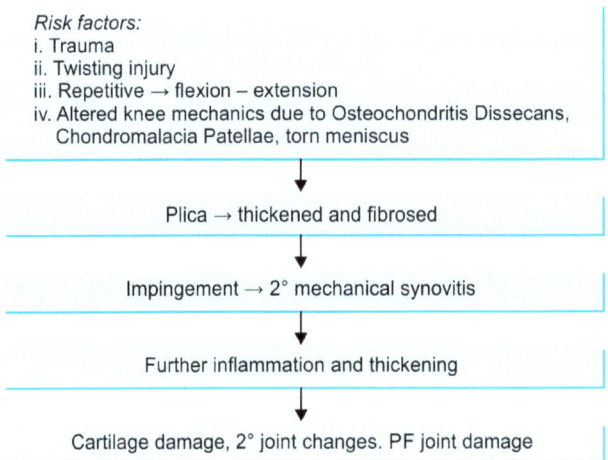

IV. CLINICAL FEATURES

1. Young age group. M = F
2. Anteromedial knee pain: Intermittent, dull aching
3. Positive theatre sign
4. Positive duvet sign → Pain ↓ by using a duvet between knees in bed
5. Mechanical → Snapping, clicking, rocking
6. Tender, palpable, thickened cord – like plica, rolls under fingers
7. Crepitus
8. Knee effusion
9. Pipkin's sign: Popping sound on knee extension from 90° flexion
10. Holding test: Examiner tries to flex extended knee against resistance → pain
11. Muscle wasting

V. INVESTIGATIONS

1. X-ray → Rule out other pathologies
2. MRI → Abnormal medial patellar plicae

VI. TREATMENT

A. Conservative: Most Cases Resolve

1. Rest
2. Activity modification
3. Pain control drugs
4. PT → Hamstring stretching, quadriceps isometric strengthening
5. Cryotherapy
6. Heat – Moist.
7. Intra-articular steroid injection

B. Operative

1. Indication: Failure of conservative treatment – 2 months
2. Arthroscopic resection of plica
3. Synovial pannus and synovitis excised
4. Intra-articular steroid at the end of the procedure
5. If 2° changes developed = Chondromalacia
   Mx = Cartilage regeneration techniques

RECURRENT DISLOCATION OF PATELLA

I. INTRODUCTION

1. Syndrome characterized by repeated acute incidents of complete lateral displacement of patella leading to degeneration of its articular surface.
2. Dislocation is <u>episodic</u> in nature with normal patellar tracking in between.

II. ETIOPATHOGENESIS

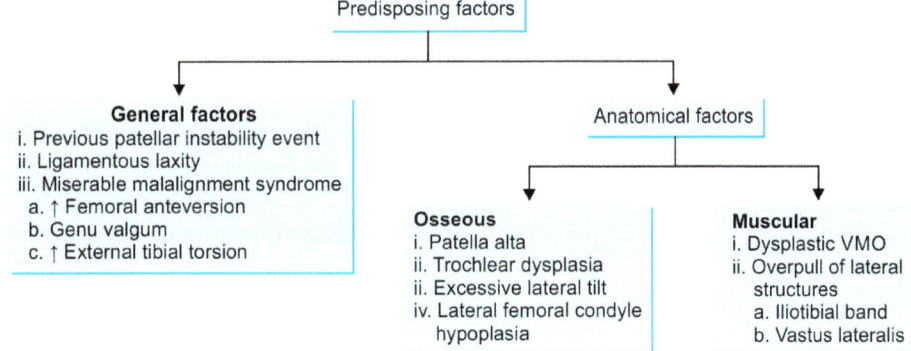

III. PATHOPHYSIOLOGY

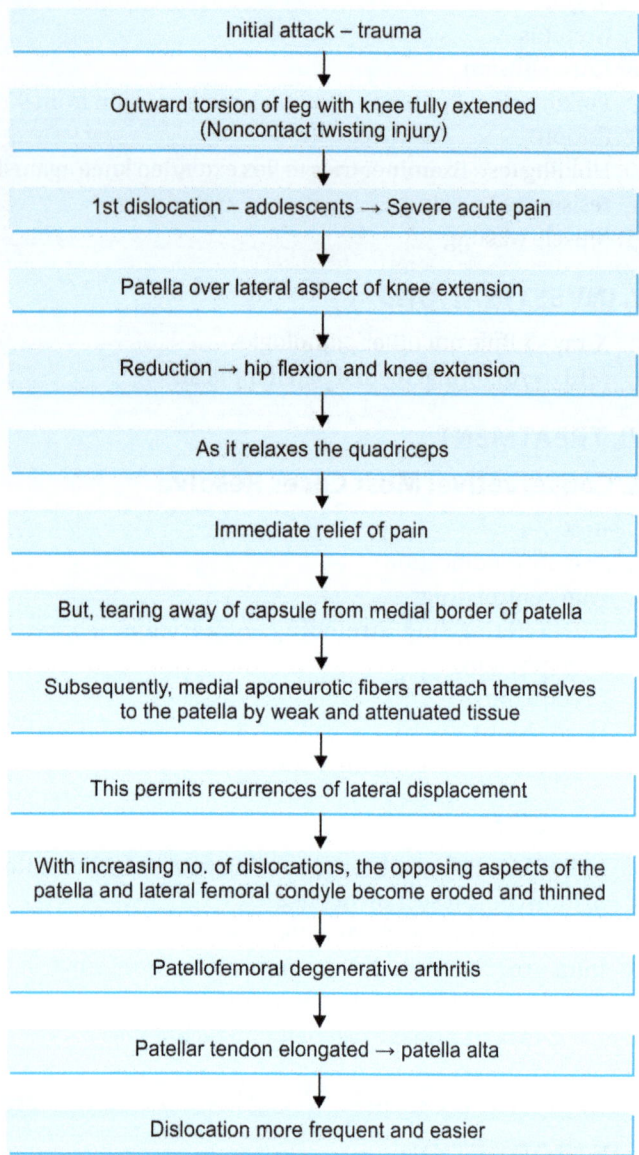

IV. CLINICAL FEATURES

1. Tenderness – at medial capsule near the medial border of patella at medial epicondyle → MPFL injury
2. Joint effusion
3. Hemarthrosis
4. Abnormal excessive passive lateral displacement of patella
5. Patellar apprehension test positive
6. Atrophy of quadriceps, especially VMO
7. Genu valgum
8. External tibial torsion
9. Genu recurvatum
10. **J–sign** = Maltracking of Patella
11. Subpatellar crepitus: Once degeneration begins
12. Iliotibial band contracture
13. Abnormal ITB attachment → limitation of knee flexion when patella is fixed in intercondylar groove
14. High riding patella
15. Torsional deformities of femur and tibia

V. RADIOLOGICAL EXAMINATION

A. AP View

1. **Q-angle:** Angle formed by a line joining ASIS to midpoint of patella and a line from midpoint of patella to TT **(Fig. 23)**.

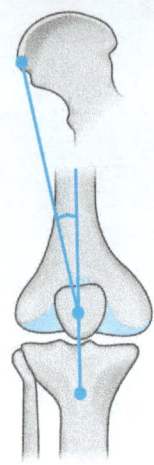

Fig. 23: Q-angle.

2. Overall lower limb alignment and version

B. Lateral Views

1. Patellar height evaluation
   i. **Blumensaat's line:** Normally the lower border of patella lies at this line extended from the intercondylar notch in 30° knee flexion.
   ii. **Insall-Salvati index (Fig. 24)**

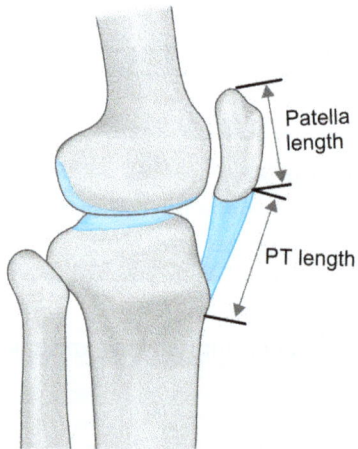

Fig. 24: Insall-Salvati index.

Patellar tendon length = 0.8–1.2 patellar length
>1.2 = Patella alta.

C. Trochlear Dysplasia Assessment

1. Crossing sign: Flattened trochlear groove. Trochlear groove lies in the same plane as anterior border of lateral condyle.

2. Double contour sign: Convex trochlear groove. Anterior border of lateral condyle lies anterior to the anterior border of medial condyle.
3. Supratrochlear spur: Arises in the proximal aspect of the trochlea.

D. Sunrise/Merchant View

1. Assessment of lateral patellar tilt
2. Lateral patellofemoral angle (LPFA) **(Fig. 25)**.

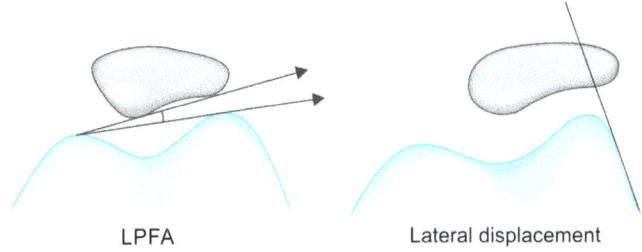

LPFA   Lateral displacement

   i. Normal >11°, opens laterally
   ii. Angle between line along subchondral bone of lateral trochlear facet + Posterior femoral condyles
3. Congruence angle = Normal = –6° (DAO in the figure)
4. Sulcus angle: Evaluate for trochlear dysplasia **(Fig. 26)**.

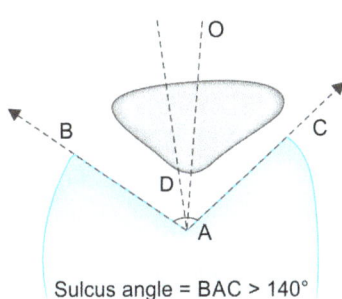

Sulcus angle = BAC > 140°

D - Lowest point on patella
AO bisects sulcus angle

E. Dejour Classification of Trochlear Dysplasia (Figs. 27A to D)

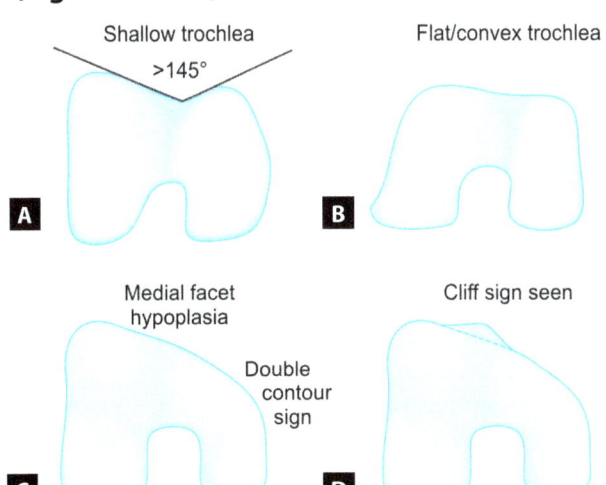

A – Shallow trochlea (>145°)
B – Flat/convex trochlea
C – Medial facet hypoplasia (double contour sign)
D – Cliff sign seen

F. CT Scan

TT – TG distance

Measures the distance between 2 perpendicular lines from the posterior cortex to the **t**ibial **t**ubercle and the **t**rochlear **g**roove.

>20 mm → Abnormal

G. MRI

1. To rule out suspected loose bodies:
   i. Osteochondral lesion
   ii. Medial patellar facet (MC)
   iii. Lateral femoral condyle
2. Tear of MPFL

VI. MANAGEMENT

A. Nonoperative

1. Closed chain short arc quadriceps exercises
2. Quadriceps strengthening
3. Core and hip strengthening to improve limb positioning and balance (hip abductors, gluteal and abdominals)
4. Patella stabilizing sleeve or "J-sleeve"

B. Operative

1. *Objective:* To align the quadriceps apparatus to a more medial position.
2. Proximal realignment procedures – Proximal to patella.
3. Distal realignment procedures – distal to patella
4. Principles based on anatomical and pathological features of cases:
   i. Isolated lateral release of extensor retinaculum is never sufficient.
   ii. If genu valgum → Correction of deformity can correct the problem.
   iii. High riding patella is managed by distal transfer of tibial tuberosity in skeletally mature.
      In skeletally immature → Medial transposition of patellar tendon.
   iv. Trochlear dysplasia → Trochleoplasty **(Albee's operation)**
   v. If no skeletal abnormality → MPFL Reconstruction
   vi. Before growth is completed → Only soft tissue procedures are permissible.
5. *Surgeries*:
   i. **Hauser:**
      a. Tibial tubercle and its attached patellar tendon are transplanted → distally and medially

b. Most effective procedure for severe repeated dislocations
c. **Fulkerson's osteotomy** is a variant
ii. **Goldthwait-Roux**
Patellar tendon is split longitudinally and lateral half is drawn medially and attached to the inner border of tibia.
iii. Tendon transplantation: Pes anserinus transfer to anteromedial distal patella → Dr DP Bakshi
iv. **Albee's operation** (Figs. 28A to C)

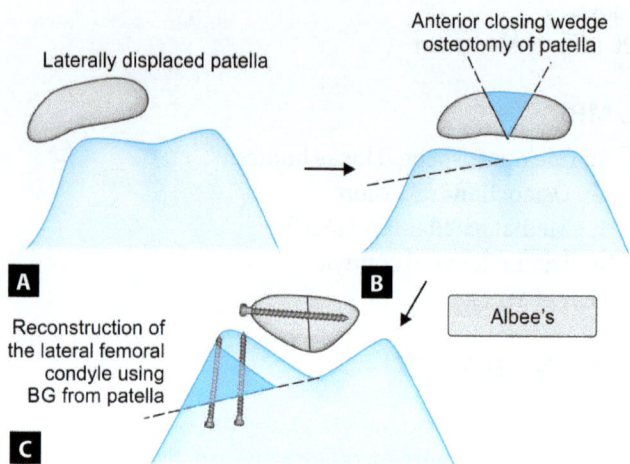

When lateral femoral condyle is shallow.
↓
Osteotomy of LFC in frontal plane
↓
Anterior fragment of bone elevated with bone graft inserted beneath.
v. Simple imbrication: Inner third of the capsule covering is freed from the patella and imbricated over the lateral 2/3rd. Lateral retinaculum is severed.
vi. **Elmslie-Trillat:**
a. Distal part of patellar tendon and tuberosity undisturbed.
b.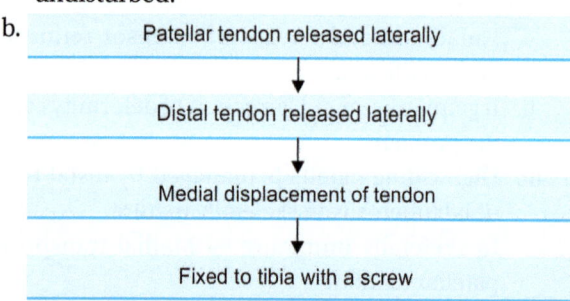
c. VM → advanced distally to increase strength during the last 10° of extension.
d. Procedure not suitable for patella alta.

OSTEOCHONDRITIS DISSECANS

I. INTRODUCTION
1. Focal idiopathic pathologic lesion affecting the subchondral bone and articular cartilage
2. Small segment of necrotic subchondral bone eventually separates as an osteochondral fragment on disease progression.
3. Types:
    a. Juvenile (physis open) at 10–15 years of age.
    b. Adult, after skeletal maturity.
4. Sites:
    a. Knee (MC): Posterolateral aspect of medial femoral condyle (MC).
    b. Capitellum
    c. Talar dome

II. ETIOLOGY
1. Trauma: Direct injury or repetitive microtrauma → Sports persons.
2. Ischemia → Circulatory obstruction by thrombi.
3. Endocrine imbalance
4. Familial predisposition
5. Epiphyseal abnormalities
6. Impingement of tibial spine
7. Mechanical factors: Association between medial condylar lesions and varus mechanical axis, lateral condylar lesions and valgus mechanical axis

III. PATHOGENESIS
Inciting factor → Disruption of focal blood supply
↓
Necrosis of subchondral bone
↓
Eventual separation of the osteochondral fragment
↓
Articular cartilage derives nourishment from synovial fluid
↓
Loose body formed, crater left behind
↓
Degenerative arthritis

IV. CLINICAL FEATURES
1. Commonly seen in adolescents and young adults
2. M:F = 3:1
3. H/O knee trauma
4. Vague, aching discomfort of several months duration
5. Pain and stiffness
6. Catching and popping
7. Palpable loose body within the joint
8. Externally rotated gait (to avoid tibial spine impingement)
9. Effusion in the knee
10. Quadriceps wasting
11. Joint line tenderness
12. Restricted range of motion
13. Wilson's test:
    i. Patient seated with knee in 90° flexion

ii. Internally rotate the knee and extend
   iii. Pain at 30° flexion
   iv. Relieved on external rotation

V. INVESTIGATIONS

1. X-ray:
   i. A-P view
   ii. Lateral view
   iii. Intercondylar notch view (defect or the loose fragment may be seen)
2. MRI – IOC, provides information regarding:
   i. Articular surface
   ii. Stability and size of the lesion
   iii. Effusion
   iv. Prognosticate healing
   v. 90% sensitivity and 95% specificity
3. Bone scan: Assess the healing activity of the lesion and may predict the results of the treatment

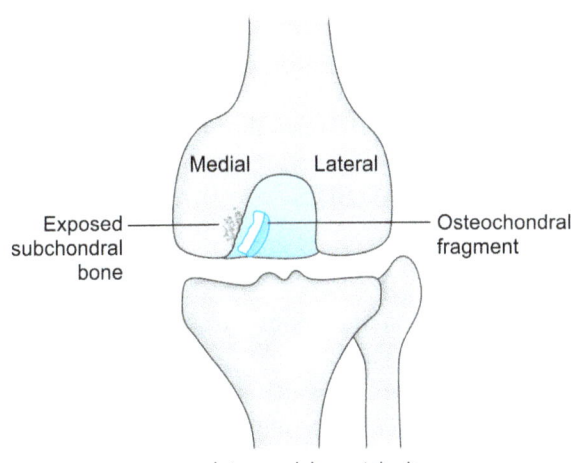

Intercondylar notch view

VI. CLASSIFICATIONS

A. Radiographic (Clanton and DeLee)

1. Type I: Depressed osteochondral fracture
2. Type II: Fragment attached by osseous bridge
3. Type III: Detached non-displaced fragment
4. Type IV: Displaced fragment

B. Arthroscopic (Guhl)

1. Grade I: Softened area covered by cartilage; stable in continuity.
2. Grade II: Partial discontinuity.
3. Grade III: Complete discontinuity, not dislocated.
4. Grade IV: Dislocated fragment with empty bed.

VII. MANAGEMENT

A. Conservative

1. Indicated in stable lesions and asymptomatic patients.
2. Usually skeletally immature patients (juvenile) without closure of physis are managed conservatively since stable lesions resolve spontaneously.
3. Modalities:
   i. Protected weight bearing
   ii. Activity restriction → Avoid sports and strenuous activities
   iii. Immobilization
   iv. Off-loading brace
   v. Physiotherapy exercises

B. Operative

1. Indications:
   i. Nonresolutions of symptoms in patients with stable lesions being managed conservatively for more than 3 months
   ii. Unstable lesions
   iii. Exposed subchondral bone
   iv. Symptomatic lesions in skeletally mature patients
2. Surgical procedures (write details from "Cartilage Injuries")
   i. Arthroscopic debridement and removal of loose bodies
   ii. Fixation of fragment
   iii. Arthroscopic subchondral drilling/microabrasions
   iv. Chondral resurfacing techniques such as OATS, allograft transplant, ACI, MACI.
   v. Total knee arthroplasty: Advanced degenerative arthritis.

OSTEOARTHRITIS OF KNEE

I. INTRODUCTION

1. Degenerative disorder of the articular cartilage.
2. Although the suffix "-itis" implies that OA is an inflammatory disorder and some evidence of synovitis is often present
   ↓
   Inflammation is not a major component of disease
3. Progressive arthropathy with heterogenous clinical presentation
   ↓
   Can occur in any synovial joint, though it commonly affects hands, knees, feet, hip and spine.
4. Results from excessive mechanical stress applied to susceptible joints predisposed due to chondrocyte dysfunction.

II. ETIOLOGY

1. *Age*:
   i. Single most strongly correlated risk factor
   ii. >80% people over 75 are affected
2. Genetic

3. *Familial*: Nodal generalized OA runs in families
4. *Joint location*: Weight bearing joints are commonly affected but the effect is differential.
5. *Trauma (intra-articular fracture)*:
   a. Produces joint incongruence and malalignment.
   b. Altered joint geometry affects the nutrition of articular cartilage and alters weight distribution.
6. *Repetitive joint use*:

   Repetitive trauma at subfracture level
   ↓
   Increased wear of cartilage
   ↓
   Increased incidence of OA in athletes

7. *Joint dysplasia, deformities, and malalignment*: Perthes, DDH, genu varum, recurrent dislocation of patella predispose to early OA.
8. Preceding crystal deposition and endocrine disorder
9. Smoking
10. *High bone density*: Stiff subchondral bone deforms less under loading → increased stress on cartilage
11. Low vitamin C and D
12. *Gender*:

    <50 years = M > F due to joint injury from accidents, sports.
    >50 years = F > M (2:1)
    Postmenopausal estrogen deficiency.

III. PATHOPHYSIOLOGY

A. Articular Cartilage

1. Water content ↑ due to ↑ water permeability
2. Alterations in proteoglycans → eventual decrease in the amount of proteoglycans
3. Normally with ageing, synthesis of keratin sulfate increases compared to chondroitin sulfate.
4. However, in a reparative response to osteoarthritic disease process,

   ↓

   Chrondrocytes revert to its chondroblastic function of synthesizing large amounts of chondroitin - 4 - sulfate.
5. The organization and orientation of the collagen fibers are lost.

B. Synovium and Capsule

1. Mild inflammatory changes → Early stages
2. As disease progresses, inflammatory changes increase and the synovium starts becoming hypervascular and thick

   ↓

C. Cell Biology

1. Increased secretion of matrix metalloproteases (MMPs)
   i. Plasmin
   ii. Aggrecanase (ADAMTS-4)
   iii. Stromelysin

   ↓

2. These are responsible for cartilage matrix digestion.
3. TIMPs (Tissue inhibitors of MMPs)

   ↓

   Control activity of MMPs
   However, during OA, there is an imbalance between TIMPs and MMPs.
4. The inflammatory cytokines are secreted by synoviocytes and are responsible for increased MMP synthesis.
   i. IL-1
   ii. IL-6
   iii. TNF-α

D. Bone

1. In an attempt to remodel , the subchondral bone → forms lytic lesions with sclerotic edges.
2. Bone cysts are formed in later stages
3. Osteophytes formation

   ↓(d/t)

   Pathologic activation of endochondral ossification
   ↓(mediated by)
   Indian hedgehog (IHH) signaling molecule.

IV. CLINICAL FEATURES

A. Symptoms

1. *Pain*:
   i. Most common and important symptom
   ii. Increases with activity
   iii. Its function limiting and decreased walking distances
   iv. May also be present at night due to " bone angina" → Intraosseous HTN and stasis
2. Activity induced swelling
3. Knee stiffness
4. *Mechanical symptoms*:
   i. Instability
   ii. Locking
   iii. Catching sensation

B. Physical Examination

1. Joint effusion
2. Quadriceps and hamstring muscle atrophy.
3. Varus deformity >>> Valgus deformity.
4. Flexion deformity
5. Antalgic gait
6. Medial joint line tenderness,
7. Bone enlargement palpable along joint line → osteophytes
8. Crepitus on joint movement
9. Restricted range of motion
10. Painful ROM especially terminal in early disease → Increases in arc with diseases progression

V. INVESTIGATIONS

1. Weight bearing → AP ⎫
   ↓   → Lateral ⎬ Radiographs

   To assess exact loss of articular cartilage and bone if any and to appreciate correctability of deformity.
2. Earliest X-ray changes = Joint spaces narrowing resulting from loss of articular cartilage
3. Radiologic changes progress with advancement of disease
   ↓
4. But, the relationship between radiological changes and clinical symptomatology is not always similar.
   ↓
5. Patient with advanced X-rays may have minimal symptoms and vice-versa.
6. Subchondral sclerosis, cysts.
7. Osteophyte formation, loose bodies.
8. Hip-knee-ankle angle → Varus deformity
9. <u>Kellgren and Lawrence</u>: Radiological class on severity of OA.

   Grade:
   0: No radiographic features of OA.
   1: Doubtful JSN + Possible osteophytic lipping
   2: Possible JSN + Definite osteophytes
   3: Definite JSN + Sclerosis, possible bony deformity + multiple osteophytes
   4: Marked JSN, severe sclerosis definite bony deformity + large osteophytes

VI. MANAGEMENT

A. Conservative

1. Fair trial of conservative treatment before considering surgical options
2. *Lifestyle modification:*
   i. High impact activities such as stair-climbing, sitting cross-legged and squatting → To be avoided
   ii. Weight reduction (BMI > 25)
       1 kg reduces 3-4 kg force across knee.
   iii. *Physical therapy:*
       a. Hamstring and quadriceps strengthening exercises
       b. Improves ROM through gentle active and passive exercises
       c. Knee braces → Hinge knee brace
       d. Additional modalities: 1. Heat
                                  2. Cold
                                  3. Ultrasound
                                  4. TENS
       e. Aerobic conditioning → Not only increased functional capacity but also decreased pain and use of meds.
       f. Use of assistive devices in opposite hands.
          ↓
          Decreased stress cross joint by 50%
          ↓
          Triples walking distance with use of cane.
   iv. *NSAIDs:* First choice drugs for treatment of patients with symptomatic arthritis.
   v. Treatment modalities with no conclusive evidence:
       a. Intra-articular injection of hyaluronic acid
       b. Devils claw extract
       c. Avocado and soyabean unsaponifiable fractions
       d. Vitamin C, D, E.
       e. Glucosamine and chondroitin sulfate

B. Operative

1. *Indications*

i. Pain affecting activities of daily living refractory to conservative management
ii. Instability
iii. Deformity
iv. Repeated acute episodes of looking effusion or hemarthrosis
    ↓
    Loose body → Osteochondral fragment, torn meniscus or osteochondral fractures.

2. *Surgical Options*

1. High tibial osteotomy
2. Unicompartmental knee replacement
3. Total knee replacement

HIGH TIBIAL OSTEOTOMY

I. PRINCIPLE

High tibial osteotomy (HTO) "unloads" the affected knee joint compartment by correcting the alignment and redistributing stresses, thus relieving pain and restoring function.

II. RATIONALE

1. Radiological progression increases four fold with varus malignment
2. The risk of progression of OA is tenfold in KL-3 knee with varus alignment
3. The adductor moment leads to progression of OA by dynamic loading of the varus knee.

III. INDICATIONS

1. Pain and disability from unicompartmental involvement (usually medial OA).
   ↓
   <4 grade Ahlback, Patellofemoral OA < 3 grade
   ↓
   In a high demand individual.

2. Age <60 and varus/valgus <15° at the knee with full extension.
3. Motivated patient who will use assistive devices and is compliant with activity limitation till healing occurs.
4. As an additional procedure to meniscal transplantation in meniscectomized knees for prevention of long term overload
5. ACL, PCL or PLC insufficiency with varus alignment or thrust.

IV. CONTRAINDICATIONS

1. Age >65 years
2. Diffuse OA
3. Tibiofemoral subluxation - lateral subluxation of tibia >1 cm
4. Medial compartment bone loss >2-3 mm
5. Medial compartment OA → Ahlback ≥4
6. Flexion contracture >15°
7. Inflammatory arthritis
8. Mediolateral insufficiency
9. Peripheral vascular disease
10. Knee ROM < 90°

V. TYPES

1. Lateral closing wedge (Coventry)
2. Medial opening wedge
3. Dual osteotomy
4. Dome osteotomy
5. Chevron osteotomy
6. Medial opening hemicallostasis:
   i. Ilizarov ring fixator
   ii. External fixator

VI. SITE

Classically, the osteotomy was performed above the level of tibial tubercle.
↓
But, concerns of Patella Baja and need of future TKR.
↓
Many surgeons therefore prefer osteotomy below tibial tubercle.

VII. PREOPERATIVE PLANNING AND ASSESSMENT OF DEGREE OF CORRECTION

1. Weight-bearing AP and lateral X-ray knee.
2. Axial views of PF joint.
3. Whole leg standing radiograph.
4. TBVA: Tibial bone varus angle. Angle between the mechanical axis (center of proximal tibia to center of ankle) of tibia and the epiphyseal axis of proximal tibia **(Fig. 29)**.
   Preoperative: TBVA > 5° → Good prognosis
5. The aim is to achieve 3-5° valgus at the knee
   Slight overcorrection to ensure shift of weight bearing force to uninvolved compartment.

   i. Under correction → Varus recurrence
   ii. Overcorrection → Lateral compartment OA

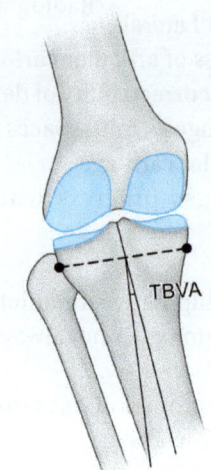

Fig. 29: Tibia bone varus angle.

6. Calculation of Wedge size (Dugdale method).
   Step 1:
   i. Draw a line from center of head to **Fujisawa point** on tibial plateau and extend distally.
   ii. Draw another line from Fujisawa point to center of ankle
   iii. This is α: The correction angle.
   iv. Fujisawa point is located at **62.5% of the tibial plateau on the lateral condyle calculated from medial side.**
   Step 2:
   i. Subtract the varus alignment due to ligament laxity (β)
   $$\beta = \frac{K \times (\Delta a)}{\text{Tibial plateau width}}$$
   JCLA → Difference between the femoral and tibial joint line Δa
   K constant → 76.4   Final correction = α − β **(Fig. 30)**
   Step 3:
   i. Center of rotation angulation (CORA)
   ii. Medial opening wedge → Fibular head
   iii. Lateral closing wedge → 2-2.5 cm distal to medial joint line
   Step 4: Size of osteotomy wedge, 1 mm wedge length for every degree of correction.

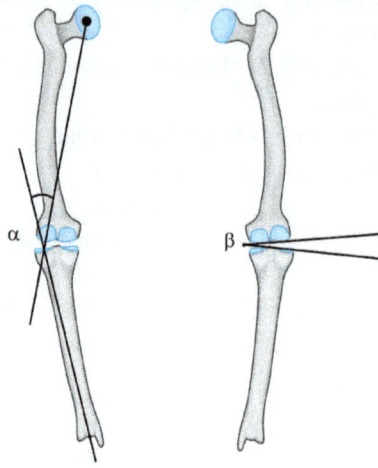

VIII. LCWO (FIG. 31)

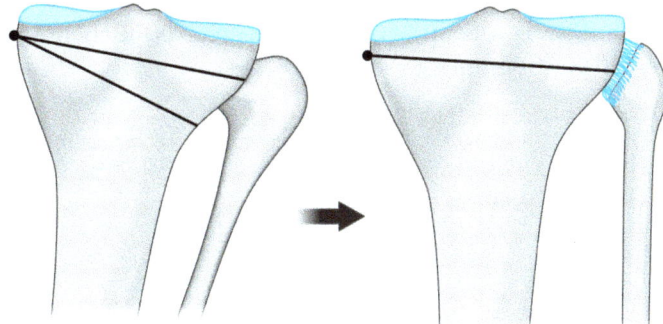

1. Most popular with longest track record.
2. Increased Patellar height: Use in patella baja
3. Decreased tibial slope → Use in ACL insufficiency
4. Shortens the limb
5. Higher union rate
6. Fixation covered with soft tissues
7. Faster rehabilitation
8. No bone graft required
9. *Disadvantages:*
    i. Peroneal nerve injury
    ii. Two cuts required
    iii. Tibiofibular joint disrupted

IX. MOWO

1. More precise, better correction
2. Restores bone stock
3. Single osteotomy cut
4. Increased tibial slope (but minimal) → **Use in PCL insufficiency**
5. Decreased patellar height
6. TKA conversion relatively easier
7. No fibular osteotomy, TF joint spared
8. No nerve dissection
9. Increased MCL tension → Good
10. May (cause) leg lengthening
11. Prolonged non-weight bearing

UNICOMPARTMENTAL KNEE REPLACEMENT

Bone preserving partial knee arthroplasty in which only 1 compartment of knee is replaced.

I. PRINCIPLE

1. UKA removes the diseased painful portion (Replacement procedure).
    ↓
    a resurfacing arthroplasty (Joint preserving)
    ↓
    thus reconstructing the bearing surfaces.
2. It restores the natural alignment of the joint and restores ligament tension and joint line.
3. Only the symptomatic compartment is tackled rather than opting for a total knee replacement.
    ↓
4. Leading to faster recovery time with minimal invasiveness.
5. Patient selection is very essential in UKR
    ↓
    Single knee compartment OA and correctable leg deformity.
    ↓
    Most Important factors.
6. Surgical goal → Slight undercorrection of the deformity of the long leg axis (compared to HTO where overcorrection is done) medial UKR: 1–4° Varus, Lateral UKR: 3–7° Valgus.
7. Correct ligament balance restored by
    ↓
    Accurate positioning of components
    +
    Inserting an appropriate thickness of bearing.
8. In high functional demand pts
    ↓
    Reconstruct ACL simultaneously or staged in addition to UKR.

II. INDICATIONS

1. Age >50
2. BMI <35, however, recently many studies have shown no adverse co-relation between high BMI and clinical outcome.
3. Low to moderate level of activity.
4. Preoperative knee ROM > 90°
5. Flexion contracture < 5°
6. Varus/valgus deformity <15° and passively correctable to neutral.

III. CONTRAINDICATIONS

1. Contralateral tibiofemoral arthritis
2. Inflammatory arthritis
3. Collateral ligament insufficiency
4. Menisectomized other compartment
5. Varus/valgus >15°, flexion contracture >10°
6. Age
7. BMI > 35
8. Patellofemoral arthritis — Relative contraindications according to the recent outcomes of UKR
9. ACL insufficiency
10. Chondrocalcinosis

IV. ADVANTAGES

1. Minimally invasive surgery
2. 1 day admission or out-patient basis (shorter hospital stay)

3. Reduced operative time
4. Less bleeding
5. Less cost
6. Greater postoperative ROM
7. Greater pain relief
8. Earlier return to activities and sports
9. Preservation of bone stock
10. Retention of cruciates → Proprioception
    ↓
    "Natural" feeling to the patient
11. Decreased postoperative morbidity and infection

V. TYPES (FIG. 32)

1. Mobile bearing (Oxford, Biomet)
2.
   Fixed bearing decreased conformity between the 2 articular surfaces
   ↓
   Higher point loading on surface
   ↓
   Higher stress within polyethylene
   ↓
   Increased of component loosening and polyethylene wear

   Mobile bearing → articular surfaces congruent over entire ROM
   ↓
   Large contact areas, better distribution of stresses
   ↓
   Decreased incidence of aseptic loosening
   ↓
   However, increased incidence of mobile tray dislocation.

VI. MODES OF FAILURE

1. Aseptic loosening (MCC)
2. Progression of OA (2nd MCC)
3. Polyethylene wear
4. Pain

VII. RECENT ADVANCES

1. *Cementless UKR:*
   i. Resurgence of interest in cementless fixation is seen as aseptic loosening is the MCC of failure of UKR.
   ii. Porous titanium and hydroxyapatite coating (Improved fixation of cementless TKR)
   ↓
   Decreased S_X time, avoidance of cementation error.
2. Domed Lateral Oxford UKA (Biomet)
   ↓
   Designed to reduce dislocation of mobile bearings seen > in lateral compartment.
3. *Robot-assisted and computer navigation:*
   i. More accurate and controlled:
      a. Lower leg alignment
      b. Soft tissue balancing
      c. Joint line maintenance
      d. Component alignment
   ii. Robot → "Semi–active": Surgeon retains the control of the procedure.

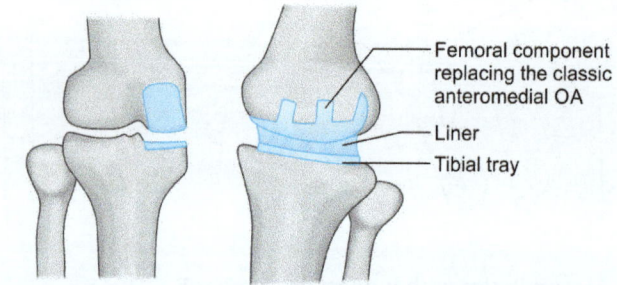

TOTAL KNEE REPLACEMENT (FIG. 33)

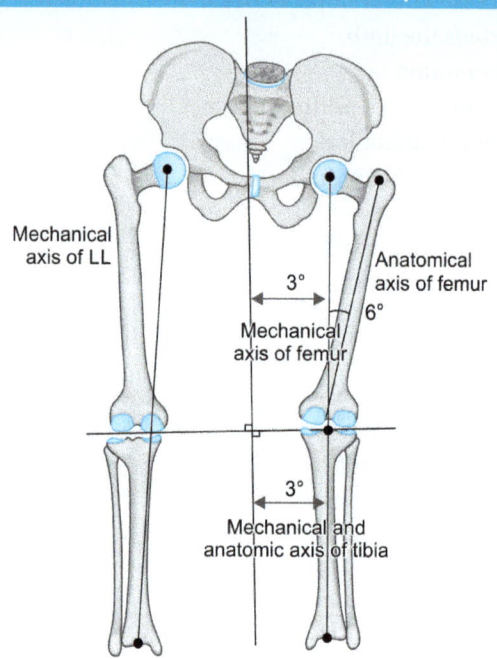

Fig. 33: Axes of lower limb.

I. BIOMECHANICAL PRINCIPLES

1. Instant centers of rotation
2. Load applied to knee
3. Screw home mechanism
4. Rotational and axial alignment
5. Patellofemoral joint mechanism

A. Instant Centers of Rotation (Fig. 34)

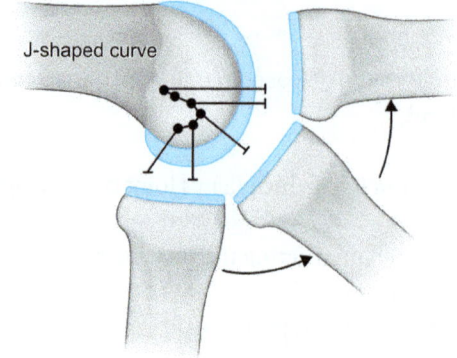

1. Knee motion is complex and includes
   ↓
   Rolling, sliding and axial motion
   ↓ (in the form of)
   Flexion and extension, adduction and abduction and IR and ER along the long axis of limb.
2. Knee flexion occurs around a varying transverse axis.
3. In the sagittal plane, the kinematic analysis reveals moving instant centers of rotation (centrodes) as the knee moves from F → E.
4. The instant centers determine the direction of velocity at the articular contact point.
5. Least resistance to sliding knee motion occurs when
   ↓
   The direction of velocity of the contact surface particle is tangent to the contact surface.
6. This occurs when the internet center lies along a line that is perpendicular to the articular surface at their contact points.
7.
If the instant center is not perpendicular to the articular surface at the contact point
↓
Direction of velocity will not be tangent to the joint surface
↓
Motion will separate or compress joint surfaces
↓
Sliding will occur, but frictional and compressive forces will be increased

B. Loads Applied to Knees (Fig. 35)

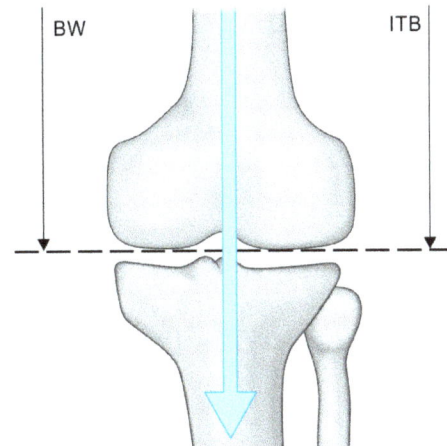

1. In the frontal plane, the BW is transmitted along a vertical line from the center of gravity and normal passes medial to persons knee.
   ↓
2. This causes the femur to tilt on the tibia
   ↓
3. Counterbalanced by a lateral force: TFL and G. Max acting through ITB
4. The sum of these forces, i.e., total load passes through the knee center.

C. Screw-Home Mechanism

1. Medial based pivoting of knee in the form of ER of tibia on femur during extension.
2. Thus in full extended knee, joint is locked, permitting standing without muscle activity.
3. As the knee flexes, the tibia rotates internally and unlocks the joint (popliteus).
4. ACL → taught in full extension, Relaxed at 45° flexion. Taut in full flexion.
5. Some portion of PCL is taut throughout flexion and extension → Important for stability.

D. Axial and Rotational Alignment of Knee (Fig. 36)

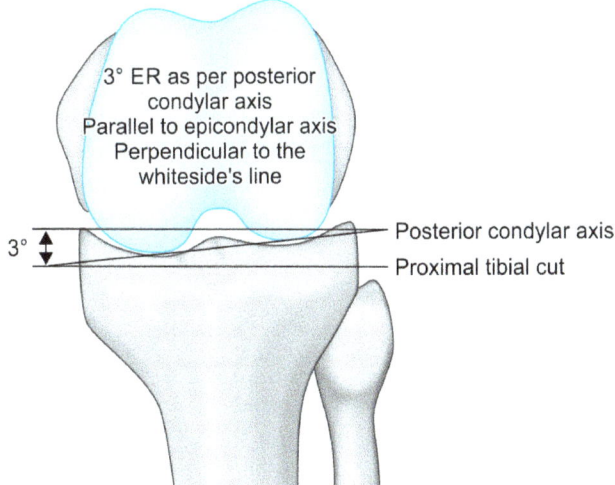

1. Normal, AA of femur and tibia → **6 ± 2° Valgus**
2. MA of LL → Center of femur head → talar dome center
3. Passing through center of knee joint = "Neutral"
   Lateral = Valgus
   Medial = Varus
4. Normal tibial articular surface → 3° Varus with respect to MA
   Femoral Articular Surface → 9° Valgus
5. However tibial cuts are taken perpendicular to MA.
6. Femoral cut (Distal) – 5–7° Valgus with respect to anatomic axis as jig is IM
   ↓
   Cuts perpendicular to MA, MA restored
7. The rotation of the femoral component
   ↓
   Balancing of flexion space + Patellofemoral tracking
8. As proximal tibia cut, perpendicular to MA and not in 3° anatomic varus,
   ↓
   Femoral component 3° ER to create symmetric flexion space.

E. Patellofemoral Joint Mechanics (Figs. 37 and 38)

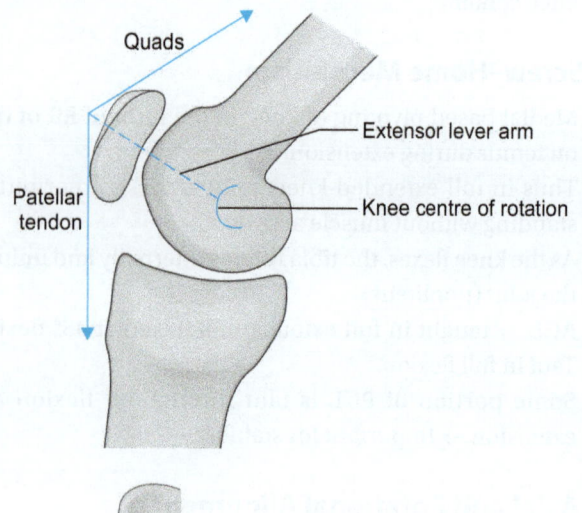

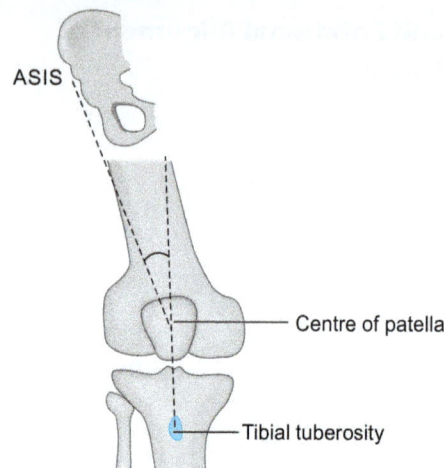

Fig. 38: Q angle.

1. Patella → increases lever arm
   ↓
   Improves quadriceps efficiency
2. Poor patellofemoral fit → increased point of pressure on patella
3. Most femoral component → lateral flange of trochlea > prominent → Better reconstruction.

II. CONTRAINDICATIONS OF TKR

A. Absolute

1. Recent or ongoing knee sepsis
2. A remote source of ongoing infection
3. Extensor mechanism discontinuity/severe knee dysfunction
4. Recurvatum deformity secondary to neuromuscular weakness
5. Presence of painless, well functional knee arthrodesis

B. Relative

1. Severely OA high I/L → Hip to be managed before knee
2. Significant atherosclerotic disease of operative leg
3. Skin condition like psoriasis on operative field
4. Recurrent cellulitis
5. Neuropathic arthropathy
6. Super obesity (BMI ≥ 50)
7. Recent UTI
8. H/O OM in proximity to knee

III. SURGICAL APPROACHES

1. The most commonly used skin incision for 1° TKR → Anterior midline incision
2. The incision may be taken slightly medial to patella to avoid it being directly over the bone.
3. Most incisions compromise the infrapatellar branch of saphenous nerve.
   ↓
   Numbness on outer aspect of knee
4. Deep to the subcutaneous level of dissection, the approaches are:
   i. Medial parapatellar retinacular
   ii. Subvastus
   iii. Midvastus
   iv. Lateral parapatellar
   v. Quadriceps sparing medial parapatellar = MIS
   vi. Extensile exposures → Quadriceps snip
      → V-Y turndown
      → Tibial tubercle osteotomy.

A. Medial Parapatellar Retinacular (Fig. 39)

1. Identify the medial aspect of patellar tendon, medial aspect of patella and quadriceps tendon lateral to VMO
   ↓
2. Arthrotomy
   ↓
3. Starting from proximal extent in a longitudinal manner curving medially along the patella.
   ↓
   3-5 mm of soft tissue cuff must be left on patella → to assist in closure.

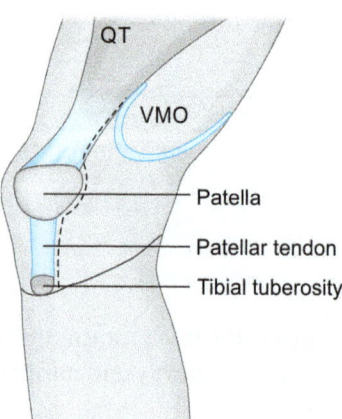

4. *Advantages:*
   i. MC used, familiar to most surgeons
   ii. Widest exposure → obese cases
   iii. 1° as well as revision TKR

5. *Disadvantages*:
   i. Access to lateral retinaculum less direct
   ii. Failure of medial capsular repair
   iii. Lateral patellar subluxation
   iv. May jeopardize patellar circulation if lateral release performed

B. Mid-Vastus (Fig. 40)

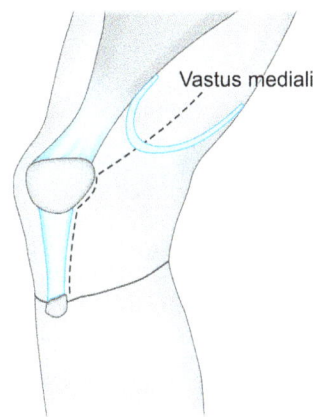

1. VM insertion of quadriceps not disrupted
   ↓
2. Accelerated rehab due to preservation of extensor mechanism.
3. Better patellar tracking as compared to medial parapatellar
4. *Disadvantages*:
   i. Less extensile: Difficulty in obese, flexion contracture
5. *Relative C/I*:
   i. ROM < 80°
   ii. Obese patient
   iii. Hypertrophic arthritis
   iv. Previous HTO

C. Sub-Vastus (Fig. 41)

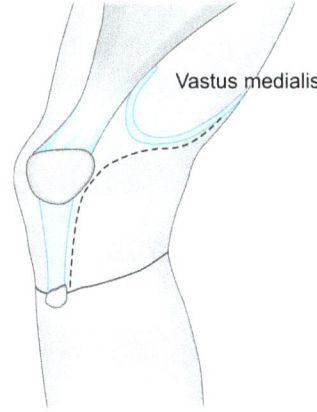

1. Muscle belly of VM is lifted off intermuscular septum
2. Patellar vascularity preserved
3. Minimal need for lateral retinacular release

Disadvantages: Potential for denervation of VMO

D. Lateral Parapatellar (Keblish Approach) (Fig. 42)

1. Used for fixed valgus deformity
   ↓
2. Direct access to lateral side
3. Preserves blood supply patella
4. Prevents lateral patellar sublux
5. *Disadvantage*:
   i. Technically demanding → Medial eversion difficult
   ii. Closure difficult

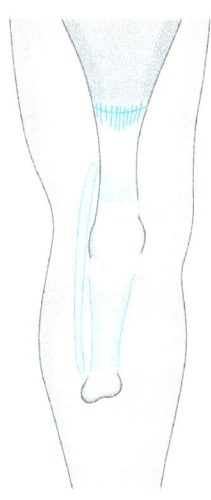

E. Extensile Approaches (Fig. 43)

1. Quadriceps snip
2. Quadriceps V-Y plasty
3. Tibial tubercle osteotomy

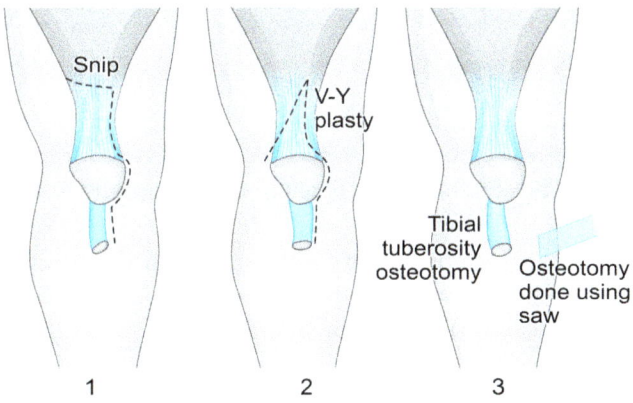

SECTION 5

Spine

ANATOMY OF VERTEBRAL COLUMN

A. CERVICAL SPINE ANATOMY

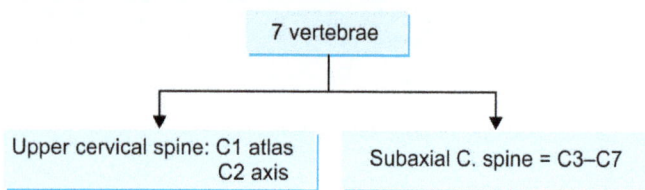

I. Bones

1. C_1, C_2, C_7: Atypical vertebrae
2. $C_3 - C_6$: Typical vertebrae

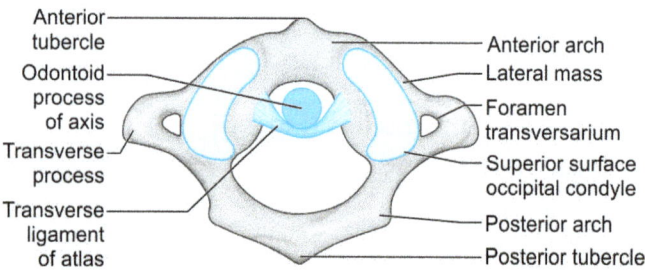

3. C_1 (Atlas) (Fig. 1):
   i. No vertebral body or spinous process
   ↓
   The vertebral body of atlas embryologically fuses to $C_2 \rightarrow$ Dens
   ii. The vertebral artery passes through the foramen transversarium and courses posteriorly within a sulcus on the superior arch of atlas.
   ↓
   iii. 15% of population, this sulcus is completely covered by anomalous ossification.
   ↓called
   iv. Ponticulus Posticus → surgical implication during screw fixation.

4. C_2 axis (Fig. 2) (Below are labels):

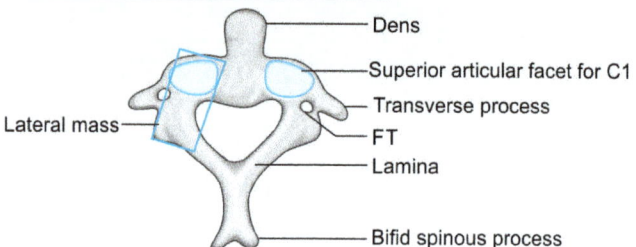

5. Vertebra prominens - C_7:
   i. Does not have a bifid spinous process.
   ii. The vertebral artery does not pass-through the foramen transversarium
   iii. Longer and larger spinous process.
6. Typical cervical vertebrae (Fig. 3):

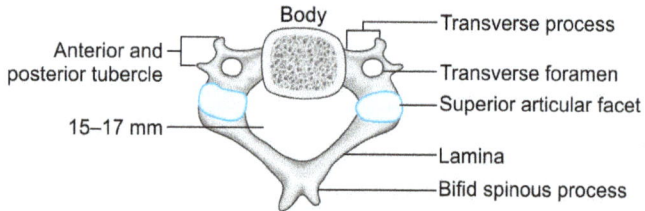

   i. Vertebral artery passes through transverse foramen (all except C_7)
   ii. Spinous process: Short and Bifid
   iii. Vertebral foramen: Triangular
   iv. Vertebral body → Small, square shaped with concave superior and convex inferior border.
   v. C_6: Palpable carotid tubercle
   ↓
   Valuable landmark for anterior approach to cervical spine.

II. Intervertebral Disc

1. It has: Annulus fibrous: Periphery
   Nucleus pulposus: Center
   2 cartilaginous end plates (superior and inferior)
2. No IVD between C_1 and C_2

3. The cervical IVD is thicker anteriorly
   ↓
   Responsible for lordotic curve

III. Joints

1. Atlanto-occipital joint: 50% F – E
   "Yes" movement
2. Atlantoaxial joint ($C_1 - C_2$): 50% axial rotation.
   "No" movement
3. Subaxial joints
   i. Intervertebral joints: Fibrocartilaginous
   ii. Uncovertebral joints **(Fig. 4)**

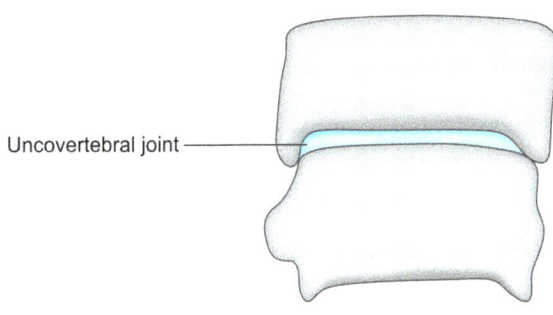

Joints at the uncinate process of Luschka
↓
Lateral aspect of IVD
↓
No articular cartilage or synovial fluid
↓
∴ Pseudojoints
   iii. Facet joints: Diarthrodial joints

IV. Ligaments

1. Tectorial membrane – Fibrous tissue from
   ↓
   Posterior border of foramen magnum → superior surface of C_1 ring.
   ↓
   Analogous to PLL in lower C. spine
2. Posterior atlanto-occipital membrane
   ↓
   Loose fibrous tissue from lower occiput → C_1 ring posterior.
   ↓
   Analogous to ligamentum flavum (lower C. spine)
3. Occipitoatlantoaxial ligament
   i. Apical (Tip of dens → occiput)
   ii. Cruciform
   iii. Alar
4. Subaxial ligaments
   i. ALL → along anterior vertebral body
   ii. PLL → along posterior vertebral body
   iii. Ligamentum flavum
        Intertransverse
        Interspinous   } connect the posterior elements
        Supraspinous

V. Nerve Roots

Eight cervical spinal nerves

VI. Blood Supply

Vertebral arteries through anterior and posterior spinal arteries.

B. THORACIC VERTEBRAE (FIG. 5)

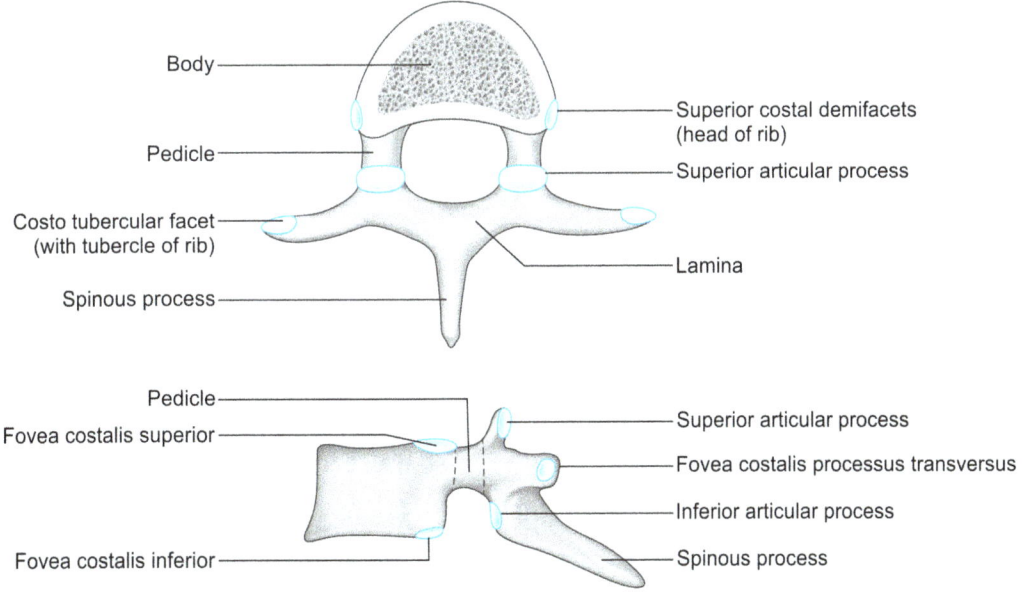

1. Heart-shaped body (viewed superiorly)
2. Vertebral foramen – round
3. Pedicles → Small in diameter (T_4 narrowest)
4. Spinout process – Long and directed downward
5. Laminae → Vertical with "Roof – tile" arrangement.
6. Intervertebral foramen → Larger, less incidence of nerve compression.
7. Body progressively increases in mass from $T_1 → T_{12}$
8. Sagittal alignment → Kyphosis. (Normal = 20–50) (Avg. 33°)
9. Peculiarity of thoracic vertebrae = costal facets

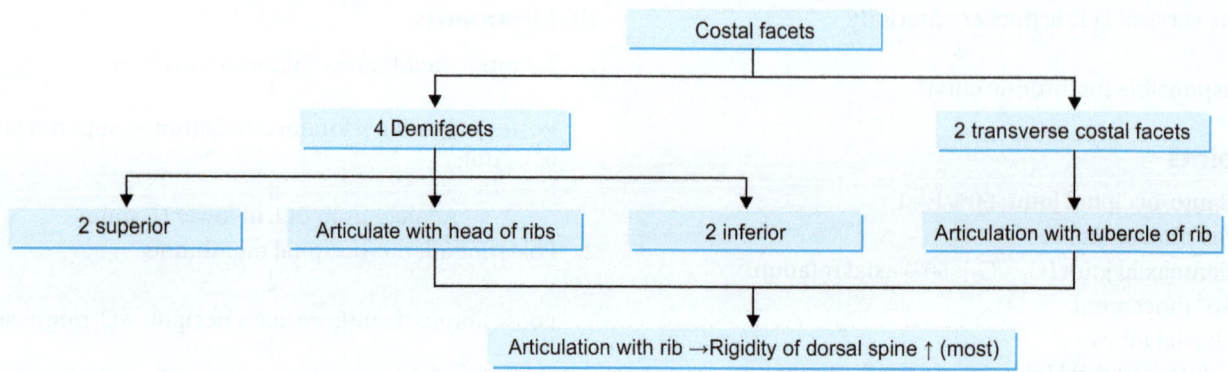

C. LUMBAR VERTEBRAE (FIG. 6)

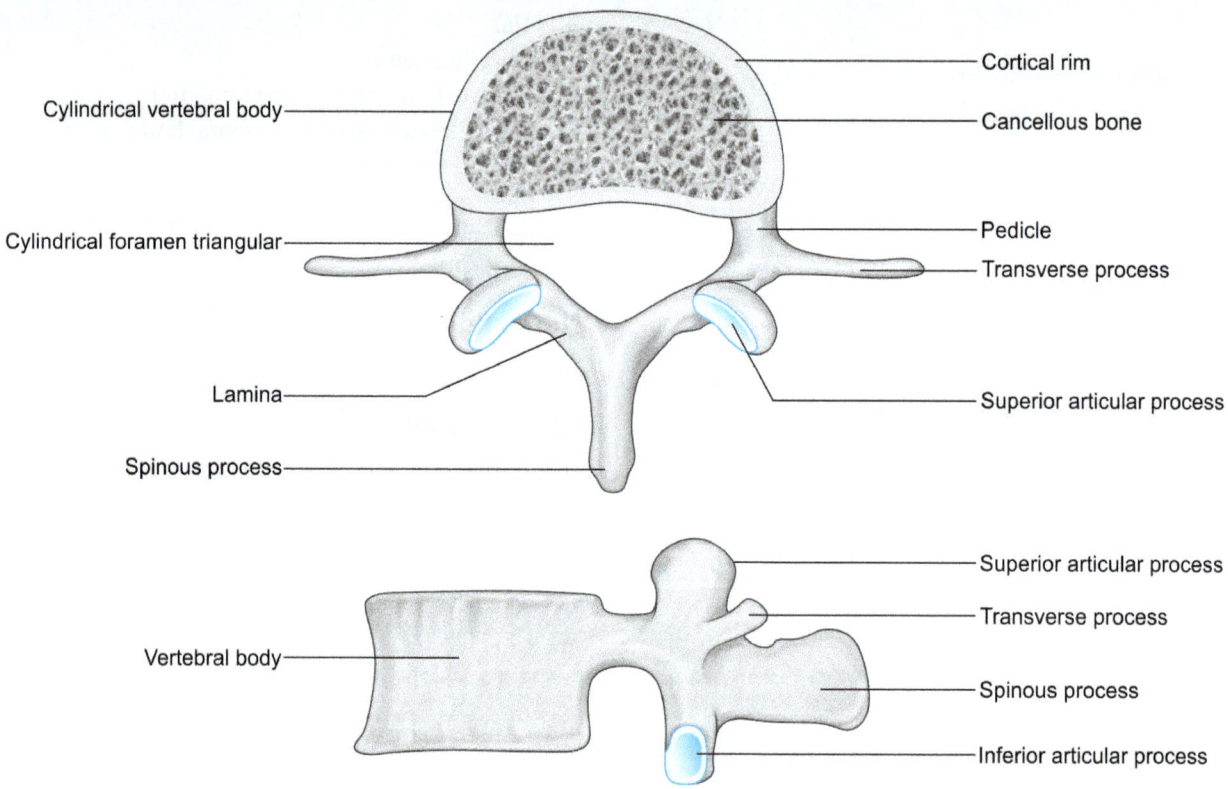

1. Distinguished by their large size - size ↑ from $L_1 \rightarrow L_5$
2. Transverse process → thin long
   ↓
   Exception → L5 → Cone - shape and large
   ↓
   Attachment of iliolumbar ligaments.
3. Pedicles longer and wider than thoracic
4. Spinous process → Horizontal and square shaped.
5. Sagittal alignment → Lumbar Lordosis
6. Apex at L3. (N) → 20 to 40 degrees.
7. Mammillary processes:
   i. Project posteriorly from superior articular facet
   ii. Separate ossification centers
   iii. Attachment for muscles = Multifidus and Intertransversarii.
8. Pars interarticularis →
   i. Mass between superior and inferior articular facets.
   ii. Site for spondylolisthesis (Scotty dog sign)
9. Zygophyseal joints → Facets become more coronal as $L1 \rightarrow L5$.
10. Nerve roots → Exit foramen under the same numbered pedicle
    (L4-L5 intervertebral foramen - L4 nerve root exits, L5 traverses.)

| Central herniation affect Traversing nerve root | Far lateral affects Exiting nerve root. |

D. GENERAL VERTEBRAL COLUMN ANATOMY

1. 33 vertebrae = 7 - Cervical
   - 12 - Thoracic
   - 5 - Lumbar
   - 5 - Sacral
   - 4 - Coccygeal

2. Sagittal alignment

   Primary curves
   Present since in utero
   i. Thoracic kyphosis (20-40°)
   ii. Sacral kyphosis

   Secondary curves
   Acquired as erect posture
   i. Cervical lordosis (20-40°)
   ii. Lumbar lordosis (30-50°)

3. Dennis 3 column theory **(Fig. 7)**

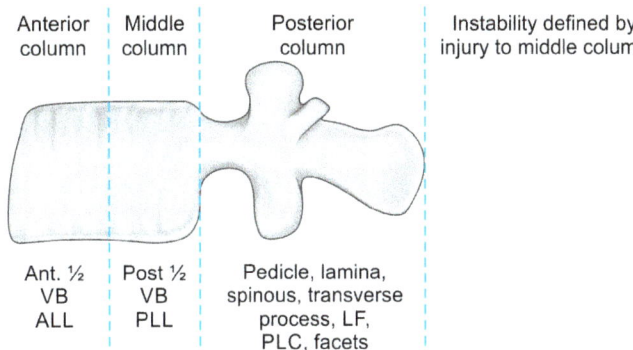

Anterior column	Middle column	Posterior column	Instability defined by injury to middle column
Ant. ½ VB ALL	Post ½ VB PLL	Pedicle, lamina, spinous, transverse process, LF, PLC, facets	

4. Blood supply:

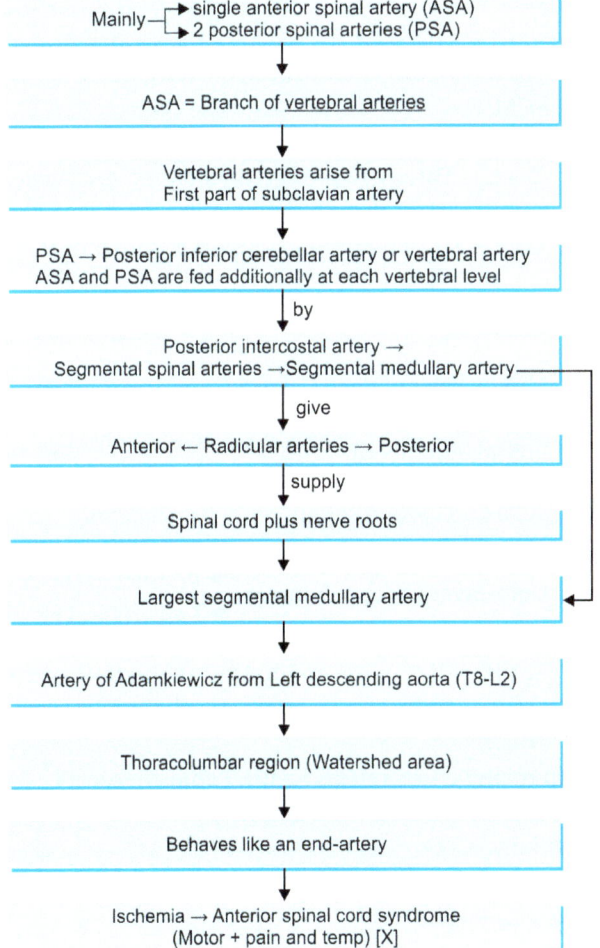

E. LIGAMENTUM FLAVUM (LF) (YELLOW LIGAMENT)

1. Series of ligaments that connect the ventral parts of laminae of adjacent vertebrae.
2. Begins at junction of axis and C_3
   ↓
   $L_5 - S_1$
3. The posterior atlanto-occipital membrane
   ↓
   Loose fibrous tissue lower end of occiput → posterior C_1 ring
   ↓
   Continues below as LF **(Fig. 8)**.

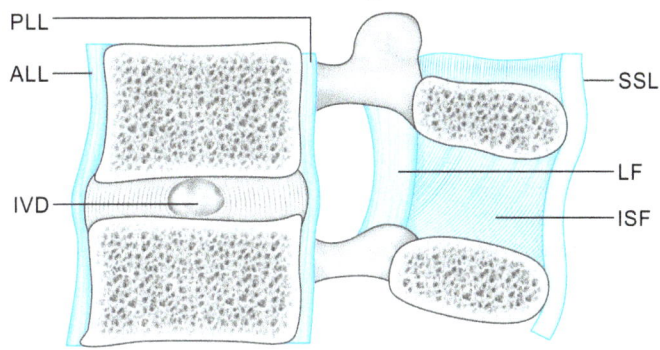

4. The gap in midline of LF → veins exit.
   ↓
   Connect internal → posterior external plexus.
5. From anterior and inferior aspect of the cephalad lamina **(Fig. 9)**.

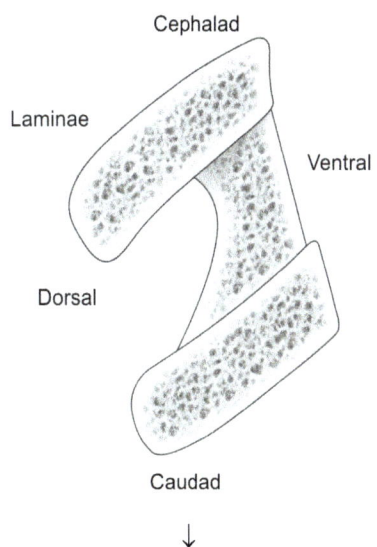

↓
Posterior and superior caudal lamina

6. LF → 80% Elastin 20% Collagen
   ↓
   With ageing elastin decreases
   ↓
   Hypertrophy of LF
   ↓
   Buckling → Spinal stenosis

7. The lateral portion of LF → Contributes to the capsule of facet joints.
8. LF thickens normally as it progresses from C_2 → Sacrum
9. Function:
    i. Maintain upright posture.
    ii. Permit and limit flexion of spine by allowing ↑ interlaminar distance.

SPINAL APPROACHES

Cervical	Dorsal	Lumbar
Anterior	Anterior	Anterior

1. Transoral
2. Retropharyngeal
3. Smith-Robinson ($C_3 - C_7$ anterior)
4. Anterolateral $C_3 - C_7$ (Bruneau and Chibaro)
5. Cervicothoracic junction ($C_7 - T_1$)
  i. Low anterior cervical approach
  ii. High transthoracic
  iii. Trans-sternal
	1. Transthoracic
	2. VATS
	3. Thoracolumbar approach
		1. Retroperitoneal
		2. Percutaneous lateral approach.
		3. Transperitoneal approach to $L_5 - S_1$
		4. Video assisted lumbar surgery

Posterior → midline 1. Occiput to C_2 2. $C_3 - C_7$	Posterior 1. Posterior midline. 2. Costotransversectomy	Posterior 1. Midline 2. Paraspinal (Wiltse) 3. Sacrum and sacroiliac jt. (Ebrahim et al.)

I. CERVICAL

A. Anterior

1. Transoral (Spetzler) (Fig. 10)

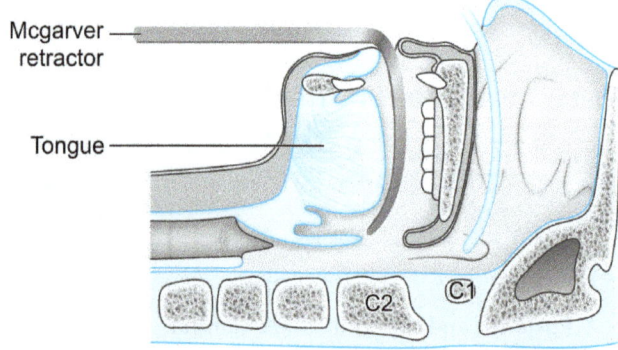

   i. Occiput to C_3
   ii. Skeletal traction with Gardner well tongs.
   iii. After palpating anterior ring of C_1
        ↓
   iv. Incision in the wall of posterior pharynx $C_1 → C_3$

2. Retropharyngeal (Mc Afee et al.)
    i. Entirely extramucosal → Less wound complications and infection.
    ii. Occiput to C_3
    iii. Right-sided transverse incision in the submandibular region with a vertical extension as required.
    iv. Carotid sheath laterally and the larynx and pharynx medially.
    v. Neurovascular structures and muscles encountered.
        1. Branches of facial nerve: Retracted
        2. Retromandibular vein: Ligand
        3. Submandibular gland: Resected.
        4. Digastric muscles: Divided
        5. Hypoglossal nerve ⎫ Retracted
        6. Superior laryngeal nerve ⎭
3. Smith-Robinson (Fig. 11)

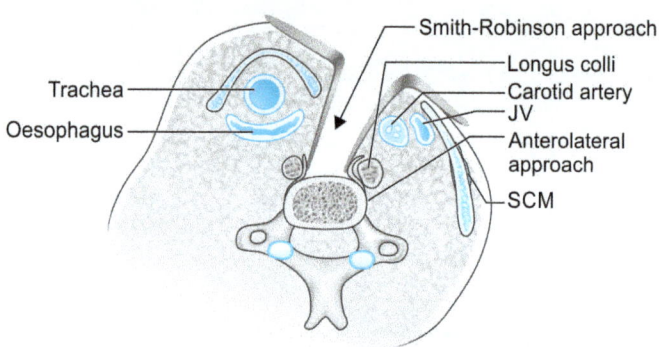

   i. Transverse incision centered over medial border of SCM.
   ii. Left-sided → ↓ risk of injury to RLN
   iii. $C_3 - C_5$: Three – four fingerbreaths above clavicle.
   iv. $C_5 - C_7$: Two – three fingerbreaths above clavicle.
   v. Skin → SC → Platysma → anterior Border of SCM
      ↓
      Superficial layer of deep C. fascia
      ↓
      Middle layer of deep C. fascia
      ↓
      Retract omohyoid ⎡→ Cephalad for below C_5
                      ⎣→ Caudad for above C_5
   vi. SCM and carotid sheath retracted – laterally
   vii. Thyroid, esophagus, trachea – medially
   viii. Deep layer of deep C. fascia ⎡→ Pretracheal fascia
                                      ⎣→ Prevertebral fascia
   ix. Longus colli → Reflect subperiosteally.
   x. Restrict dissection medial to uncinate process → prevents injury to sympathetic chain and vertebral artery.
4. Anterolateral → Same as Smith-Robinson except, Plane is between SCM laterally and carotid sheath medially.
5. High transthoracic – Peri-scapular incision. Remove 3rd rib → $C_6 - T_4$ interval

6. Transsternal approach
   Vertical incision from suprasternal notch to just below xiphoid process.
   ↓
   Split sternum using Gigli saw
   ↓
   $C_4 - T_4$

7.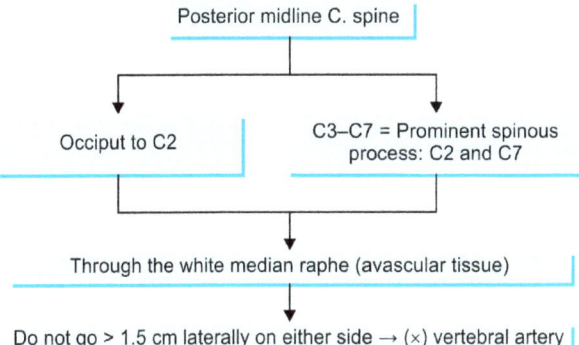

II. THORACIC SPINE
A. Anterior

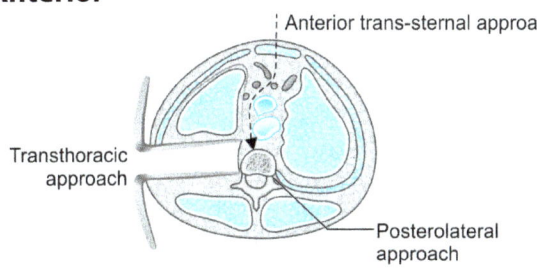

1. Trans thoracic – (**Fig. 12**)
   i. Direct access $T_2 - L_2$
   ii. Left-sided thoracotomy incision preferred
   ↓
   Heart retracted anteriorly
   iii. Right sided → Liver obstacle to exposure
   iv. Level of incision → At or above the level involved segment in the intercostal space.
   ↓
   Rib at the level removed
   Advantages:
   i. Ease of exposure
   ii. Rib graft
   v. If multiple levels involved
   ↓
   Ribs of the proximal level resected.
   ↓
   Because of normal thoracic kyphosis,
   ↓
   Dissection is easier proximal to distal.
   vi. Incise the parietal pleura and reflect it to expose the spine.
   ↓
   Plane developed between aorta and VB, after retraction of lungs.

   vii. Anterior approach is hazardous with complications > post approach.
2. VATS
3. Thoracolumbar → Curvilinear incision, Resect 10th rib, transpleural.

B. Posterior

1. Posterior midline:
   i. Prone position
   ii. Confirm level using C-arm
   iii. Standard midline longitudinal exposure with reflection of the erector spinae laterally up to the tip of transverse process.
2. Costotransversectomy (**Fig. 13**)

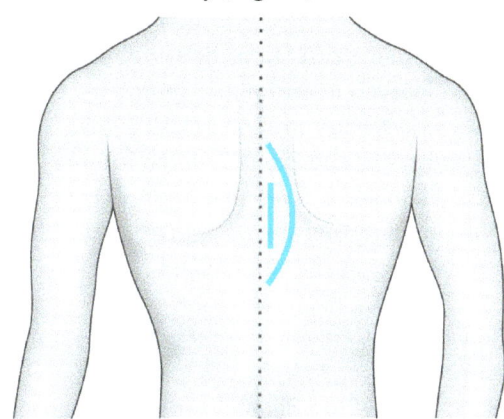

   i. For direct access to the transverse processes and pedicles.
   ii. Incision = Straight, long incision 5 cm lateral to spinous process or curved incision with apex lateral to midline.
   Skin → subcut → trapezius → lumbosacral fascia
   ↓
   Sharp dissection of paraspinal muscles from their insertion on the ribs. Resect 5 cm of the rib, at the most prominent posterior angle and transverse process. (**Fig. 14**)
   ↓
   Retract the parietal pleura anteriorly.
   ↓
   After completion of the spinal procedure, wound is filled with saline and lungs inflated to check for air-leaks.

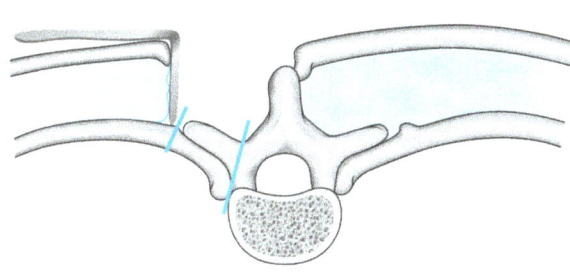

III. LUMBAR

A. Anterior

1. Retroperitoneal (L_1-L_5) **(Fig. 15)**

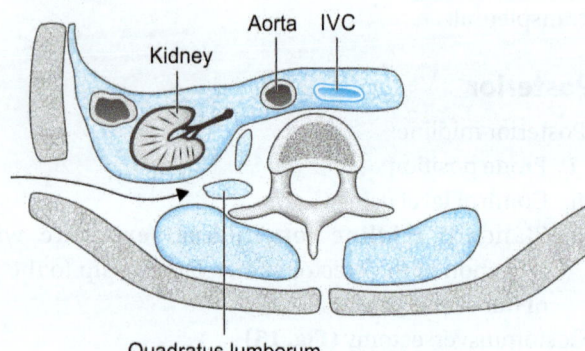

i. For extensive resection, debridement, grafting at multiple levels in the lumbar spine
ii. Lateral decubitus position (R) (side down)
iii. To avoid liver and the IVC which is more difficult to repair than aorta, if vascular injury occurs.
iv. Oblique flank incision → depending on the level of Lumbar spine to be approached,
↓
Between 12th rib and the superior aspect of the iliac crest.
v. Skin → SC → external oblique → Internal oblique → transverse abdominis.
↓
Protect peritoneum and reflect it anteriorly
↓
Elevate psoas muscle bluntly of the vertebra and retract laterally.
vi. Major dissection in this approach is behind the kidney in the potential space between the renal fascia and the quadratus lumborum and psoas muscle **(Fig. 16)**.

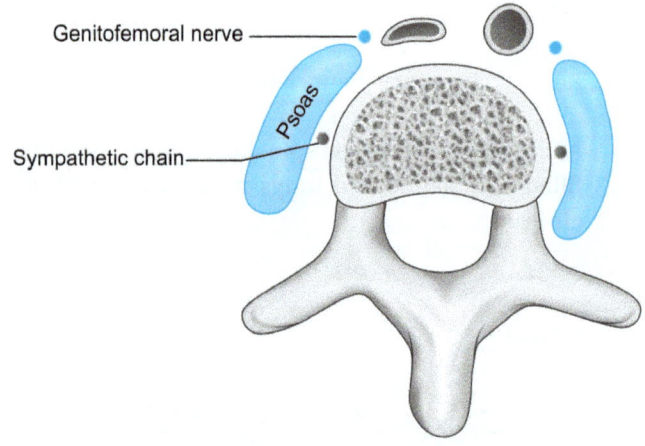

2. Percutaneous lateral approach to lumbar spine:
   i. XLIF: Extreme lateral interbody fusion.
   ii. ALIF: Anterior lumbar interbody fusion

3. Anterior transperitoneal (L_5-S_1)
   i. Indications:
      - L_4 - L_5 ⎫
      - L_5 - S_1 ⎬ fusion
   ii. Position: Supine, Trendelenburg.
   iii. Incision: Midline longitudinal or transverse Pfannenstiel **(Fig. 17)**

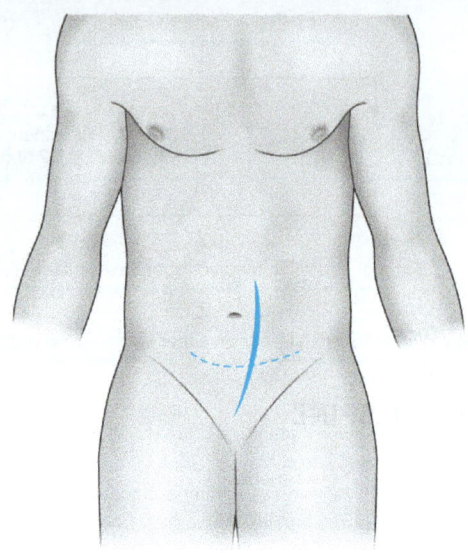

Transverse Pfannenstiel is cosmetically superior and gives excellent exposure:

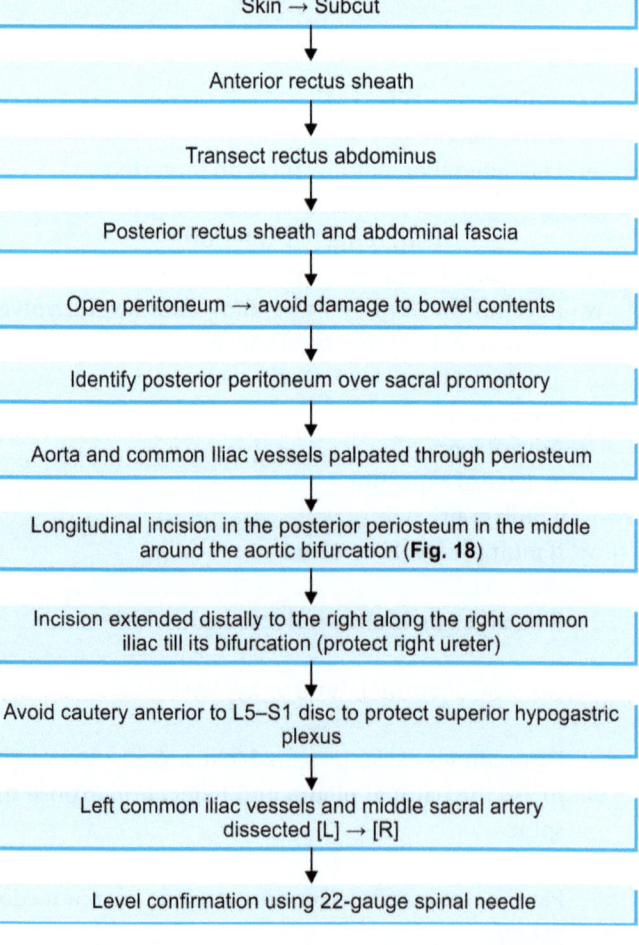

Skin → Subcut
↓
Anterior rectus sheath
↓
Transect rectus abdominus
↓
Posterior rectus sheath and abdominal fascia
↓
Open peritoneum → avoid damage to bowel contents
↓
Identify posterior peritoneum over sacral promontory
↓
Aorta and common Iliac vessels palpated through periosteum
↓
Longitudinal incision in the posterior periosteum in the middle around the aortic bifurcation **(Fig. 18)**
↓
Incision extended distally to the right along the right common iliac till its bifurcation (protect right ureter)
↓
Avoid cautery anterior to L5–S1 disc to protect superior hypogastric plexus
↓
Left common iliac vessels and middle sacral artery dissected [L] → [R]
↓
Level confirmation using 22-gauge spinal needle

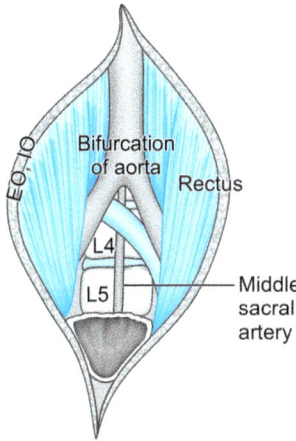

B. Posterior

1. Posterior midline → L₁ - L₅
   Prone, abdomen hanging free → ↓ IV pressure → ↓ Blood loss
   (Collapse of epidural venous plexus)
   Skin → SC → lumbodorsal fascia → tip of SP
   ↓
   Subperiosteally explore the posterior elements from distal to proximal using electrocautery.
2. Paraspinal (Wiltse)
   i. Posterior midline incision.
   ii. Dissect up to lumbodorsal fascia
       ↓
   iii. Fascial incision 2 cm laterally to midline.
       ↓
       Plane between multifidus and longissimus (Sacrospinalis group)
       Useful in removing far - lateral disc herniation, decompressing "far - out syndrome", inserting pedicle screws.

INTERVERTEBRAL DISC: ANATOMY, PHYSIOLOGY AND PROLAPSE

I. ANATOMY

1. *Fibrocartilaginous structure*:
   i. Water (85%)
   ii. Collagen (10-20%)
   iii. Proteoglycan
2. *Consists of*:
   a. Annulus fibrosus
   b. Nucleus pulposus
   c. End plates **(Fig. 19)**

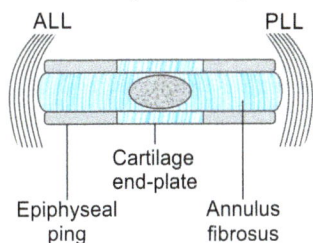
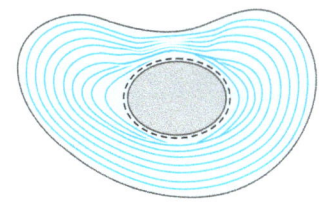

i. Annulus Fibrosus

1. Obliquely oriented, type I collagen arranged in lamellae (thick: anterior and lateral, thin-posterior)
2. High tensile strength → prevents intervertebral distraction
3. High collagen/low proteoglycan ratio

ii. Nucleus Pulposus

1. Gelatinous
2. Notochord remnant.
3. Type II collagen.
4. 88% water
5. Low collagen/high proteoglycan ratio
   ↓
   Hydrophilic → react with water and resist compression
   ↓
   Maintain vertebral height.
6. Aggrecan → Proteoglycan responsible for high water content of disc.

iii. End Plates
   → Bony
   → Cartilaginous
1. Bilayer of cartilage → separates IVD from vertebral body.
2. Growth plate of VB in childhood
   ↓
   Adults → thin, avascular layer of hyaline cartilage.

II. FUNCTION OF DISC

1. Allows spinal motion and provide stability.
2. Links adjacent vertebral bodies
3. Responsible for 25% of vertebral height.
4. Supports axial load of the body.
5. Shock absorbing system
6. Assists in maintaining normal curve of each spinal region.

III. BLOOD SUPPLY

1. Avascular - capillaries terminate at end plates
2. Diffusion of nutrients through pores.

IV. NERVE SUPPLY

1. DRG gives sinuvertebral nerve
2. Innervates the superficial fibers of AF
3. No nerve fiber beyond superficial layer.

V. BIOMECHANICS

1. Creep - allows deformity over time.
2. Hysteresis - allows energy absorption with repetitive axial compression.
3. Stresses: AF → Tensile
   NP → Compressile
   ↓
   Intradiscal Pressure
   Position dependent → Sitting > standing > lying supine

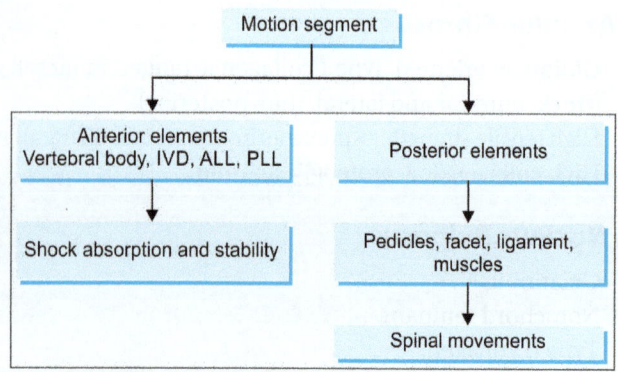

1. Basic functional unit of spine.
2. 2 adjacent vertebrae and intervening soft tissues.
3. Actively controlled by muscles
   Passively → ligaments

VI. DISC AGING (DEGENERATION)

Decrease in:
1. Water content → due to break-up of aggrecan
2. Nutritional transport
3. Absolute no. of viable cells
4. Proteoglycans
5. pH

Increase in:
1. Keratin/chondroitin sulfate ratio
2. Lactate
3. Degradative enzyme activity
4. Density of fibroblast-like cells
→ No change in absolute quantity of collagen.

SPECTRUM OF DEGENERATIVE SPINE DISEASE

1. Internal disc disruption
2. Disc herniation
3. Degenerative spondylolisthesis
4. Spinal stenosis
5. Adult spinal deformities

I. Pathophysiology

Internal disc disruption
↓
Disc herniation
↓
Decreased intervertebral space (loss of disc height)
↓ uneven stress on annulus
Overloading of facet joints, ligament instability.
↓
Instability of motion segment
↓
Attempt to stabilize by osteophyte formation and ligament hypertrophy
↓
Spinal stenosis
Kirkaldy – Willis
Dysfunction → Instability → Stability

II. Etiology

1. Repetitive mechanical stress (activities)
2. Sedentary lifestyle
3. Obesity
4. Traumatic injury
5. Tobacco
6. Genetic factors

III. Disc Herniation

1. Lumbar > cervical
2. $L_5 - S_1$ MC, $C_5 - C_6$ MC
3. Age = 30–40 years
4. M:F = 3:1

IV. Anatomic Classification (Fig. 20)

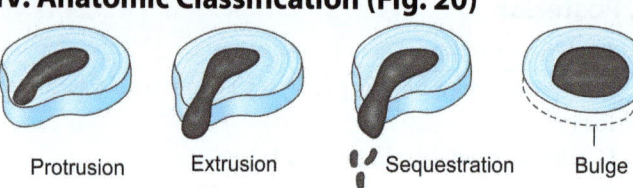

1. *Protusion:* Herniated portion of disc covered with thin layer of annulus
2. *Extrusion:* Nucleus pulposus herniated through AF → but continuous with disc space.
3. *Sequestration:* NP herniates through AF → No longer continuous with disc space.
4. *Bulge/prolapse:* >50% circumferential herniation (Generalized) with covering of annulus.

V. Location

1. Central ⎯ Back pain
            ⎯ Cauda equina
2. Paracentral (posterolateral)
   i. Most common → 90–95%
      ↓
   ii. As PLL is weakest here
   iii. Affects traversing nerve root in lumbar region
3. Forminal (Far lateral, extra foraminal)
   Exiting nerve root (**Fig. 21**).

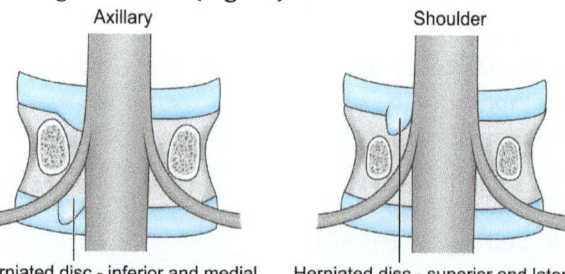

CERVICAL SPONDYLOSIS

I. INTRODUCTION

1. Spondylosis refers to age related degenerative changes in the spinal column.

2. Most patients are > 40 years
3. 3 main symptom complexes:
   i. Axial neck pain → Pain along the spinal column and its related paraspinal musculature.
   ii. Cervical Radiculopathy → Pain radiating to the arm with sensory or motor changes in radicular distribution
   iii. Cervical Myelopathy → Developmental of long tract signs as a result of degenerative changes at the cervical spinal column.

II. PATHOPHYSIOLOGY

1.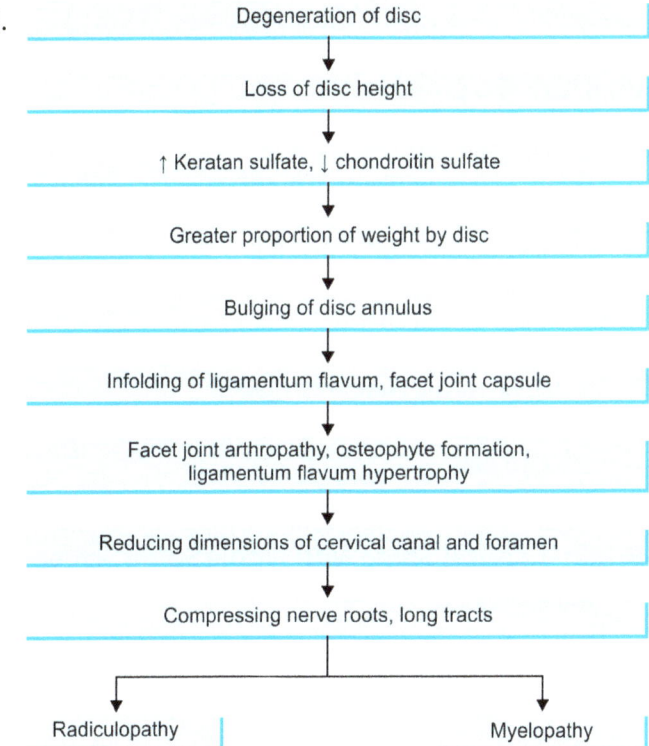

2. Kirkaldy-Willis theory of disc degeneration
   Dysfunction → Instability → Stability

III. ETIOLOGY

A. Radiculopathy

1. Disc Herniation
2. Double Crush syndrome - A combination of cervical root compression and distal nerve compression.
   Nerve root compression leads to ↓ axoplasmic flow → Predisposes to peripheral entrapment syndromes in the downstream nerves.
3. Intra and extraspinal tumors
4. Cysts → Synovial, meningeal

B. Myelopathy

1. Congenital and acquired stenosis
2. Ossified posterior longitudinal ligament (OPLL)
3. Ossified ligamentum flavum (OLF)
4. Epidural abscess
5. Trauma
6. Cervical Kyphosis
7. Cervical tumors

IV. CLINICAL FEATURES

A. Symptoms

1. Neck pain
2. Radicular arm pain
3. Gait and balance abnormalities
4. Fine motor control is affected:
   i. Handwriting
   ii. Manipulate buttons, zippers
5. Poor hand grip
6. Proximal group of muscles > distal
7. Difficulty in rising out of chair/going up stairs
8. UL affected more than LL → Central cord syndrome

B. Examination

i. Restricted neck extension (↓ROM)
ii. LMN signs at the level of lesion and UMN signs below level of lesion
iii. Radiculopathy signs: Dermatomyotomal distribution of neurological symptoms - Numbness, motor weakness, Hyper/hyporeflexia.
   1. *Reflexes*:
      i. C5-Biceps
      ii. C6-Brachioradialis
      iii. C7-Triceps
      iv. L4-Knee
      v. S1-Ankle
   2. Dermatomes (**Figs. 22 and 23**)

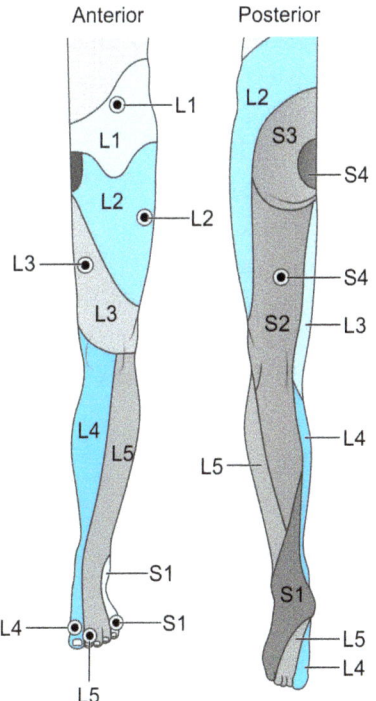

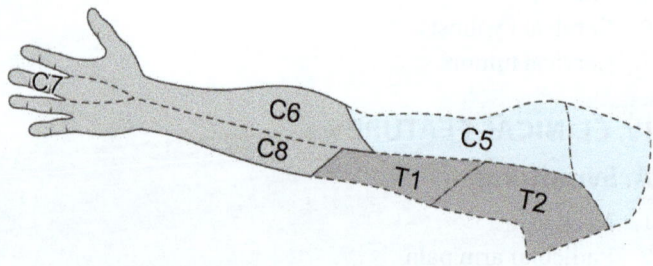

3. Myotomes

Upper limb myotomes		Lower limb myotomes	
Shoulder abduction	C5	Hip flexion	L1, 2
Elbow flexion	C5, 6	Hip extension	L5, S1
Elbow extension	C7	Knee flexion	L5, S1
Wrist extension	C7	Knee extension	L3, 4
Wrist flexion	C8	Ankle dorsiflexion	L4
Finger extension	C7	Ankle plantarflexion	S1, 2
Finger flexion	C8	1st metatarsal extension	L5
Finger abduction	T1		

iv. *Myelopathic signs*:
1. Weakness of upper and lower limbs
2. Myelopathic hand
3. Loss of manual dexterity
4. Finger escape sign: Fingers kept in extension and adduction →
   Little finger abducts spontaneously due to weakness of intrinsic muscles
5. Grip and release test +: Fails to make fist and release 20 times in 10 seconds.
6. Loss of proprioception (Dorsal column affected) → +ve Romberg test
7. Upper motor neuron signs:
   i. Spasticity → Clasp-knife
   ii. Inverted radial reflex
   iii. Hoffman reflex +ve
   iv. Clonus (>3 beats)
   v. Babinski +ve → Dorsiflexion of great toe
8. Bowel and Bladder abnormalities
9. Wide based spastic myelopathic gait

v. *Special tests*:
1. Spurling's sign
2. Shoulder abduction test – relieves symptoms
3. Lhermitte's sign → Cervical flexion ⎫
4. Reverse Lhermitte's sign → Cervical extension ⎬ Electric shock like sensations that extension Radiate down the spine and extremities
5. Upper limb tension tests

V. CLASSIFICATION OF MYELOPATHY

1. Nurick Classification
   1. Based on gait and ambulatory function

Nurick Classification	
Grade 0	Root symptoms only or normal
Grade I	Signs of cord compression; normal gait
Grade II	Gait difficulties but fully employed
Grade III	Gait difficulties prevent employment, walks unassisted
Grade IV	Unable to walk without assistance
Grade V	Wheelchair or bedbound

VI. RADIOLOGY

A. Radiology Radiography

1. Loss of cervical lordosis → Straightening or kyphosis
2. Kyphosis angle
3. Disc space narrowing
4. End plate sclerosis
5. Osteophyte formation
6. Facet arthrosis
7. Flexion extension views → Instability
8. Torg ratio (Pavlov's ratio) = $\dfrac{\text{Spinal canal diameter}}{\text{Mid-cervical body diameter}}$
   (Lateral X-ray)
   Canal Stenosis → < 0.8

B. MRI–Cervical Spine with Whole Spine Screening

1. Disc herniation
2. Hypertrophy, buckling of ligamentum flavum
3. Degree of cord compression
4. Cord edema
5. Myelomalacia → Bright signal in cord on T2 images
6. Cervical canal and foraminal stenosis
7. Visualization of soft tissue
8. Syrinx formation
9. Tandem stenosis → Cervical + Lumbar canal stenosis **(Fig. 24)**
10. Compression ratio =
    (Axial) $\dfrac{\text{Smallest anteroposterior diameter of spinal cord} \times 100}{\text{Largest transverse diameter of spinal cord}}$

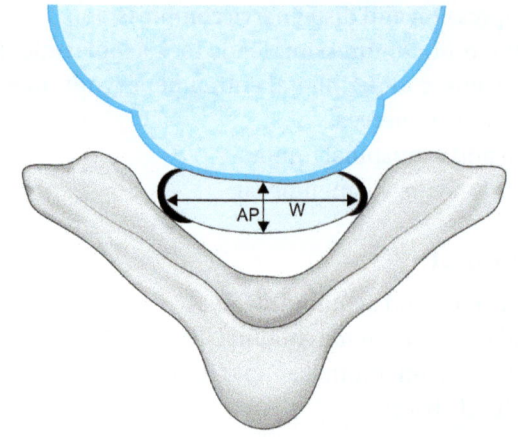

C. CT Scan

1. Assessment of bony anomalies.
2. Angiography: Preoperatively to identify course of vertebral artery.
3. Myelography: Replaced by MRI. Indicated when MRI is contraindicated

VII. TREATMENT
A. Conservative

Mild disease with no functional impairment

1. Medications → NSAIDS, Pregabalin, Gabapentin, Methylcobalamin, Nortriptyline
2. Physiotherapy → Neck strengthening, balance and gait training
3. Cervical Traction
4. Selective nerve root steroid injections → Pure radiculopathy symptoms

B. Surgical

1. *Indications*:
    i. Balance and gait abnormalities
    ii. Fine motor difficulty
    iii. Intractable pain
    iv. Degree of cord compression
    v. Patients with rapid neurologic deterioration
    vi. Severe cervical kyphosis
    vii. Cervical instability
2. *Approach and options*:
    i. Posterior approach:
        a. Multilevel laminectomy
        b. Laminectomy + Fusion
        c. Laminoplasty
    ii. Anterior approach:
        a. Anterior cervical discectomy + fusion (ACDF) - 1 level disease
        b. Anterior Cervical Corpectomy + fusion with strut graft (ACCF) - 2 or more levels
        c. Corpectomy + anterior column reconstruction with anterior cervical plating
    iii. Circumferential – Both anterior and posterior

	Anterior approach	Posterior approach
Advantages	1. Direct decompression 2. Stabilization with arthrodesis 3. Correction of deformity 4. Good axial pain relief	1. Less loss of motion 2. Familiarity 3. Less bracing needed 4. Avoids grafts complications
Disadvantages	1. Technically demanding 2. Loss of motion 3. Graft complications 4. Need for postoperative bracing 5. Adjacent segment degeneration	1. Indirect compression 2. Postoperative instability 3. Inconsistent axial pain results.
Preferred in	1. One-two level disease 2. Pre-op uncorrectable kyphosis 3. Focal anterior pathology 4. Disc Herniation	1. Three or more level disease 2. Obese patient → Difficulty in anterior approach 3. Surgeon experience and preference 4. Developmental Stenosis 5. OPLL 6. Focal posterior compression (ligamentum flavum) 7. Previously operated anterior approach 8. Elderly 9. Comorbidities

iv. **Laminoplasty:**
   a. Posterior elements are preserved by making a hinge.
   b. Fusion-less surgery → No loss of motion
   c. Indications:
      1. Younger patient < 70 years
      2. Minimal kyphosis (<15°) to Lordosis
      3. Smoker/risk of nonunion
      4. Types → i. Open door, ii. Modified French door
   d. Contraindications:
      1. >15° kyphosis
      2. Segmental instability
      3. Severe axial neck pain
      4. Previous posterior surgery done

v. Foraminotomy → Anterior or posterior→ unilateral pure radiculopathy

vi. Cervical disc arthroplasty → Single level disease with no arthrosis

VIII. COMPLICATIONS
A. Anterior Approach

1. Dysphagia
2. Recurrent laryngeal nerve palsy
3. Superior laryngeal nerve palsy
4. Horner's syndrome:
    i. Ptosis
    ii. Miosis
    iii. Anhidrosis

5. Durotomy (CSF leak)
6. Airway obstruction from edema, hematoma
7. Injury to vertebral artery
8. Graft complications like fracture, dislodgement.

B. Posterior Approach
1. Wound complications (Infection)
2. CSF leak
3. Instability postoperative
4. Vertebral artery injury
5. C_5 motor root palsy
6. Pulmonary complications
7. Venous thromboembolic events

SPONDYLOLYSIS AND SPONDYLOLISTHESIS

I. INTRODUCTION
1. Forward translation of one vertebra on another in sagittal plane of the spine → Spondylolisthesis
2. Spondylolysis: Defect in the par interarticularis of lumbar vertebra
   ↓
   Region between the superior and inferior articular process of the vertebra.

II. CLASSIFICATION
A. Wiltse
I. *Dysplastic/congenital (20%)*:
   i. Only at $L_5 - S_1$ → Aplasia/dysplasia of facet joint
   ii. No pars IA defect.
   iii. Associated with spina bifida
   iv. F > M, strict genetic predisposition
   v. Symptoms begin → adolescent growth spurt
II. *Isthmic (50%)*:
   A - Lytic - stress fracture
   B - Healed - Elongated, intact
   C - Acute fracture.
     i. Due to repetitive cyclical extension and torsion of spine
     ii. R.F → Gymnasts, football, dancing
     iii. L5 - S1 → MC site L5 Pars defect
     iv. M > F, 1ST - 2nd decade of life < 15 years
III. *Degenerative*:
   i. Intersegmental instability of long duration → Incompetence of facet joints.
   ii. Etiopathogenesis - 2 theories

   Sagittal facet theory → **Disc degeneration theory**
   ↓   ↓ Disc height loss → Facet
   Facet orientation   overload → Accelerated
   facilitates intra-   arthritis 2° remodeling
   translation forces   → Anterolisthesis

   iii. >45 years, most common L4 - L5 > L5 - S1 (6 times), F > M (6 times)
IV. *Traumatic* - Fracture of the vertebra → not through pars (pedicle, laminae, etc.)
V. *Pathologic* → Local - Metastasis
              → Systemic - RA, OI
VI. *Iatrogenic*:
   Post - Sx → Posterior Elements

B. Meyerding – % of Slip
I <25%
II 25–50%
III – 50–75%
IV 75–100%
V Spondyloptosis

III. CLINICAL FEATURES
1. Wide spectrum
2. Maybe asymptomatic → Spondylosis
3. Onset of dysplastic and isthmic → Childhood and Adolescence
4. Onset of Degenerative → >50 years
5. Low back pain → Most consistent symptom
6. Neurogenic claudication
7. Radiating pain
8. Postural deformity, transverse abdominal crease
9. Hamstring tightness
10. Paraspinal muscle spasm
11. Step-off palpated
12. Tenderness at the level. Rotatory → instability
13. Neurologic deficit
14. EHL weakness → L_5 MC radiculopathy
15. Quadriceps
    ↓Knee reflexes L_4
16. Cauda Equina - Rare
17. ↓ Lumbar flexion and extension.
18. Altered gait → Trendelenburg, Crouch
19. Popliteal angle - Hamstring tightness
20. Phalen–Dickson sign → Hip and knee flexed position
    ↓
    Lumbosacral kyphosis, hyperlordotic, upper lumbar, waddling gait.
21. Stork (One leg hyperextension test)
    Pain → Spondylolysis (+)
22. Buttocks: Flat, heart shaped in severe due to sacral prominence.
23. SLRL, cross SLRT ±
24. Scoliosis → muscle spasm

IV. RADIOLOGY
A. X-ray
1. Oblique LS → Scotty dog sign = Spondylolysis (**Fig. 25**)

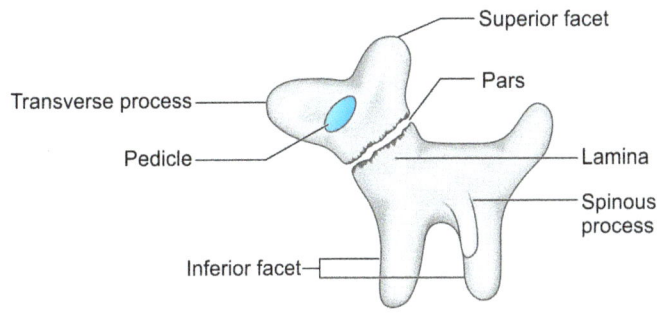

2. Lateral X-ray → % → Meyerding
3. Slip angle = In dysplastic spondylolisthesis **(Fig. 26)**

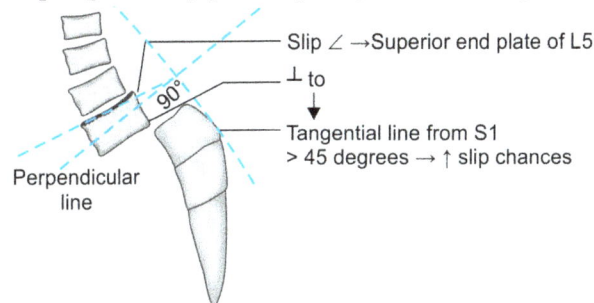

4. Flexion - Extension → spinal instability
   ↓
   >4 mm translation
   > 15° rotation.
5. AP → Inverted Napoleon hat sign
6. Pelvic incidence = pelvic tilt + sacral slope **(Fig. 27)**

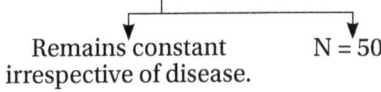

Remains constant   N = 50
irrespective of disease.

7. Degenerative spondylolisthesis → Facet arthropathy, ↓ Disc height, osteophytes.

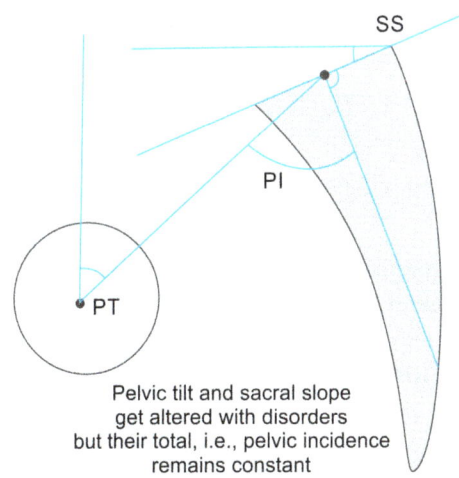

B. CT

1. Better delineate anatomy of pars defect
2. Surgery planning

C. MRI – Neural Elements

1. Canal/foramen stenosis
2. Nerve root impingement
3. LF hypertrophy, buckling

V. MANAGEMENT

Depends on → Age
→ Extent of slip
→ Severity of symptoms

A. Conservative

1. Rest
2. NSAIDs
3. Activity modification → weight
4. PT → Abdo and back strength exercises (Hamstring)
5. Lumbar corset.
6. Degenerative → Epidural steroids

B. Operative

1. *Indications*:
   i. Failed conservative management × 6 months
   ii. Neurological deficit
   iii. Radicular pain with nerve root comp. not responding to nonsurgical
   iv. Dysplastic and Isthmic → High grade slip, ↑↑ Lumbosacral kyphosis ↑ slip angle
   v. Cauda Equina.
2. *Goals of surgery*:
   i. To relieve pain
   ii. Stabilize spine
   iii. Maximize patient function
3.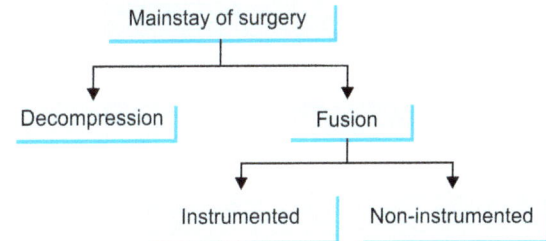

   i. Fusion → PLIF, TLIF, ALIF → Revision Cases and MIS Techniques   Bone Grafting
   ii. Dysplastic/Isthmic → Pars interarticularis repair
      Screws
      Tension wiring
      Sublaminar hooks
      or
      $L_5 - S_1$ Posterolateral fusion
   iii. Spondyloptosis → Gaines procedure
      Resection of L_5, $L_4 - S_1$ fusion

VI. COMPLICATIONS

1. Pseudoarthrosis
2. Adjacent segment disease
3. SSI
4. Neurodeficit → L_5 MC
5. Dural tear
6. Hardware failure
7. Slip progression

LUMBAR CANAL STENOSIS

I. INTRODUCTION
1. Narrowing of the vertebral canal, lateral recess and/or intervertebral foramina.
2. Most commonly occurs as a result of chronic degenerative changes at the lumbar motion segment.

II. ETIOPATHOGENESIS
A. Pathoanatomy
1. Normal lumbar canal cross sectional area = 150–200 mm^2
2.

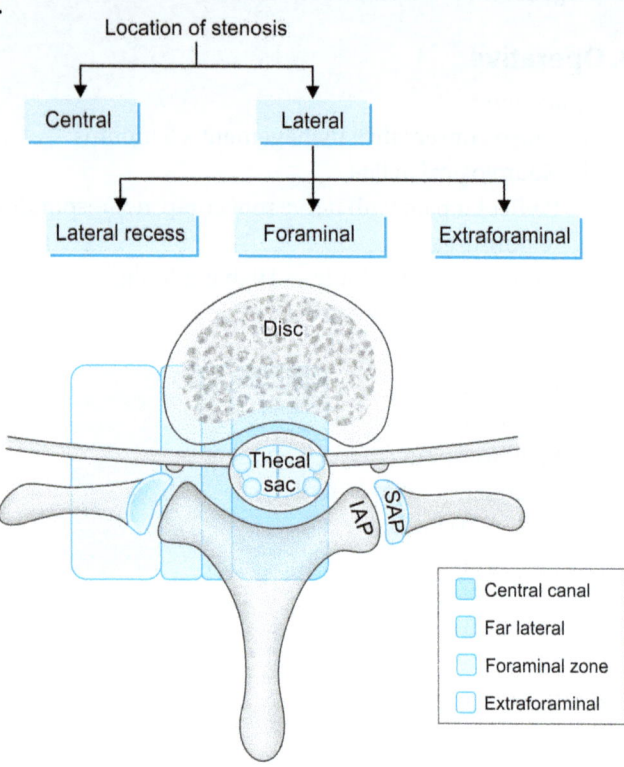

B. Etiological Classification
Etiological Classification of Lumbar Spinal Stenosis

- **Congenital/Development**
1. Degenerative—age related
2. Achondroplasia
3. Congenital small spinal canal
4. Congenital meningeal cysts
5. Osteoporosis

- **Acquired**
1. Degenerative—age related
2. Degenerative spondylolytic/spondylolisthesis
3. Degenerative scoliosis
4. Ankylosing spondylitis
5. Rheumatoid arthritis
6. Pseudogout
7. Acromegaly
8. Diffuse idiopathic skeletal hyperostosis (DISH)
9. Iatrogenic—Postdiscectomy/laminectomy/fusion, scarring/fibrosis postchemonucleolysis
10. Malunited vertebral fractures
11. Spinal infections with abscess bone collapse
12. Paget's disease
13. Fluorosis
14. Pseudogout

- **Combined**

C. Pathophysiology
1. Kirkaldy-Willis theory

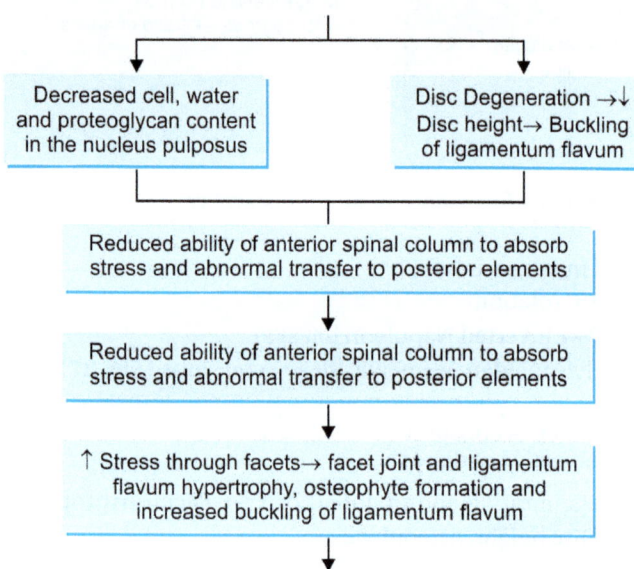

III. CLINICAL FEATURES
A. Symptoms
1. Back Pain
2. Leg pain
3. Difficulty in walking long distances due to pain
4. Numbness and heaviness in the legs

B. Examination
1. Neurogenic Claudication
2. Pain ↑ on extension and ↓ on flexion
3. Tenderness → Over lumbar spinous process and facet joints
4. Decreased sensations → Dermatomal
5. Weakness → ↓ Power ±
6. Findings in LCS are usually non-specific and vague.
7. Root tensions signs are usually negative
8. Can present rarely as Cauda Equina Syndrome

IV. INVESTIGATIONS
A. Radiograph
1. Loss of lumbar lordosis
2. Disc space narrowing
3. Osteophytes
4. Degenerative scoliosis
5. Degenerative spondylolisthesis
6. Flexion and Extension views → Instability

B. MRI
1. Investigation of choice
2. Ligamentum flavum hypertrophy
3. Facet joint arthropathy
4. Disc degeneration and herniation
5. Compression of lateral recess and/or foramen
6. Mid sagittal lumbar canal diameter
    < 10 mm → Absolute LCS
    10-13 mm → Relative LCS
7. Cross section area of thecal sac < 100 mm^2
8. Nerve Root Sedimentation sign + → Absence of nerve root sedimentation to the dorsal aspect of the Dural sac, thus leading to compression and symptoms.

V. TREATMENT
A. Conservative
1. Treatment is started with conservative therapy as first line, unless there is neurological deficit/Bowel, Bladder involvement.
2. Life style modification
    i. Avoid lifting heavy weights
    ii. Avoid floor level activities
    iii. Weight loss
3. Physiotherapy → Back and Core strengthening exercises
4. Pain medications → Paracetamol, NSAIDS, muscle relaxants and opioids
5. Adjunct medications → Vitamin B12, Pregabalin, Nortriptyline

B. Operative
1. Indications:
    i. Neurological deficit
    ii. Bowel and bladder involvement
    iii. Failure of conservative therapy after treatment for 5-6 months.
2. Neural Decompression → Complete laminectomy, removal of >50% of facets.
3. Instrumentation done along with decompression in cases of spinal instability.

CAUDA EQUINA SYNDROME

I. INTRODUCTION
1. Cauda Equina Syndrome (CES) is caused by the compression of the nerve roots within the thecal sac, present distal to the termination of the spinal cord.
2. Diagnosis must be made clinically.
3. Patient presents with low back pain accompanied by the following:
    i. Perineal Anesthesia or 'saddle' anesthesia
    ii. Flaccid paraparesis—sensory loss or weakness involving lower lumbar roots (asymmetric radiculopathies)
    iii. Loss of bowel/bladder control (urinary retention)
4. Delay in the diagnosis and management can lead to permanent disability of varying degrees including urinary retention, impotence (in males).

II. Anatomy
1. Conus medullaris:
    i. Terminal end of spinal cord
    ii. Present at end lower end plate of L1 vertebrae body or at the level of L1-L2 disc
    iii. Disc herniation at this level causes Conus medullaris syndrome (UMN lesion)
2. Cauda Equina:
    i. Collection of the nerve roots L1-S3 enclosed within the meningeal coverings, each exiting at their respective neural foramina.
    ii. Compression of these nerve roots leads to Cauda Equina syndrome (LMN lesion)

III. ETIOLOGY
1. Lower lumbar disc herniation
2. Lumbar spinal stenosis
3. Spondylolisthesis
4. Epidural hematoma
5. Infections
6. Primary and metastatic neoplasms
7. Trauma
8. Iatrogenic
9. Spinal anesthesia

IV. CLASSIFICATION
A. Tandon and Sankaran described three variations of CES (T and S groups)
    1. Rapid onset without a previous history of back problem
    2. Acute bladder dysfunction with a history of low back pain and sciatica

3. Chronic backache and sciatica with gradually progressing CES often with canal stenosis
B. Clinically, CES can be grouped as follows:
1. CESS (CES suspected or suspicious = bilateral radiculopathy without CES)
2. CESI (CES incomplete = sphincter problems with objective evidence of CES but voluntary control of micturition)
3. CESR (CES retention = patient paralysed, with insensate bladder with incontinence)

V. CLINICAL FEATURES
1. Low back pain - M/C symptom
2. Unilateral > Bilateral leg pain (radiculopathy)
3. Saddle anesthesia

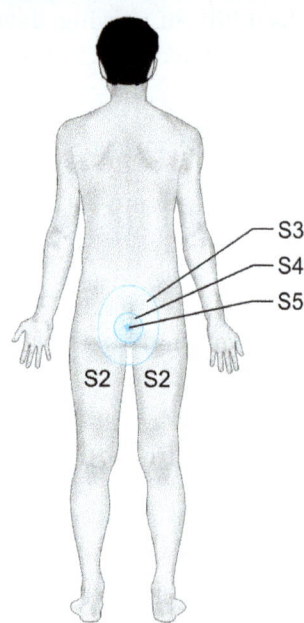

4. Asymmetric sensory changes in the lower limbs
5. Bladder dysfunction leading to urinary retention
6. Sexual dysfunction (Impotence in males)
7. Bowel dysfunction (rarely)
8. O/E:
   i. U/L or B/L motor weakness in lower limbs
   ii. Decreased anal sphincter tone
   iii. U/L or B/L sensory changes in the lower limbs (asymmetric)
   iv. Decreased or absent lower extremity DTR
   v. Decreased or absent BCR
   vi. Decreased or absent Anal wink test (Anal wink test is reflex contraction of anal sphincter upon stimulation the adjacent skin)

VI. RADIOLOGY
1. Radiographs: A/P and Lateral views
   i. Usually normal
   ii. May be helpful in evaluation of fractures leading to CES (rare)

2. MRI:
   i. IOC
   ii. Should be done early if CES is suspected on clinical examination
   iii. CES is a clinical diagnosis, MRI confirms the cause and is important for surgical planning
   iv. Degree of neural compression
   v. Disc prolapse
   vi. Epidural abscess or hematoma
   vii. Space occupying lesion within the neural canal
   viii. Tumors causing compression of the neural structures
3. Urodynamic studies:
   i. Pre-operative and post-operative Post Void Residual Volume (PVR)
   ii. Can detect subtle bladder dysfunction
   iii. They should not delay the decompression
   iv. Normal value of PVR is 50–100 mL

VII. MANAGEMENT
1. Surgical Decompression → Treatment of choice
2. Timing of surgery:
   i. As early as possible, as prognosis becomes more and more guarded with delay
   ii. Preferably within 24–48 hours
3. Technique:
   i. Discectomy with/without instrumentation
   ii. Discectomy and fusion with instrumentation
   iii. Laminectomy with/without posterior instrumentation

VIII. PROGNOSIS
1. CES is an emergency condition and should be managed promptly
2. Delay in diagnosis and management can lead to lifelong devastating complications including urinary retention, impotence (in males)
3. Even with early surgery neurologic recovery is variable
4. There are improved outcomes in bowel and bladder function and resolution of motor and sensory deficits when decompression performed within 48 hours of the onset of symptoms
5. Prognostic factors:
   i. Presence of saddle anesthesia or bladder dysfunction is associated with worse outcomes
   ii. Surgical decompression after 48 hours is associated with worse outcomes

SCOLIOSIS

I. DEFINITION
(by Scoliosis Research Society)
1. "Abnormal lateral curvature of spine measuring >10° on radiograph"
   ↓
2. Associated with rotation of vertebra and thus a 3-dimensional deformity.

II. CLASSIFICATIONS

Scoliosis

I. Nonstructural
1. Postural
2. Compensatory

II. Transient structural
1. Sciatic
2. Hysterical
3. Inflammatory

III. Structural

Structural

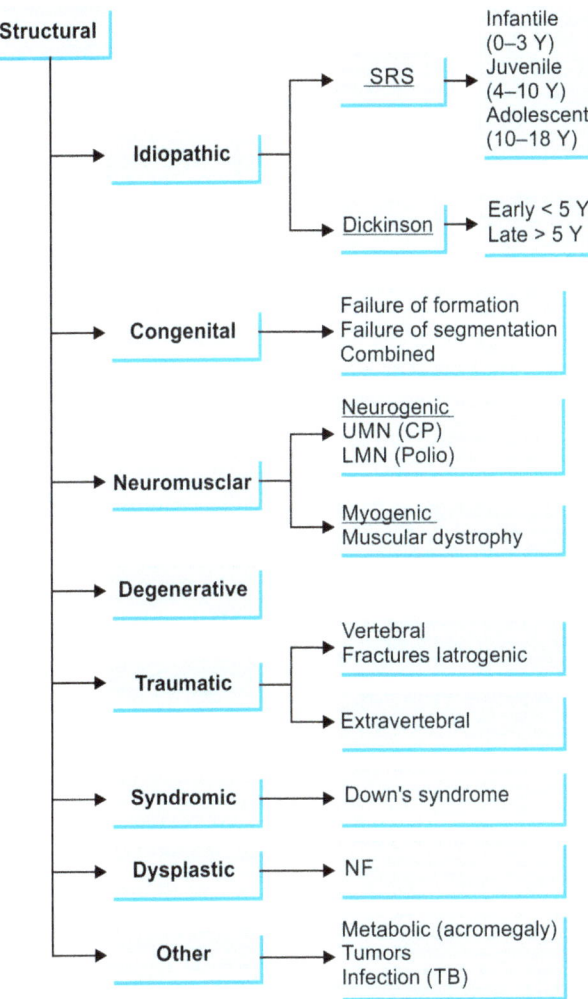

A. Idiopathic

a. **Infantile** *(80-90% - self-resolving)*:
1. 0–3 y
2. Mainly left thoracic
3. Associated with:
   i. DDH
   ii. Congenital heart defect
   iii. Plagiocephaly
   iv. Mental deficiency
4. Risk of progression: < 6 months → low (90% resolve)
   (Increases with) ↓ >1 year → high

   i. >37° Cobbs method
   ii. Associated with complications and 2° curve
   iii. Rib vertebral angle difference (RVAD) (Mehta's angle) **(Fig. 28)**
      a. >20° → Progressive
      b. Measured at apical vertebrae
      c. Angle between vertical line drawn at center of vertebra and line along neck of ribs.

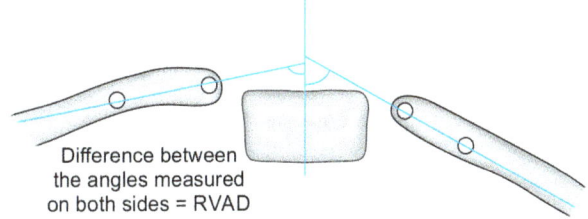

Difference between the angles measured on both sides = RVAD

5. Conservative: Observation→ Cobbs angle <30, RVAD <20
6. Flexible curve → Cobbs >30 and RVAD >20
   i. TSLO
   ii. Risser casting – 3 point bending correction
   iii. Cotrel and Morel → Derotation of rib cage
7. Surgery: Cobbs angle >50
   i. <8 years → Instrumentation only
      Non-fusion: Growing rod construct
      a. Distraction:
         1. VEPTR: Vertical expandable prosthetic titanium ribs
         2. MAGEC: Magnetic Expansion Control (using external remote control)
      b. Guided growth:
         1. Shilla
         2. Modified Luque Trolley
   ii. 8-11 years → Anterior + posterior fusion with or without instrumentation (to prevent crankshaft phenomenon)
      a. Crankshaft → In skeletally immature patients, progression of deformity with ↑ rib prominence inspite of posterior fusion due to continued anterior column growth.
      b. Winter's formula → Shortening of height in cm = 0.7 × number of vertebral bodies fused × number of years of growth remaining.
   iii. >11 years and closed TRC → Posterior fusion and instrumentation.

b. **Juvenile** *(75% Progressive)*:
1. 4-9 years
2. Right Thoracic → 6: 1
3. Risk of progression → High (6°/year at puberty)
4. Surgery same as infantile
   Rule out other diagnosis. For example → Café au lait → NF

Rx.
  i. Observation → Cobbs <20°
  ii. Milwaukee bracing = 20–49°
  iii. Surgery → >50°
c. **Adolescent:**
  1. 10–18 years
  2. MC type of scoliosis
  3. M:F → 1:6
  4. Right thoracic → 8:1
  5. Etiological factors:
      i. Genetics → Positive family history
      ii. Neuromuscular factors
      iii. Hormonal and metabolic dysfunction (↓ melatonin and disturbed calmodulin = ↓ muscle contractility)
      iv. Consequence of bipedal posture.
  6. *Risk of progression*:
      i. Curve magnitude: >25° before skeletal maturity → ↑↑ progression
      ii. Remaining skeletal growth **(Fig. 29)**

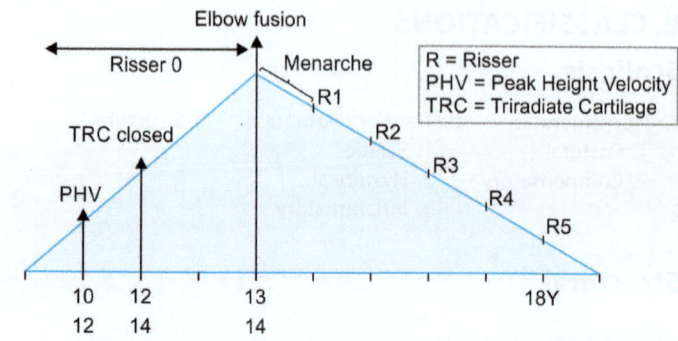

  1. <12 years at presentation
  2. Tanner < 3 for females
  3. Risser (0–1)
     0 → covers first 2/3rd of pubertal growth spurt. Correlates with greatest velocity of skeletal linear growth.
  4. Open TRC
  5. Peak growth velocity → Best predictor of curve progression
  6. Thoracic >Lumbar
  7. Double >single
  8. Girls >boys

7. **Classification (Fig. 30):**

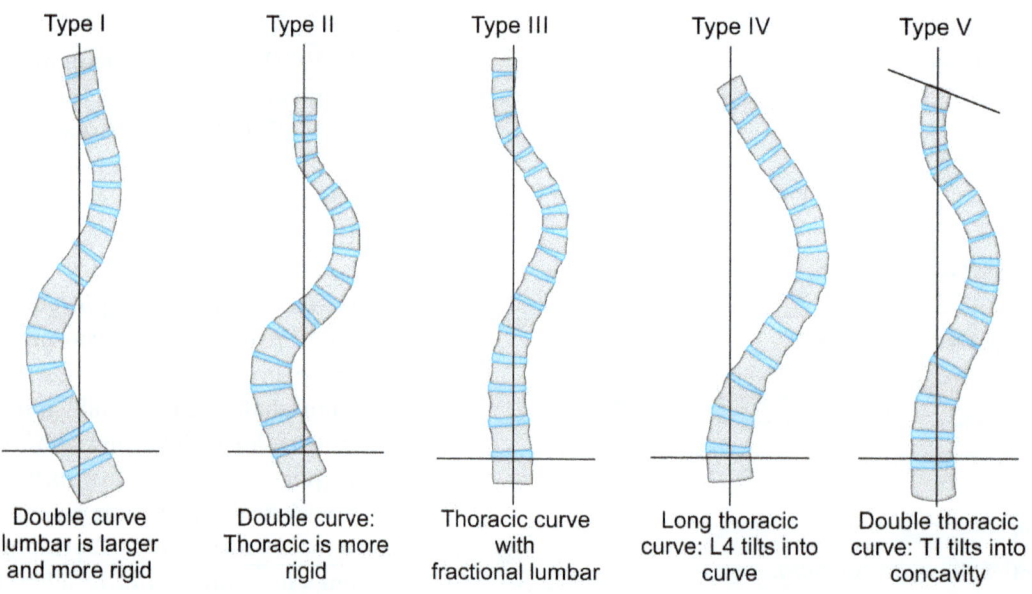

Fig. 30: King's classification.

  i. Kings
  ii. Lenke's
      I. Curve Type [Proximal thoracic (PT), Main Thoracic (MT), Thoracolumbar-Lumbar (TL/L)]
          i. Main Thoracic (MT)
          ii. Double Thoracic (PT, MT)
          iii. Double Major (MT, TL/L)
          iv. Triple Major (PT, MT, TL/L)
          v. Thoracolumbar-Lumbar (TL/L)
          vi. TL-L – MT (Lumbar > Thoracic)
      II. Lumbar Modifier (Coronal):
          A. CSVL between pedicles
          B. CSVL touching apical body
          C. CSVL completely medial
      III. Thoracic modifier (sagittal):
          Hypo (–) → <10 degrees

Normal (N) → 10–40 degrees
Hyper (+) → >40 degrees

8. **Pathophysiology (Fig. 31):**

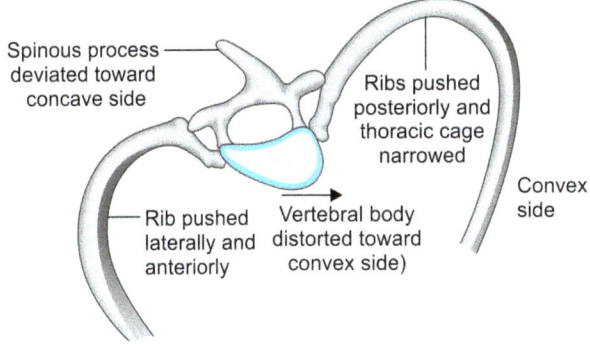

9. **Clinical presentation:**
   i. Deformity → MC presenting symptom
   ii. Pain - Rare
   iii. Level of shoulder, scapula, pelvis → Asymmetry
   iv. Trunk arm distance asymmetry
   v. Spinal balance: Hypokyphotic in sagittal plane. Compensatory curve plumb line.
   vi. **Adam's** forward bending test: Persistence suggestive of structural curve
   vii. LLD
   viii. Midline skin defects → Hairy patch or nevi.
   → Signs of spinal dysraphism
   ix. Rib prominence
   x. Café au lait spots → NF
   xi. Asymmetric abdominal reflexes → r/o syringomyelia
   xii. Scoliometry → <7° - normal.

10. **Radiology:**
    i. PA, Lateral
    ii. Flexibility → (R) and (L) Bending, traction and push - prone imaging films,
    iii. **Stagnara** view - to eliminate rotational component of curve.
    iv. Radiographic parameters to assess maturity.
       a. PBH - Rissers
       b. Hand and wrist → Sanders
       c. Olecranon - Sauvegrains
    v. Angle calculation → Cobbs **(Fig. 32)**

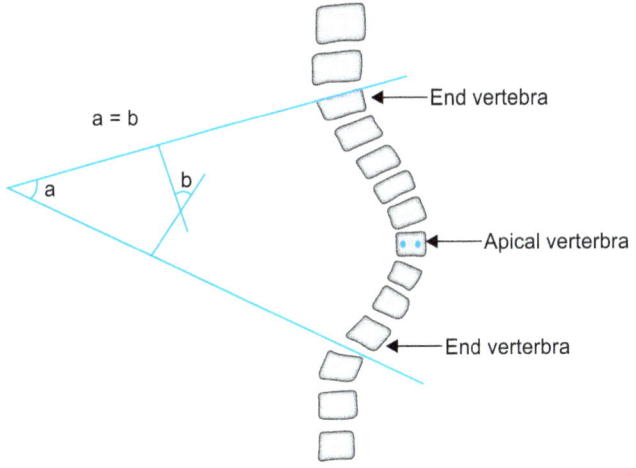

vi. Vertebral rotation → Nash and Moe **(Fig. 33)**

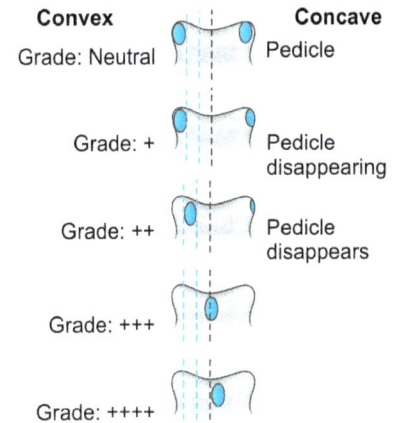

Pedicle	Convex	Concave
Grade: Neutral	No asymmetry	No asymmetry
Grade: +	Migrates within first segment Early distortion	May start disappearing Early distortion
Grade: ++	Migrates to second segment	Gradually disappears
Grade: +++	Migrates to middle segment	Not visible
Grade: ++++	Migrates past midline to concave side of vertebral body	Not visible

vii. Coronal and sagittal balance
↓
C_7 → posterosuperior border of S_1

viii. MRI → to rule out intraspinal anomalies
Indications:
1. Atypical curve → Left sided
→ Short angular
→ Apical kyphosis
2. Rapid progression
3. Excessive kyphosis
4. Structural abnormality
5. Neurologic symptoms or pain
6. Foot deformities
7. Asymmetric abdominal reflexes

ix. PFT → > 50° curves

11. **Treatment:**
Based on → Skeletal maturity
→ Magnitude of deformity
→ Curve progression

A. **Conservative:**
1. <20° → Observation
↓
Serial radiographs 6 monthly till <u>Skeletal Maturity</u>
↓
a. Risser 4
b. 2 years post menarche
c. <1 cm change height at 6 month follow-up

2. Bracing:
   i. Indications:
      a. Cobbs → 20–45° (Risser 0, 1, 2)
      b. Flexible deformity in skeletally immature.
   ii. Goal → Stop progression, not to correct deformity
   iii. 16 hours/day
   iv. Curve with apex above T_7 → Milwaukee brace (CTLSO brace)
      ↓
      3 point fixation principle.
   v. Apex at or below T_7 → Boston (underarm)
   vi. Success → < 5° Progression
   vii. Failure → ≥ 6° or absolute > 45° → Surgery
   viii. Poor prognosis:
      a. Hypokyphosis
      b. Male
      c. Obese
      d. Poor in brace correction
      e. Noncomplaint

B. **Operative:**
   1. Surgical options:
      Posterior fusion and instrumentation:
      i. Principles:
         a. Fuse above and below end vertebrae
         b. Selective → 1° curve
            (2° resolves after primary correction)
      ii. Cobbs > 50°
      iii. Gold standard: Thoracic and double major
      iv. Suitable for all idiopathic

      Anterior spinal fusion: Best for TL and L with normal sagittal profile.

      Anterior + posterior:
      i. Large and stiff curve > 75°
      ii. In young patient → prevent crankshaft phenomenon
      iii. Intraoperative neuromonitoring essential
   2. Indications of surgery:
      a. Failure of conservative management
      b. Curve >50
      c. Pain uncontrolled
      d. Thoracic lordosis
      e. Cosmetic deformity
   3. **Complications:**
      a. Neurologic injury
      b. Pseudoarthrosis
      c. Infection
      d. Crankshaft phenomenon
      e. Flat back syndrome
      f. SMA syndrome
      g. Hardware failure

4. **Methods of reduction:**
   a. Axial translation technique
   b. Rod rotation technique
   c. Vertebral column manipulation
   d. Severe deformity → Osteotomy
      1. Ponte–facet based
      2. Pedicle subtraction osteotomy
      3. Vertebral column resection.

PEDICLE SCREW

INTRODUCTION

1. The pedicle screw system traverses and fixes all the 3 columns of the vertebrae 3 column stability.
   ↓
   Stabilizes the ventral and dorsal aspects of spine.
2. Most common technique in spinal stabilization
3. Does not require intact dorsal elements → Can be used after laminectomy, traumatic disruption of laminae, spinous, and/or facets.

I. INDICATIONS

1. Unstable spinal fractures
2. Degenerative disc disease
3. Spondylolisthesis
4. Post-laminectomy } Spinal instability
5. TB spine
6. LCS → Potential instability
7. Augmenting anterior strut grafting → Tumor / Infection
8. Correction of deformities

II. DISADVANTAGES

1. Requires extensive tissue dissection.
2. Can result in dural or neural injury.
3. Postoperative imaging studies → Obscures by the implant.
4. Rigid fixation can accelerate.
   ↓
   Adjacent motion segment degeneration
5. Steep learning curve
6. Costlier than other methods of spinal stabilization.

III. SCREW PROPERTIES (FIG. 34)

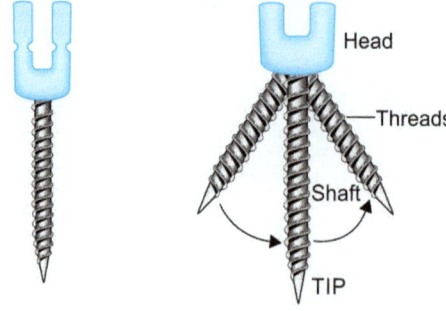

1. *Types*:
   i. Polyaxial
   ii. Monoaxial
   iii. Uniaxial
   iv. Reduction screw
   v. HA coated screw
2. *Shaft*:
   i. Cylindrical
   ii. Tapered (Conical)
3. Tapered screws → fit the pedicle geometry better than cylindrical screws
   +
   Improved bone compaction
   ↓
   They contact more fresh bone with each turn thread.
4. Variable pitch Pedicle Screw: Better purchase in bone.
   Large pitch → distal shaft → Cancellous bone
   Smaller pitch → Proximal Shaft → Cortical bone
5. Polyaxial head → Allows angulation in multiple directions to facilitate rod attachment.
6. Pedicle screws → Superior biomechanical stability compared to other segmental constructs.

   Excellent longitudinal   Torsional and sagittal
   Compression - distraction. stability.
7. *Diameters*:
   i. Core diameter → Bending screw resistance. (Fatigue strength)
   ii. Thread diameter → Pull-out strength.

IV. PEDICLE SCREW INSERTION

   i. Intersection technique
   ii. Pars interarticularis
   iii. Mamillary process
1. **Entry points (Fig. 35)**

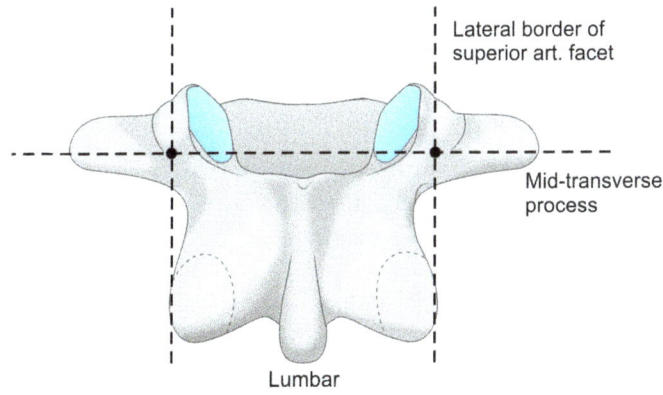

Lumbar

Lateral border of superior articular Facet.
Mid-transverse process.

2. Entry points more cephaled in proximal thoracic levels
3. Sagittal pedicle angle → T_1 → 0°
   T_8 → 10°
   T_{12} → 0°
4. Lordotic lumbar spine → Rostral angulation for upper lumbar vertebra.
   L_4 → 0°
   L_5 → Caudal angulation (5-10°)
5. Coronal pedicle angle - T_1 = 15°
   L_1, T_{12} = 5°
   L_5 = 15°

Goal: Avoid medial penetration → Spinal elements
                    Inferior → Nerve roots

The two screws must provide coverage but stay entirely within the cortex **(Fig. 36)**.

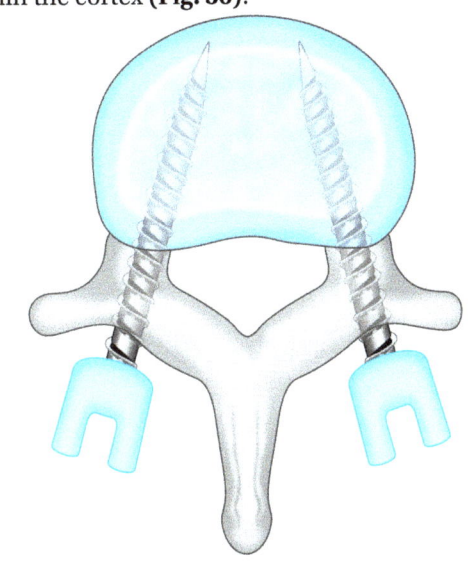

V. COMPLICATIONS

1. Neurological: Spinal cord/nerve root injury
2. Dural tear: CSF leak/fistula
3. Vascular: Aortic injury
4. Visceral: Pleural/lung injury
5. Local:
   a. Pedicle fracture
   b. Screw fracture
   c. Screw pull out

LATERAL MASS FIXATION FOR CERVICAL SPINE

I. INTRODUCTION

1. The lateral mass is the body junction between the superior and the inferior articular processes.
2. Roy–Camille et al. introduced LMF in 1964.

II. INDICATIONS

1. Trauma: Unstable fracture
2. Reconstruction:
   i. Tumors
   ii. Infection
   iii. Inflammatory → RA

3. Degenerative:
    i. Combined with posterior decompression.
    ii. Adjunct multilevel fixation
4. Pediatric spine: Congenital malformations
5. Scoliosis

III. FIXATION TECHNIQUE (FIG. 37)

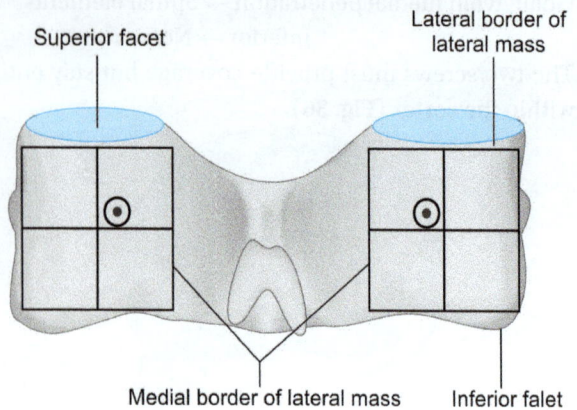

1. Superior facet
2. Lateral border of lateral mass
3. Medial border of lateral mass
4. Inferior facet
    These 4 landmarks form a square
    ↓
    Equally divided by a horizontal and vertical line
    Two techniques:
    a. Magerl
    b. Roy-Camille **(Fig. 38)**

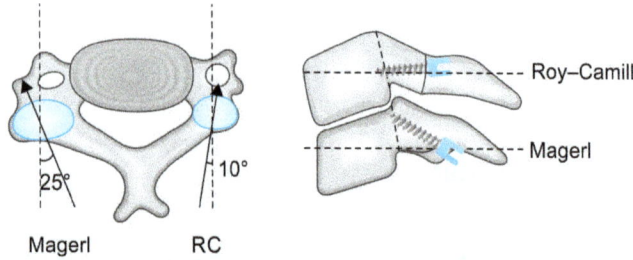

a. Magerl:
    1. 1 mm medial and cranial to the midpoint
    2. Lateral angulation → 25–30°
    3. Sagittal inclination → 20°
b. Roy-Camille:
    1. Entry: Midpoint of lateral mass
    2. Lateral angulation → 10°
    3. Sagittal inclination → 90° to lateral mass surface
       Magerl trajectory is longer the RC
       ↓
       Screws directed → Laterally: Prevent injury to vertebral artery
       ↓
       Superiorly → Prevent injury to the spinal nerve and its dorsal ramus.

IV. COMPLICATIONS
1. Nerve root injury
2. Vertebral artery injury
3. CSF leak → Dural tear
4. Facet joint violation
5. Pseudoarthrosis
6. Fracture of LM while inserting.

V. DISADVANTAGES
1. Dependent on amount of bone and its quality.
2. Only posterior tension band, not 3 columns.
3. Fracture of LM while inserting.

VERTEBROPLASTY AND KYPHOPLASTY

A. VERTEBRAL BODY COMPRESSION FRACTURE
1. Most common osteoporotic fractures.
2. Result in severe and disabling pain
3. ↓ Quality of life:
    i. Prolonged immobilization
    ii. Kyphosis
    iii. Pulmonary deterioration (↓ VC)
    iv. Depression
    v. Loss of independence.
    vi. Chronic back pain
    vii. ↑ Mortality rates
    viii. Increased tendency to fall
    ix. Shift of sagittal balance
    x. Stooped posture
4. Majority of the fracture will heal spontaneously and are clinically silent. (Silent vertebral fracture)
5. 25–33% of fractures become painful and gradually pain reduces over 6–12 weeks

B. VERTEBROPLASTY

I. Introduction
1. VP first described by Galibert in 1987 is a minimally invasive image-guided procedure involving the injection of bone cement in VB fracture.
   ↓
2. Improves pain and stability.
3. Cement most commonly used → PMMA.

II. Rationale
1. Fractures that fail to heal get filled with fluid typically near the superior end plate in the anterior region.
   ↓
2. True intravertebral 'Pseudoarthrosis' formation.
   ↓
3. Fluid gradually replaced by air and surrounding bone gets necrosed and hematopoietic stem cells → Marrow edema and fibrosis.

4. The intravertebral pseudoarthrosis is associated with dynamic mobility due to presence of cleft filled with air/fluid.
5. On supine extension radiograph, 90% of OP vertebral fractures are mobile.
6. The intervertebral cleft is responsible for spinal instability, but provides an opportunity to restore height by cement augmentation.
7. The cement sets and provides the vertebral body with requisite strength under compressive forces.

III. Indications

1. Failed conservative management in symptomatic acute osteoporotic vertebral fracture.
2. Symptomatic osteoporotic VB fracture that is progressively collapsing on imaging.
3. Symptomatic OVB fracture → Dynamic mobility.
4. Metastatic disease
5. Multiple myeloma
6. Painful aggressive hemangiomas
7. Osteonecrosis (Kummel disease)
8. Paget disease
9. Langerhans cell histiocytosis
10. Osteogenesis imperfecta
11. Spinal pseudoarthrosis
12. Intravertebral vacuum phenomenon
13. Painful Schmorl's nodes.

IV. Contraindications

1. Asymptomatic VF
2. VF improving on conservative care
3. Disruption of posterior VB wall
4. Tumor extension into spinal canal
5. Ankylosing spine
6. Uncorrectable coagulopathy
7. Active local or systemic infection
8. Severely compressed VB fracture → Relative C/I

V. Assessment and Workup

1. VF can occur with minimal or no trauma.
2. Typically (but not always) associated with acute onset of severe back pain.
3. Pain: Midline, localized to level of fracture, typically not radicular.
4. Pain may radiate bilaterally to the anterior abdomen in a belt-like fashion.
5. X-ray ⤷ First investigation for diagnosis
   ⤷ Supine extension for mobility
6. CT scan → Posterior wall integrity
7. MRI → to rule out other diagnosis, tumors, cord involvement, etc.

VI. Technique

1. Position: Prone
2. Anesthesia: Local
3. Approach: Unipedicular/Bipedicular
4. Bipedicular approach → Useful when suspecting vascular malformation, so that one can confirm by injecting contrast initially.
5. Extrapedicular approach may be used for thoracic vertebra where the pedicles are smaller (Fig. 39).
6.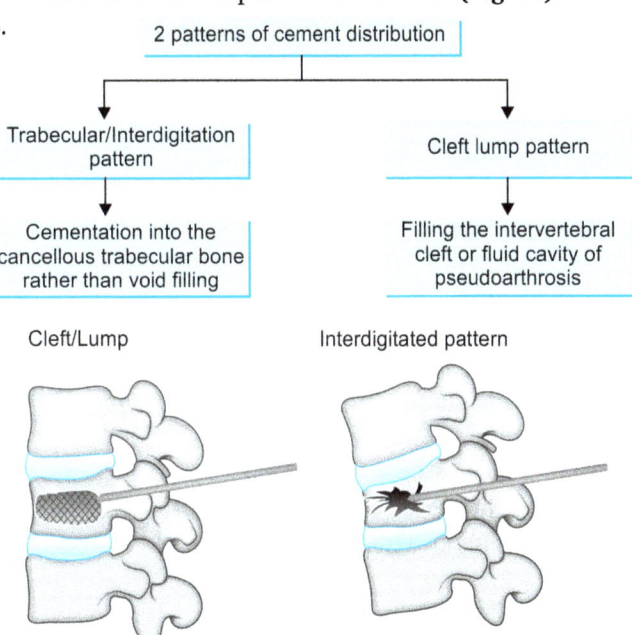
7. Average cement → 4 mL
8. Complete filling of the VB under pressure from end plate to end plate must be avoided to prevent cement leakage.

VII. Complications

1. Extradural extravasation of bone cement
2. Neurological compromise
3. Formation of cement emboli

C. KYPHOPLASTY

I. Introduction

1. Minimally invasive image guided procedure
   ↓
2. Involves inflating a balloon inside the vertebra
   ↓
3. Restore vertebral body weight
   ↓
4. Bone cement injected
   ↓
5. The inflation of balloon inside the VB potentially ameliorates the cement extravasations

II. Indications

1. Painful fractures with a back pain score of 4 points or more on a 0–10 scale not responding to conservative treatment for 6 weeks.
2. Compression fracture due to OP → Osteolytic metastatic tumors (D_5 – L_5 levels), multiple myeloma.
3. Junctional lesions: "Adjacent vertebra" of a fractured and treated one at the level of D_{12} or L_1 in severely OP patients. Preventive treatment as it has been found that at D_{12} – L_1 level if one of the other one shows a fracture within 18 months.

III. Contraindications

1. Age < 21 years
2. Previous vertebroplasty of same vertebra
3. Pedicular fracture
4. Severe disease:
    i. Radicular pain
    ii. Neurological deficit
    iii. Evident spinal cord compression
5. Patients on uninterruptible anticoagulation therapy
6. Allergy to cement
7. Nonambulatory before fractures (relative)
8. Fractures due to 1° bone tumors, osteoblastic metastasis and high energy trauma.

IV. Technique

1. Short admission of 24 hours
2. Success depends on uniform expansion of the vertebral body that can be stabilized by intraosseous cement
3. Two most important parameters

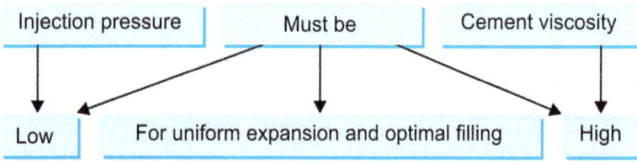

4. Position – Prone
5. Anesthesia → GA
6. Correct level and pedicle localized by ↓ C-arm
7. 11-gauge needle biopsy is advanced into the fractured vertebral body by transpedicular approach
8. Working cannula inserted, needle removed
9. Inflatable balloon tamp introduced under the collapsed end plate.
10. Balloon tamps inflated under C-arm
    ↓
11. Pressure measured through in-built manometer
12. Maximum fracture reduction achieved
13. Inflation is stopped when balloon reaches the cortical wall or obtains the "balloon kissing" position
    ↓
14. Two balloons touching each other in the vertebral body center.
15. Cement is prepared and loaded in syringes
16. At semisolid state (3–5 min) after mixing, cement inserted
17. At cement setting, the cannula is removed and wound closed

V. Complications

1. Minor:
    i. Bradycardia
    ii. Desaturation
2. Serious:
    i. Pulmonary embolus
    ii. Extravasation to epidural space
    ↓
   Push cement only in semi solid state and remove cannula in rotating maneuver

VI. Pros and Cons

1. Disadvantage → Costly
2. Advantage → Pain relief immediate

VIDEO-ASSISTED THORACIC SURGERY

INTRODUCTION

1. Minimally invasive thoracic surgery
   ↓
2. Performed using a small video camera mounted on a fiberoptic thoracoscope (5 mm or 10 mm) and other elongated endoscopic instruments.
   ↓
3. Finds its applications in diseases of the spine in orthopedics
4. Adequate exposure to all the levels of thoracic spine (T_2-L_1)

I. TECHNIQUE (FIG. 40)

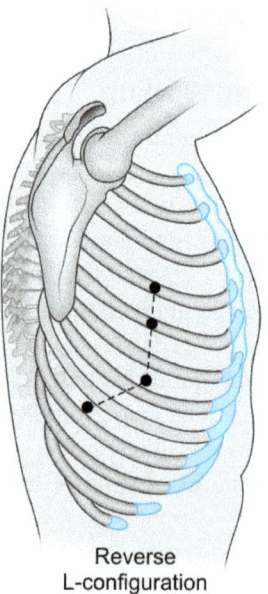

Reverse L-configuration

1. Position = Lateral decubitus
2. GA
3. Single lung ventilation.
4. Collapse of ipsilateral lung
5. CO_2 insufflation not needed as in abdomen because thoracic cage gives rigid support.
6. 1 cm incisions are taken for portal placement
   ↓
   Anterior, middle and posterior axillary lines.
7. Initially trocar in 7th IC space
   ↓
   Posterior axillary line
8. 10 mm, 30° end-viewing scope placed through trocar for direct visualization of the vertebral body and disc.
   ↓
9. 2-3 working ports are now made in AAL/MAL (Anterior and middle axillary line)
10. Reverse L – arrangement can be moved cephalad or caudad depending on the level of thoracic spine affected.

II. INDICATIONS

1. Thoracic discectomy
2. Anterior release of stiff thoracic scoliotic deformities
3. Drainage of paraspinal abscess due to TB, pyogenic infection
4. Bone grafting of the thoracic vertebral space can also be done
5. Tumors
6. Fractures
7. Non-orthopedic:
   i. Pneumothorax: Mechanical pleurodesis.
   ii. Diagnostic: Lung, LN biopsy
   iii. Pleural effusion drainage
   iv. Lobectomy for lung Ca

III. ADVANTAGES

1. ↓ Acute pain
   ↓
2. ↓ Need for analgesic, epidural catheters
3. Shorter hospital stay:
   ↓
   Overall cost.
4. ↓ Blood loss
5. Better cosmesis
6. ↓ Chest tube duration
7. Improved quality of life.
8. ↓ Long-term thoracotomy pain
9. ↓ Postoperative shoulder dysfunction
10. Earlier return to activities.

IV. DISADVANTAGES

1. Learning curve high
2. Presence of thoracic surgeon must
3. May need conversion to open thoracotomy.

V. COMPLICATIONS

1. Intercostal neuralgia
2. Atelectasis
3. Excessive epidural blood loss (up to 2,500 mL)

VI. CONTRAINDICATIONS

1. Inability to tolerate single lung ventilation
2. Pleural disease
3. Previous surgeries

MINIMALLY INVASIVE SPINE SURGERY

INTRODUCTION

Broad term to describe a variety of spinal surgical techniques which are a promising alternative to traditional open surgical procedures.

I. PRINCIPLES

1. To decrease muscle crush injuries during retraction.
2. Avoid injury to the Osseo-tendinous attachments → essential for spinal stability
3. Maintain integrity of dorsolumbar fascia.
4. Limit bony resection.
5. Avoid injury to neurovascular supply of muscle compartments by using known anatomic planes.
6. Decrease size of surgical corridor to coincide with area of the surgical target site.

II. ADVANTAGES

1. Small incision → cosmetically better.
2. Muscle splitting instead of muscle cutting.
   ↓
3. ∴ ↓↓ Soft tissue trauma and blood loss.
   ↓
   Shorter hospital stay
   ↓
   Faster recovery
4. ↓↓ Postoperative pain
5. ↓ Infection rate
6. ↓ Adjacent segment disease

III. TYPES

1. MIS Lumbar discectomy (microscopic microdiscectomy, endoscopic, laser)
2. MIS Lumbar fusion
   ↓
   i. TLIF → transforaminal lumbar interbody fusion
   ii. XLIF → Extreme lateral lumbar interbody fusion
   iii. DLIF → Direct, OLIF (oblique lateral)
   iv. ALIF → Anterior [laparoscopic (transperitoneal), retroperitoneal]
3. Video assisted Thoracic Surgery
4. Video assisted Lumbar Surgery

5. Vertebroplasty
6. Kyphoplasty
7. Intradiscal electrothermotherapy (65°C for 17 min, collagen shrinkage, destruction of nociceptor fibers)

IV. INDICATIONS

In principle, the indications of MISS are like open surgeries
↓
After trial of conservative treatment
↓
When exact source of the pain/dysfunction can be pin - pointed.

1. Degenerative disc disease – leg pain > back pain, radicular
2. Herniated IV discs
3. Spinal instability
4. Scoliosis
5. Spinal stenosis
6. Trauma
7. Osteoporotic fractures.
8. Biopsy
9. Degenerative ← Spondylolisthesis
↓
Isthmic

V. DISCECTOMY (FIG. 41)

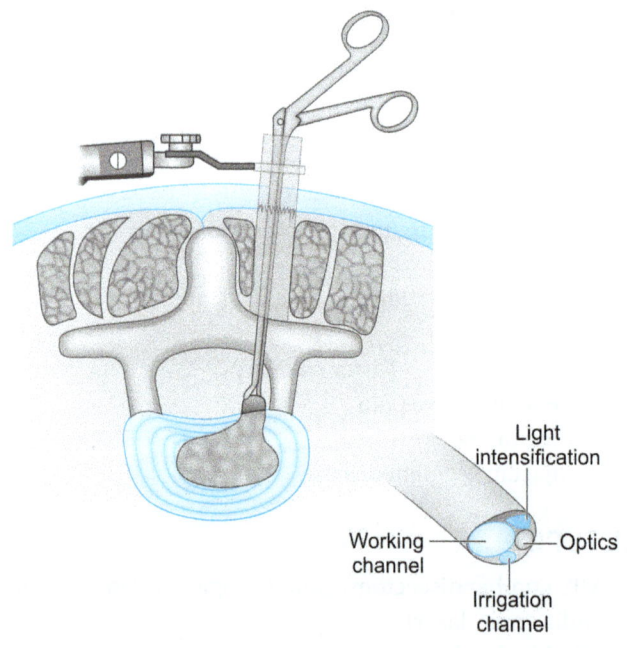

1. General anesthesia
2. Position – Prone – abdomen free
3. Pressure points appropriately padded
4. Spinal level localization → Image intensifier
↓
5. Incision 1–1.5 cm lateral to midline
6. Retractors – (Tubular, McCulloch)
7. Lumbodorsal fascia opened using a blunt guide wire
↓
First tubular retractor
↓
Sequential tubular retractors (usually 16 mm used)
↓
Laminectomy performed using high speed burr
↓
LF opened up, nerve root retracted medially
↓
Whitish, shiny avascular extruded disc
↓
Removed using pituitary rongeur

VI. DISADVANTAGES

1. High learning curve
2. Inadequate decompression
3. ↑ OT time
4. Difficult to address migrated disc fragments

DURAL TEAR

I. INTRODUCTION (FIG. 42)

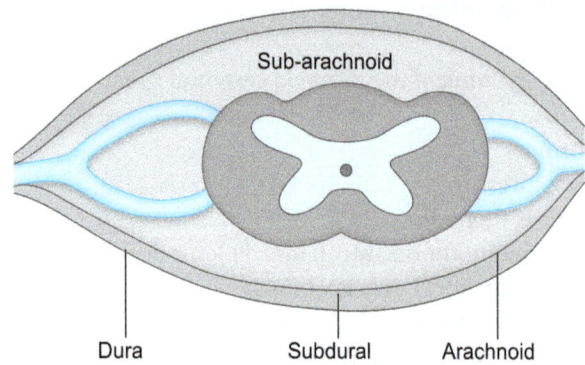

1. Spinal cord covered by 3 layers of meninges:
   i. Dura mater: Outer most layer
   ii. Arachnoid mater: Transparent, contains CSF in subarachnoid space
   iii. Pia mater: Inner most
2. Dural tear is a breach in the integrity of the dural layer.
↓
Almost always involves the arachnoid
↓
CSF leak

II. RISK FACTORS

1. Revision surgery – Fibrosis
2. Ossified LF ⎫
3. Ossified PLL ⎭ Adherent
4. Infections ⎫
5. Elderly ⎭ Weakened dura
6. Spinal stenosis → Folding of redundant dura under LF → Caught

7. Failure to recognize congenital malformations
8. For example, spina bifida occulta
9. Inexperienced surgeon
10. Diabetes
11. Chronic steroid used
12. Smoking
13. Preexisting deformities:
    i. Scoliosis
    ii. Kyphosis
14. Multilevel spine surgery (>3)
15. Exostosis (osteophytes)

III. SEQUELAE OF UNREPAIRED TEARS

1. CSF fistula
2. Pseudomeningocele
3. Meningitis
4. Epidural abscess
5. Delayed wound healing

IV. SYMPTOMS

1. Postural headache - resolves on recumbency
2. Nausea, vomiting
3. Diplopia, blurred vision
4. Tinnitus, vertigo
5. Hypotension.

V. INVESTIGATIONS

1. Lab → β_2 transferrin
2. MRI.

VI. MANAGEMENT

1. Operative field → Unobstructed, dry, well-exposed.
2. Dural suture of a 4-0 or 6-0 gauge tapered or reverse cutting needle (**Fig. 43**).

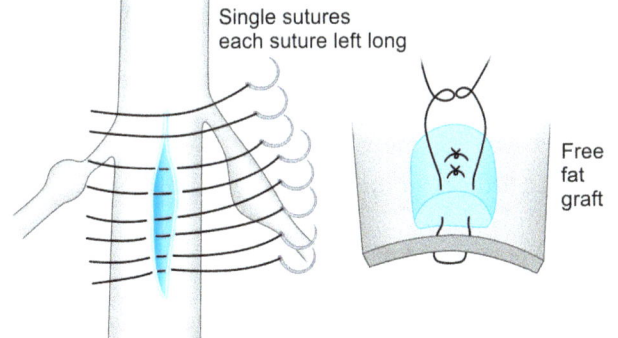

3. Large leak → Free fat or fascial graft
4. Fibrin glue
5. All repairs must be tested → reverse Trendelenburg position or Valsalva maneuvers.
6. Paraspinal muscles and overlying fascia
   ↓
   Closed in 2 layers → Watertight
7. Use of drain only if integrity of the wound closure questionable
   ↓
   If used → keep passive
8. Bed rest in supine position for 4-7 days
9. Foot end elevation
10. Acetazolamide (500 mg BD) for 7 days
    ↓
    Chemical drain → ↓CSF production in the choroid plexus by ⊗ Carbonic anhydrase.

SOMATOSENSORY–EVOKED POTENTIALS

1. "Evoked potentials" are the measurements of the electrical potentials produced in response to
   ↓
   Stimulating the nervous system (evoked)
   ↓
   By sensory, electrical magnetic or cognitive stimulation.
2. Evoked potentials → used to detect conduction disturbances in CNS
3.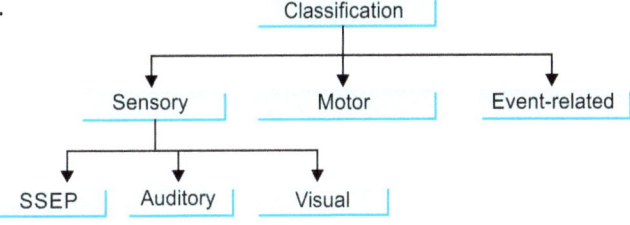
4. SSEP is the response to electrical stimulation of peripheral nerves.
5. Stimulation of any nerve is possible, but most commonly (signal initiation)
    i. Median
    ii. Ulnar
    iii. Posterior tibial - behind ankle
    iv. Peroneal
6. SSEP monitors the integrity of the dorsal column sensory pathways of spinal cord (**Fig. 44**).

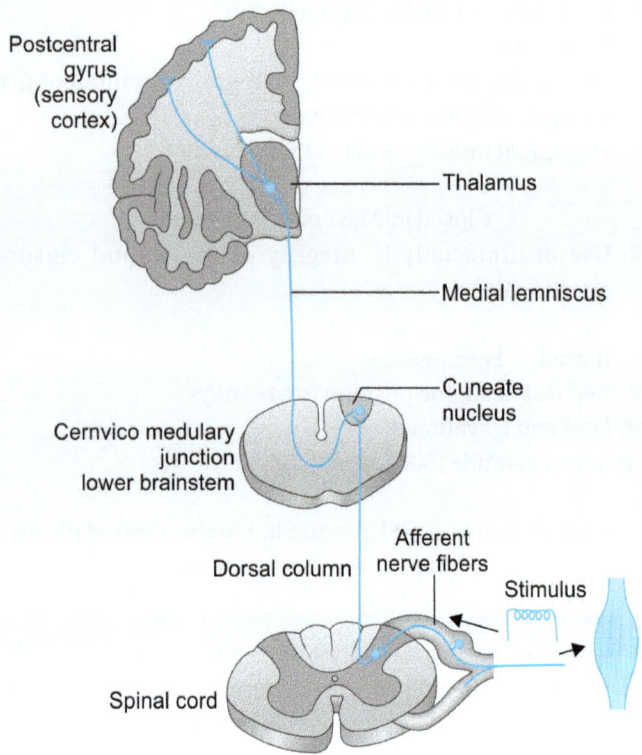

7. Brief electrical impulses are delivered to the peripheral nerve
↓
Cathode proximal to anode
↓
Stimulus cannot selectively activate sensory fibers
↓
∴ Small muscles twitch seen → Confirmation of stimulus
8. Recording ┬ Transcranial
             ├ Spinal cord
             └ Afferent nerve
9. Uses:
    i. Real-time monitoring intra-operatively in spine surgeries (e.g., scoliosis)
    ↓
    Loss of signal during distraction (50% decrease in amplitude and 10% decrease in latency) mandates immediate removal or adjustment of device.
    Advantage → unaffected by anesthetics
    Disadvantage → not reliable for integrity of motor pathways.
    ii. Diagnosis of demyelinating disorders (transverse myelitis, MS)
    iii. Nonorganic sensory loss or malingering.
    iv. Diabetic peripheral neuropathy
    v. Usually normal in radiculopathy
    vi. To identify anatomic level of dysfunction
    vii. Brachial plexus surgeries → during exploration

NERVE ROOT BLOCKS/EPIDURAL STEROIDS

Outpatient procedure commonly used for treating radicular lower limb pain.

I. RELEVANT ANATOMY (FIG. 45)

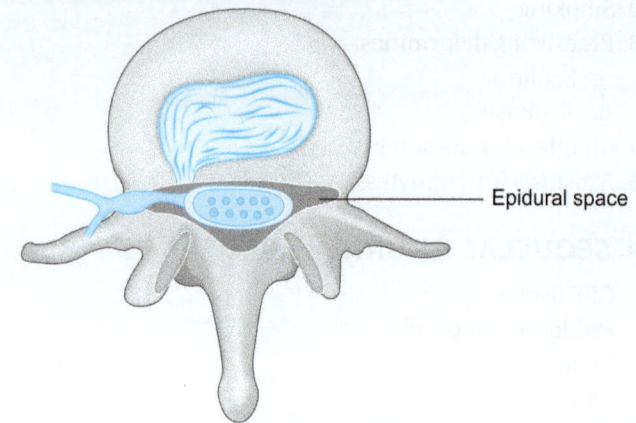

The narrow space between the vertebral canal and the outer covering of the spinal cord → Epidural space

II. USE

Patient unresponsive to traditional analgesic, rest and impairment of activities of daily living.
1. Radicular pain due to prolapsed IVD
2. Spinal stenosis (Central, Lateral)

III. INJECTION DRUGS

1. Steroids → Triamcinolone: 80 mg
   Methylprednisone: 40–80 mg
2. Local anesthetic → Lignocaine (2%)

IV. RATIONALE

Mechanical compression of neural elements
↓
Structural and chemical injury to nerve roots
↓
Edema, venous congestion → (leakage of neurotoxins phospholipase, leukotriene b)
↓
Further compression and ischemic neuritis.

1. Steroids:
    i. Potent anti-inflammatory
    ii. ↓ Leukocyte migration
    iii. Inhibition of cytokines
    iv. Membrane stabilization
2. Local anesthetics:
    i. Pain relief
    ii. Reversible nerve blockade
    iii. Blocks sodium channels (MOA)

3. Nonionic contrast agents (iohexol–omnipaque)
   i. Reduces risk of intravascular/subarachnoid injection
   ii. Confirmation of correct location of injecting

V. TECHNIQUE

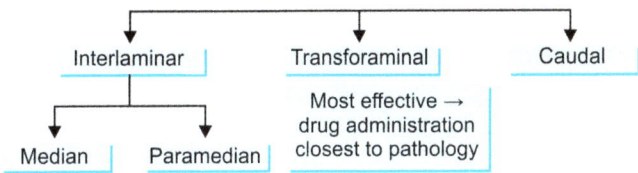

1. Consent
2. IV access → Analgesics, antibiotics
3. Position → Prone on radiolucent table
4.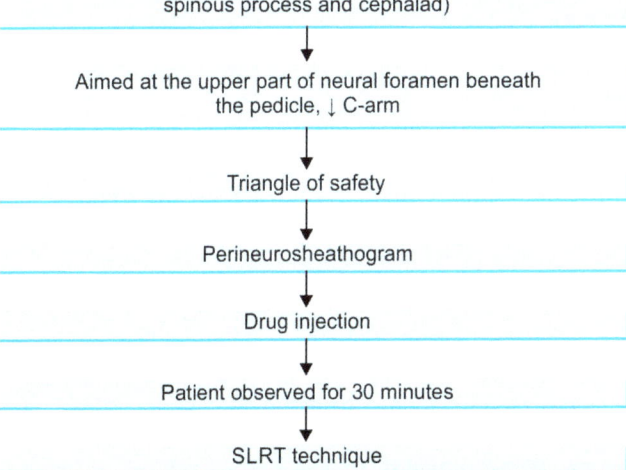

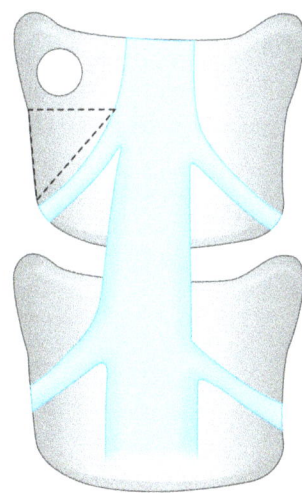

VI. COMPLICATIONS

1. Epidural hematoma
2. Temporary neurological deficit
3. Epidural abscess
4. Chemical meningitis
5. Retinal hemorrhage
6. Anaphylaxis

SPINAL FUSION METHODS

I. INTRODUCTION

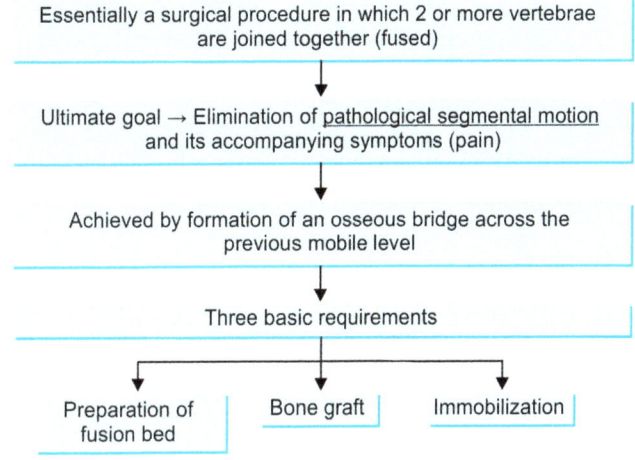

II. INDICATIONS

1. Degenerative disc disease
2. Spondylolisthesis → (Degenerative, Isthmic)
3. Spinal trauma
4. Infection – tuberculosis
5. Tumors
6. Scoliosis

III. TYPES

A. Interbody
B. Posterolateral

A. Interbody

i. Removal of IVD (discectomy) + Replacement with bone graft and/or a device (cage) → to maintain alignment and disc height.

ii.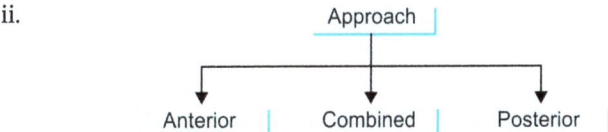

iii. Lumbar
   1. ALIF PLIF   1. PLIF
   2. DLIF, XLIF   2. TFIF ┌→ Open
   3. OLIF MIS   └→ MIS
iv. Cervical
   1. Anterior cervical discectomy and fusion (ACDF)
   2. Anterior cervical corpectomy and fusion (ACCF)
   3. Posterior cervical decompression and fusion
v. Remove pain generators.
vi. Large surface area for fusion (80%: Load, 90%: Surface area)
vii. Compression force through graft.
viii. Correction of coronal and sagittal alignment

- ALIF – Anterior abdominal incision
  1. Types — Transperitoneal
           — Retroperitoneal
  2. Advantage: No trauma to paraspinal muscles
  3. Disadvantage: Risk of injury to abdominal organs
  4. Contraindications:
     i. Calcified aorta
     ii. Prior vascular reconstruction surgery
     iii. Prior intra-abdominal surgery
     iv. History of severe pelvic inflammatory disease
     v. Prior anterior spinal surgery
- DLIF/XLIF:
  1. Through psoas muscle
  2. Advantage: No trauma to PS muscle and abdominal organs
  3. Disadvantage:
     i. $L_5 - S_1$ not accessible
     ii. ⊗ Sympathetic plexus → retrograde ejaculation
- OLIF → Anterior to psoas
  Advantage → Gives access to $L_5 - S_1$

Advantages of Anterior Approaches
1. No need for nerve root extraction and entry into the vertebral canal.
   ↓
2. ∴ Eliminating epidural scarring and perineural (fibrosis)
3. Larger graft placement
4. In kyphotic cervical spine → Anterior
   Posterior → inadequate decompression
5. Preservation of posterior stabilizing structures — Facet capsules
                                                    — IS, SS, LF Ligaments
                                                    — Laminae
6. No muscle disruption and postoperative atrophy

- PLIF 3 surgical steps
  ↓
  Laminectomy/Laminotomy → Discectomy
  ↓
  Bone grafting → Fusion
- TLIF:
  1. Anterior column support (+)(+)
  2. Posterior fixation (+)(+) **(Fig. 46)**

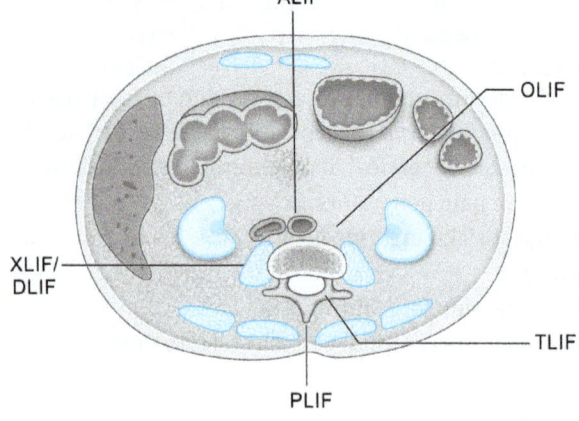

Posterior–disadvantages
1. Poor visualization of disc space
2. Suboptimal restoration of disc height
3. Nerve root injury

B. Posterolateral Fusion – Bone Graft Between Transverse Processes

Bone grafts used	Devices
1. Cancellous autograft	**Cages**
2. Cortical autograft	↓
3. Vascularized autograft	Titanium
4. Allograft	PEEK
5. Bone Marrow Aspirate	Zero-profile
6. Demineralized Bone Matrix	Banana
7. Bone Morphogenic Protein	Bullet
8. Ceramics	

Spinal instrumentation is almost always used with fusion

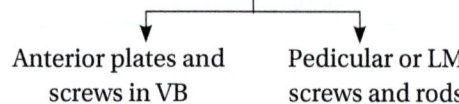

Anterior plates and screws in VB   Pedicular or LM screws and rods

IV. COMPLICATIONS
1. Pseudoarthrosis
2. Adjacent segment disease
3. Deformity
4. Failed back syndrome.

ROLE OF PHYSIOTHERAPY IN LOW BACK PAIN

INTRODUCTION
1. Low back pain: Discomfort or pain below the posterior costal margins and above the gluteal folds.

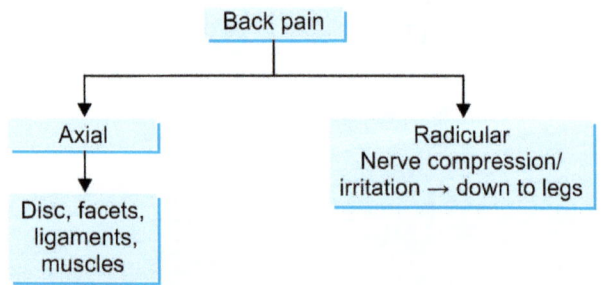

2. Most of the cases of back pain Mx conservatively.
3. Rest for not >3 days

I. RATIONALE FOR PT
1. Weak low back muscles
2. Poor posture
   ↓
   Paraspinal muscle spasm
   ↓
   Pain
   PT → Prevents recurrence of these episodes

II. PT ARMAMENTARIUM

1. Patient counseling
2. Exercise:
   i. Lumbar stabilization
   ii. Strengthening exercises
   iii. ROM
   iv. Stretches
   v. Aerobic conditioning
3. Spinal manipulation (manual therapy)
4. Posture correction
5. Local ultrasound
6. TENS
7. Heat and cryotherapy

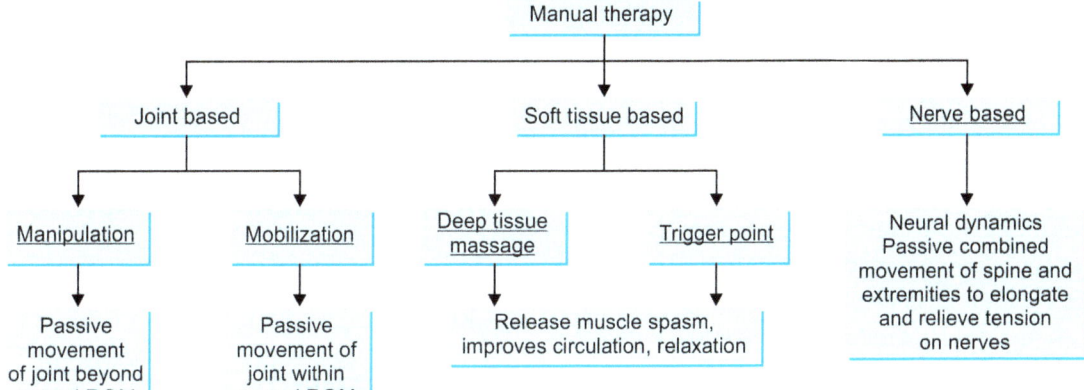

Mckenzie

Mechanical diagnosis and therapy

↓

Categorize patients complaints not on anatomical basis → But clinical presentation

4 Steps = Assessment → Classification – Rx → Prevention

Centralization → Symptom movement from distal to proximal → Good signal.

Traction

Traction → Mechanical
          → Core

Exercise → Core Strengthening → Multifidus and Transversus abdominis

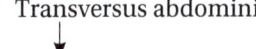

Extension exercises:
i. Strengthening → muscle work against force
ii. Endurance
iii. Co-ordination and stabilization → ↓ Recurrence of back pain

FAILED BACK SYNDROME

I. DEFINITION

A condition where there is a failure to improve satisfactorily following back surgery.

II. CLASSIFICATION

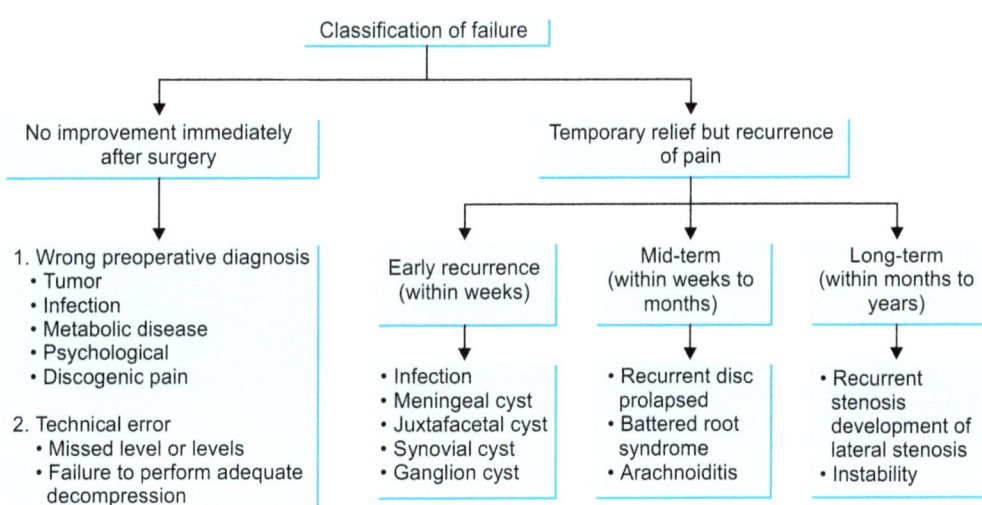

III. EVALUATION

1. Patients' history
2. Physical examination
3. Detailed neurological evaluation
4. Nonorganic signs of Waddell
   i. *Superficial tenderness*: Tenderness to light touch or pinch over a wide area of lumbar skin
   ii. *Nonanatomic tenderness*: Deep tenderness over a wide area that crosses the over non-anatomic boundaries.
   iii. *Axial loading*: The examiner presses downward on the patient's head while they are standing → lumbar pain.
   iv. *Distraction test:* The patient reports pain on SLR test in supine position and the pain markedly decrease on performing the distracted SLR when the examiner extends the knee with the patient sitting.
   v. *Regional sensory disturbance*: A glove and stocking-like pain that does not follow a dermatomal pattern.
   vi. *Regional weakness:* Weakness that cannot be explained on neuroanatomical basis.
   vii. *Overreaction:* Exaggerated painful response to a stimulus that is not reproduced when the same stimulus is given later.
   >3/5 → Significant
5. Examination of:
   a. SI joint
   b. Hip
   c. Knee joint

IV. RADIOGRAPH

Spine → AP
       → Lateral
1. Dynamic view → to check instability
2. Pelvic and hip X-ray

V. MRI, MYELOGRAM, CT

1. Level of prior surgery
2. Dural ectasia or CSF leak
3. Discitis/lysis
4. Arachnoiditis
5. Dynamic instability

VI. HEMATOLOGICAL INVESTIGATION

1. CBC ⎫
2. ESR ⎬ Infection
3. CRP ⎭

VII. MANAGEMENT

Conservative—Counselling
               Pharmacological therapy
               Physical therapy
Surgical:
1. Treat the underlying cause
2. Nerve root blocks
3. Decompression: In case of inadequate decompression
4. Fusion → Instability

SECTION 6

Shoulder

SHOULDER INSTABILITY/RECURRENT SHOULDER DISLOCATION

Instability is a pathological condition that presents as pain or discomfort and is associated with excessive humeral head translation relative to the glenoid during active shoulder movement.

I. ANATOMY AND BIOMECHANICS

GH stability → Static factors / Dynamic factors

A. Static

1. Glenoid labrum
   i. Deepens the concavity of bony glenoid.
   ii. Increases contact between humerus head and glenoid from 25 → 75%
   iii. Acts as a "chock-block" to prevent the humerus head to slip over to labrum.
2. Glenoid version
   Change in version causes change in the net joint reaction force (directional)
3. Negative intra-articular pressure
   Suction effect resists displacement.
4. Adhesion-cohesion
   Minimal amount of synovial fluid facilitates sliding motion, but limits the two surfaces from being pulled apart.
5. Capsuloligamentous structures
   Reciprocally tighten and loosen during rotation of arm → *Checkrein* mechanism. (GHL—Glenohumeral ligament)
   i. Superior GHL → Restricts inferior and posterior translation in adducted arm.
   ii. Middle GHL → Prevents anterior and posterior translation in 60-90° abduction.
   iii. Inferior GHL: Three components:
      a. Anterior band
      b. Posterior band
      c. Axillary pouch

Acts like a hammock → passive restraints to excessive humeral head translation.

B. Dynamic Stabilizers

1. Rotator cuff:
   a. Supraspinatus
   b. Infraspinatus
   c. Teres minor
   d. Subscapularis
2. Long head of biceps brachii
   Center the humeral head to glenoid in terminal rotational motion.
3. Scapular rotators → Trapezius, latissimus dorsi, levator scapulae, rhomboids, serratus anterior.
4. Proprioception
   Ruffini nerve endings and Pacinian corpuscles
   ↓
   Protective mechanism against capsular failure **(Fig. 1)**.

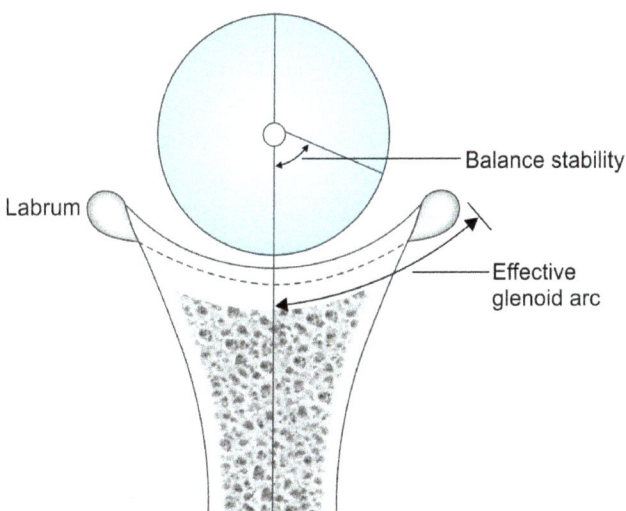

Fig. 1: Mechanics of GH stability is dependent on net joint reaction force and shape of glenoid cavity.

Glenohumeral joint will not dislocate as long as the net humeral reaction force is directed within the effective glenoid arc.

II. ASSOCIATED INJURIES WITH RECURRENT SHOULDER DISLOCATION

A. Labral and Cartilage
1. *Bankart:* Avulsion of anterior labrum and anterior band of IGHL from anterior inferior glenoid 80–90% in TUBS.
2. *HAGL:* Humeral avulsion of glenohumeral ligament
3. *GLAD:* Glenoid labral articular defect.
4. *ALPSA:* Anterior labral periosteal sleeve avulsion.

B. Fractures and Bone Defects
1. *Bony bankart:*
   a. Anterior inferior glenoid fracture
   b. 50% patients of recurrent dislocations
   c. Defect >13.5–25%: *Critical bone loss*
   ↓
   Stability cannot be restored with soft tissue reconstruction alone, require bony procedure to restore bone loss.
2. *Hill Sach's (HS):*
   a. Chondral impaction injury on posterosuperior humeral head due to contact with glenoid rim.
   b. Present in 80% recurrent dislocation and 25% recurrent subluxations.
   c. Not clinically significant if does not engage the glenoid
   d. *Pathophysiology:*
      1. Anteriorly directed force on the arm when the shoulder is ABER
      2. *"On track versus Off track"* concept
         A. Hill Sach's defect is "off-track" and will "engage" on the glenoid if
         ↓
         HS defect > Glenoid articular track
         B. Hill Sach's is "on-track" and will "not- engage" if → HS < Glenoid
3. *GT fracture:* Anterior dislocation >50 years
4. *LT fracture:* Posterior dislocation
5. *Nerve injuries:* Axillary nerve: transient neuropraxia
6. *Rotator cuff tears:*
   30% in > 40 years
   80% in > 60 years

III. ARTHROSCOPIC ANATOMY
Shoulder arthroscopy is a process of examination and possible intervention of a pathology in the joint using a fiber-optic instrument.
A. *Position:* Beach–chair or lateral decubitus
B. *Portals:*

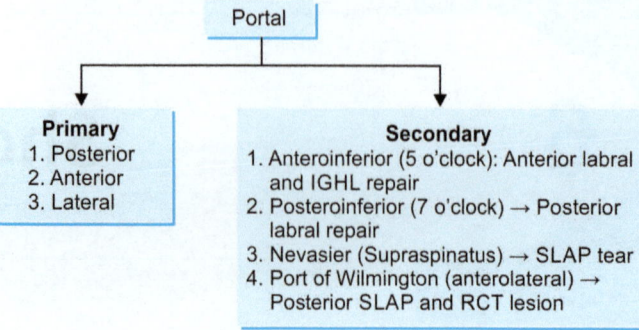

Primary
1. Posterior
2. Anterior
3. Lateral

Secondary
1. Anteroinferior (5 o'clock): Anterior labral and IGHL repair
2. Posteroinferior (7 o'clock) → Posterior labral repair
3. Nevasier (Supraspinatus) → SLAP tear
4. Port of Wilmington (anterolateral) → Posterior SLAP and RCT lesion

   i. *Posterior portal:*
      1. Established first → viewing portal
      2. "Soft spot" → 2 cm medial and 2 cm inferior to the posterolateral corner of acromion
      3. The axillary nerve and the posterior circumflex humeral vessels are safe as they are caudal to teres minor.
      Risk: Portal too inferior: Axillary nerve ⊗
         Portal too medial: Suprascapular nerve ⊗
   ii. *Anterior portal (Inside-out and Outside-in technique)*
      1. Made in the rotator interval
      2. Just lateral to the tip of the coracoid process and inferior to the anterolateral acromial border.
      3. The rotator interval is seen arthroscopically as a triangle **(Fig. 2)**.

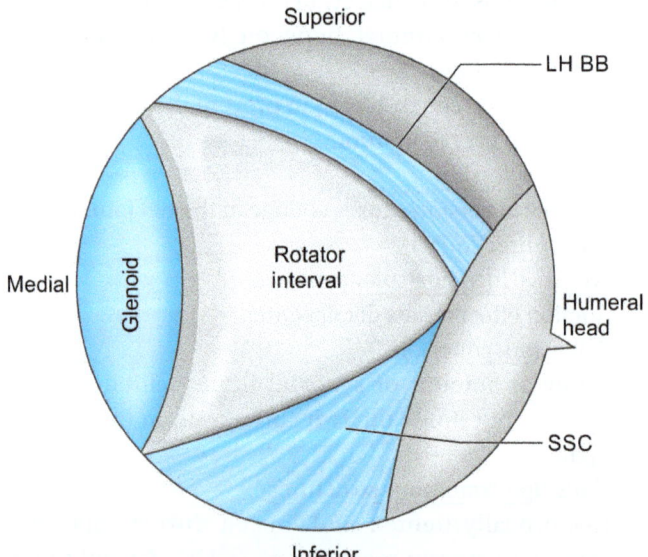

      4. All anterior portals must be lateral to the coracoids process to avoid injury to the brachial plexus and axillary vessels which are medial to coracoid process.
   iii. *Lateral portal:*
      1. 3–5 cm lateral to the lateral margin of the acromial border.
      2. May change based on intraarticular anatomy.

C. *Diagnostic arthroscopy:*
1. Diagnostic arthroscopy of shoulder starts with → identification of the intraarticular portion of LHB and its origin at the supraglenoid tubercle.
2. The LHB traverses obliquely over the humeral head and exits the GHJ beneath the transverse HL.
3. The glenoid labrum is continuous peripherally with the joint capsule and periosteum of the scapular neck.
4. Centrally, it is attached to the hyaline cartilage of the glenoid fossa **(Fig. 3)**.

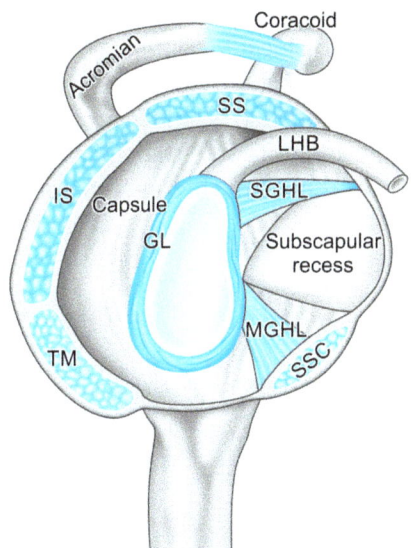

Fig. 3: Anatomy surrounding the glenoid.

5. Labrum
   - Above glenoid equator
     i. Triangular or meniscoid
     ii. Drapes over articular margin
     iii. Mobile attachment
   - Below glenoid equator
     i. Rounded
     ii. Firm attachment to articular surface
6. Internal surface of GH capsule ↓ Discrete thickenings ↓
7. SGHL: Obscured by the LHB
8. MGHL: Best visualized arthroscopically in mid portion where it crosses subscapularis tendon.
9. IGHL: Three components:
   - Anterior band
   - Posterior band
   - Axillary pouch

   Best visualized in abducted position
10. Bankart lesion injury → MGHL, anterior band of IGHL and anterior GL
11. *Buford complex* → Complete absence of anterosuperior labrum with a cord like MGHL arising at the biceps origin.

→ If Buford complex is mistaken for labral avulsion and reattached to glenoid → painful restriction of movement.
12. Articular cartilage over glenoid → thick in periphery, thin in center.
13. "Bare spot" in the center of glenoid → used as reference for arthroscopic measurement of glenoid bone loss in recurring instability
14. Articular surface of humeral head is normally seen smooth except on the posterolateral aspect that is devoid of articular cartilage → "bare area" must not be confused with Hill Sach's lesion
15. *Bursoscopy:* Subacromial space seen by arthroscope placed in the subacromial bursa.

IV. TYPES OF GLENOHUMERAL (GH) INSTABILITY

A. Based on Degree of Instability
1. GH instability/dislocation → Complete dissociation of articular surfaces.
2. Subluxation → Incomplete separation of GH surfaces without dislocation.

B. Circumstances
Matsen's TUBS and AMBRII

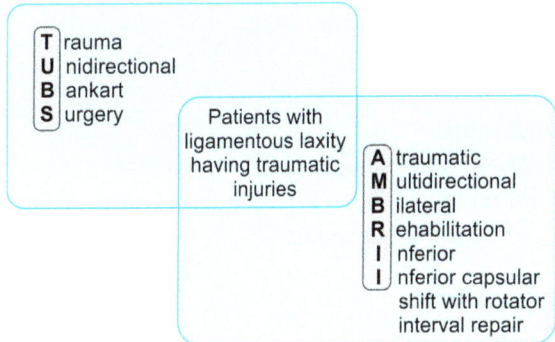

C. Stanmore Instability Classification (Fig. 4)

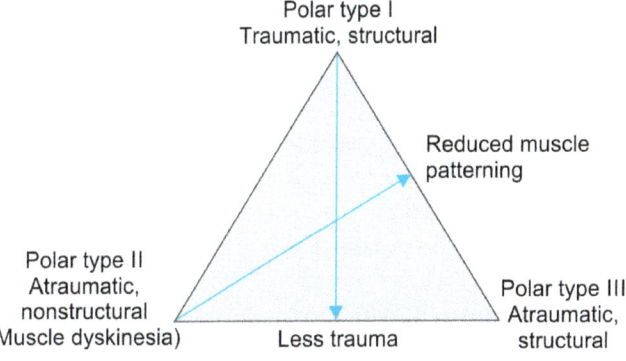

Fig. 4: Stanmore classification is based on proportion of trauma and inherent muscle structure causes of instability.

D. Direction

1. *Anterior (>80%):*
   a. Subcoracoid
   b. Subclavicular
   c. Subglenoid
   d. Intrathoracic (rarely)
2. *Posterior:*
   a. Subacromial
   b. Subspinous
3. *Inferior:* Luxatio erecta

V. CLINICAL EVALUATION

A. History

1. Age at which the symptoms of instability started: determines likelihood of having recurrent instability.
2. Mechanism of initial injury.
3. Position of the upper limb during incident
   ↓
   Anterior instability → *ABER* (abduction and external rotation)
   Posterior instability → force is applied to arm when it is in front of chest

B. Physical Examination

1. Atrophy or asymmetry of shoulder on inspection.
2. Axillary/brachial plexus injury
   ↓
   Regimental badge sign
3. Tenderness
   i. Anterior instability → posterior capsule
   ii. Multidirectional → medial angle of the scapula due to muscle compensation.

C. Special Tests

1. *Anterior instability:*
   i. *Anterior apprehension test:* Arm abducted to 90° in supine or sitting position.
   ↓
   Slowly externally rotated while anterior stress is applied to humerus
   ↓
   Facial expression → Apprehension
   ii. *Relocation test* → with the arm in position that produces apprehension, a posteriorly directed force is applied on proximal arm.
   ↓
   Reduces the subluxation by pushing the humeral head back toward the center of the glenoid
   ↓
   Relief to the patient

   iii. *Surprise test:* The posterior force applied by the examiner in the relocation test is suddenly stopped
   ↓
   Apprehension returns.
   iv. *Anterior and posterior drawer test:*
   Arm is abducted to 60° and the shoulder is subluxated anteriorly and posteriorly after stabilizing the scapula.
   GRADE I: Translation of humeral head to glenoid rim
   GRADE II: Translation of HH over glenoid rim that reduces back spontaneously
   GRADE III: Dislocation without spontaneous reduction.
   v. *Load and shift test:* Stabilize scapula, then "load" HH by pushing it toward glenoid followed by shifting the humeral head in anterior, inferior and posterior direction.

2. *Posterior instability:*

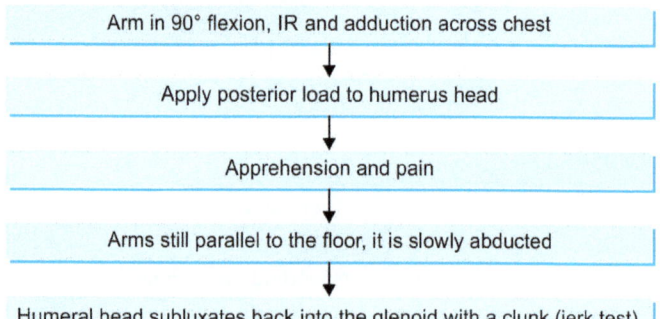

3. *Inferior instability:*
   Sulcus test: Arm kept on the side of the body → pull the arm down toward the foot
   ↓
   Sulcus/Dimple is noted between the humeral head

VI. INVESTIGATIONS

A. *X-ray:* — True AP (Grashey view)
   Axillary view

1. *Grashay view:*
   a. X-ray in the plane of the scapula, unlike standard AP where it is in the plane of thorax
   ↓
   b. Erosion or fracture of anterior glenoid
   c. IR view → Hill sach's lesion on the posterolateral aspect of HH
2. *Axillary view:*
   a. Patients arm in abduction cassette placed on superior aspect of shoulder
   ↓
   X-ray passed through axilla, toward I/L coracoids.
   b. Anteroinferior glenoid lesion

3. *West point view:* Axillary lateral view, in prone, shoulder 90° abduction and elbow bent and hanging over the table.
↓
Work-up of suspected glenoid bone loss
4. *Stryker notch view:* Variant of AP with arm abducted and ER. Beam 10° cephalad
↓
Hill Sach's lesion in humeral head.

B. *CT scan:*
1. Glenoid bone loss, bony Bankart
2. Glenoid version, hypotension, erosion
3. 3D CT: Qualification of bone loss **(Fig. 5)**

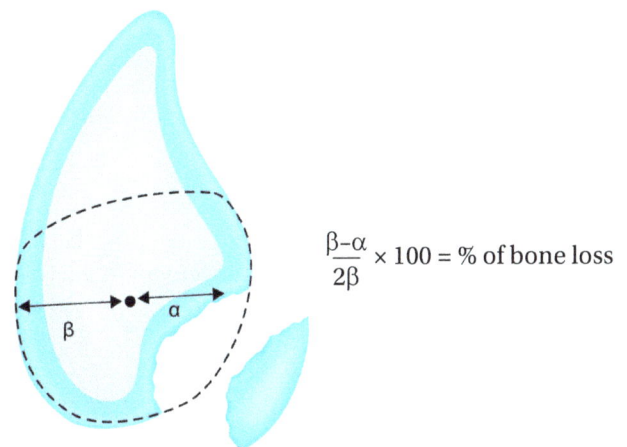

$\frac{\beta-\alpha}{2\beta} \times 100 = \%$ of bone loss

C. *MRI*:
1. Capsule ligament complex integrity.
2. *Perthes lesion:* Variant of Bankart *torn labrum*, still attached to *scapular neck* by *medially striped* but *intact periosteum*
3. *ALPSA:* Anterior labral periosteal sleeve avulsion
↓
Medialized Bankart lesion where the avulsed labrum pulled medially
↓
Heads on the glenoid neck at a more medial and inferior level.
4. *J-sign: Humeral avulsion of the glenoid labrum (HAGL)* causing effusion of the anteroinferior capsule.
D. *Examination* ↓ *Anesthesia and arthroscopy*
↓
Demonstration of unsuspected plane of instability in multidirectional instability.
↓
Dx arthroscopy in the same anesthesia identifies intra-articular pathologies that require intervention.

VII. TREATMENT
1. Traumatic anterior dislocation is the MCC of shoulder instability.

2. *Nonoperative:*
   A. Acute reduction + immobilization
      i. Kocher's maneuver
      ii. Stimsons
      iii. Traction—counter traction
      Followed by physiotherapy after 3 weeks.
   B. Anterior atraumatic subluxation ⎫
   C. Posterior instability   ⎬ rehabilitation
      i. Dynamic stabilizing mechanisms →
         a. Muscle strength
         b. Co-ordination and training
      ii. Optimal neuromuscular control of periscapular muscles
      iii. Improving proprioception
3. *Operative:*
   A. *Indications:*
      i. Irreducible dislocation
      ii. Open or recurrent dislocations
      iii. Traumatic anterior instability
      iv. Failed nonoperative Mx
      v. Young age
      vi. Significant glenoid or Humeral bone defects
   B. *Groups:*
      Group 1—Bankart repair
      Group 2—Bristow and Latarjet (bony procedure to augment bone defect)
      Group 3—Putti-Platt and Magnuson-Stack (historical)
      i. **Bankart repair:**
         1. Capsular reattachment procedure
         2. Anatomic reconstruction of the avulsed capsule and labrum at the glenoid labrum → suture anchors
         3. Indications:
            • First time traumatic shoulder dislocation with Bankart lesion in athlete < 25 years
            • High demand athlete
            • <25% glenoid bone loss
            • Remplissage augmentation with Bankart
            ↓
            Hill sach's "off track"
         4. Open Bankart repair
            i. Revision stabilization following failed arthroscopic Bankart
            ii. Humeral avulsion of GH ligament (HAGL) **(Fig. 6)**

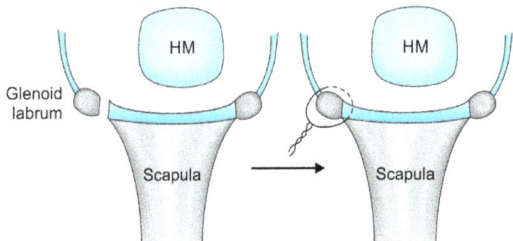

Fig. 6: Bumper effect of Bankart repair.

ii. **Latarjet**
  1. Indicated in chronic bone deficiency with > 25% glenoid bone loss
     ↓
     Inverted pear deformity
  2. Transfer of coracoid bone along with

     Conjoint tendon   Coracoacromial ligament
     • Biceps (SH)
     • Coracobrachialis
  3. *Triple effect* (Fig. 7)

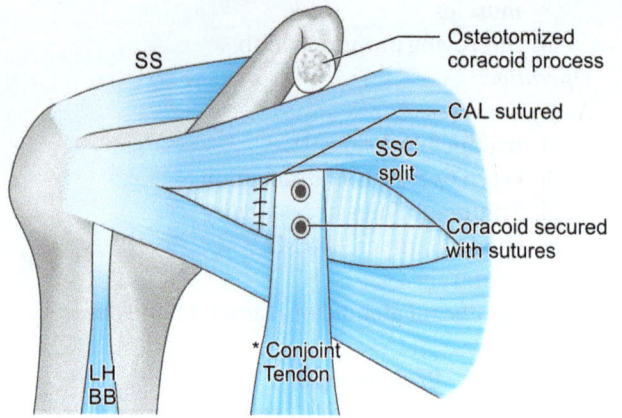

  i. Bony: AP diameter of glenoid ↑, ↑ Glenoid track
  ii. Sling: Conjoint tendon on top of Subscapularis
  iii. Capsule reconstruction: Using coracoacromial ligament
  4. If glenoid loss > 40%: Iliac crest graft.
     ↓
     Eden-Hybinette procedure
iii. *Putti–Platt*

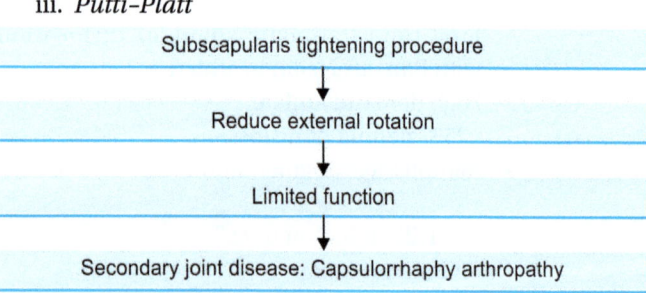

FROZEN SHOULDER

I. INTRODUCTION
A pathological condition characterized by an *idiopathic, progressive, painful* loss of active and passive shoulder motion.

II. CLASSIFICATION (LUNDBERG)
1. *Primary:* No underlying cause
   Risk factors: DM, hypo/hyperthyroid, Dupuytren's disease.
2. *Secondary:*
   i. Post-traumatic
   ii. Post-surgical

III. PATHOPHYSIOLOGY

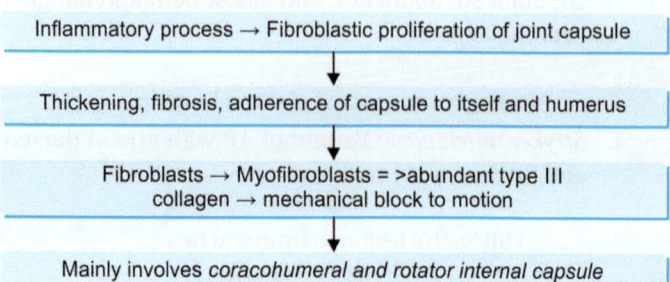

IV. CLINICAL STAGES (FIG. 8)
1. *First 3 months*
   Pain and minimal loss of motion
2. *Freezing/painful (3–9 months)*
   Pain and progressive loss of motion
3. *Frozen/stiff (9–15 months)*
   Pain subsides
   Almost complete loss of motion
4. *Thawing (15–24 months)*
   Minimal pain → Progressive improvement ROM

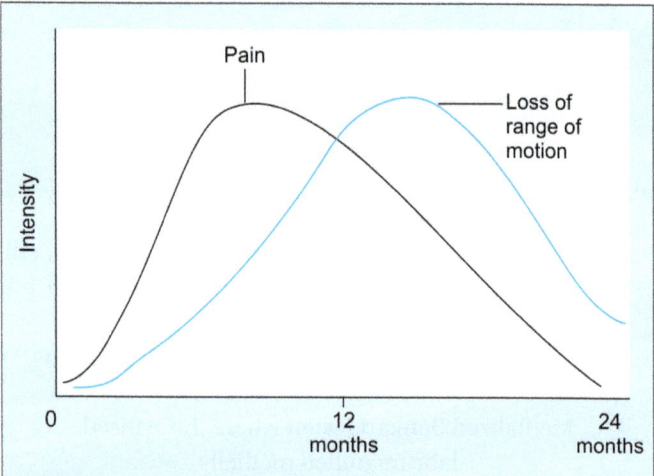

V. ARTHROSCOPIC STAGING (NEVIASER)
1. Patchy fibrinous synovitis
2. Capsular contraction and fibrinous adhesions
3. ↑ Contraction, resolving synovitis
4. Advanced capsular contraction and poor negotiation of arthroscope

VI. CLINICAL PRESENTATION
1. Purely clinical diagnosis
2. Insidious onset shoulder pain and night pain
3. ↓ ROM, ER: Most common, but global restriction
4. Pain and loss of ROM is variable depending on the time of presentation (Fig. 8)
5. 40–60 years, female > male
6. Symmetric loss of active and passive ROM

VII. INVESTIGATIONS

1. X-ray:
   i. May show osteopenia
   ii. Excludes other diagnosis
2. MRI:
   i. Synovitis
   ii. Capsular thickening. Loss of capsular recess.

VIII. DIFFERENTIAL DIAGNOSIS

1. Calcific tendonitis
2. RC tendinopathy
3. GH arthritis

IX. TREATMENT

A. Conservative

1. Pain control → NSAIDs
2. *Physical therapy:*
   i. Pain-free stretching
   ii. Pendulum exercises
   iii. Shoulder elevation exercises
   iv. Hand to back
3. Heat and cryotherapy
4. Local ultrasound
5. TENS
6. Intra-articular steroid injections

B. Operative

1. *Manipulation under anesthesia (MUA):*

   Indication: Failure of nonoperative Rx.
   Must be done after freezing stage when pain has settled.
   ↓
   Otherwise, injury to capsule
   ↓
   Loss of ROM (2°)
   MUA → Gentle and controlled →
   avoid injury to bony and soft tissues.

2. *Arthroscopic capsule release:*
   i. After extensive therapy has failed (6 months)
   ii. Posterior release: ↑ IR and adduction
   iii. Coracohumeral ligament and rotator interval released

X. RECENTLY

FROST Trials from UK → Physiotherapy, MUA and Arthroscopic release → Same outcome at 12 months of treatment.

ROTATOR CUFF DISEASE

I. INTRODUCTION

Full spectrum of shoulder joint disorder involving RC.
1. Subacromial and subcoracoid *impingement*
2. Calcific tendinitis.
3. Rotator cuff tears
4. Rotator cuff arthropathy

Neer Stages of Impingement
   i. Edema, hemorrhage <25 years
   ii. Fibrosis, tendinosis 25–40 years
   iii. Bone spurs and tendon rupture >40 years

II. ANATOMY

Muscles	Origin	Insertion	Function	Innervation
Supraspinatus	Supraspinous fossa of scapula	GT—superior facet	Initiates shoulder abduction up to 15°	Suprascapular nerve
Infraspinatus	Infraspinous fossa of scapula	GT—posterior facet	External rotation	Suprascapular
Teres minor	Lateral border of scapula	GT—inferior facet	External rotation	Axillary
Subscapularis	Subscapular fossa (internal surface) of scapula	Lesser tubercle	Internal rotation	Subscapular

Long head of biceps—functional part.

III. ETIOLOGY—PATHOGENESIS

1. *Chronic impingement*: Most common typically starts on the *bursal* surface or within the tendon.
2. *Chronic degenerative tear*: Aging
   i. Intrinsic degeneration
   ii. Older patients
   iii. Usually involves *SIT* muscles
3. *Trauma*—Repetitive microtrauma (overuse)
   High velocity trauma
4. *Developmental:*
   Bigliani classification—Shape of acromion
   i. Flat 3%
   ii. Curved 24% } Percentage of tears
   iii. Hooked 73%
5. Iatrogenic

IV. NATURAL HISTORY

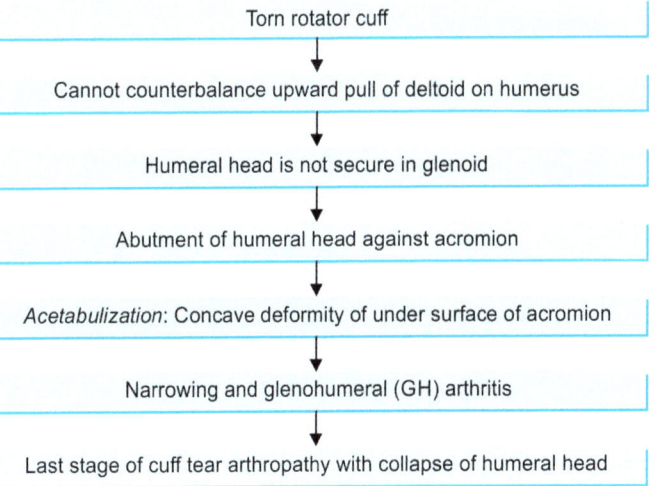

Hamada and Fukuda classification of rotator cuff arthropathy (AHI: acromiohumeral interval)
Grade 1: AHI ≥ 6 mm
Grade 2: AHI ≤ 5 mm
Grade 3: AHI ≤ 5 mm + acetabulization
Grade 4: GH arthritis
    Grade 4A: GHA without acetabulization.
        AHI > 7 mm
    Grade 4B: GHA with acetabulization.
        AHI ≤ 5 mm
Grade 5: GH collapse

V. CLASSIFICATION

A. Duration
1. Acute
2. Chronic

B. Degree
1. Partial
2. Complete

C. Etiology
1. Traumatic
2. Degenerative

D. Ellman
Partial thickness tear—%:
    Grade I: <3 mm (<25%)
    Grade II: 3-6 mm (25-50%)
    Grade III: >6 mm (50%)
    Location:
A = Articular
B = Bursal
C = Intratendinous

E. Goutallier
Fatty infiltration:
0—normal
1—some fatty streaks
2—muscle > fat
3—muscle = fat
4—fat > muscle

F. **Patte's:** *Supraspinatus tendon retraction* **(Fig. 9)**

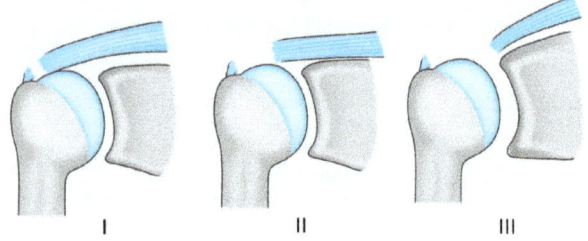
I   II   III

I–Proximal stump near bony insertion
II–At humeral head
III–At glenoid or more proximal

G. **Ellman:** Full thickness tear **(Fig. 10)**

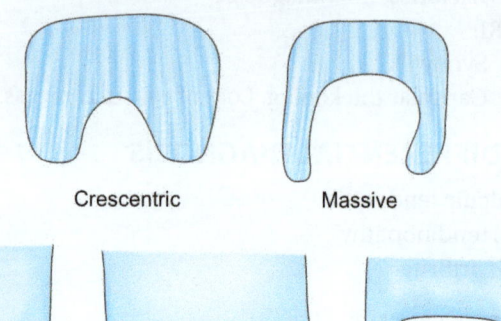

Crescentric   Massive
L-shaped   Reverse-L   Trapedoidal

VI. CLINICAL PRESENTATION
A. History of trauma ±
B. *Symptoms:*
   1. *Pain:*
      i. Insidious and deltoid region
      ii. Exacerbated by overhead activities
      iii. *Night pain*
      iv. Acute → traumatic
   2. *Weakness:*
      i. Loss of active ROM
      ii. Intact passive ROM
   3. Catching, popping, and clicking
   4. Restricted activities of daily living
C. *Physical examination:*
   1. Muscle atrophy
   2. Neer's, Hawkins, painful arc test → *Impingement*
   3. Empty can/Jobe's, drop arm test—SS
   4. External rotation lag sign—IS
   5. Hornblower's test—T. Minor
   6. Belly press/bear hug
      Lift off   } SSC
      Gerbers

VII. INVESTIGATIONS
A. X-ray
   1. True AP: Glenohumeral joint
   2. AP in internal rotation: Hill Sachs
   3. AP in external rotation: GT and proximal humeral physis
   4. *Axillary*: Glenoid rim, acromion, and coracoids
   5. Rule out other diagnosis
B. *MRI*: Diagnosis standard for RC pathology
        Medial biceps tendon subluxation
                ↓
            Indicative of *SSC* tear

VIII. TREATMENT

A. *Considerations*:
   1. Age
   2. Activity level
   3. Severity of symptoms
   4. Patient requirements
   5. Type of tear
B. *Conservative*: First-line Rx for most tears.
   1. Rest
   2. Activity modification
   3. Pain control: NSAIDs
   4. Physiotherapy: Stretching and strengthening exercises
   5. Subacromial corticosteroid injections
C. *Operative*: Failure of conservative (at least 6 weeks)
   i. *Samilson and Binder criteria*
      1. Physiological age <60 years
      2. Clinically and arthroscopically demonstrable full thickness tear
      3. Failure of nonoperative Rx: 6 weeks
      4. Need overhead elevation
      5. Full passive ROM
      6. Ability and compliance
   ii. *Objectives*:
      1. Closure of cuff defect
      2. Eliminating impingement
      3. Preserving origin of deltoid
      4. Preventing postoperative adhesions: PT
   iii. *Modalities*
      1. Mini–open
      2. Arthroscopic
   iv. *Subacromial decompression and rotator cuff debridement alone*
      1. Indications → Low grade PASTA (partial articular supraspinatus tendon avulsion)
   v. *Rotator cuff repair*:
      1. Acute full thickness tear
      2. Bursal—side > 3 mm (>25%)
      3. PASTA > 50%
         Techniques:
            i. Single row
            ii. Double row
            iii. Transosseous
   v. *Tendon transfer*–Massive RCT:
      1. Pectoralis major
      2. Latissimus dorsi
   vi. *Reverse total shoulder arthroplasty*:
      1. Indicated in GH arthritis
      2. Low demand
      3. Deltoid intact.

LONG HEAD OF BICEPS BRACHII RUPTURE

I. PATHOANATOMY

1. Origin → Supraglenoid tubercle and superior labrum.
2. Transverse humeral ligament stabilizes it within the bicipital groove.
3. Also stabilized by the biceps sling

   i. Fibers of the subscapularis
   ii. Supraspinatus
   iii. Coracohumeral
   iv. Superior glenohumeral ligaments
4. Functions → Dynamic stabilizer of the shoulder joint → Prevents upward migration of humeral head → reduces impingement.

II. ETIOPATHOLOGY

1. Male > Female
2. Age group 40-60, middle age
3. Risk factors: Parachutists, heavy weight lifting, and high contact sports
4. *Elderly*:
   i. Attrition of tendon from friction of coracoacromial arch or AC osteophytes
   ii. Repeated steroid injections into bicipital groove
5. Young → Traumatic
6. Associated with SLAP tear

III. CLINICAL FEATURES

1. Young → Feeling a "snap" at the time of injury.
2. Indirect injury often occurs via powerful contraction of the biceps against isometric position.
3. Acutely → Severe pain and swelling with feeling of loss of strength especially in elbow flexion and shoulder external rotation.
4. This is followed by a few weeks of mild-to-moderate pain, followed by resolution of the pain and restoration of normal function.
5. Degenerative → Painless or dull pain
6. Tenderness at bicipital groove
7. ROM → Full
8. Negligible loss of flexion and supination → Short head still attached
9. Popeye deformity
10. Speed test positive
11. Yergason test positive

IV. RADIOLOGY

1. Shoulder: RC arthropathy
2. Rule out other injuries
3. MRI: Absence of tendon in groove

V. MANAGEMENT

1. Rest, ice, compression, and limb elevation
2. NSAIDs
3. Physiotherapy
4. Patients may be treated nonoperatively since most will become asymptomatic after 4-6 weeks
5. *Surgical management:*
   - Young
   - Active population (<50 years) → requiring powerful supination activities (carpenters)
   - Chronic rotator cuff pathology
6. Tenodesis → young active patients
7. Tenotomy → elderly patients
8. Open or Arthroscopic
9. Acromioplasty and coracoacromial ligament excision → As rupture of the long head of the biceps ↑ risk of subacromial impingement syndrome resulting from the pull of short head of the biceps onto the humeral head.

REVERSE SHOULDER ARTHROPLASTY

I. INTRODUCTION

1. Reverse shoulder arthroplasty (RSA) is a type of shoulder arthroplasty that uses a convex glenoid hemispheric ball and a concave humerus articulating cup to reconstruct the glenohumeral joint.
2. It was introduced in 1987 by Professor Paul Grammont as a treatment option for rotator cuff arthropathy in the elderly.

II. HISTORY AND EVOLUTION OF RSA

1. Rotator cuff muscles encircle the humeral head, and compress it against the glenoid, → providing a fulcrum on which the deltoid can lever to elevate the arm.
2. When rotator cuff is lost → humeral head displaces superiorly, with loss of a functioning fulcrum.
3. Deltoid contraction is unable to raise the arm as the head does not rotate on the glenoid.
4. Humeral head displacement toward the coracoacromial arch leads to a painful acromial erosions and glenohumeral arthritis.
5. Total shoulder replacement in these cuff deficient cases is associated with a high rate of failure because of a "rocking horse" phenomenon which leads to eccentric glenoid loading and failure.
6. Consequently, hemiarthroplasty was the most appropriate treatment option for patients with arthritis secondary to a rotator cuff deficiency.
7. Although pain improved, there was limited improvement in function and the results were compromised by glenoid and acromial bone erosion.
8. To prevent the proximal humeral migration, constrained and semi-constrained implants were tried but all of these failed because of excessive stress on the constraints causing implant loosening.
9. To compensate for the rotator cuff deficiency, the ball and socket articulations were reversed by Grammont.

III. PRINCIPLE

1. Medialization of the center of rotation
2. Retensioning of the deltoid by distalizing the humerus
3. A constant center of rotation leading to an inherently stable implant
4. A semi-constrained prosthesis with a larger arc of motion.

A. Medialization of Centre of Rotation

1. The centre of rotation (COR) is medialized compared to an anatomic shoulder, the RSA confers stability at the bone-implant interface.
2. Movements occur around the fixed COR, this helps to convert the compressive and shear forces into a largely compressive vector.
3. There is reduction in the magnitude of the peak forces generated in both compression and shear across the shoulder joint throughout the ROM in reverse total shoulders.

B. Retensioning of the Deltoid

1. Medialization of COR leads to an increased lever arm of deltoid leading to increased efficiency/power of deltoid in abducting/overhead elevation of arm.
2. RSA also distalizes the deltoid insertion thus increasing its length and thus its tension and efficiency.
3. The orientation of the muscle fibers becomes more vertical, and muscle recruitment changes such that all three sub-regions of the deltoid become primary shoulder abductors

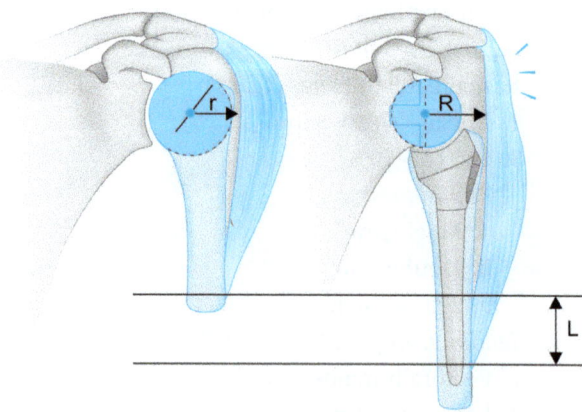

Medialization of COR and lengthening of deltoid

4. These changes in muscle recruitment for abduction come at a cost → As the posterior deltoid is recruited to

become an abductor, its external rotation moment arm is lost, contributing to the external rotation deficit seen following RSA.

C. An Inherently Stable Shoulder
The minimization of shear forces conferred by a constant, medial COR leads to an inherently stable shoulder.

D. A Semi-constrained Prosthesis
1. A semi-constrained prosthesis is achieved by utilizing a relatively larger glenosphere relative to the humeral cup component.
2. The humeral component must be deep enough to allow inherent stability in a cuff-deficient shoulder, but shallow enough to minimize impingement and shear forces generated in extremes of motion.

IV. INDICATIONS
1. Cuff-tear arthropathy
2. Massive rotator cuff tear with pseudoparalysis
3. Severe inflammatory arthritis with a massive cuff tear
4. Proximal humeral fractures in the elderly → 3-4 part fractures, age > 65.
5. Failed total shoulder arthroplasty
6. Absence of tuberosities (failed hemiarthroplasty for fracture/nonunion)
7. Absence of cuff (failed hemiarthroplasty for cuff-tear arthropathy)
8. Instability
9. Proximal humeral non-union
10. Reconstruction after tumor removal

V. PATIENT CHARACTERISITICS
1. Low functional demand
2. Physiological age > 65-70
3. Sufficient glenoid bone stock (otherwise needs bone graft build up)
4. Working deltoid muscle → intact axillary nerve

VI. CONTRAINDICATIONS
1. Non-functioning deltoid muscle
2. Axillary nerve damage
3. Glenoid vault deficiency precluding baseplate fixation
4. Active infection
5. Neuropathic joints (relative C/I off lately)
6. Severe osteoporosis especially in the glenoid

VII. SURGICAL TECHNIQUE
1. Approach: Deltopectoral
2. Position: Beach chair with free movement of the limb
3. Superficial dissection: Plane between deltoid and pectoralis major, preserving and retracting the cephalic vein laterally.
4. Deep dissection: Identify the rotator interval and open it. Tenotomize the long head of biceps.
5. Subscapularis is tenotomized close to the musculotendinous junction or osteotomy of lesser tuberosity is performed, the subscapularis is repaired at the end of the procedure in an attempt to provide an anterior envelope and increased stability.
6. Humeral head typically osteotomized, respecting the greater and lesser tuberosities, in around 20° of retroversion → More retroversion is gaining popularity as it may improve postoperative external rotation.
7. This exposes the glenoid. The labrum is excised and the capsule is released circumferentially.
8. Glenoid preparation
    i. The exact positioning and orientation of the guidewire for the reamer are crucial.
    ii. Upward tilting must be avoided to prevent glenoid component loosening.
    iii. Inferior notching can be avoided by positioning of the glenoid component as low as possible.
    iv. Ream the glenoid until the "smiley face" is achieved, with bleeding cancellous bone inferiorly and hard sclerotic bone superiorly. This confirms adequate inferior tilt of the baseplate.
    v. Impact the baseplate and secure it with screws. The peripheral screws are ideally placed in the "pillars" of densest cortical bone—the coracoid base, inferior pillar, and scapular spine.
    vi. Dry the Morse taper and impact the glenosphere onto baseplate
9. Humeral preparation
    i. Ream and broach technique is used.
    ii. Position of the implant is in 20-30° retroversion
    iii. If cementing is deemed necessary because of a previous surgical procedure, fracture, osteoporosis, rheumatoid arthritis, or degenerative cysts, place a cement restrictor or a cortical bone plug from the resected humeral head 2 cm inferior to the tip of the prosthesis.
    iv. Trial stem with humeral concave plate is placed followed by reduction with gentle traction, internal rotation and forward elevation of the arm.
    v. Check for stability and final implantation is done.
10. Tuberosity repair: Tuberosities are fixed onto the implant, though not essential for the functioning of the prosthesis

VIII. COMPLICATIONS
1. Glenoid component loosening → MC mechanism of failure
2. Humeral stem loosening
3. Instability
4. Dislocation
5. Prosthetic joint infection
6. Periprosthetic fractures

7. Deltoid muscle dysfunction (d/t injury to axillary nerve)
8. Stiffness
9. Acromial stress fractures (d/t over lengthening of deltoid)
10. Scapular spine fractures (common in osteoporotic patients)
11. Scapular notching
    i. Occurs due to impingement of medial humeral rim during adduction
    ii. Risk factors:
        a. Superiorly placed glenoid component
        b. Superior tilt of glenoid component
        c. Medialization of centre of rotation
        d. High BMI
    iii. Use of a more varus stem with a neck-shaft angle of 135° (rather than 155°) and a lateralized glenosphere reduces notching rates.

SECTION 7

Foot and Ankle

ARCHES OF THE FOOT

I. DEFINITION
Structures formed by the tarsal and metatarsal bones, giving the characteristic curvature of the plantar surface of the feet.

II. FUNCTION
1. Supports the body weight—proportional distribution
2. Shock absorbers
3. Works like a lever or springboard to propel the body forward during locomotion
4. Adapts to uneven surfaces
5. Plantar concavity protects the plantar vessels and nerves from compression
   That is why, Flat foot → Compression → Metatarsalgia.

III. TYPES

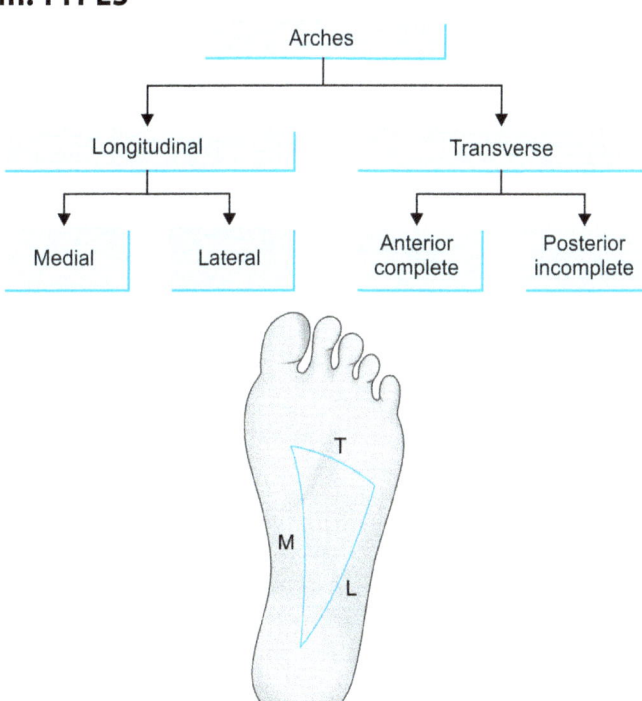

Fig. 1: M: medial longitudinal arch; L: lateral longitudinal arch; T: transverse arch.

IV. PARTS
A. Medial Longitudinal Arch (MLA) (Fig. 2)

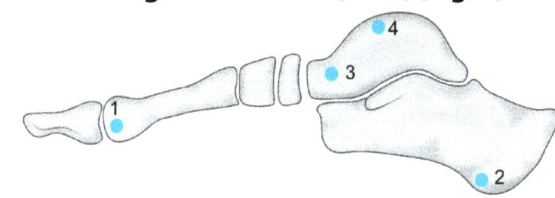

Fig. 2: Parts of medial longitudinal arch.

1. Anterior pillar: 1st–3rd MT heads
2. Posterior pillar: Medial tubercle of calcaneus
3. Keystone: Talus
4. Summit: Superior articular surface of talus
5. Nine bones: 3 MT, 3 cuneiforms, navicular, talus calcaneum.

B. Lateral Longitudinal Arch (LLA)
1. Anterior pillar: 4–5th MT heads
2. Posterior pillar: Calcaneum
3. Keystone: Cuboid
4. Summit: Subtalar articular surface
5. Four bones: MT-2, Cuboid, calcaneum.

Difference between MLA and LLA:

MLA	LLA
1. Resilience	1. Rigidity
2. Higher	2. Less
3. ↑ Mobile	3. ↓ Mobile
4. Propulsion	4. Receiving and supporting weight

C. Transverse Arch

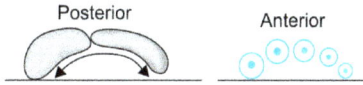

Fig. 3: Transverse arch-.

1. Anterior:
   i. Heads of all MTs
   ii. Complete: Standing position 1st and 5th MT heads touch the ground.
2. Posterior:
   i. Incomplete
   ii. Base of all MT, three cuneiforms and cuboid.
   iii. Half-dome: Completed when foot placed together.

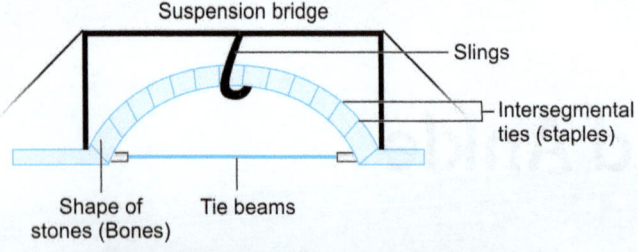

Fig. 4A: Analogy of foot arches to a bridge.

V. FACTORS MAINTAINING THE ARCHES (FIGS. 4A AND B)

1. Bones
2. Suspension bridge
3. Slings
4. Intersegmental ties (staples) (cement)

	Sling	Tie-beam	Staples
1. Medial longitudinal arch	Tibialis anterior and posterior	Plantar fascia	Deltoid ligament. TP insertion
2. Lateral longitudinal arch	Peroneus longus, brevis	Flexor digiti minimi Extensor digiti minimi	Long and short plantar ligament
3. Transverse	*Medial:* Tibialis anterior *Lateral:* Peroneus longus peroneus tertius	Peroneus longus tendon	Dorsal interossei Deep transverse ligament

VI. DEFORMITIES

1. *Pes planus*:
   a. Flexible
   b. Rigid
2. Pes cavus
3. CTEV
4. Equinovalgus.

BLOOD SUPPLY OF TALUS

1. The talus is 60% covered by articular cartilage → limited space for blood vessels.
2. No muscles originate from or insert into the talus.
3. Therefore, the vascular supply is dependent on fascial structures to reach the talus.
   ↓
   Capsular disruptions → Osteonecrosis.
4. Talus is supplied by three main arteries of the leg.

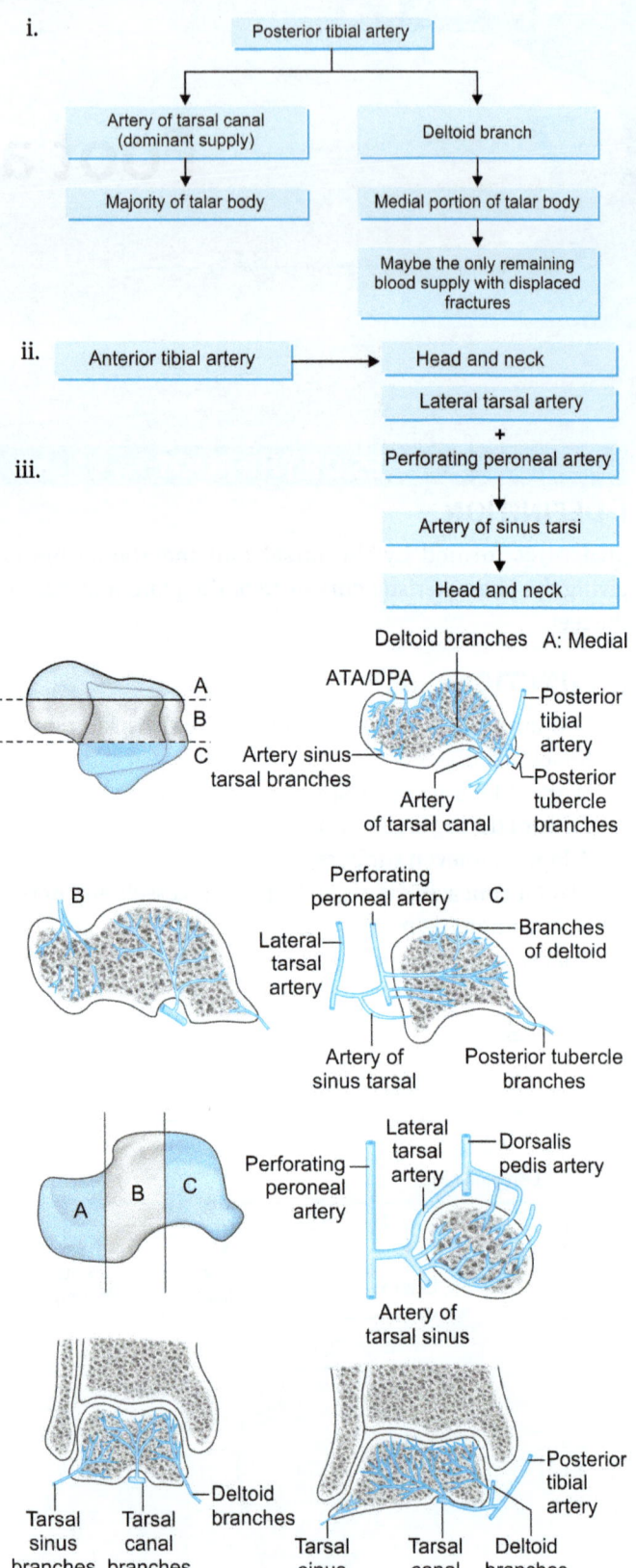

Fig. 4B: Blood supply of talus.

5. Wildenauer described the critical anastomotic sling of vessels in the tarsal sinus and tarsal canal, lying inferior to neck of talus.

6. With tarsal sinus and tarsal canal
↓
Anastomotic vessels perforate the inferior neck
↓
1° blood supply to body of talus.

7. Tarsal sinus is bounded
   i. Inferiorly → Calcaneus
   ii. Posteriorly → Body of talus
   iii. Anteriorly → Talar head and neck
8. The tarsal canal lies between the talus and calcaneus just behind and below the tip of medial malleolus (**Fig. 5**).

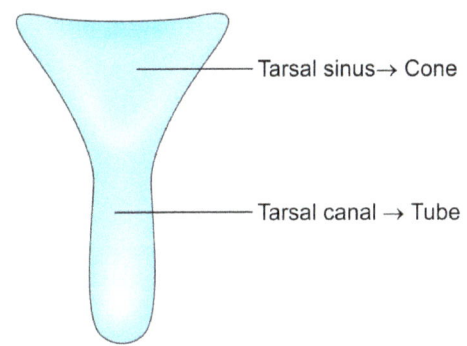

Fig. 5: Funnel shaped tarsal canal and tarsal sinus.

9. *Clinical application:*
   i. Deprivation of single source of blood supply (BS) usually does not cause necrosis.
   ii. Severity of injury α extent of vascular interruption α AVN
   iii. Types (Hawkins)
      I. Type I: Minimally displaced neck fracture. 1 source of BS ⊗ → AVN unlikely.
      II. Type II: Neck fracture + Subtalar dislocation. 2 BS sources ⊗: 50% AVN
      III. Type III: Neck, subtalar + Ankle joint dislocation. All 3 sources ⊗: 95% AVN
      IV. Type IV: Neck fracture + Subtalar + Ankle + Talonavicular joint dislocation
         Severe disruption of blood supply → AVN almost certain.
   iv. Earliest evidence of AVN: **Hawkin's sign**
      Sign of preserved bone → Subchondral lucency, best seen on mortise X-ray at 6–8 weeks.
   v. Premature weight bearing in presence of dead bone → Collapse.
   vi. *Investigations:* MRI, bone scan
   vii. Non-weight-bearing and immobilization for months
   ↓
   Revascularization and replacement by creeping substitution.

TARSAL TUNNEL SYNDROME

I. INTRODUCTION

1. Compression neuropathy of the posterior tibial nerve as it passes through the fibro-osseous tunnel beneath the flexor retinaculum on the medial side of the ankle (**Fig. 6**).
2. From superior to inferior, behind the MM (**T**om, **D**ick **A**nd **V**ery **N**ervous **H**arry).

T: Tibialis posterior
D: FDL
AVN: Post tibial art, vein and nerve
H: FHL.

3. Course and muscles supplied by PTN

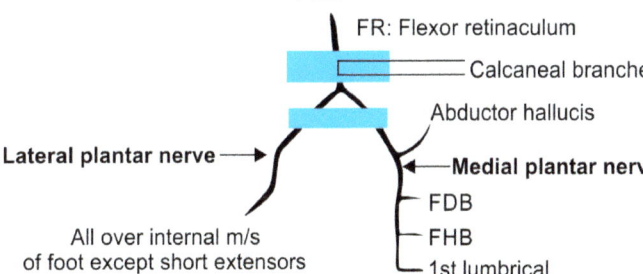

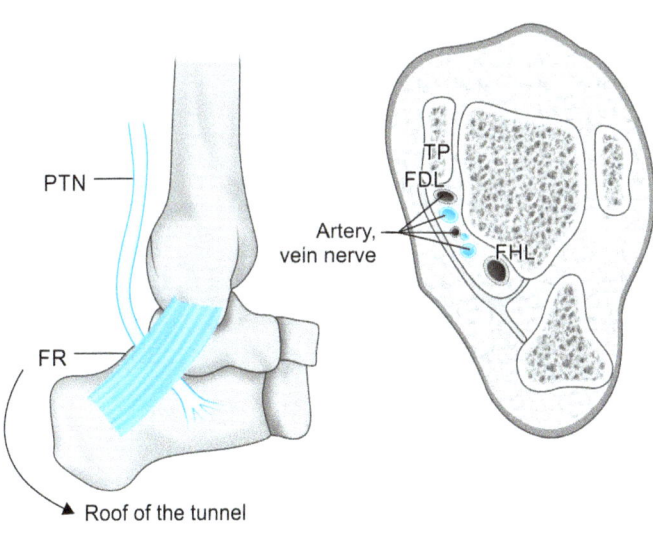

II. ETIOLOGY

A. Intrinsic

1. SOL: Ganglia, lipoma and enlarged veins
2. Osteophytes (degenerative)
3. Hypertrophic retinaculum
4. Post-traumatic hemorrhage:
   i. Adhesions
   ii. Perineural fibrosis.

B. Extrinsic
1. Varus, valgus deformities of foot
2. Direct trauma
3. Contributive footwear
4. Post-surgery scarring.

III. PATHOGENESIS AND CLINICAL FEATURES (FIG. 7)

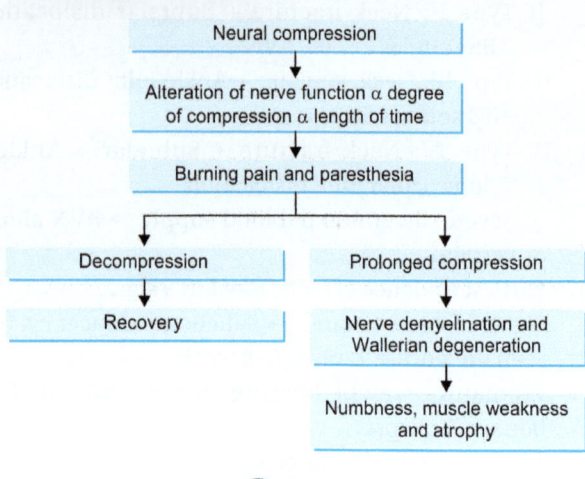

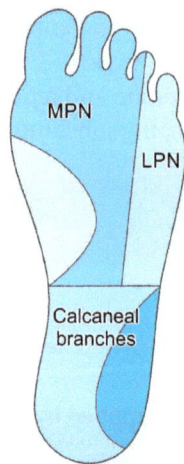

Fig. 7: Area supplied by posterior tibial nerve. (MPN: medial plantar nerve; LPN: lateral plantar nerve)

1. MC symptom → **Nocturnal** burning pain
   ↓
   Awakens patient.
   Causes them to hang leg over edge of bed and shake it.
2. Tingling numbness
3. Increases on standing and walking
4. Decreases on removing shoes and with rest.
5. Hallmark → sensory loss in area of distribution of medial and lateral plantar nerves
   ↓
   Decreased 2-point discrimination and hypoesthesia
6. Tinel sign ±
7. Tenderness over tarsal tunnel.
8. In advanced stage → Muscle weakness
   ↓
   Poor prognosis

IV. INVESTIGATIONS
1. Radiographs demonstrate structural abnormality
2. MRI—space-occupying lesion
3. EMG and NCV—to differentiate between TTS versus S1 compression

V. TREATMENT
A. Conservative: Local steroids → Temporary
B. Operative
   1. Surgical decompression
   2. Incision: Curvilinear, 1 cm posterior to medial malleolus
   3. NVB isolated, flexor retinacular divided, and nerve freed.
   4. Post-surgery exercises started immediately to decrease post operation fibrosis.
   5. If nerve tumor → Excise.
   6. For good outcome, do early surgical decompression if conservative treatment fails.
   7. Positive Tinel's sign: Good outcome.

TARSAL COALITION

I. INTRODUCTION
Structural anomaly between two or three tarsal bones leading to a **rigid pes planus**.

Two types based on etiology:
1. Congenital/developmental (more common)
2. Acquired
   i. Trauma
   ii. Degenerative
   iii. Infection
   Prevalence: 1%

II. PATHOPHYSIOLOGY
i. *Embryology*:

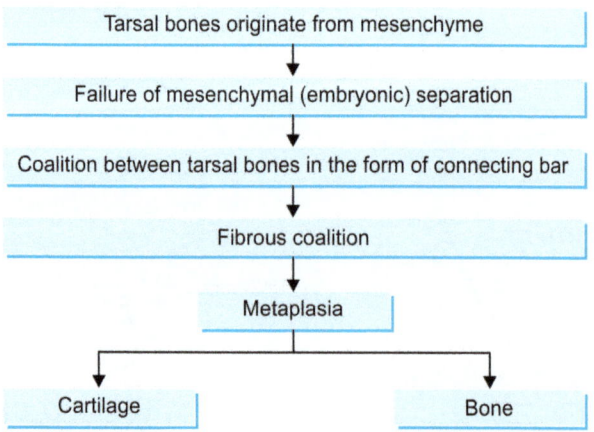

ii. *Gait mechanism*:
Normal subtalar joint rotates 10° internally during stance phase.
In presence of coalition → IR does not occur.

iii. *Deformity:*
   1. Flattening of longitudinal arch
   2. Abduction of forefoot
   3. Valgus hindfoot
   4. Peroneal spasticity (aka = peroneal spastic flat foot)
iv. *Pain generator theory:*
   1. Microfractures at coalition bone interface
   2. Increased stress on other hindfoot joints
   3. Ossification of previously fibrous or cartilaginous coalition
   4. Secondary chondral damage or degenerative changes.
v. *Associations:*

Nonsyndromic	Syndromic
Autosomal dominant	1. Fibular hemimelia 2. Carpal coalition 3. Craniosynostosis 4. Apert, Pfeiffer, Crouzon syndrome

III. CLASSIFICATION

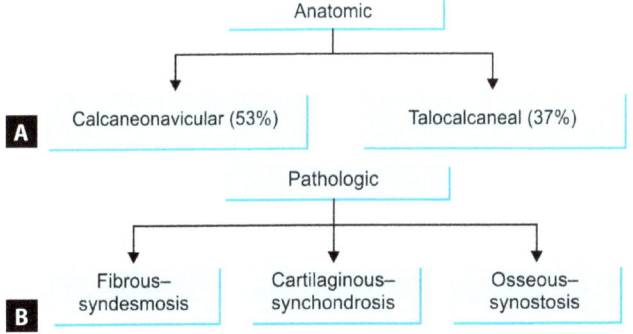

IV. PRESENTATION

A. Symptoms

1. *Asymptomatic:* 75% patients asymptomatic–incidental diagnosis
2. History of prior recurrent ankle sprains
3. *Age of onset:*
   Calcaneonavicular = 8–12 years
   Talocalcaneal = 12–15 years
4. *Pain:*
   i. Location:
      a. Calcaneonavicular: Sinus tarsi
      b. Talocalcaneal: Distal to MM, medial foot
   iii. Onset of pain correlates with age of ossification of coalition
   iv. Worsens with activity
   v. Calf pain: Due to peroneal spasticity.

B. Physical Examination

i. Inspection:
   1. Hindfoot valgus
   2. Forefoot abduction
   3. Pes planus

ii. ROM:
   1. ↓ Subtalar motion
   2. Heel cord contractures
   3. Arch of foot does not reconstitute upon toe standing. (Hindfoot remains in valgus, does not swing into varus on toe standing)
iii. Special test:
   1. Reverse Coleman block test
   2. Evaluates for subtalar rigidity

V. INVESTIGATIONS

1. Coalition in not visible before 10 years as sufficient ossification has not occurred.
2. Views:
   i. AP view foot
   ii. Standing lateral foot view
   iii. 45° Internal oblique view → CN coalition
   iv. Harris heel view
3. Findings (**Figs. 8A to C**):

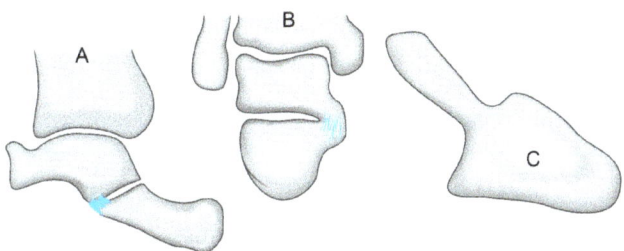

Figs. 8A to C: Tarsal coalition: (A and B) Talocalcaneal; (C) Ant eater sign of calcaneonavicular.

   i. Calcaneonavicular: "Ant-eater sign"—Elongated anterior process of calcaneus
   ii. Talocalcaneal
      a. Talar beaking on lateral radiograph
         ↓
         Result of ↓ subtalar motion
      b. C-sign: C-shaped arc formed by the medial outline of the talar dome and posteroinferior aspect of the sustentaculum tali
      c. Dysmorphic sustentaculum: Enlarged and rounded
4. *CT scan:*
   1. Rules out additional coalitions
   2. Determines size, location, and extent
   MRI:
   1. Rule out inflammatory changes
   2. Fibrous or cartilaginous coalition

VI. TREATMENT

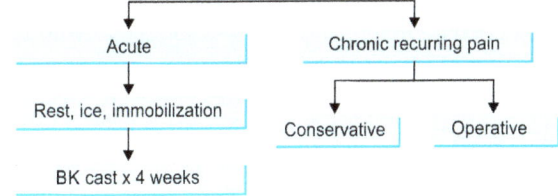

A. Conservative

1. *Indication:* Minimal pain and deformity
2. Whitman plate, arch support, molded shoe
   ↓
   Relieves stress on tarsus, ↓ symptoms
   ↓
3. If these fail, short-leg walking cast for up to 6 weeks
4. If surgical treatment required, it is best postponed till age of 12 years.

B. Operative → Open
       ↘ Arthroscopic

1. **Coalition resection** with interposition graft ± correction of associated deformity.
   (Hindfoot Valgus → Calcaneal osteotomy + hell cord lengthening)
   Indication: Involves < 50% joint surface area.
2. **Subtalar arthrodesis:**
   Indication: If coalition involves > 50 joint surface area in TC coalition
3. **Triple arthrodesis:** Advanced coalition that fails resection.

FLAT FOOT

INTRODUCTION

A condition characterized by the loss of the medial longitudinal arch of the foot.

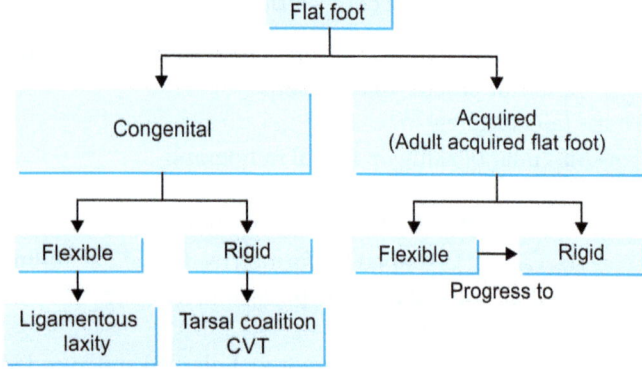

A. FLEXIBLE FLAT FOOT

I. Etiopathology

Generalized ligamentous laxity.

II. Clinical Features

1. Asymptomatic: Incidental finding
2. Arch pain
3. Standing: Foot flat: Medial border of foot touches the floor.
4. Heel raise test: Medial arch is formed
5. Hindfoot: Valgus
6. Forefoot: Abduction
7. Tight heel cord.

III. Radiograph

1. Weight-bearing X-rays
2. Talar head coverage: AP view
3. ↑ Meary's angle: Lateral view
4. Oblique views: For ruling out tarsal coalition.
5. Plantar flexed lateral view: For ruling out CVT.

IV. Treatment

1. Asymptomatic → Observation → can improve spontaneously by 8 years of age.
2. Whitman arch support
3. Physiotherapy → Stretching exercises: Tendoachilles and Peroneii
4. Tendoachilles lengthening → For tight heel cord
5. Evan's calcaneal lengthening osteotomy → Failure of conservative management.
6. Lateral column is lengthened → Forefoot abduction corrected.
7. Sliding calcaneal osteotomy
8. Grice procedure → Extra-articular arthrodesis by using bony struts lateral to the talocalcaneal joint.
9. Arthroeresis → Insertion of silicone implant in the subtalar joint to restrict valgus.

B. ADULT ACQUIRED FLAT FOOT/POSTERIOR TIBIAL TENDON INSUFFICIENCY (PTTI)/ CHRONIC PROGRESSIVE FOOT DEFORMITY

I. Etiopathophysiology

Risk factors
   i. Hypertension
   ii. Diabetes Mellitus → Charcot's joint
   iii. Obesity
   iv. Elderly
   v. Steroids
   vi. Inflammatory arthropathy → Mid-tarsal joints
   vii. Secondary to trauma

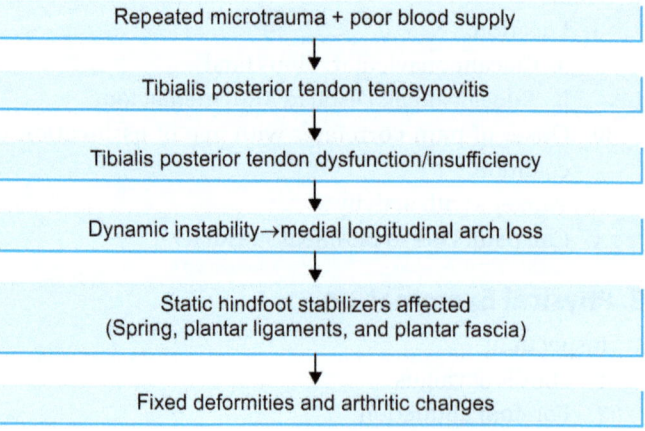

II. Stages: Classification

Johnson and Storm

Stage	Disorder
I	Tendon inflamed, but intact
II	Tendon dysfunctional, arch collapses. Passively correctable
III	Fixed deformity + Subtalar arthritis
IV	III + Ankle arthritis

III. Clinical Features

1. Female > male, 6th decade
2. Pain and weakness → medial side foot
3. Progressive collapse of medial longitudinal arch
4. Flexible → Passively correctable deformity
5. Rigid → Not correctable
6. Tenderness → Posterior to medial malleolus
7. Hindfoot → Valgus
8. Forefoot → Abduction
9. "Too many toes" sign
10. Tibialis posterior motor weakness
11. Single heel rise test:
    Patient lifts normal foot off the ground and affected foot heel is raised.
    Inability to perform → Positive test.

IV. Radiology

i. *Radiograph*:
   1. Weight-bearing X-rays → Anteroposterior and lateral foot, ankle mortise
   2. ↑ Talonavicular uncoverage
   3. ↑ Simmon's angle → Talo-1st MT angle } AP view
   4. ↑ Meary's angle (>4°) → Talo-1st MT angle (lateral view)
   5. ↓ Calcaneal pitch **(Fig. 9)**

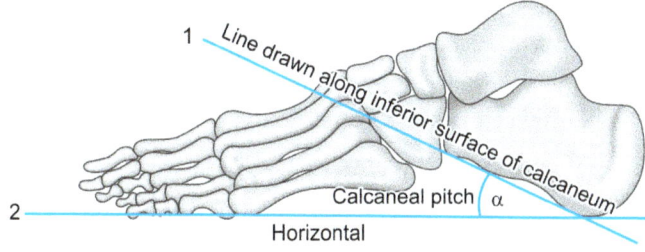

   6. Subtalar arthritis
   7. Talar tilt → mortise view → due to deltoid ligament insufficiency

ii. MRI → Posterior tibial tendon degeneration.

V. Management

1. Ankle foot orthosis:
   i. Initial treatment for stages II, III, IV
   ii. Low demand elderly
2. Walking cast immobilization → Stage I
3. In-shoe orthosis - custom molded → Stage II

Longitudinal arch support and medial heel lift:

4. Tenosynovectomy
5. Lateral column lengthening: For talonavicular uncoverage
6. Medial column arthrodesis
7. Tendoachilles lengthening
8. Deltoid ligament reconstruction/repair
9. Flexor digitorum longus transfer
10. Triple arthrodesis → Stage IV with correctable ankle valgus
11. Tibiotalocalcaneal arthrodesis → Stage IV with rigid hindfoot + tibiotalar and subtalar arthritis.

HALLUX VALGUS (BUNION)

I. INTRODUCTION

"Bunio" → Turnip
1. A deformity in which the large toe is deflected laterally.
2. A bony prominence develops secondarily over the medial aspect of the 1st head and neck.

II. ETIOLOGY

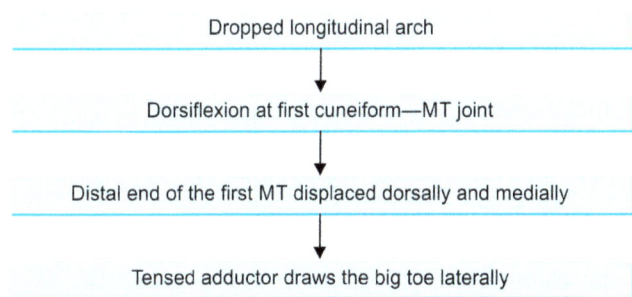

Other Factors

1. Hypermobility of 1st ray (ligamentous laxity)
2. Narrow footwear
3. Heredity
4. Contracture of TA
5. ↑ 1st MT length.
6. Metatarsus adductus
7. Pes planus
8. RA
9. Cerebral palsy.

III. PATHOLOGY (FIG. 10)

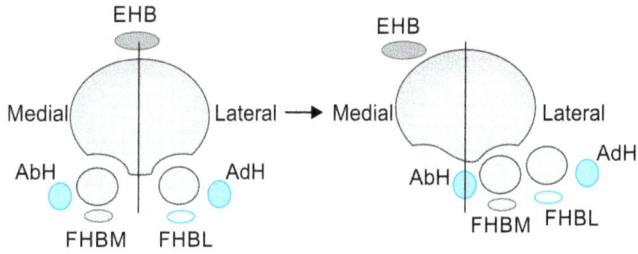

Fig. 10: Pathological displacements in hallux valgus.

1. The large toe is displaced laterally and rotated along its long axes
   ↓
   Nail tends to face medially
2. The conjoined tendon of abductor hallucis and medial tendon of insertion of the FHB, with its contained sesamoid bone → laterally.
3. Abduction of great toe is ineffective.
4. The soft tissue structures on the lateral side, conjoint tendon of the adductor and FHB and the lateral capsule → contracted
5. The sesamoid bone in this (lateral) tendon → Enlarged and displaced between the interval of 1st and 2nd MT.
6. Continuous pressure over the medial bony prominence: adventitious bursa.
7. Degenerative arthritic changes: 1st MTP
   ↓
8. Narrow and rigid joint (hallux rigidus).

Associated Pathology
1. 2nd toe displaced dorsally by great toe
   ↓
   Develops hammer toe deformity and dorsal callosity
2. The transverse arch is flat
3. Heads of middle metatarsal prominent
   In the sole → Calluses.

IV. INVESTIGATIONS (RADIOGRAPH)
1. Lateral displacement of large toe
2. Degenerative arthritic narrowing
3. MTP joint spurs
4. Lateral displacement of sesamoid
5. Medial exostosis
6. Abducted and shortened first MT.

V. CLASSIFICATION
1. *Intermetatarsal angle:* Angle between the first and second metatarsals
   i. <13°: Mild
   ii. >20°: Severe
   iii. 13-20: Moderate
2. *Hallux valgus angle*: Between long axis of the first MT and proximal phalanx
   i. <30°: Mild
   ii. >40°: Severe
   iii. 30-40: Moderate

VI. CLINICAL PICTURE

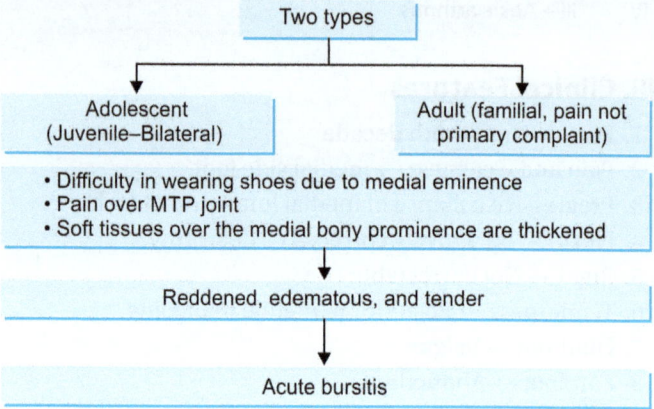

VII. TREATMENT
A. Conservative
1. Indicated for mild deformities
2. Stretching exercises
3. Toe separators
4. Shoe with enlarged toe position to accommodate the bunion
5. Acute bursitis:
   - Ice, moist compresses
   - Infected: Incision and drainage, antibiotics
6. Intra-articular injection of and steroids.

B. Operative
I. Mild deformity with congruent MTP joint:
   1. *Silver procedure:* Medial eminence resection.
   2. *Akin osteotomy:* Closing medial wedge proximal phalange osteotomy.
   3. Distal soft tissue reconstruction-McBride procedure (Fig. 11)

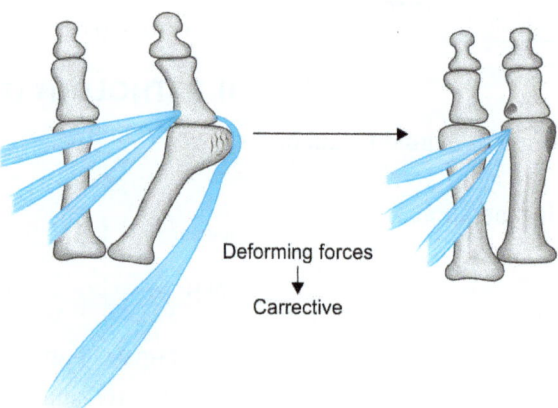

Fig. 11: McBride procedure.

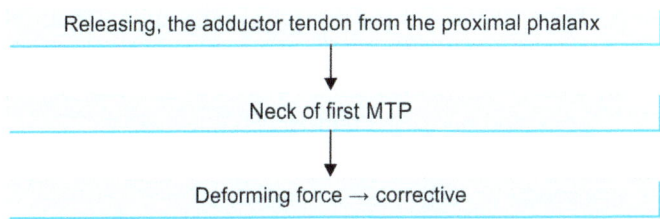

II. Mild deformity with incongruent MTP joint:
   1. *Chevron osteotomy:* V-shaped osteotomy of distal MT in coronal plane head shifted laterally.
   Ideally for young with moderate deformity.
   2. *Mitchell procedure:* Step-cut osteotomy in addition to medial eminence resection. Proximal to site of chevron osteotomy.
   Corrects associated metatarsus adductus.
III. *Moderate deformity:* Requires more proximal osteotomies
   1. *Scarf osteotomy:* Mid-shaft Z-cut osteotomy.
   2. *Akin procedure:* When deformity is at IP joint closed medial wedge osteotomy of proximal phalanx.
   These are combined with soft tissue release procedure.
IV. Severe deformity.

1. Modified Lapidus Procedure

a. Corrective metatarso–cuneiform joint fusion, after wedge resection + DSTR
b. *Indications:*
   i. Failed surgically managed cases
   ii. Neuromuscular
   iii. Inflammatory
   iv. Advanced OA of 1st MTP joint.

2. Arthroplasty of 1st MTP Joint

i. *Keller's procedure:* Resection arthroplasty: Medial eminence removal + proximal end of phalanx excision + soft tissue balancing.
ii. *Mayo/stone procedure:* Partial resection of MT head.
iii. Resection of a portion of both phalanx and MT
   Disadvantages:

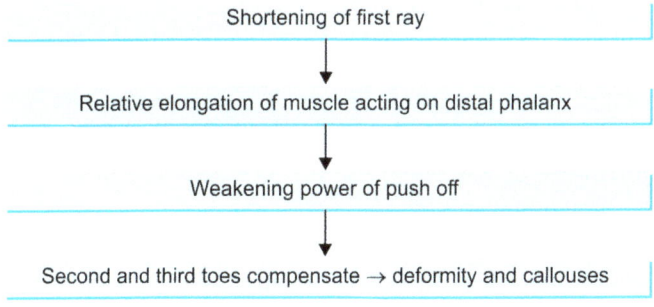

iv. Therefore, inserting flexor implant as a spacer (Swanson)

3. Arthrodesis of 1st MTP Joint

i. Salvage procedure
ii. *Position:*
   Men: 15–20° extension
   Women: 15–25° extension: Medium heels
   35–40° extension: High heels.

RETROCALCANEAL BURSITIS/HAGLUND

I. INTRODUCTION

Achilles tendonitis comprises of three disorders affecting the Achilles tendon:
1. *Insertional Achilles tendonitis:* Pain and tendon thickening at insertion of Achilles tendon.
2. *Retrocalcaneal bursitis (RCB):* Inflammation of the bursa between the anterior aspect of the Achilles and posterior aspect of the calcaneus.
3. *Haglund deformity:* Enlargement of the posterosuperior tuberosity of the calcaneus.

II. ETIOPATHOLOGY

1. *Age:*
   i. Insertional Achilles tendonitis: Middle aged and elderly
   ii. RCB and Haglund: Young patients
2. *Mechanism:* Repetitive trauma → Inflammation → Cartilaginous metaplasia → Bony metaplasia.

III. CLINICAL FEATURES

A. Symptoms

1. "Startup pain": Worse in morning or after inactivity.
2. Posterior heel pain, swelling, burning, and stiffness
3. Shoe wear pain due to direct pressure
4. Progressive bony enlargement of calcaneus at insertion site.

B. Examination

1. Midline tenderness at Achilles insertion site
2. Pain with dorsiflexion
3. Hindfoot abnormalities
4. Wasting of gastrosoleus muscle
5. *Neurovascular examination:* Ability to tip toe walk.

IV. RADIOLOGY

1. *Radiographs:* Lateral foot shows bone spur and intratendinous calcification
2. Haglund deformity
3. *MRI:* Gold standard for soft tissue.

V. LABORATORY FINDINGS (UNDERLYING DISEASES)

1. *Crystal arthropathy:* Uric acid levels
2. *Inflammatory arthropathy:* ESR, CRP, and rheumatoid factor
3. *Enthesopathy:* HLA-B27

VI. TREATMENT

A. Conservative: First Line of Management
1. Activity modification
2. Shoe wear modification
3. Physical therapy with eccentric training
4. Gastrocnemius-soleus stretching
5. Heel sleeves and pads
6. *Ankle foot orthosis:* About 6-9 months
7. Avoid steroid injections due to risk of Achilles tendon rupture

B. Surgical
1. Retrocalcaneal bursa excision
2. Debridement of diseased tendon
3. *Calcaneoplasty:* Calcaneal bony prominence resection
   Indications: Failure of conservative management and <50% of Achilles needs to be removed.
4. Suture anchor repair
5. Tendon augmentation or transfers (FDL, FHL, or PB)
   Indicated when >50% of Achilles tendon insertion must be removed during thorough debridement.

POST-POLIO RESIDUAL PARALYSIS

I. INTRODUCTION
Poliomyelitis → Infectious disease → caused by neurotropic virus.

II. CLINICAL MANIFESTATIONS
1. Asymptomatic infection (90-95%)
2. Abortive poliomyelitis (minor illness) (4-8%)
3. Nonparalytic poliomyelitis
4. Paralytic poliomyelitis (<1%)

III. PHASES OF SYMPTOMATIC DISEASE

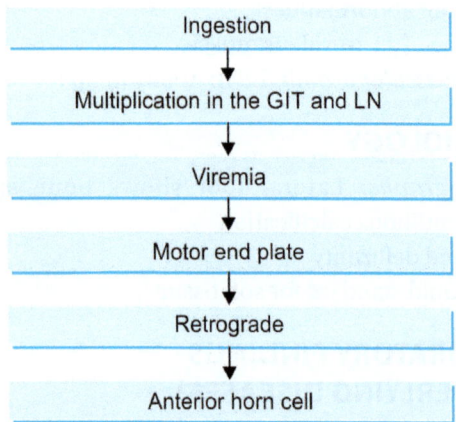

i. *Acute (5-10 days):* Stage of onset of paralysis 2-3 days after fever begins.
   a. *Preparalytic:* Fever, headache, neck rigidity, painful spasm, m/s tenderness.
   b. *Paralytic:* If brainstem affected (bulbar polio) respiratory muscle paralysis.
ii. *Convalescent phase (up to 18 months):* Spontaneous recovery
iii. *Chronic phase:* Residual paralysis.

IV. FEATURES OF PARALYTIC POLIO
1. Asymmetric, patchy, LMN flaccid paralysis
2. Nonprogressive
3. No sensory loss
4. History of acute paralytic illness
5. Signs of residual weakness.
6. Signs of nerve damage on EMG
7. A period of partial or complete functional recovery after acute paralytic polio followed by an interval of stable neuromuscular function (≥15 years).

V. CAUSES OF PROGRESSIVE DEFORMITY
1. Muscle imbalance → Due to flaccid paralysis, antagonists dominate
2. Unrelieved muscle spasm → Protective for pain
3. Growth disturbances → LLD
4. Gravity and posture → Paralyzed muscle, no posture
5. Bony deformities → Long-standing contractures

VI. NATURAL HISTORY OF PARALYTIC POLIO
1. 30%: Recover completely in few weeks/months
2. 30%: Mild paralysis
3. 30%: Moderate to severe paralysis
4. 10%: Die or respiratory paralysis

VII. CLINICAL EXAMINATION
i. *Hip:*
   1. Flexion, abduction, external rotation deformity
   2. Paralytic dislocation.
ii. *Knee:*
   1. Flexion deformity
   2. TRIPLE deformity (PERF)
      a. Posterior subluxation
      b. External rotation
      c. Flexion
   3. Valgus/valgus deformity
   4. Callus on knee
   5. Recurvatum
iii. *Foot:*
   1. Equinovarus
   2. Equinovalgus
   3. Calcaneovarus and calcaneovalgus.
   4. Claw toes
   5. Cavus

iv. *Spine:*
  1. Neuroparalytic scoliosis
     ↓
  2. Pelvic obliquity → LLD
  3. Rib hump
v. *Upper limb:*
  1. Dislocated shoulder
  2. Elbow recurvatum
vi. *Gait:*
  1. Hand to knee
  2. Trendelenburg
  3. Short limb
  4. Foot drop

VIII. GENERAL PRINCIPLES OF MANAGEMENT

1. Correction of soft tissue contractures
   ↓
   Strengthening of unaffected muscles, stretching of shortened muscles
2. Range of motion exercises of joints
3. Appropriate use of orthosis and splints, gait and walking aids.
4. Early correction of deformities not amenable to conservative management by soft tissue release procedures.
5. *Restoring muscle balance:* Tendon transfers
6. Adequate compensation for equalizing the leg length:
   - Footwear modifications
   - Limb lengthening
7. *Stabilization of joints:*
   - Arthrodesis
   - Soft tissue plications
8. Correction of bony deformities at early stage
9. Eliminate external supports.

IX. TIMING OF SURGERY

1. Wait for at least 1.5 years after paralytic attack
2. Tendon transfers in skeletally immature >5 years → 10–11 years
3. Extra-articular arthrodesis = 3–8 years
4. Triple arthrodesis > 10 years
5. Ankle arthrodesis > 18 years

DEFORMITIES OF FOOT AND ANKLE IN POLIO

1. *Foot and ankle:*
   Most dependent parts
   ↓
   Therefore, subjected to significant amount of deforming forces
2. *MC deformities:*
   i. Equinus
   ii. Equinovarus
   iii. Equinovalgus (MC)
   iv. Calcaneus
   v. Calcaneovarus
   vi. Calcaneovalgus
   vii. Claw toes
   viii. Cavus deformity and claw toes
   ix. Dorsal bunion

Peabody Classification (⊗: Affected)

i. Limited extensor invertor insufficiency [Tibialis anterior (TA) ⊗]
ii. Gross extensor invertor insufficiency
   A = Tibialis anterior + Long toe extensors ⊗
   B = A + Tibialis posterior ⊗
iii. Evertor insufficiency (Peronei ⊗)
iv. *Triceps surae insufficiency*

a. Limited extensor invertor insufficiency:
   TA ⊗ → Equinus (cavus), planovalgus
   Treatment: EHL → base of 1st MT + plantar fasciotomy
b. Gross extensor invertor insufficiency:
   A: TA + (EHL + EDL) ⊗ = Equinus, equinovalgus
   Rx Peroneus longus → 1st cuneiform
   B: TA + EHL + EDL + TP → Equinovalgus
   Rx Peroneus longus + peroneus brevis → dorsum of foot
   If fixed deformities (A or B): Triple arthrodesis
c. Evertor insufficiency:
   Peroneii ⊗ → Varus
   Rx mild, moderate: EHL → base of 5th MT severe → EHL → Base of 5th MT
   +
   Tibialis anterior → cuboid
d. Triceps surae insufficiency:
   1. Calcaneo-varus: Peronei ⊗
      Rx = TP + FHL → Calcaneum
   2. Calcaneo-valgus: [TP (weak) ⊗]
      Rx = Peronei → Calcaneum
   3. Calcaneo-cavus: Both TP and peronei strong
      Rx = Transfer both to calcaneum
   4. Plain calcaneus:
      Rx Posterior transfer of TA through IO membrane + EHL → Dorsum of foot.

CLAW TOES

I. INTRODUCTION

Hyperextension of MTP joints and flexion of both the interphalangeal joints.

(Hammer toe → MTP extension, DIP extension, PIP flexion)

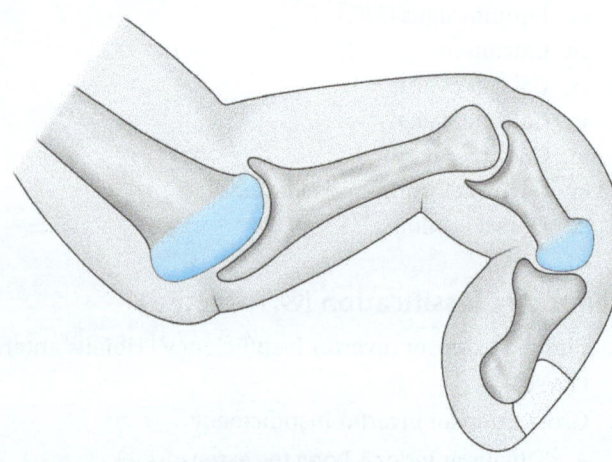

Fig. 12: Claw toe.

II. ETIOPATHOGENESIS

Etiology
i. Synovitis
ii. Trauma
iii. Missed compartment syndrome
iv. Neuropathic claw foot
v. Talipes cavus
vi. Poliomyelitis

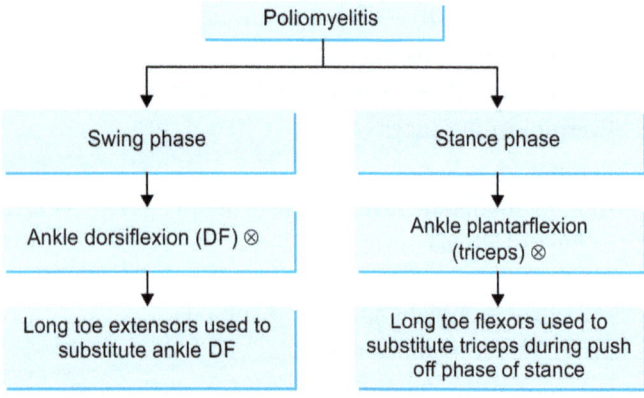

III. CLINICAL FEATURES
1. Irritation of flexed PIP by shoes: Erythema
2. Painful callosities at MT heads and tip of toe
3. Eventually clawing becomes permanent
4. Malformed nail
5. Metatarsalgia
6. Painful for MTP joint due to synovitis
   ↓
   following persistent hyperextended position and instability

IV. TREATMENT

A. Nonoperative
Taping and shoe modification → 1° R_x, provides plantar padding, sling to hold pip parallel to ground.

B. Operative Principles
1. Foot deformity must be corrected before surgery for clawing
   ↓
   As clawing correction may be unnecessary after foot deformity correction
2. In swing phase clawing
   ↓
   Restore active DF of ankle and correct equines deformity
3. In stance phase → Restore active ankle plantarflexion and correct cavus

C. Indications
1. Persistence of clawing after correction of foot deformities
2. Pain due to clawing.

D. Contraindications
1. Poor vascularity to the toe
2. Poor skin quality.

E. Options
A. *For lateral toes:*
  1. Dorsal capsulotomy of MTP joint
     +
     Lengthening of exterior tendon by Z-plasty
     +
     Divide FDL at its insertion
     ↓
     Capsulotomy of IP joint → Correct deformity
     ↓
     Reattach FDL to the proximal phalanx
  2. **Girdlestone-Taylor tendon transfer**

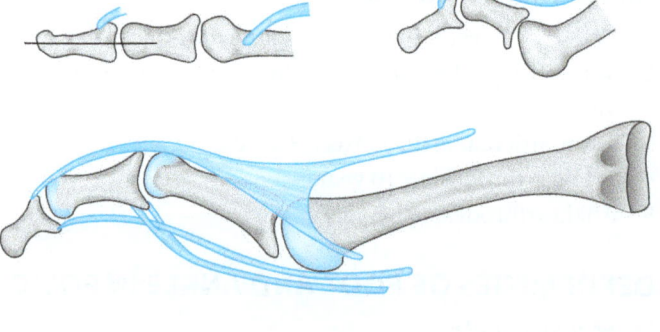

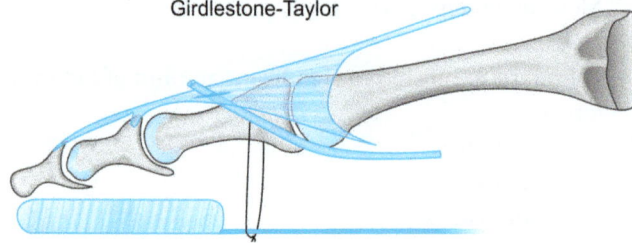

Girdlestone-Taylor

i. Long toe flexors

$\xrightarrow{\text{TRANSFER}}$ Dorsal expansion of extensor Tendons

ii. Enable long toe extensors to act as intrinsic muscles of foot → Active MTP flexion and IP extension (more useful in swing phase clawing)

B. *For great toe:*
   i. *Modified jones:*
      1. Division of EHL over proximal phalanx
      2. EHL: Neck of 1st MT
      3. Arthrodesis of IP joint
      4. Distal slip attach to soft tissue **(Fig. 13)**

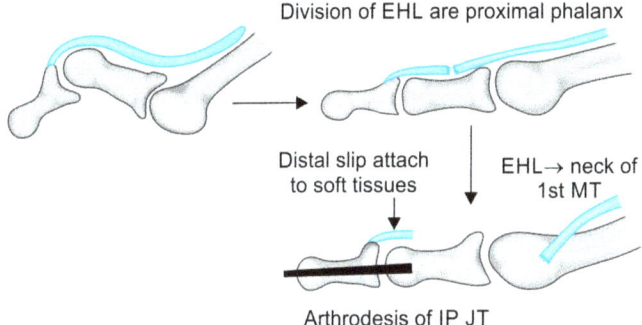

   ii. *Dickson-Diveley:* EHL → FHL (medial side of 1st MT head) 1,3,4 same as above **(Fig. 14)**

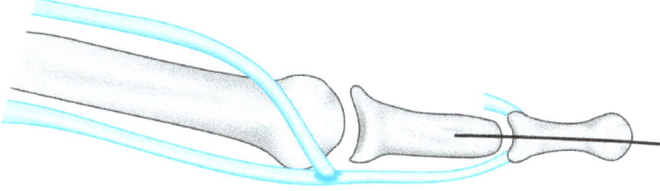

Fig. 14: Dickson-Diveley procedure.

TRIPLE ARTHRODESIS

I. DEFINITION

Fusion procedure of the three joints of the hindfoot and midfoot.
1. Talonavicular
2. Calcaneocuboid.
3. Talocalcaneal (subtalar).

II. INDICATIONS

1. End-stage arthritis:
   i. Rheumatoid arthritis
   ii. Post-traumatic
   iii. Degenerative
2. Charcot's arthropathy
3. Tarsal coalition
4. Cavus foot
5. CTEV: Late and neglected
6. End-stage flat foot deformities
7. Lateral ankle instability
8. Ankle equines
9. Ruptured TP tendon with advanced foot collapse
10. *Neuromuscular disease*:
    i. Cerebral palsy
    ii. Polio
    iii. Charcot-Marie-Tooth
    iv. Friedreich's ataxia.

III. CONTRAINDICATIONS

1. Age < 12 years:
   i. Limits growth of foot.
   ii. Bone cartilaginous → Talus AVN, fibrous union
2. Ankle arthritis
3. Active infection
4. Arterial insufficiency.
5. *Chronic smoking:* Nonunion
6. Patients managed with bracing, soft tissue procedure

IV. GOALS (FIG. 15)

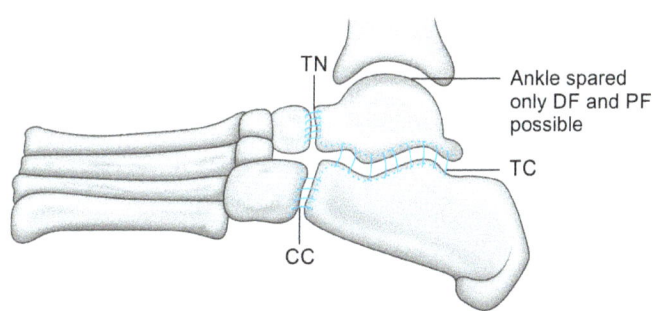

Fig. 15: Triple arthrodesis.

1. To obtain well-aligned and plantigrade stable foot
2. Pain free
3. To eliminate deforming forces
4. To arrest progression of deformity
5. Ability to wear shoes.

V. TECHNIQUE

1. *Approach:* Ollier (classical) and two incision technique (new)
2. *Ollier:* From tip of lateral malleolus across the sinus tarsi to the dorsal part of TN joint (single)
3. Obvious potential hazard to vital NV structures and extensor tendons
4. There, two incision technique

Lateral	Medial
Straight incision 1 cm inferior to tip of fibula → extending distally over the anterolateral border of calcaneus and cuboid. ↓ Exposes CC and ST joint.	From MM to naviculocuneiform joint distally. Exposes TN joint and fixation for ST joint.
↓	↓
Neurovascular and tendon structures at risk	

Lateral	Medial
1. Sural nerve	1. Deltoid artery
2. Artery of sinus tarsi	2. Artery of tarsal canal
3. Peroneal tendons	3. Long saphenous vein
4. EDB muscle belly	4. Distal insertion

5. Mid-tarsal joint surface resection first followed by subtalar: ↑Soft tissue relaxation and better exposure of ST joint.
6. Anatomic dissection: Minimal bone resection and rigid internal fixation
    i. Screws
    ii. Cancellous
    iii. Staples
7. Complete removal of TN articular cartilage as most common complication is TN joint non-union.
8. According to the specific deformities bone grafting/or wedge resection can be done to achieve normal alignment. For example, Lambrinudi → fixed equinus deformity
9. Subtalar joint, 4° valgus compared to ground
10. Drain → ↓ Hematoma, wound complications
11. *Postoperative:* Above knee cast with window for wound inspection.
    PT: Knee ROM, NWB mobilization
    Partial → 8 weeks
    Full WB → 3–4 months, union confirmed.

VI. COMPLICATIONS

1. *Wound complications:*
    i. Dehiscence
    ii. Infection
    iii. Necrosis
    iv. Eschar
2. Persistent/reversed deformity
3. Nonunion
4. Persistent pain
5. Pseudoarthrosis
6. *Talus AVN:* Vascular disruption
7. Early OA of ankle.

SECTION 8

Orthopedic Diseases

OSTEOGENESIS IMPERFECTA

I. INTRODUCTION

1. Genetic disorder of connective tissue characterized by:
   i. Long bone fracture
   ii. Skeletal deformity
   iii. Blue sclera
   iv. Deafness
   v. Fragile opaque teeth (Dentinogenesis imperfecta)
2. **Type I collagen** formation defect
3. *Pattern of inheritance:*
   i. Autosomal dominant
   ii. Autosomal recessive
   iii. Sporadic
4. *Incidence:* 1 in 10,000

II. ETIOPATHOGENESIS

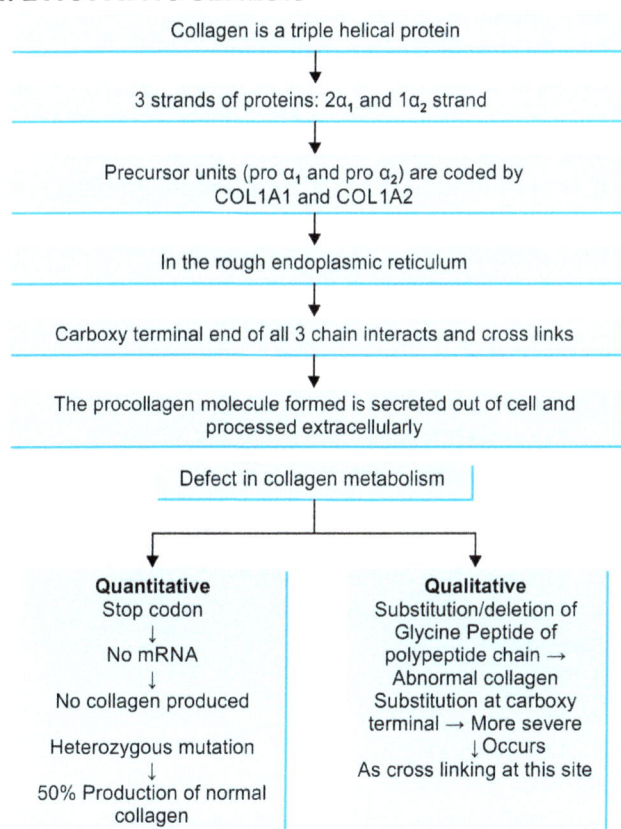

III. CLASSIFICATION (VAN DIJK AND SILLENCE)

Type	Inheritance	Sclera	Features
I	AD	Blue	Mildest form, presents at preschool age. Deafness – 50%
II	AR	Blue	Lethal in prenatal period
III	AR	Initially blue, white in adulthood	Progressively deforming. Most severe survivable form. Short stature. Fracture at birth
IV	AD	Normal	Moderate severity. Hearing normal. Bowing bones, vertebral fracture

Addition:

V. AD: Calcification of interosseous membrane (RU, TF) Congenital antero-lateral radial head dislocation Hypertrophic callus > fracture.
VI. Moderate severity, like IV.
VII. AR: Rhizomelia and coxa vara.

IV. CLINICAL FEATURES

1. Degree of severity varies with type of disease.
2. Most severe form (II): Multiple fractures at delivery.
   ↓
   Fatal → Intracranial hemorrhage
   → Respiratory insufficiency due to incompetence of rib cage.
3. Bone fragility: Exceptional feature.
4. Growth arrested due to multiple epiphyseal micro-fractures
   Multiple fractures: Saber shin
   Bowing of long bones.
5. Spine deformity: Scoliosis or kyphosis occurs in most cases.
6. Blue sclera
7. Poor dentition, blue/brown/opalescent > caries, breaks easily.
8. Bruck's syndrome: Multiple joint contractures + Bone Fragility.
9. UMN features, Apnea due to Basilar invagination
10. Trendelenburg gait due to coxa vara.

V. RADIOLOGY

1. Osteopenia
2. Olecranon fracture – presenting feature in type I
3. Flaring of metaphysis
4. Extreme bowing due to multiple fractures
5. Wormian bones in skull
6. Spine: Scoliosis, kyphosis
7. Protrusio acetabuli
8. V: Hyperplastic callus and calcification of IOM

VI. LABORATORY

1. Calcium and phosphorous: Normal
2. ALP ↑
3. Confirmation → Genetics analysis
   ↓
   COL1A1, COL1A2
4. Biopsy → Collagen analysis

VII. TREATMENT

A. Medical

1. Mainstay of treatment.
2. **Pamidronate**: Prevents resorption.
3. 6–9 mg/kg body weight →
   i. Decrease bone pain
   ii. Fracture rate
   iii. Increased prepubertal growth
   iv. Increased BMD
   v. Vertebral height
4. S/E → Minor: Nausea, vomiting, flu-like symptoms
   Major: Seizures, hypocalcemic tetany
5. Recent research exploring role of:
   i. Denosumab
   ii. Bortezomib
   iii. Growth hormone
   iv. Gene therapy
   v. BM transplant

B. Surgical Management

1. *Goals:*
   i. To correct deformity which decreases function
   ii. Prevent fracture and refracture
   iii. Correct LLD
   iv. Restore anatomical axes of long bones
   v. Facilitating ambulation
   vi. Providing internal splinting of long bones.
2. *Intramedullary rods:*
   i. Rush rods
   ii. Double rush rods
   iii. Elastic nails
   iv. Elongating rods **(Fassier–Duval rods)**
3. Plates and screws → Contraindicated → Stress risers → fractures
4. External immobilization → Contraindicated → leads to ↓ BMD (30%)
5. However, Age < 2 years → Fracture → Immobilization
6. Skeletal traction contraindicated → Cut through bone → Growth plate injury
7. **Sofield and Miller** = Realignment osteotomy with rod fixation **(Fig. 1)**.

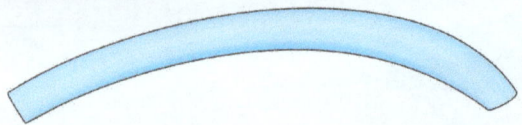
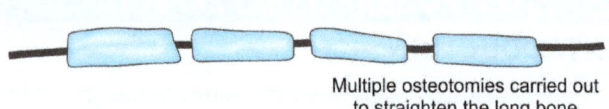

Multiple osteotomies carried out to straighten the long bone

8. Maintain bisphosphonate free period around time of IM nailing. Interferes with osteotomy healing more than fracture healing.
9. *Basilar invagination:*
   i. Anterior decompression + Posterior fusion
   ii. Indication → >45 degrees

CEREBRAL PALSY (STATIC ENCEPHALOPATHY)

I. INTRODUCTION

1. Nonprogressive upper motor neuron disease due to injury to the immature brain.
2. MCC of chronic childhood disability.
3. Result of a brain lesion, therefore, the spinal cord and muscles are structurally and biochemically normal with disorders developing as secondary manifestations.
4. Brain lesion must be fixed and nonprogressive. ∴ All progressive neurodegenerative disorders are excluded from the definition.
5. Incidence: 2–3/1,000.

II. ETIOLOGY

A. *Prenatal:*
   1. Maternal infections and toxins (TORCH)
   2. *Drugs:* Cocaine, heroin, marijuana
   3. Alcohol
   4. Rhesus blood group incompatibility (Rh -ve mother)
   5. Maternal health: Renal failure, infections
   6. Placental abnormalities
B. *Perinatal:*
   1. Anoxia
   2. Premature delivery
   3. Low birth weight
   4. Neonatal sepsis
   5. Cardiac SX for Rx of severe congenital HD

C. *Postnatal:* Although older children with brain damage were traditionally excluded from CP, it is not clinically relevant from orthopedic standpoint.
   1. Infectious meningitis
   2. Near drowning ⎫ Hypoxia leading to developing
   3. Suffocation ⎭ brain damage.
   4. Brain trauma (motor vehicle accident)

III. CLASSIFICATION

A. Physiological
B. Functional (GMFCS)
C. Anatomic

A. Physiological

1. **Spastic**: MC
   i. Velocity dependent increased muscle tone and hyperreflexia
   ii. Slow restricted movements due to simultaneous contraction of agonist and antagonist muscles.
   iii. Results from damage to pyramidal system, particularly the motor cortex of the brain.
   iv. Disinhibition of pathologic reflex arcs leads to increased tone in extremities
   v. Most amenable to operative Rx.
2. **Hypotonic (Floppy)**
   i. Abnormal decreased tone.
   ii. Precedes spastic or ataxic for 2–3 years as the child matures.
3. **Dystonia**
   i. Increased tone which is not dependent on velocity
   ii. Tone → in spasticity: Clasped knife.
   iii. Tone → in dystonic → lead-pipe → tone does not decrease with prolonged stretching.
   iv. Due to disruption of the basal ganglia.
   v. Myelination is required for development of dystonia → ∴ typically occurs later in life than spasticity (5–10 years).
4. **Athetoid**
   i. Abnormal slow writhing movements.
   ii. Involuntary
   iii. More exaggerated as pt. tries to complete a purposeful motion
   iv. Basal ganglia ⊗
   v. Speech is garbled and difficult to understand. Intelligence maybe normal.
   vi. Usually result of neonatal kernicterus
5. **Ataxic**
   i. Cerebellar lesion
   ii. Inability to co-ordinate m/s movements
   iii. Unbalanced, wide based gait
6. **Mixed**
   Mixed Spastic + Athetoid, involves entire body

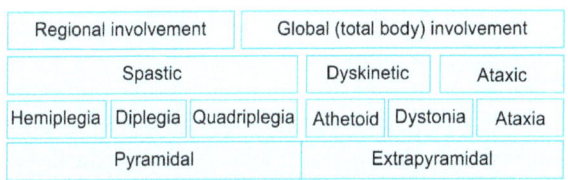

B. Anatomic
1. *Quadriplegic:* Total body involvement, nonambulatory
2. *Diplegic:* Legs > arms, ambulatory. IQ maybe normal
3. *Hemiplegic:* Arms and legs of one side of the body. Spasticity [+]. Will eventually walk, irrespective of Rx.

C. Functional—Gross Motor Function Classification Scale (GMFCS)
Levels:
  I. Near normal gross motor function, independent ambulatory.
  II. Walks independently, but difficulty with uneven surfaces, minimal ability to jump.
  III. Walks with assistive device.
  IV. Severely limited walking ability, primary mobility is wheelchair
  V. Nonambulatory with global involvement, dependent in all aspects of care.

IV. CLINICAL EVALUATION

A. History
1. *Perinatal:*
   i. Birth weight
   ii. Gestational age
   iii. Complications
   iv. Ventilator assistance or hospitalization.
2. *Growth and development:*
   a. Evaluation of motor milestones:
      i. Head control: 3–5 months
      ii. Sitting: 6–9 months
      iii. Crawling: 9 months
      iv. Standing: 10–12 months
      v. Walking: 12–18 months
   b. Preferential use of one hand or early handedness, dragging one leg when crawling → spastic hemiparesis.
   c. Prior medical treatment.
3. *Functional status:*
   i. Poor eyesight
   ii. Delayed speech development
   iii. Seizures

B. Physical Examination
1. *Muscle Tone*
   i. Child should be relaxed (even sitting in the mother's lap) and the extremities brought through full range of motion.
   ii. Spasticity feels like tightness in the m/s, which become tighter, the quicker the limbs are passively moved.

iii. Greater ROM can be achieved by slowly and gently stretching the joints.
iv. **Tardieu test**: Measure of spasticity. When assessing hamstring spasticity, the angle at which a "grab" of resistance occurs when quickly extending the knee with the hip in flexion, is compared with amount of extension possible when the knee is stretched slowly **(Fig. 2)**.

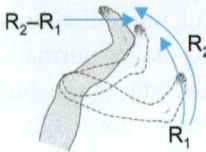

R_2-R_1 = Dynamic component
R_2-R_1 = High → amenable to botulinum
R_2-R_1 = Low → M/S contracture, not spasticity

R_2 = Passive ROM → slowly (normal way) R_1 = as fast as possible.
R_2-R_1 = Dynamic component, spasticity.
R_2-R_1 = High → spasticity → amenable to botulinum
R_2-R_1 = Low → muscle contracture, not spasticity.

v. Passing the child a toy reveals spastic hemiplegia → fine motor activities.

2. Reflexes

i. ↑ Deep tendon reflexes
ii. Clonus [+] - Quick passive DF of ankle
iii. Hemiparesis → Asymmetric reflexes.
iv. Infantile reflexes normally disappear by 3–6 months → retained in CP.
v. Moro's/startle reflex → Normally disappeared by 4 months → Retained,
Infants head dropped back into extension with the infant supine.
↓
Arms and legs extend abruptly.
vi. Parachute reflex → holding the child in the air and lowering him quickly headfirst.
↓
Children older than 5 months will reach out with both arms protect themselves.
Children with CP will not. Hemiplegia → only one arm.
vii. Persistence of tonic neck reflex beyond infancy.

3. Balance and Sitting

Note whether the child can sit unsupported without use of hand.

4. Gait (Fig. 3)

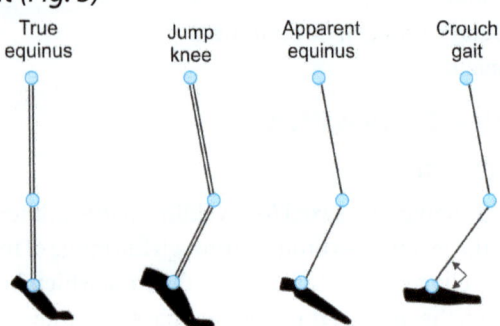

i. Jump knee gait
ii. True equinus
iii. Apparent equinus
iv. Crouch knee gait
v. Stiff knee gait
vi. Rotational deformities affecting gait

i. *Jump knee gait*
Increased hip flexion with slight DF of ankle at initial contact
↓f/b
Rapid knee extension + Plantar flexion during midstance
↓
Resultant hip and knee joint extension reactions giving the appearance of the person jumping from one knee to another.

ii. *True and apparent equinus:*
1. Equinus – one of the MC deformities in CP.
2. Excessive plantar flexion relative to tibia
3. Equinus → Planovalgus
   → Cavovarus
4. True equinus deformity → Forefoot makes initial contact and persists throughout the stance phase Toe-Toe gait.
5. Apparent equinus → Initial contact of forefoot occurs because of excessive hip and knee flexion.
6. True Equinus → Calf spasticity ++ → PF at ankle. Hip and knee relatively normal.
7. Apparent Equinus → If any surgical procedure that weakens the calf muscles is done, it will cause crouch gait. Therefore, differentiation between true and apparent equinus is very important
R_X → Iliopsoas and hamstring resection.

iii. *Crouch gait:*
1. ↑ Hip flexion   Knee flexion   ↑ Ankle DF
   ↓   ↓   ↓
   Iliopsoas, RF   Hamstrings   Weak or lengthened calf m/s

iv. *Stiff knee gait:*
1. MC gait pattern in spastic CP
2. Stiff knee → spastic rectus femoris (Duncan-Ely test)
3. Decreased foot clearance
   ↓ compensated by
Circumduction of involved limb, ER of foot. Pelvic elevation or trunk lean away from affected side.

v. *Rotational abnormalities:*
1. MC → Femoral anteversion and tibial torsion.
2. Increased femoral anteversion → MCC intoeing gait.
3. Tibia and foot rotational deformities typically are in same direction.
   Intorsion → equinovarus
   Extorsion → planovalgus
4. R_X to be delayed till skeletal maturity to avoid recurrence

5. Spine
  i. Scoliosis: Presence and flexibility.
  ii. Spinal balance and shoulder height.
  iii. Pelvic obliquity
  iv. Resting head posture.
  v. Hamstring contracture → ↓Lumbar lordosis

6. Hip
  i. Contractures → Flexion → ↑ Lumbar Lordosis
      → Adduction → Scissoring gait
  ii. Hip instability and dislocations → Galeazzi test

7. Foot and Ankle
  i. Equinovarus and planovalgus
  ii. Hypertonicity, callouses
  iii. Toe-toe gait, absent heel strike
  iv. **Silverskoid test**: Gastrocnemius v/s soleus contracture DF at ankle joint with knee in extension and at 90° flexion.
  Increased DF with knee flexion → Gastrocnemius contracture.
  Equal DF → Soleus or both.

V. PRINCIPLES OF MANAGEMENT
A. General
1. Counselling of parents for slow progress of RX effectiveness.
2. Reducing disabilities.
3. Improving learning, self-dependency, and socialization.

B. Treatment of Spasticity in CP
1. Passive stretching f/b splinting.
2. **Oral medications**
   i. **Baclofen**
      a. GABA agonist
      b. Primarily acts on spinal cord → ↓spasticity, clonus and hyperreflexia.
      c. Dose 2.5-10 mg/day
      d. Intrathecal administration avoids cognitive impairment.
   ii. **Dantrolene sodium**
      a. Acts on skeletal m/s opposed to other drugs which act on neurotransmitter system.
      b. Decrease release Ca^{2+} ions from sarcoplasmic reticulum during m/s contraction.
      c. Dose: 6-8 mg/day.
      d. S/E - Hepatotoxicity → Monitor LFT.
   iii. **Tizanidine**
      α2-adrenergic agent → decrease tone through hyperpolarization of motor neurons.
3. **Botulinum toxin**
   i. Competitive inhibitor of presynaptic cholinergic receptors.
      ↓
   ii. ∴ Inhibits release of Acetyl Choline
   iii. Produced by clostridium botulinum.
   iv. Effects are reversible, hence injection to be repeated every 3-4 months.
   v. *Dose:* 10-12 U/kg. Never exceed 400 U in single setting.
   vi. Type A → BOTOX®
       Type B → MYOBLOC®
   vii. Appropriate candidate → where reduction of spasticity in a limited number of m/s can provide a meaningful benefit in care, comfort, and activity.
   viii. Reduces spasticity in focally affected m/s.
   ix. ∴ Affected m/s can be stretched; antagonists can be rebuilt by PT, improved joint balance.
   x. Surgeon can assess possible benefits of surgery.
   xi. Botox can also be used in conjunction with surgery or serial casting and splinting.
   xii. Used to maintain joint motion during rapid growth when child is too young for surgery.
   xiii. Useful in dynamic contractures, less in static.
   xiv. MC used in Gastrocnemius.
4. **Selective dorsal rhizotomy (SDR)**
   i. Neurosurgical treatment preformed through laminoplasty.
   ii. Dura opened → Dorsal rootlets (T_{12} - S_1) identified
       ↓
       Resection of rootlets with abnormal response to stimulation (40-60%)
   iii. Age: 4-8 years, ambulatory spastic diplegia
   iv. C/I → Athetoid CP, dystonia
   v. Falling out of favor as subsequent surgery is required.

C. Operative
1. Releasing/lengthening of spastic muscles.
2. Tendon transfers to supplement weak muscles. Replace lost muscle function.
3. Stabilization of unstable joints.
4. Bony osteotomes

Soft Procedures/Releases
1. To improvise function in a child from 3 to 5 years with spasticity and voluntary muscle control.
2. Tenotomies → for continuously active muscle → hip adductors.
3. Tendon lengthening for continuously active muscle → hamstrings, TA.
4. Tendon transfers for muscle firing out of phase → RF, T. Posterior.

Bony Procedures/Deformity Correction
1. Later childhood/adolescence.
2. Static contractures
3. Progressive joint breakdown
4. SEMLS surgery:
   a. Single event, multi-level surgery.
   b. To limit multiple surgery, anesthesia and increase rehabilitation.
   c. Successful when combined with gait lab assessment.
   d. Simple lengthening can cause deteriorations in gait when other contractures are "uncovered"
   e. SEMLS: Avoids iatrogenic complications.

D. Management of Hip Deformities in CP
1. Child born with CP → Normal hips
   ↓
   Abnormal forces by spastic muscles
   (Usually adductors, flexors, hamstrings)
2. Asymmetrical spasticity → windblown deformity
3. If child walks by 30 months → no hip instability

Radiographs
i. Acetabular index
   Angle between → Hilgenreiner's line and line along acetabular roof.
   Normal <28°
ii. Reimers migration index **(Fig. 4)**

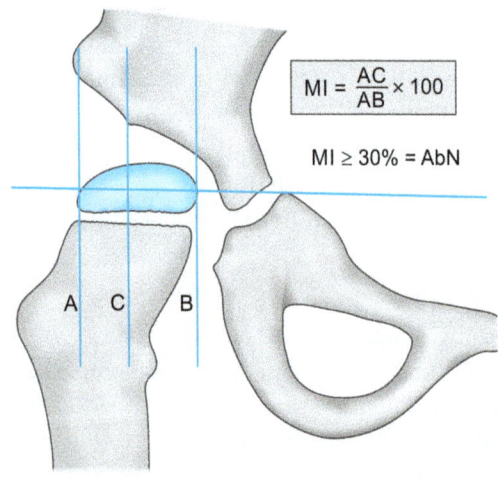

MI = AC/AB × 100
MI ≥ 30% → Abnormal
A = Outer limit of epiphysis
B = Inner limit of epiphysis
C = Perkins line

iii. Increased neck shaft angle and persistent anteversion.

Management
Nonsurgical → Described earlier

Surgical:
1. *Adductor tenotomy ± flexor release:*
   a. MC procedure in CP
   b. Indications:
      1. Abduction < 30° in flexed hip and knee.
      2. MI ≥ 20% with progression
   c. Medial approach
   d. Muscle released – Adductor longus and brevis, Gracilis
   e. Combined with iliopsoas release.
2. *Correction of rotational deformities:*
   a. Soft tissue procedures → Not satisfactory.
   b. Derotation osteotomy → Procedure of choice
   c. Indication (Gait abnormal)
      IR > 60°
      Femoral Anteversion = 45°
   d. Hip subluxation or Coxa Valga
      ↓
      Varus derotation osteotomy (VDRO)
3. *Dislocated hip:*
   a. Single stage → Open reduction
   b. Soft tissue lengthening
   c. Femoral shortening with osteotomy
   d. Pelvic osteotomy → Periacetabular
      ↓
      San Diego
4. *Painful dislocated hip:*
   a. Hip arthrodesis
   b. Femoral head resection
   c. Interpositional arthroplasty
   d. Valgus redirectional osteotomy

E. Management of Knee Deformities in CP
1. Hamstring lengthening in distal part → MC procedure
2. Flexion deformity of knee + crouch gait → Supracondylar extension osteotomy **(Fig. 5)**

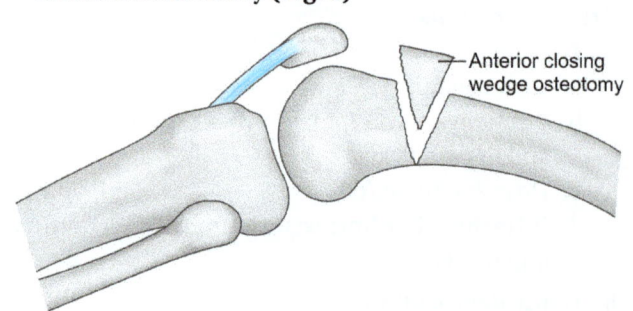

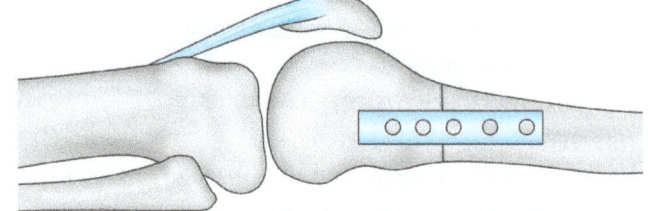

F. Management of Foot and Ankle

1. *Complains of:*
   a. Pain
   b. Frequent falls
   c. In/out toeing
2. Foot deformities (can be divided into)
   ↓   ↓   ↓   ↓
   Forefoot   midfoot   hindfoot   2 columns
                                   i. Medial
                                   ii. Lateral
3. Relative length of each column and alignment of each segment assessed.
4. Foot deformity in CP
   ↓
   Dynamic muscle imbalance
   ↓due to
   a. Spasticity
   b. Abnormal motor control
   c. Impaired balance.
5. *Three levels:*
   i. Dynamic soft tissue imbalance
   ii. Flexion deformity, muscle length fixed, but no skeletal changes
   iii. Structural skeletal deformity.
6. *Three MC malalignment patterns:*
   i. Equinus (MC)
   ii. Equinoplanovalgus
   iii. Equinocavovarus
7. Typically in spastic CP
   Ankle PF → Overactive
   DF → Ineffective
   i. **Equinus:**
      1. Clinical features:
         a. Forefoot callosities
         b. Toe walking, absent heel strike
         c. Compensatory hyperextended knee with heel contact
         d. Silverskoid test
      2. Treatment:
         Nonoperative (level 1):
         a. Serial manipulation and casting younger child, mild equinus
         b. Botulinum toxin A
            Intramuscular inj → gastrocnemius
         c. Articular/hinged AFO
         d. Solid AFO

Operative

Level II deformity → Soft tissue procedures release, lengthening or transfer musculotendinous unit **(Fig. 6)**.

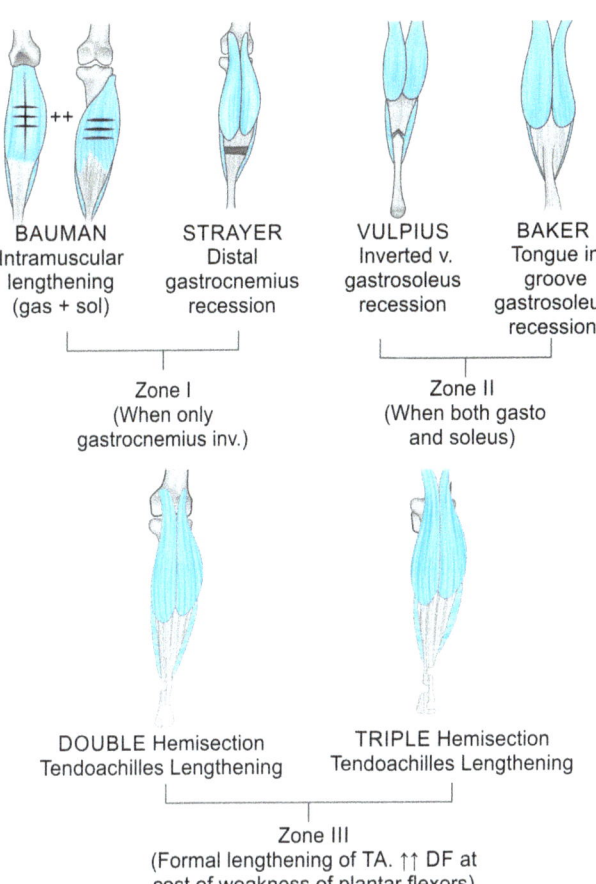

BAUMAN — Intramuscular lengthening (gas + sol)
STRAYER — Distal gastrocnemius recession
VULPIUS — Inverted v. gastrosoleus recession
BAKER — Tongue in groove gastrosoleus recession

Zone I (When only gastrocnemius inv.)
Zone II (When both gasto and soleus)

DOUBLE Hemisection Tendoachilles Lengthening
TRIPLE Hemisection Tendoachilles Lengthening

Zone III (Formal lengthening of TA. ↑↑ DF at cost of weakness of plantar flexors)

ii. **Equinocavovarus**

Level 1 → IM Botulinum toxin: A → plantar flexors and invertors.

Level 2 →
1. Fractional lengthening of ankle plantar flexors ± FHL, FDL
2. Split transfer of tibialis anterior.
3. Sequential release of plantar fascia.

Level 3 →
a. Lateral closing wedge osteotomy for hindfoot varus → Dwyer's
b. Lichblau's → Calcaneocuboid arthroplasty
c. Triple arthrodesis

CLEIDOCRANIAL DYSOSTOSIS

I. INTRODUCTION

1. Congenital developmental disorder
2. Membranous bones fail to ossify sufficiently, particularly in the calvarium (skull) and the clavicles, where fibrous tissue replaces the bones.

II. ETIOPATHOGENESIS

1. 1/1 lakh
2. All ethnicities
3. **AD**, **RUNX2** gene (Runt related transcription factor)
4. Short arm of **Chromosome 6**
5. Mutation causes error in **osteoblast differentiation**

III. CLINICAL FEATURES

1. Partial or complete absence of both the clavicles
2. Abnormality of skull bones.
3. Difficult to D_X at birth presentation – early teens
4. Proportionate dwarfism.
5. Complete absence of clavicle (10%) ∴ Rare
   ↓
6. Hypermobility of shoulders allows the patient to touch both the shoulders together in front.
7. Usually clavicles → Hypoplastic, lateral part poorly developed
8. Absence of clavicular portion of trapezius and anterior fibers of deltoid → clinically insignificant.
9. Scapula → Small, deformed, winged
10. Spina bifida occulta
11. Deficient ossification of pubic bones → Clinically insignificant
12. Well-marked frontal, parietal and occipital bossing.
13. Synostosis of the metopic suture. ⎫
14. Large anterior fontanelle. ⎬ Arnold head
15. Shortened middle phalanges of hand
16. Mild hydrocephalus
17. Small maxilla, relatively large mandible → prognathous
18. Delayed dentition
19. Conduction deafness.

IV. IMAGING

A. X-ray Chest

1. Absent/hypoplastic clavicles
2. Rudimentary pectoral stubs of clavicle
3. Bell-shaped chest

B. X-ray PBH

1. Coxa vara
2. Delayed closure of symphysis pubis
3. Open fontanelles
4. Visible suture lines beyond regular

C. X-ray Skull

1. Open fontanelles
2. Visible suture lines beyond regular age of suture closure.
3. Supernumerary teeth
4. Dental crowding
5. Wormian bones in occipital and parietal bones
6. Hypoplasia of maxillary bones

V. TREATMENT

1. Normal life expectancy.
2. Therefore, treatment if any → Conservative.
3. Dental procedures for retained deciduous teeth.
4. Orthodontic measures.
5. Craniofacial S_X → Correct skull defects including surgical closure of fontanelles.
6. ENT procedures → Recurrent sinus and middle ear infections.
7. Hypoplastic clavicle does not require any surgery since there is no functional impairment.
8. Rarely, clavicular remnant may press on brachial plexus requiring **surgical decompression**.
9. Active surveillance for dental, ENT and skeletal complications.
10. Valgus intertrochanteric osteotomy for Coxa Vara if neck-shaft angle <100°.

ACHONDROPLASIA

I. INTRODUCTION

1. Congenital skeletal dysplasia characterized pathologically by defective endochondral ossification.
2. Most common form of short limb dwarfism.
3. Most common nonlethal skeletal dysplasia

II. ETIOLOGY

1. Autosomal dominant with full penetrance.
2. Sporadic mutation in >80% followed by autosomal dominant.
3. Gene on chromosome 4
4. Mutations in fibroblast growth factor receptor 3 gene (FGFR-3)
5. Glycine to arginine substitution at 380 position on chr. 4.
6.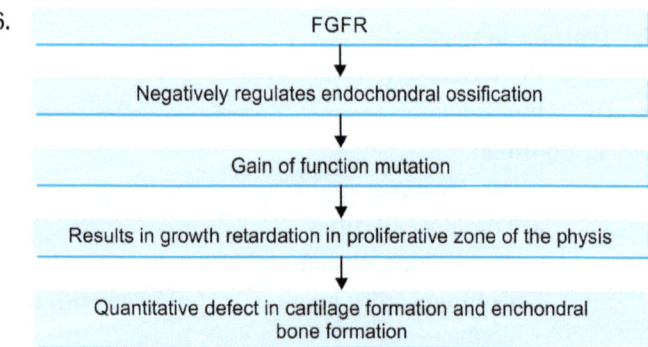
7. ↑ Risk with ↑ paternal age.

III. CLINICAL FEATURES

1. F > M
2. Short limbs compared to normal trunk length
3. Rhizomelic shortening → Proximal limb shortening (Humerus and Femur)
4. Frontal bossing
5. Head → Brachycephalic
6. Depressed nose bridge, maxillary hypoplasia, and mandibular prominence
7. Dental crowding
8. Trident hands

9. Spinal deformities:
    i. Thoracolumbar kyphosis
    ii. Lordosis
    iii. Scoliosis
10. Spinal canal stenosis:
    i. Neurogenic claudication
    ii. Paresthesia and numbness
11. Waddling gait
12. Genu varum
13. Flexion contractures of elbow
14. Subluxation of radial head
15. Ligamentous laxity
16. Recurrent otitis media
17. Hearing loss
18. Normal intelligence
19. Normal sexual development (remember Tyrion Lannister)
20. Apnea and sudden death → Foramen magnum stenosis

IV. RADIOLOGICAL FEATURES

1. Squared iliac wings
2. Champagne glass pelvis
3. Flaring of metaphysis of long bones
4. Diaphysis of long bones are thick owing to the subperiosteal new apposition.
5. Genu varum
6. Dental abnormalities:
    i. Delayed loss of 1° tooth
    ii. Delayed appearance of 2° teeth
    iii. Peg like teeth
    iv. Misalignment of teeth and jaws
7. Spinal canal stenosis → Short pedicles, thick facets, and ligamentum flavum

V. TREATMENT

A. *Spine:*
   1. Thoracolumbar kyphosis:
       i. 90% improve → Observation
       ii. Bracing → when there's persistent vertebral wedging >3 years
       iii. Surgical →
           a. Kyphosis > 50°
           b. Posterior fusion with anterior strut corpectomy
   2. Lumbar stenosis:
       i. Physiotherapy, nerve root blocks and weight loss
       ii. Surgical → Multilevel laminectomy and fusion when conservative therapy fails and severe affection.
   3. Surgical decompression of foramen magnum.
B. Limb:
   1. Genu varum → Femoral or tibial osteotomies (based on CORA)
   2. Coxa vara → Valgus osteotomy

SPRENGEL DEFORMITY

I. INTRODUCTION

1. Also called as congenital high scapula, Sprengel's shoulder, undescended scapula, or congenitally elevated scapula.
2. Common congenital anomaly of the shoulder.
3. Consists of permanent elevation of the shoulder girdle due to a failure of descent of the scapula from its embryonic position.
4. Characterized by a small and undescended scapula often associated with scapular winging and scapular hypoplasia.
5. M:F – 1:3

II. ETIOLOGY

1. Defect of incomplete segmentation and failure of fusion of the bony elements.
2. Interruption of embryonic subclavian blood supply.
3. Omovertebral connection between superior medial angle of scapula and cervical spine (30–50%).

III. PHYSICAL EXAMINATION

1. High riding medially rotated scapula
2. Loss of long medial border
3. Equilateral triangle like shape
4. Shoulder abduction most limited due to loss of normal scapulothoracic motion and glenoid malpositioning
5. Forward flexion limited as well
6. Periscapular muscles – varying degrees of developmental defects – fibrosis
7. From the superior angle, a sheet or band-like structure extends upward to attach to the transverse processes of several cervical vertebrae.
8. Part of syndrome: Klippel Feil syndrome
9. Scoliosis: Thoracic.

IV. CLASSIFICATION

A. **Cavendish:**
   1. Very mild: Not seen when dressed
   2. Mild: Seen when dressed
   3. Moderate: 5 cm elevation, obvious
   4. Severe: Up to occiput.
B. **Rigault (X-ray) Superomedial border:**
   1. T2–T4
   2. C5–T2
   3. Above C5

V. MANAGEMENT

A. Observation
Indication: No severe cosmetic concerns or loss of shoulder function

B. Surgical
1. **Surgical correction**
   Indications:
   i. Severe cosmetic concerns or functional deformities (abduction <110–120 degrees)
   ii. Age of child ideal for surgery: 3–8 years
   iii. ↑ Risk of neurological insult after the age of 8
2. Preoperative planning: MRI or CT to identify omovertebral bar
3. *Procedures:*
   i. *Woodward procedure:*
      a. Detachment and reattachment of medial parascapular muscles at spinous process origin to allow scapula to move inferiorly and rotate into more shoulder abduction.
      b. Modified Woodward includes resection of superomedial border of scapula in conjunction with surgical descent.
   ii. *Schrock, Green procedure:* Extraperiosteal detachment of paraspinal muscles at the scapular insertion and reinsertion after inferior movement of scapula with traction cables.
   iii. Clavicle osteotomy: To avoid brachial plexus injury performed for severe deformity in conjunction with above procedures.
   iv. *Bony resection:* Extraperiosteal resection of proximal scapular prominence for cosmetic concerns, may be done with other procedures or alone.

KLIPPEL-FEIL SYNDROME

I. INTRODUCTION

Congenital disorder characterized by defect in the formation or segmentation of the cervical spine during embryological development.

II. ETIOPATHOLOGY

1. *Associated abnormalities:*
   i. Congenital scoliosis
   ii. Sprengel deformity (30%)
   iii. Renal aplasia
   iv. Deafness
   v. Congenital heart disease
2. 1 in 40,000 births
3. Fusion and rigidity of C. spine → Susceptible to injury and fracture from insignificant trauma

III. CLINICAL FEATURES

1. Short neck
2. Limited neck motion } Triad
3. Lowered hair line
4. Neurological signs and symptoms
5. High scapula
6. Jaw anomalies
7. Torticollis
8. Scoliosis

IV. RADIOLOGY

1. Two or more vertebrae → Fusion [Subaxial or craniocervical (occiput to C2)]
2. Basilar invagination → Dens above McRae's line
3. Atlantoaxial instability - Atlantodens interval (ADI) >5 mm
4. Cervical canal Stenosis → <13 mm
5. Degenerative changes in cervical spine
6. Intervertebral space calcifications
7. MRI - To look for spinal anomalies → affected spinal cord, brainstem
8. CT: Assess bony pathoanatomy of region.

V. MANAGEMENT

A. *Observation: Asymptomatic patients*:
   1. Participation in contact sports
      i. Allowed: Subaxial fusion of 1–2 vertebrae
      ii. Not allowed: Fusions C2 and above, long fusions
B. *Surgical decompression and fusion*:
   1. Basilar invagination
   2. Chronic pain
   3. Myelopathy
   4. Associated atlantoaxial instability
   5. Adjacent level disease if symptomatic

DUCHENNE MUSCULAR DYSTROPHY

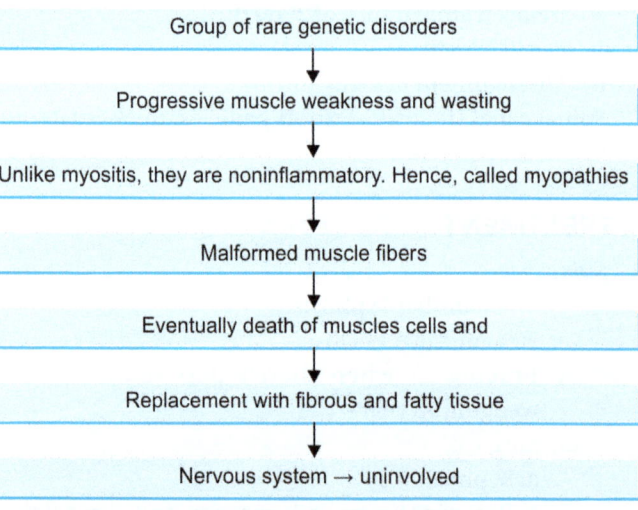

Walton's classification of progressive muscle dystrophy.
I. *Pure muscular dystrophy*:
   a. X-linked recessive inheritance:
      1. Duchenne type (severe)
      2. Becker (Benign)
      3. Emery-Dreifuss
   b. AR:
      1. Scapulohumeral–"limb-girdle"
      2. Early onset in childhood–"Duchenne-like"
      3. Congenital

c. AD:
      1. Facioscapulohumeral
      2. Scapuloperoneal
      3. Late-onset proximal
      4. Distal (adult)
      5. Distal (infantile)
      6. Ocular
      7. Oculopharyngeal
II. *Dystrophies with myotonia (myotonic m/s dystrophies):*
   1. Myotonia congenita
   2. Dystrophia myotonica
   3. Paramyotonia congenital

I. INTRODUCTION
1. Most common muscle dystrophy.
2. 1:3,500 male births
3. **X-LR (Xp21)** → failure to code **dystrophin gene**
   ↓
   Required for stability of cell membranes of cardiac and skeletal muscle cells
   ↓
   Muscle fiber damage → replacement by fat and fibrous tissue.

II. CLINICAL FEATURES
1. *Age:* 3–6 years, Insidious onset
2. The key role of orthopedic surgeon is to diagnose the disease early so that birth of another affected child in the family is avoided
3. Symmetrical weakness
4. Proximal muscle involvement first followed by distal muscles.
5. Chiefly affecting the glutei, quadriceps and tibialis anterior giving rise to wide-based stance and gait with foot in equinus, forward tilted pelvis, lordotic back and extended neck.
6. Calf muscles → Bulky → Pseudohypertrophy → Replacement by fat
7. **Gower's sign**: Child gets up on his own legs
   ↓
   d/t weakness of gluteus maximus and thigh muscles (quadriceps)
8. UL weakness follows 3–5 years after clinical onset.
9. Facial, cardiac and axial muscles then affected.
10. By age 10, child becomes dependent on wheelchair,
    ↓
    Deterioration of posture
    ↓
    Scoliosis
11. Cardiopulmonary failure is the usual cause of death < 30 years.
12. Intellectual level ↓

III. LABORATORY FINDINGS
1. ↑ Creatine excretion,   ↓ Creatinine excretion
   (N) 2 mg/kg/24 h   (N) 22 mg/kg/24 h
2. Normal creatine is made from glycine and other amino acids in liver and deposited in muscles.
3. Creatine → loss of phosphate → Creatinine
4. When muscles are destroyed → Not capable of storing creatine → excreted, not converted to creatinine.
5. ↓ Creatinine excretion more important than ↑ Creatine excretion
   ↓
   As this occurs in a lot of other conditions such as hyperthyroidism.
6. ↑ Sr. Creatine phosphokinase and Sr. Aldolase → diagnostic
7. These enzymes escape from muscle fibers because of degeneration and increased muscle membrane permeability.
8. CPK more specific than aldolase
   ↓   ↓
   Skeletal muscles   Muscles + liver, blood cells
9. 24-hour urinary creatine excretion
   ↓
   Quantitative assessment of progression
10. *EMG:* Individual motor unit potentials decrease in size during voluntary contraction and number and rate of unit firings.
11. *Genetic testing:* DNA PCR identify defective gene and carriers.
12. *Muscle biopsy (for confirmation):* Muscles with 50% strength more likely to give positive result than the one with end stage disease.
13. Vastus lateralis commonly biopsied.
14. Dystrophin analysis

IV. PATHOLOGY
A. Gross Appearance
1. Enlarged gastrocnemius look like fatty tumors, not muscles.
2. Other muscles small → color varies from yellowish to pinkish gray
3. Pale translucent appearance → resembles fish flesh → depends on relative amount of fat and fibrous that replaces muscles.

B. Microscopy
1. Most significant histological feature.
   ↓
   Loss of muscles fibers due to segmental necrosis and fragmentation of fibers.
   ↓
2. Phagocytosis and proliferation of histiocytes
3. Sarcolemmic nuclei enlarged with increase in interstitial connective tissue.

Orthopedic Diseases

4. No regeneration is evident.
5. Motor and sensory nerve fibers are not damaged. CNS (N)
6. Myocardial fibrosis
7. Immunofluorescent/ELISA for dystrophin content.

V. TREATMENT

1. No definite Rx till date and ultimately proves fatal for affected person.
2. Principles of Rx → Achieving stabilization and balance so as to enable the patient with muscle dystrophy to ambulate independently or with little support over longer period than would otherwise be possible.

A. Medical Therapy

1. **Corticosteroids** through their anti-inflammatory action → Preserve muscles strength and increase duration of ambulation. S/E → Osteoporosis, increased fractures, cataract.
2. Glutamine and creatine
3. Aminoglycosides (Gentamycin)
   ↓
   ↑ Muscles power when defect is in stop codon.
   ↓
   Aminoglycosides lead to readthrough of these stop codons

B. Physical and Sx Therapy

1. To maximize the duration of ambulation.
2. Prevent the complications of immobilization once child loses the power to move independently
3. *Physiotherapy:*
   a. Instruction on exercises
   b. Stretching
   c. Walking with crutches
   d. Gait training with braces.
4. The contractures must be treated at an early stage by stretching and splinting at night.
5. During the day, strong, long steel brace with drop ring locks.
6. Long lace surgical high shoes
7. Heel cord released by subcutaneous tenotomy
8. Toe-to-groin casts with knees in extension and ankles in 10° DF.
9. **Yount procedure**: ITB release. Large rectangular segment of the band with a corresponding portion of intermuscular septum removed.
10. Tibialis posterior retains considerable power for long periods → transferred by the inter osseous route to the 3rd cuneiform to reinforce dorsiflexors.
    ↓
    Postoperative encouraged to walk immediately
    ↓
    Immobilization rapidly weakens them.

11. **Management of scoliosis:**
    i. NM type of scoliosis → curves long and associated with pelvic obliquity.
    ii. Curve progression is the rule and can be up to 90°.
    iii. Role of corset or plastic jacket is limited as it does not prevent progression and ↓ pulmonary function.
    iv. >30° → Instrumentation and spinal fusion.
    v. Preoperative forces (FVC) >35% → good results.
    vi. Preoperative cardiac and pulmonary function evaluation.
    vii. But if affected lifespan <2 years, spinal surgery contraindicated.
    viii. Family counselling
12. **Gene therapy:** Difficulties with viral vectors and associated immunological responses.

GOUT

I. INTRODUCTION

Chronic hereditary disorder of uric acid metabolism
↓
Deposition of monosodium urate crystals
↓
In articular, periarticular, and subcutaneous tissue
↓
Leading to recurrent attacks of acute arthritis
↓
Most common inflammatory joint disease in men ≥ 40 years

II. PATHOPHYSIOLOGY/ETIOPATHOGENESIS

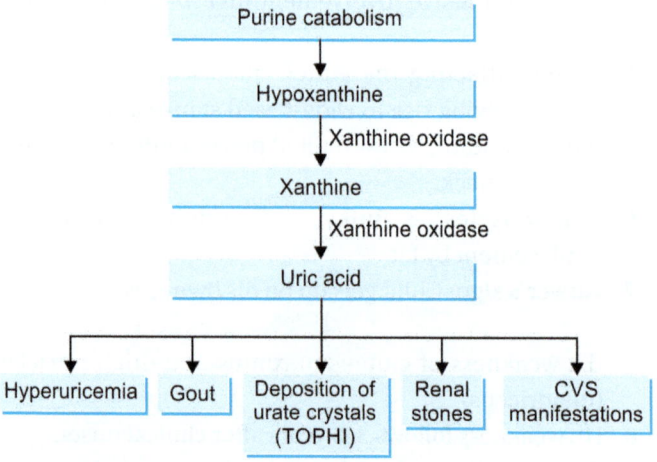

Purine catabolism
↓
Hypoxanthine
↓ Xanthine oxidase
Xanthine
↓ Xanthine oxidase
Uric acid
↓
Hyperuricemia | Gout | Deposition of urate crystals (TOPHI) | Renal stones | CVS manifestations

1. Hereditary
2. Sex: M >> F
3. Age: 2nd to 4th decade
4. Diet: Rich in purines – Meat, fish, alcohol.
   Gout 1° – Idiopathic
   2° – Associated with high metabolic turnover disease (chemotherapy, psoriasis, leukemia)

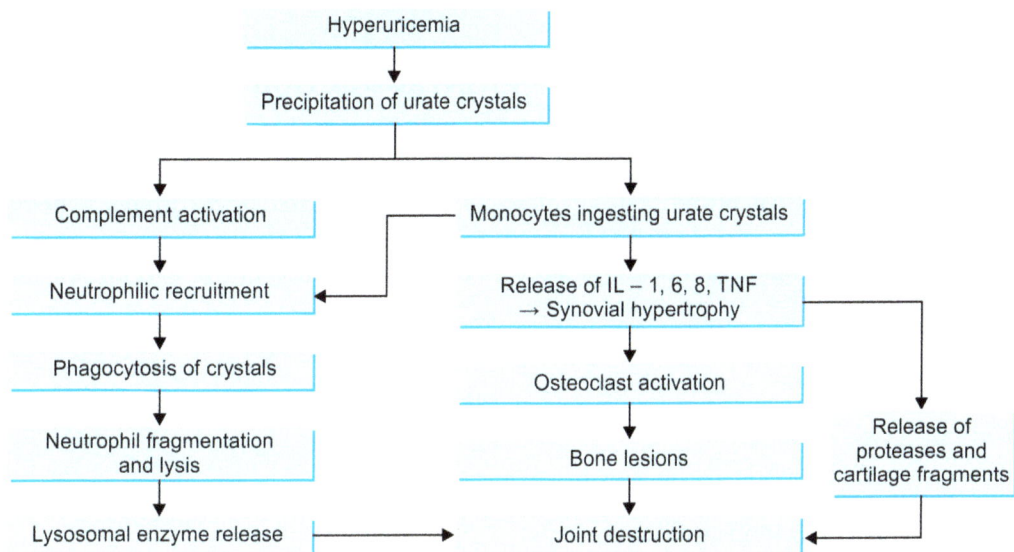

III. STAGES

1. Asymptomatic hyperuricemia
2. Acute gout
3. Intercritical gout
4. Chronic tophaceous gout

IV. CLINICAL FEATURES

A. Acute

1. "Podagra" or pain – 1st MTP joint
2. Sudden onset, usually at night
3. Throbbing, crushing, excruciating pain
4. Joint → warm and red
5. 1 or more joints → 1st MTP, knee, ankle, wrist.
6. After 1st attack → 50%: No symptoms
   50%: More attacks

B. Chronic

1. Frequency of attack ↑ : Chronic pain
2. Large subcutaneous tophi → Ear pinna, eyelids, nose and joints.
   ↓
   Yellow, sometimes discharge, a chalky material
3. Urate crystals in kidney → renal disease
4. Joint deformities, loss of ROM.

V. INVESTIGATIONS

1. *Radiograph:*
   i. Punched out periarticular erosion with sclerotic overhanging.
   ii. Soft tissue crystal deposition.
2. *Lab:* Serum uric acid → Elevated, but not diagnostic, BUN, creatinine, urine uric acid.
3. **Synovial fluid analysis: Diagnostic**

   Monosodium urate crystals
   i. Thin, tapered, needle shaped (intracellular) **(Fig. 7)**
   ii. Negatively birefringent.

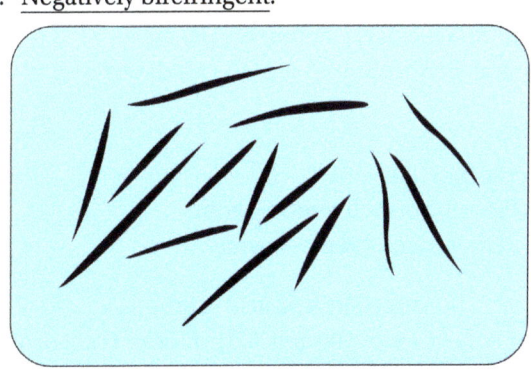

VI. DIFFERENTIAL DIAGNOSIS

i. Pseudogout: CPPD, chondrocalcinosis
ii. Psoriatic arthritis
iii. OA, RA, septic arthritis
iv. Cellulitis

VII. TREATMENT

A. Goals

i. Terminate acute attack
ii. Prevent future flairs
iii. Reduce crystal induced inflammation
iv. Prevent disease progression and complications
v. Correct metabolic cause

B. Drugs

Acute	Chronic
• NSAIDs	• Allopurinol
• Colchicine	• Probenecid
• Corticosteroids	• Febuxostat

Acute

1. *NSAIDs:*
   i. Indomethacin (50 mg TDS) – first line of treatment.
   ii. Inhibits urate crystal phagocytosis by decreasing migration of granulocytes.
   iii. ↓ Pain and inflammation. (also naproxen, ketorolac)
2. *Colchicine:*
   i. Indicated in acute attacks if patient has h/o peptic ulcers
   ii. MOA: Binds to intracellular protein tubulin → prevents its polymerization
   ↓
   Inhibition of leukocyte migration
   ↓
   Also inhibits synthesis and release of leukotrienes
   iii. 1 mg orally f/b 0.25 mg 3 hourly till symptoms controlled or ADR → diarrhea, vomiting.
3. *Corticosteroids:*
   i. Indications:
      a. NSAIDs and Colchicine C/I
      b. NSAIDs ineffective
   ii. Intra-articular: Depomedrol 80 mg
   iii. Oral: Prednisone 40 mg QID × 4 days, taper

Chronic

1. Allopurinol (300 mg)
   i. First line of Rx in chronic gout.
   ii. ⊗ Xanthine oxidase enzyme
   ↓
   Prevents uric acid synthesis
2. Probenecid (250–500 mg BD): Blocks reabsorption of urate from proximal tubule.
   ↓
   ↑ Uric acid excretion

Newer Drugs

1. *Febuxostat:* For chronic gout – Inhibits xanthine oxidase
2. *Lesinurad:* Selective Uric acid resorption inhibitor (URAT-1 ⊗)
3. *Rasburicase:* Recombinant urate oxidase → ↑ Uric acid metabolism
4. IL-1 blockers

C. Lifestyle Modifications

1. Restrict purine rich foods – red meat
2. Stop alcohol consumption.
3. Balance weight: Diet and exercise
4. Drinking plenty of water.

D. If Surgery, Principles are

1. Avoid LA → impairs local blood supply
2. Incision parallel to blood vessels
3. Sharp dissection
4. Pressure dressing

HEMOPHILIA

I. INTRODUCTION

1. Hereditary coagulation disorder
   ↓
   Characterized by occurrence of hemorrhages
   ↓
   Spontaneously or insignificant trauma.
2. **X-LR** → Males
3. Types

Hemophilia		
A	B	C
• Factor VIII • Classic hemophilia	• Factor IX • Christmas disease	• Platelets + factor VIII • Von Willebrand's

II. COAGULATION PATHWAY (FIG. 8)

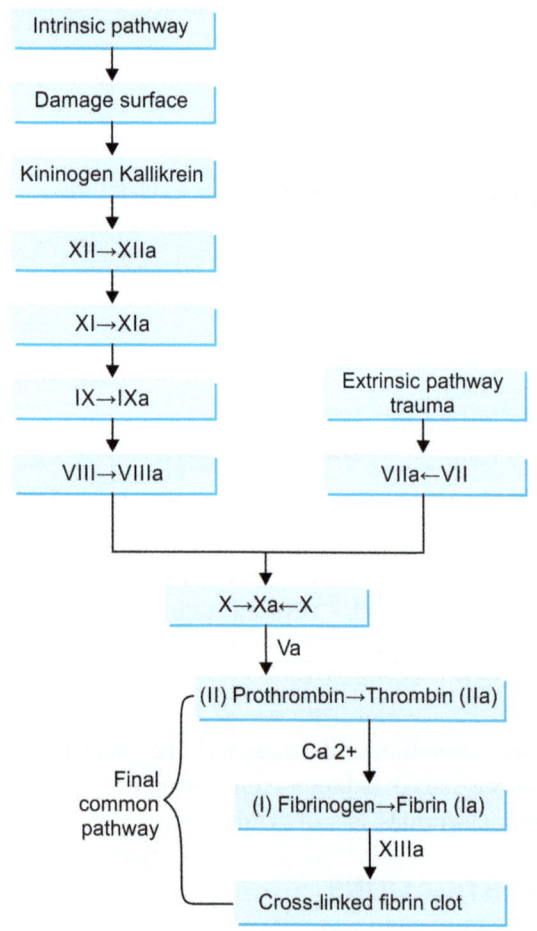

III. ORTHOPEDIC MANIFESTATIONS

1. Hemophilic arthropathy (MC = knee, ankle, elbow)
   i. Hemarthrosis
   ii. Synovitis
   iii. Cartilage destruction
   iv. Joint deformity and arthritis (end stage)

2. Hematoma (Pseudotumor) → Intramuscular
   → Subcutaneous
   i. Psoas hematoma resembles acute appendicitis
   ii. Iliacus hematoma → compresses femoral nerve
       ↓
   Presents with paresthesia of L_4 distribution

3. Leg length discrepancy: Due to epiphyseal overgrowth.
4. Fractures: Generalized osteopenia
5. Compartment syndrome.

IV. PATHOPHYSIOLOGY

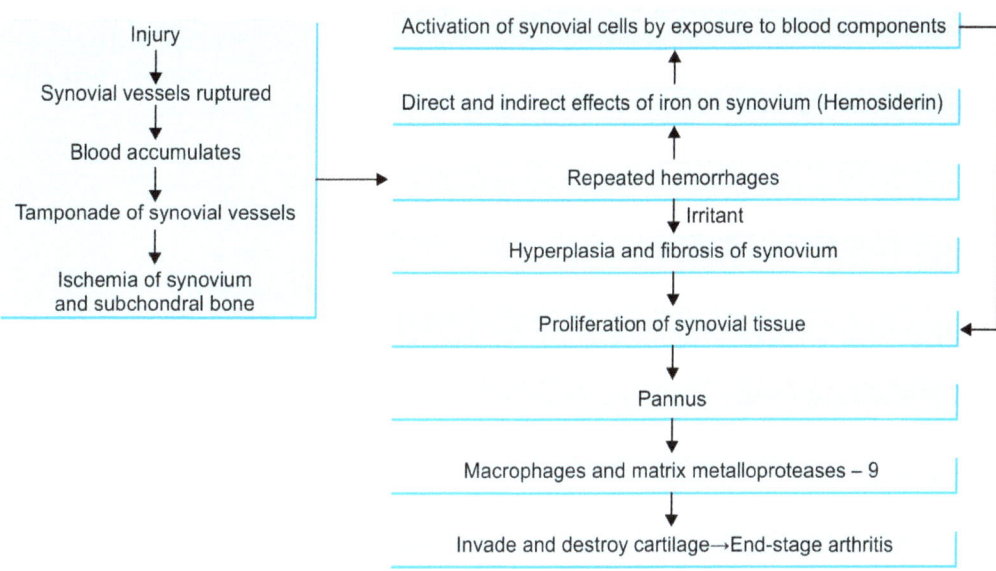

V. CLINICAL MANIFESTATIONS

i. *History:*
  1. Male gender
  2. Family history [maternal uncle]
ii. *Symptoms:*
  1. Recurrent or severe bleeding
  2. Frequency and severity of bleeding indirectly proportional to Factor VIII levels
     Factor VIII activity:
     a. Mild (>5%): Hemorrhage secondary to trauma. Rare spontaneous bleeding.
     b. Moderate (2-5%): Occasional spontaneous bleeding.
     c. Severe (<1%): Frequent spontaneous bleeding.
  3. Mucocutaneous bleeding: Gums, nose, easy bruising.
iii. *Physical examination:*
  1. Pallor
  2. Joint effusion: Swelling
  3. Redness and bruising
  4. Soft tissue contractures
  5. Muscle atrophy: Quadriceps
  6. Warmth [+]
  7. Tenderness
  8. ↓ ROM → deformities (flexion deformity of knee)
  9. Focal neurological deficits.
  10. Muscle pain d/t Intramuscular bleeding

VI. INVESTIGATIONS

i. *Radiograph:*
  A. General findings:
    1. Epiphyseal overgrowth
    2. Generalized osteopenia
    3. Pathological fractures
    4. Irregularities in joint space
    5. Joint effusion
  B. *Specific* (**Fig. 9**):

Jordan's sign – Squaring of patella and femoral condyles

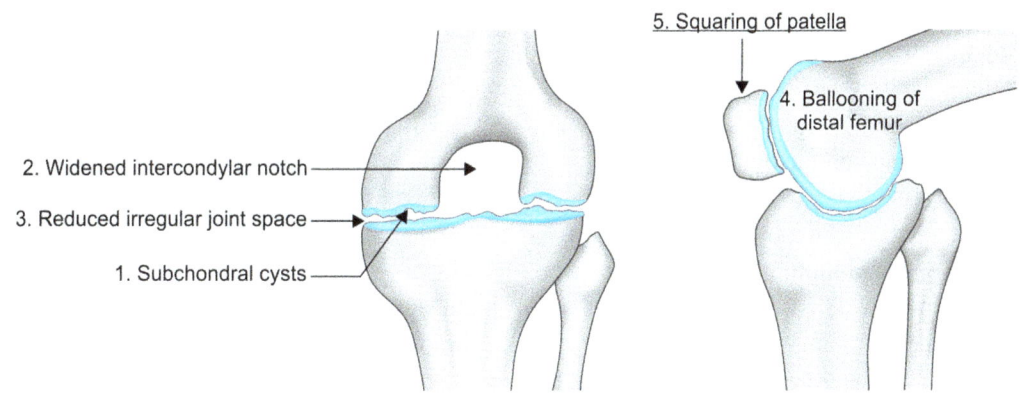

C. Arnold–Hilgartner grading (X-ray)
Stage:
1. Soft tissue swelling
2. Periarticular osteoporosis
3. Subchondral cysts, widened notch squaring of patella
4. Narrowing of joint space
5. Severe arthritis of affected joint, contractures.
   i. MRI: Pseudotumors, cartilage status
   ii. USG: Effusion vs pseudotumor
   iii. Lab:
      1. ↑ aPPT, [N] PT
      2. Specific factor assays → VIII, IX
      3. Bethesda assay

VII. MANAGEMENT

A. Prevention of Manifestations

1. Multidisciplinary approach → Hematologist, orthopedician and physiotherapist

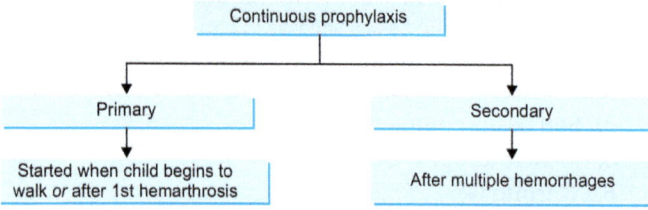

B. Conservative

1. *Replacement therapy:*
   i. Factor VIII: Costly
   ii. Factor IX: FFP
   iii. Cryoprecipitate: Risk of HIV, hepatitis B, C transmission
   iv. Levels required during:
      a. Physiotherapy: 20%
      b. Acute hematoma: 30%
      c. Acute hemarthrosis ⎫
      d. Soft tissue surgery ⎬ 40–50%
      e. Bone surgery → 100% 1st week, more than 50% 2nd week
2. *Pain management:*
   i. COX – 2 inhibitors and opioids
   ii. NSAIDs and aspirin → Gastric bleeding
   iii. Intramuscular injections C/I: Bleeding → Hematoma
3. *Physiotherapy:*
   i. Start slowly → progress gradually
   ii. Isometric exercises
   iii. No clinical gain → if painful movement
   iv. Splints, orthotics → to immobilize bleeding or painful joints, joint contracture
4. Compressive bandages

C. Operative Principles

1. *Synovectomy:*
   i. Recurrent hemarthrosis not responding to medical management
   ii. Synovectomy → Surgical = Arthroscopic/open
                    → Chemical = Rifampicin/Tetracycline
                    → Radionuclide (synoviorthesis)
                      (Colloidal phosphorous – 32)
2. Supracondylar osteotomy → Severe knee flexion deformity
   ↓
   a. Serial casting
   b. Hamstring release
3. Total joint arthroplasty:
   i. Factor replacement 100%
   ii. Indication: End-stage arthritis
   iii. Presence of factor inhibitors → C/I to surgery
   iv. Multiple procedures in single setting
   v. Vessels must be ligated, not cauterized
4. Arthrodesis: Arthropathy of ankle.
5. Fractures:
   i. Closed POP casts → risk of compartment syndrome
   ii. Rigid internal fixation preferred
6. Achilles tendon lengthening:
   ↓
   Bleeding in calf → Achilles' tendon contractures
   ↓
   Equinus deformity
7. Hemophilic Pseudotumor (Hemophilic cyst):
   i. Massive hemorrhage in muscle, extending till periosteum of bone
   ↓
   Fails to coagulate → Feeder keeps filling the cyst with blood
   ↓
   Fibrous wall forms around it.
   ii. Osseous pseudotumors → Uniformly expansile lytic lesions
   iii. Rx: Static → Observation
   iv. Progressive → Neuro, vascular manifestations
   ↓
   v. Surgery > replacement therapy
   ↓
   Excision
   vi. Radiation therapy for inaccessible pseudotumors.

PAGET'S DISEASE (OSTEITIS DEFORMANS)

I. INTRODUCTION

1. Idiopathic chronic bone remodeling disorder affects widespread noncontiguous areas of skeleton.

2. Exaggerated rates of bone resorptive and osteogenic activity
   ↓
   Bony thickening and deformity
3. Monostotic or polyostotic
4. Femur > Pelvis > Tibia > Skull > Spine

II. ETIOPATHOLOGY

1. Primary cellular abnormality → ↑↑ Osteoclastic bone resorption + ↑ Vascularity and fibrosis.
2. Trabeculae – Thinned, Haversian canals – Enlarged.
3. Periosteal and endosteal new bone formation → Thicken the cortex
4. Osteoblastic repair and osteoclastic destruction take place at the same time → disorderly and disorganized.
5. Therefore, 3 phases:
   i. Lytic phase: Intense osteoclastic resorption
   ii. Mixed phase: Resorption and compensatory bone formation
   iii. Sclerotic phase: Osteoblastic bone formation predominates
   (All three phases may co-exist in the same bone)
6. Hypothesized viral infection:
   i. Paramyxovirus
   ii. Respiratory syncytial virus
7. Hereditary: 40% autosomal dominant

III. CLINICAL FEATURES

1. 5th decade, M > F
2. Most commonly → Asymptomatic: Incidental finding
3. Bone Pain → fractures, stress fractures
4. Bowing of lower limbs
5. Backache, Radiculopathy ±
6. Progressive deafness → Otosclerosis
7. Cardiac: High output heart failure

IV. RADIOLOGY

A. Radiographs

1. Coarsened trabeculae → Blastic appearance of bone
2. *Lytic phase:*
   i. Lucent areas with expansion and thinned, intact cortices
   ii. **"blade of grass"** or **"flame-shaped"** lucent advancing edge
3. Mixed phase → Combination of lysis + sclerosis with coarsened trabeculae
4. Sclerotic phase → Bone enlargement with cortical thickening and sclerosis
5. Remodeled cortices → Loss of distinction between cortices and medullary cavity
6. Long bone bowing
7. Looser's zones
8. Fractures
9. Hip and knee osteoarthritis
10. Cotton wool Skull: Osteitis circumscripta
11. Paget's secondary sarcoma:
    i. Cortical bone destruction and sunray appearance
    ii. Soft tissue mass

B. Bone Scan

1. Accurately marks site of disease
2. Intensely hot in lytic and mixed phase

V. LABORATORY

1. Alkaline Phosphatase (ALP): ↑↑ (up to 10 times normal)
2. State of remission when ALP normalizes
3. Urinary Hydroxyproline: ↑ > 1 g/day (Marker of collagen breakdown)
4. Serum Calcium and Phosphorus: Normal

VI. HISTOLOGY

1. Mosaic pattern appearance → Irregular broad trabeculae in woven bone along with disorganized cement lines.
2. Large osteoblasts – Multiple nuclei/cell
3. Virus-like inclusion bodies in osteoclasts

VII. DIFFERENTIALS

1. Metastatic bone disease
2. Multiple myeloma
3. Lymphoma
4. Hyperparathyroidism
5. Fibrous dysplasia

VIII. MANAGEMENT

A. Asymptomatic/inactive/incidental: Observation
B. Active disease: Primarily medical management
   1. *Goals:*
      i. Suppression of active disease
      ii. Relief of pain
      iii. Prevention of deformity, especially of large weight-bearing bones
      iv. Counteracting high-output cardiac dysfunction
      v. Reducing the tendency to fracture
      vi. Preventing and correcting hypercalcemia
      vii. Reducing the probability of sarcomatous transformation
   2. **Bisphosphonates:** 1st line of treatment:
      i. Inhibit osteoclastic resorption
      ii. Alendronate and Risedronate: Oral
      iii. Zoledronic acid: IV (5 mg)

3. Calcitonin: 2nd choice:
   i. 100 IU/day
   ii. SC or IM
4. Teriparatide: Contraindicated → Risk of transformation to osteosarcoma

C. *Surgical*:
1. Management of fractures:
   i. Non-operative treatment: ↑ Complication rate
   ii. IM nailing: Maybe unsuitable due to bowing
2. Correction of bone deformities → Metaphyseal osteotomy and plate fixation
3. Total hip and knee replacement
   i. Risk of severe bleeding
   ii. Malalignment in TKR
4. Spinal surgery
5. Ablative therapy for malignant lesions

OSGOOD-SCHLATTER DISEASE

I. INTRODUCTION

Osteochondrosis or traction apophysitis of the tibial tubercle (Fig. 10).

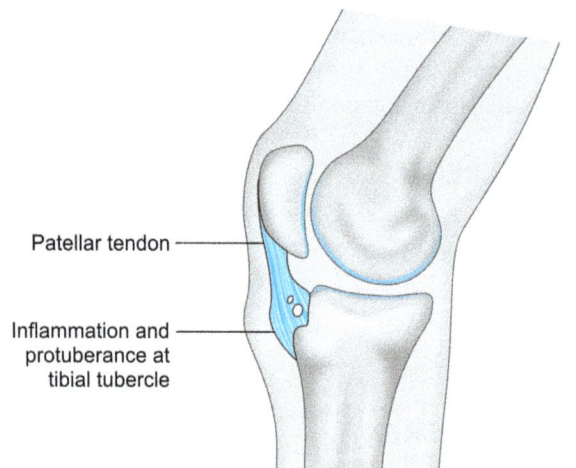

II. ETIOLOGY

1. Repeated microtrauma at the insertion of patellar tendon.
2. Single violent trauma against a tightly contracted quadriceps
3. RF: Children about the rapid growth period of puberty → Playing
4. Jumpers and Sprinters

III. PATHOPHYSIOLOGY

1. Tibial tubercle: 2° ossification center
2. Age < 11 years: Tubercle cartilaginous
3. 11–14 years: Apophysis appears
4. 14–18 years: Apophysis fuses with tibial epiphysis
5. 18 years: Epiphysis and apophysis fuse with rest of tibia

IV. CLINICAL FEATURES

1. M > F
2. Boys: 12-15 years. Girls: 8-12 years
3. Bilateral
4. *Symptoms:*
   i. Anterior knee pain
   ii. Exacerbated by kneeling, jumping, running
   iii. Swelling
5. *Examination:*
   i. Enlarged tibial tubercle
   ii. Tenderness
   iii. Resisted knee extension → Painful
   iv. Quadriceps – atrophy

V. INVESTIGATIONS

1. *X-ray:* Irregularity and fragmentation of tibial tubercle
2. *MRI:*
   i. Soft tissue swelling
   ii. Thickening and edema → Inferior patellar tendon

VI. TREATMENT

A. *Conservative* – 90% cases – first line
1. Rest
2. NSAIDs
3. Ice – Cryotherapy
4. Activity modification
5. Strapping and sleeves → decrease tension on the apophysitis
6. Quadriceps stretching
7. Severe symptoms → not responding to simple conservative measures
   ↓
   Cast immobilization × 6 weeks
   Complication → Wasting

B. *Operative*:
1. Drill holes through tibial tuberosity into the main bone → forms channels through which rapid revascularization occurs.
2. Peg of bones from adjacent area of tibia inserted through drill holes → immobilizing bone graft
3. Ossicle excision: Refractory cases
4. In skeletally mature with persistent symptoms.

VII. PROGNOSIS

Self-limiting → but does not resolve till growth halted.

CARPAL TUNNEL SYNDROME

I. DEFINITION

Compressive neuropathy of the median nerve at the level of wrist.

II. PATHOPHYSIOLOGY (FIG. 11)

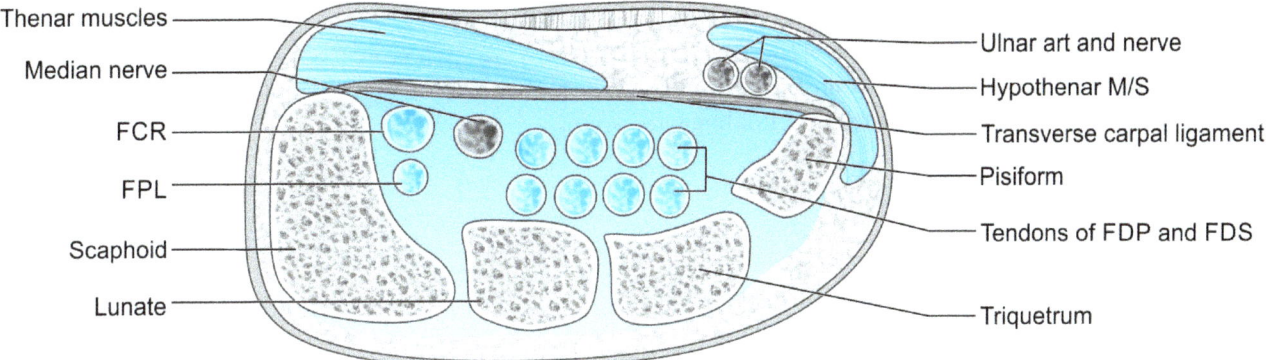

Borders:
1. Radially = Scaphoid tubercle, trapezium
2. Ulnarly = Hook of hamate and pisiform
3. Roof = Transverse carpal ligament
4. Floor = Proximal carpal row

III. ETIOLOGY

i. Idiopathic: Most common.
ii. Factors ↑ volume of carpal tunnel.
   A. Factors outside nerve:
      1. Altered fluid balance:
         i. Hypothyroidism
         ii. Pregnancy
         iii. Renal failure
         iv. Myxedema
         v. Acromegaly
      2. Inflammatory conditions: RA, SLE, Gout, amyloidosis
      3. Tumors and tumor-like: Ganglion, PVNS, lipoma
      4. Hematological disorders: Hemophilia, vW disease
      5. Post-traumatic: Traction neuropathies
   B. Factors within nerve:
      1. Tumor and tumor-like: Schwannoma, lipoma
      2. Persistent median artery (thrombosis)
iii. Extrinsic factors altering contour of tunnel:
   1. Acute distal radius fracture
   2. Acute fracture – dislocation, complex carpal injuries
   3. Chronic wrist injuries
   4. Malunited distal radius fracture
iv. Exertional/overuse
v. Neuropathic factors:
   1. DM
   2. Alcoholism
   3. Nutritional deficiency

IV. PATHOPHYSIOLOGY

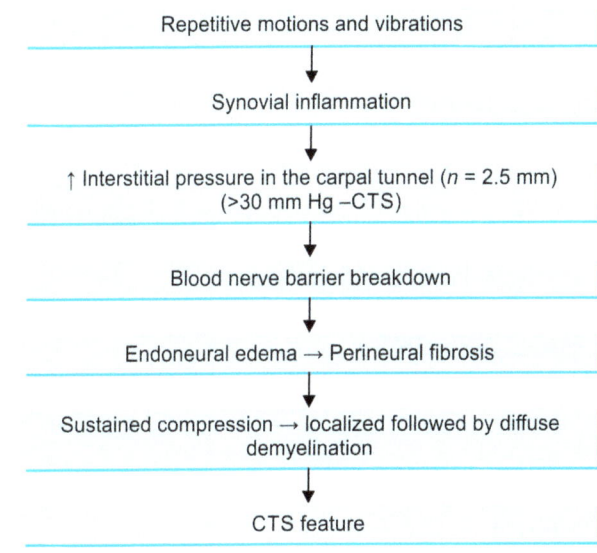

V. CLINICAL FEATURES

Middle age, F > M
A. *Symptoms* (**Fig. 12**):

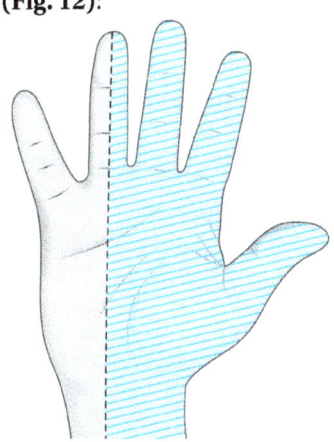

1. Pain
2. Paresthesia
3. Numbness and tingling } Radial 3½ digits
4. Clumsiness

5. Pain is insidious and nocturnal → awakens patient from sleep. Patient shakes wrist vigorously
B. *Signs/examination*:
1. Thenar atrophy, dry skin, swelling, color changes
2. Self-administered hand diagram – Most specific
3. Durkan's test: Carpal tunnel compression test. Most sensitive → Pressing thumb over CT, holding for 30 seconds ≥ symptoms
4. Phalen's test: Wrist volar flexion ≥ 60 seconds
5. Reverse phalens.
6. Tinel's sign → Tapping median nerve over CT
7. Gilliat: Tourniquet test
8. Sensory test:
   i. Semmes: Weinstein monofilament test (most sensitive)
   ii. 2-point discrimination (>5 mm)
   iii. Tuning fork.

VI. INVESTIGATIONS

Diagnosis is clinical:
i. X-ray → Fractures malunion. Carpal tunnel view – bony cause
ii. MRI → Cross section of carpal tunnel, soft – tissue structures
iii. EMG/NCV → Prolonged latency, slow conduction velocity ↑ insertional activity, fibrillation

VII. MANAGEMENT

A. *Conservative–First line Rx*:
1. NSAIDs
2. Rest
3. Night splints
4. Activity modification
5. Steroid injections → transient improvement
B. *Operative*:
1. Indications:
   i. Failure of nonoperative management
   ii. Acute CTS following DER fracture
2. Open or endoscopic
3. **Transverse carpal ligament release**

VIII. COMPLICATIONS OF SURGERY

1. Progressive thenar atrophy ⎫
2. Lumbrical muscles weakness ⎬ Injury to median nerve
3. Incomplete division of TCR ⎭

TENNIS ELBOW/LATERAL EPICONDYLITIS

I. DEFINITION

A chronic, symptomatic, degenerative condition that affects the common extensor muscle at their origin leading to tendinosis and inflammation.

II. PATHOANATOMY (FIG. 13)

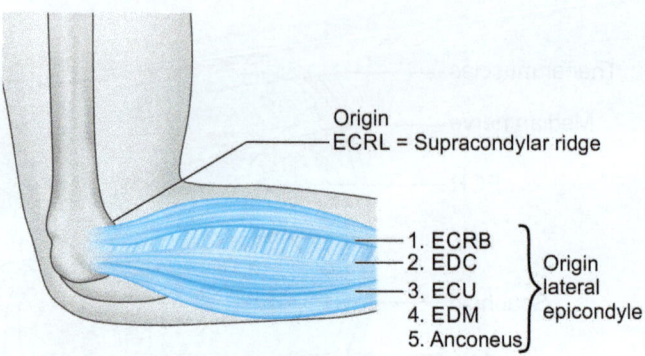

- Origin:
  – ECRL: Supracondylar ridge
- Ligament: LUCL
- Nerve: PIN enters supinator just distal to radial tunnel
- Differential diagnosis: Radial tunnel syndrome

III. ETIOLOGY AND PATHOPHYSIOLOGY

i. *Demographics*:
1. Males = Females
2. Age = 35–50 years
3. Up to 50% tennis players affected
ii. *Risk factors*:
1. Tennis → Poor swing technique
   →Heavy racket
   →Incorrect grip size
   →High string tension
2. Laborer's → Utilizing heavy tools.
3. Repetitive gripping or lifting tasks. Wrist extension and pronation-supination.
iii. *Pathophysiology*:

Repetitive microtrauma
↓
Microtear → origin of **ECRB**
→ **STAGE 1**
Acute inflammatory response
↓
Resolves completely
→ **STAGE 2**
Sustained stage 1 or recurrence
↓
Angiofibroblastic hyperplasia → High concentration of fibroblasts, unorganized collagen
→ **STAGE 3**
Partial/Complete tendon rupture
→ **STAGE 4**
Stage 3 + fibrosis, soft tissue calcification

IV. CLINICAL FEATURES

1. Pain – outer aspect of elbow
    i. On gripping – with wrist extension activities
    ↓
2. Decreased grip strength.
    Examination:
    i. Point tenderness: ECRB insertion at Lateral Epicondyle (Few mm distal to tip)
    ii. Provocative Cozen's test: Resisted wrist extension
    iii. Maudsley's test: Long finger extension
    iv. Mill's maneuver: Pronate forearm, wrist full flexion and elbow extended → Pain.
3. Morning stiffness

V. INVESTIGATIONS

1. Diagnosis clinical
2. X-ray: Rule out avulsion fracture, loose bodies, OA, OCD
3. MRI: Degenerative tear of ERCB
4. NCS: Exclude PIN entrapment

VI. TREATMENT

i. *Principles*:
   1. Pain control
   2. Preservation and restoration of movement
   3. Regaining grip strength
   4. Return to function
   5. Prevent recurrence

ii. *Conservative (85% patients)*:
   1. Rest
   2. Brace → Orthotic band/strap → 10 cm distal to L/E decreased tension over muscle attachment
   3. Local ultrasound, ice massage, ECSWT
   4. Physiotherapy
   5. Local steroid injection → PRP injection
   6. Manipulation under anesthesia → to convert partial → complete tear
   7. Percutaneous ultrasonic tenotomy

iii. *Operative (>1 year of conservative trial)*:
   1. Extensor slide: Partial release of extensor origin
   2. Open or arthroscopic
   3. Cortical bone curetted to expose cancellous bone → ↑ Vascularity
   4. Postoperative immobilization: 6 weeks
   5. Complications
      - ECRL release = wrist extension weakness
      - LUCL ⊗ → Instability
      - Radial nerve ⊗

DUPUYTREN'S CONTRACTURE

I. DEFINITION

Thickening and hypertrophic fibroplasia of the palmar aponeurosis and its extensions into the digits.
↓
Occurring in the form of nodules and cords
↓
Flexion contractures of finger joints

II. ETIOPATHOGENESIS

1. Autosomal dominant
2. *Risk factors:*
    i. Diabetes mellitus
    ii. Alcoholism
    iii. HIV infection
    iv. Antiepileptic drugs
    v. Rheumatoid disease
3. *Dupuytrens diathesis:*
    i. B/L involvement
    ii. Ledderhose's: Plantar fascia
    iii. Peyronie's: Dorsal fascia penis
    iv. Garrod: Knuckles
4. Local ischemia at microvascular level.
    ↓
5. Increase in myofibroblasts and fibroblasts: Nodule formation
    ↓
6. These organize themselves along lines of stress.
    ↓
7. Myofibroblasts have intracellular actin filaments along the long axis of the cell.
    ↓
8. Adjacent fibroblasts connect to each other via extra-cellular fibronectin to create contracted tissue ≥ cord formation
9. Type III > I collagen
10. 2 fibrotic structures

Nodule	Cord
• Vascular	• Collagen – rich
• ↑Fibro and myofibroblasts	• Avascular } Relatively
	• Acellular
	• Normal fascial bands become pathological cords

11. Stages by (Luck):
    i. Proliferative: Myofibroblast proliferation – Nodule formation
    ii. Involutional: Fibroblasts align along tension lines → produce collagen → cord formation.
    iii. Residual: Myofibroblasts disappear (acellular). Fibrocytes predominant. Dense collagen rich scar.

III. PATHOANATOMY

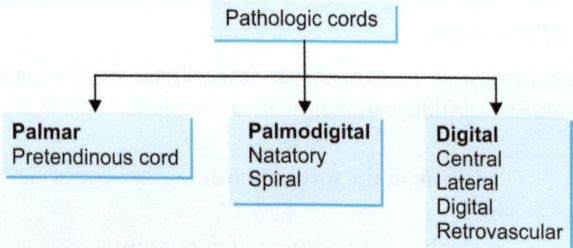

i. **Spiral cord (Fig. 14):**

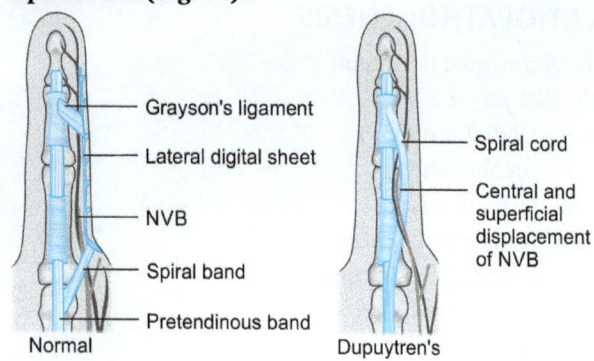

1. Most important
2. Causes PIP contracture
3. Travels under NVB and displaces it centrally and superficially
4. Components = Pretendinous band, spiral band, lateral digit sheet, Grayson's ligament

ii. Pretendinous cord: MCP contracture + skin pitting
iii. Natatory: Web space contracture
iv. Retrovascular: DIP hyperextension contractures

IV. CLINICAL FEATURES

1. M:F = 2:1. More severe in males
2. 5th – 7th decade
3. Ring > Small > Middle > Index
4. Caucasians ++

A. Symptoms
1. ↓ROM → Restricted activities of daily living.
2. Painful nodules.

B. Examination
1. Pitting of skin.
2. Hueston's table top test: Palm flat on table. MCP or PIP contracture
3. Thinning of SC fat
4. Firm nodules - tender
5. Painless cords → flexion contractures
6. Rule out ectopic associations

V. TREATMENT

A. Conservative
Limited role:
1. Physiotherapy - ROM exercises, heat, local USG
2. Custom splint, braces
3. Local injections:
   i. Corticosteroids
   ii. Clostridium histolyticum collagenase
   ↓
   Lysis and rupture of cords. Contractures < 5°

B. Operative
1. Percutaneous needle aponeurotomy: Mild cases
2. Surgical resection (fasciectomy)
   Indications:
   i. MCP contractures > 30°
   ii. PIP contractures
   Technique:
   i. Partial: Removal of all diseased tissue only in involved digits.
   ii. Open palm (McCash): Leaves a transverse skin incision open at distal palmar crease. ↓ hematoma, stiffness.
   iii. Total/Radical Fasciectomy: Excision of all palmar and digital fascia. Not done now.
3. Surgery resection with skin graft: Severe recurrent disease
4. Salvage: Arthrodesis, Amputation indicated in chronic advanced disease.

MADELUNG DEFORMITY

I. DEFINITION
Congenital dyschondrosis of the volar and ulnar aspect of the distal radius physis leading to asymmetric growth.

II. ETIOPATHOGENESIS
1. Henry and Thorburn etiology classification:
   i. Idiopathic or 1°
   ii. Post-traumatic
   iii. Dysplastic ⟶ 1. HME
   iv. Chromosomal/Genetic (Turner's)
       2. Olliers disease
       3. Achondroplasia
       4. Leri–Weill Dyschondrosteosis *SHOX* gene ⊗ Mesomelic dwarfism + Madelung
2. AD
3. Pathophysiology:
   i. Repetitive microtrauma/dysplastic arrest
   ↓
   Disruption of ulnar volar physis of DER
   ↓
   Excess radial inclination and volar tilt
   Ulnar carpal impaction
   ii. Vicker's ligament: Pathological radio–lunate ligament tethering growth of DER.

III. CLINICAL FEATURES

A. *Symptoms*:
   1. Females > Males = 4:1
   2. B/L > 50%
   3. Symptoms → Adolescence = 10–14 years girls
   4. Pain in the wrist
   5. ↓ ROM
   6. Progressive deformity: Cosmetic concern

B. *Examination*:
   1. Radial and volar displacement of hand
   2. Restricted DF, pronation and radial deviation
   3. Median nerve irritation maybe present
   4. Protrusion of lower end of ulna abutting the carpus
   5. In advanced disease = Complete dislocation of DRUJ

IV. INVESTIGATIONS

i. *Radiography* (Fig. 15):

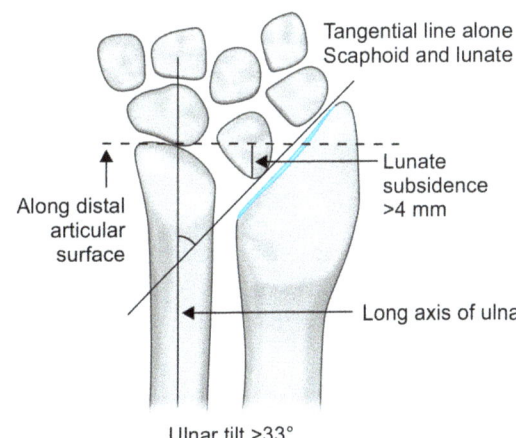

1. Ulnar tilt > 33°
2. Lunate subsidence – 4 mm } Diagnostic
3. Palmar carpal displacement ≥ 20 mm
   Distance between longitudinal axis of the ulna and the most volar point on the surface of lunate or capitate → palmar carpal displacement >20 mm (Lateral X-ray) (Fig. 16)

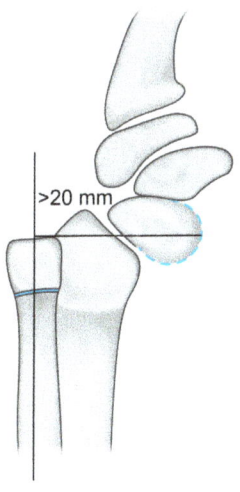

- *Other features*:
  1. Widened IO space
  2. True shortening of radius
  3. "Flame - like" lesion → focal osteopenia → site of attachment of Vickers ligament.
  4. Carpal wedging → Apex is lunate
ii. MRI = Vickers ligament
iii. CT scan = Surgical planning

V. TREATMENT

A. *Conservative: Mild deformity and symptoms*:
   1. Rest
   2. NSAIDs
   3. Sugar tong type splint

B. *Operative*:
   i. Indications:
      1. Significant wrist pain
      2. ↓ ROM → ADL affected
      3. Cosmetic concern
   ii. Physiolysis with Vickers ligament release:
       In skeletally immature, when deformity has not fully developed
   iii. Radial dome osteotomy with/without ulnar shortening:
       1. Approach → Modified Henry.
       2. Fixation → K wires, plates, screws, Ex. fix
       3. Patients suffer from ulnar sided wrist pain due to +ve ulnar variance (Fig. 17).

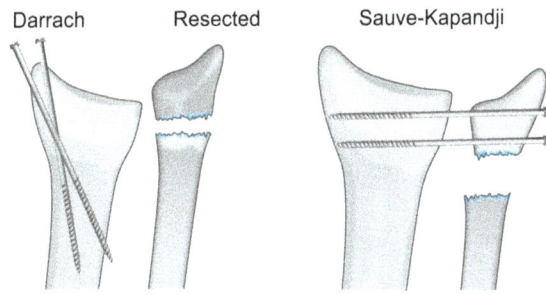

   iv. DRUJ arthroplasty – Controversial
   v. Salvage = Wrist arthrodesis. Recurrent, failed cases

VI. COMPLICATIONS

1. Recurrence
2. Nonunion
3. Continued ulnar impaction
4. Premature growth arrest

DEQUERVAIN'S TENOSYNOVITIS

I. INTRODUCTION

1. Chronic inflammation of the tendons of the abductor pollicis longus and the extensor pollicis brevis (APL and EPB) where they lie over the styloid process of the radius.
2. Also known as tenovaginitis, washerwoman's sprain

II. PATHOANATOMY (FIG. 18)

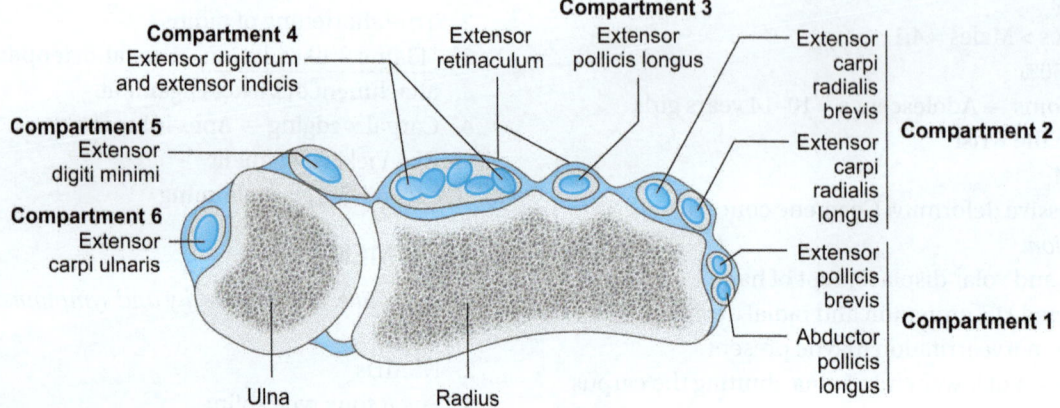

III. PATHOPHYSIOLOGY

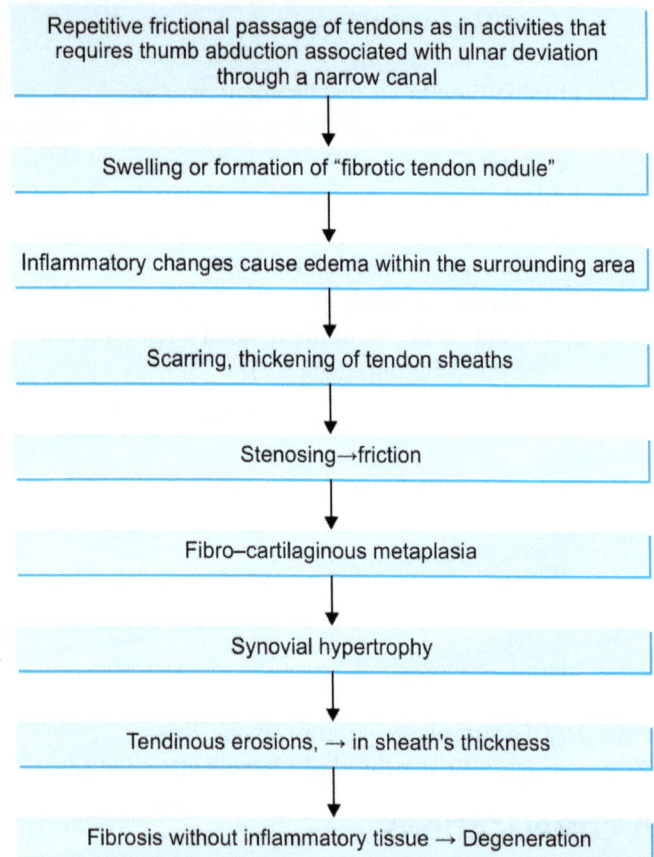

IV. ETIOLOGY

1. Idiopathic
2. RA
3. Pregnancy
4. Recent trauma
5. Occupational
6. Malunited radius fractures
7. Bony exostosis
8. *Associated conditions*:
    i. CTS
    ii. Trigger finger
    iii. Epicondylitis

V. CLINICAL FEATURES

1. F > M
2. 40–60 years
3. Dominant wrist more common
4. *Triad*:
    a. Tenderness over radial styloid
    b. Swelling over 1st extensor compartment
    c. Positive Finkelstein's test
5. Crepitus with movements of involved tendons may be palpable
6. **Finkelstein test:** Ulnar deviating the partially flexed wrist, with thumb in opposition → severe pain

VI. DIFFERENTIAL DIAGNOSIS

1. Intersection syndrome
2. CMC joint arthritis
3. Scaphoid fracture
4. Radial styloid fracture
5. Scaphotrapeziotrapezoid arthritis
6. Lindberg syndrome → Anomalous connection between FPL and index FDP

VII. RADIOLOGY

1. Clinical diagnosis
2. X-ray - Rule out arthritis and fractures
3. USG → ↑ in APL, EPB sheath's thickness.

VIII. TREATMENT

A. *Medical treatment*:
    1. Nonsteroidal anti-inflammatory drugs
    2. Local ointments
    3. Splints
    4. Physiotherapy
    5. Ice packs

B. Injection of local steroids in the synovial sheath (Dexamethasone preparations)
C. *Surgical*:
   1. For recurrent disease or resistant one that does not respond to conservative treatment.
   2. Surgical release of 1st dorsal compartment through a radial longitudinal or transverse incision aims at decompression of the twin tendons.
   ↓
   Excision of thickened sheath

IX. COMPLICATIONS
1. Radial superficial nerve laceration, neuroma formation
2. Volar tendon subluxation.
3. Hypertrophic scarring
4. Tendinous adhesions
5. CRPS

WRIST ARTHRODESIS

Wrist arthrodesis is a salvage procedure involving wrist joint fusion providing a pain free, stable wrist in a maximum functional position.

I. INDICATIONS
1. Post-traumatic wrist arthritis
2. Rheumatoid arthritis
3. Septic arthritis
4. Scapholunate advanced collapse (SLAC)
5. Scaphoid NU advanced collapse (SNAC)
6. Severely comminuted intra-articular fracture.
7. Segmental bone loss → Tumor resection (GCT)
   Trauma
8. Stabilization of paralytic wrist and hand (for tendon transfers)
9. Spastic hemiplegia: Correction of wrist flexion deformity
10. Crystalline arthropathy
11. Severe carpal instability
12. Failed limited arthrodesis
13. Failed total arthroplasty
14. Kienbock's disease

II. POSITION
1. Dorsiflexion: 10–20° → Allows maximal grip strength.
2. Long axis of the 3rd metacarpal aligned with radius long axis
3. Neutral to 5° ulnar deviation
4. If B/L → position determined by pt. needs
5. Cast immobilization preoperatively will help patient decide

III. METHOD (FIG. 19)

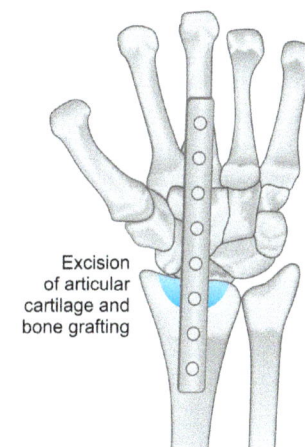

Excision of articular cartilage and bone grafting

1. Approach: Dorsal
2. Denude the radiocarpal and intercarpal joint surfaces of cartilage.
   ↓
   Fill gaps with cancellous BG
3. If severe bone loss → Corticocancellous grafts
4. If positive ulnar variance → Proximal row carpectomy.
5. Radioulnar joint not included
   ↓
   Pronation/supination possible
6. Fixation: 3.5 mm Recon. Plate with carpal bend → Distal radius to 3rd MC.
7. Detach ERCB insertion → mobilize over the plate → incorporating in capsular closure → Prevents wound dehiscence.
8. Postoperative: Volar splint × 3 weeks union by 3 months.

IV. CONTRAINDICATIONS
1. Open physis of distal radius
2. Elderly patient with sedentary lifestyle
3. Quadriparetics → use their motors, for modified grasp and transfer techniques
4. Neurologic disorders causing major sensory deprivation of hand
5. Patients who would benefit more from tendon transfers and wrist arthroplasty

V. COMPLICATIONS
1. Painful/irritation hardware: Removal
2. Tendon adhesions: Adhesiolysis
3. Early wound dehiscence and swelling
4. DRUJ pain and instability
5. MCP joint stiffness
6. Carpal tunnel syndrome
7. Reflex sympathetic dystrophy
8. Nonunion, pseudoarthrosis
9. Persistent pain
10. Donor site morbidity
11. Fracture of healed fusion
12. Intrinsic contracture

KIENBOCK'S DISEASE

I. INTRODUCTION
1. Kienbock's disease is the avascular necrosis of the lunate which can lead to progressive wrist pain and abnormal carpal motion.
2. Most common in males → 20-40 years old

II. PATHOPHYSIOLOGY
1. History of trauma: ↑ Risk
2.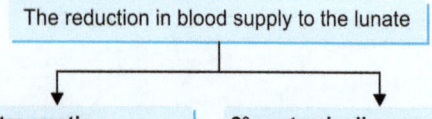
5. Blood supply to lunate (Gelberman): Three variations
    i. Y-pattern
    ii. X-pattern
    iii. I-pattern – 31% of patients → highest risk for avascular necrosis (Fig. 21)

3. *Biomechanical factors*:
    i. Ulnar negative variance → ↑↑ Radio-lunate contact stress
    ii. Decreased radial inclination
    iii. Repetitive trauma
4. Zapico types: Based on the shape of lunate:
    i. Type I lunate:
        a. Angle greater than 130° (proximal apex or crest)
        b. Weakest with a greater potential for bone fatigue and stress fracture
        c. Seen in ulna negative wrists
    ii. Type II lunate 100—seen with ulna zero
    iii. Type III lunate:
        a. Two distinct facets on proximal surface (one for radius and other for TFCC)
        b. Seen with ulna plus (Fig. 20)

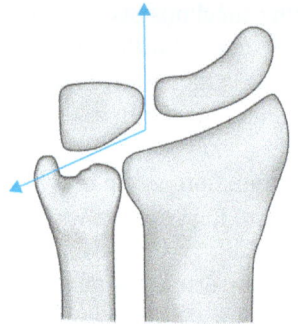
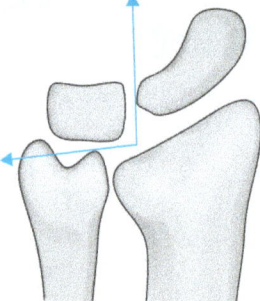
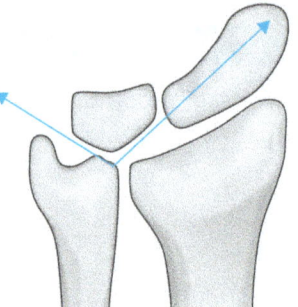

Type-I–Trapezoid   Type-II–Rectangular   Type-III–Pentagonal

IV. RADIOLOGY

A. Radiograph
1. The lunate in later stages → flattened and fragmented.
2. The carpal height ratio → Carpal collapse
3. The ratio of the height of the carpus to the height of the third metacarpal (Youm's index) → abnormal following carpal collapse.
4. A scaphoid ring sign can be seen following carpal collapse suggesting a rotary subluxation of scaphoid.

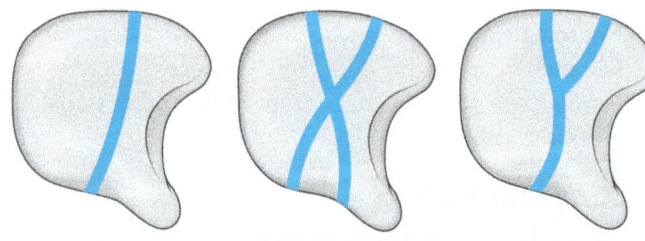

III. CLINICAL FEATURES
A. *Symptoms*:
  1. Dorsal wrist pain
  2. Activity related
  3. More in dominant hand
B. *Physical examination*:
  1. Wrist swelling +
  2. Tenderness → radiocarpal joint
  3. ↓ Range of motion
  4. ↓ Grip strength

B. CT
Most useful once lunate collapse has already occurred:
1. Extent of necrosis
2. Trabecular destruction
3. Lunate geometry

C. MRI
1. Best for diagnosing early disease
2. Rule out ulnar impaction
3. Decreased T1 signal intensity
4. ↓ vascularity of lunate

V. LICHTMAN CLASSIFICATION

Stage	Description
Stage I	No visible changes on X-ray, changes seen on MRI
Stage II	Sclerosis of lunate
Stage IIIA	Lunage collapse, no scaphoid rotation
Stage IIIB	Lunate collapse, fixed scaphoid rotation
Stage IV	Degenerated adjacent intercarpal joints

- Vascularized bone graft
- *Technique*:
  - Transfer of pisiform
  - Transfer of distal radius on a vascularized pedicle of pronator quadratus
  - Transfers of branches of the first, second, or third dorsal metacarpal arteries
  - 4 + 5 extensor compartment artery (ECA)

VI. MANAGEMENT

Stage of disease	Treatment suggested
I	Immobilization for 3 months (surgery as in stages II and IIIa-optional)
II and IIIa, negative or neutral variance	• Radial shortening osteotomy • Ulinar lengthening • Capitate shortening
II and IIIa positive ulna variance	• Revascularization with scaphocapitate pinning (or external fixation) • Capitate shortening • Radial wedge osteotomy • Joint leveling + Revascularization
IIIb	• STT fusion (or scaphocapitate fusion) + excision of lunate and tendon anchovy • Proximal row carpectomy
IV	• Total wrist fusion • Proximal row carpectomy • Total wrist arthroplasty • Wrist denervation

THORACIC OUTLET SYNDROME

Neurovascular disorder resulting from compression of the brachial plexus and/or subclavian vessels traversing the superior aperture of chest.

I. PATHOANATOMY

1. Boundaries of thoracic outlet:
   i. Posteriorly: T1 vertebral body
   ii. Laterally: First rib and costal cartilage
   iii. Anteriorly: Manubrium sterni
2. Interscalene triangle **(Fig. 22)**

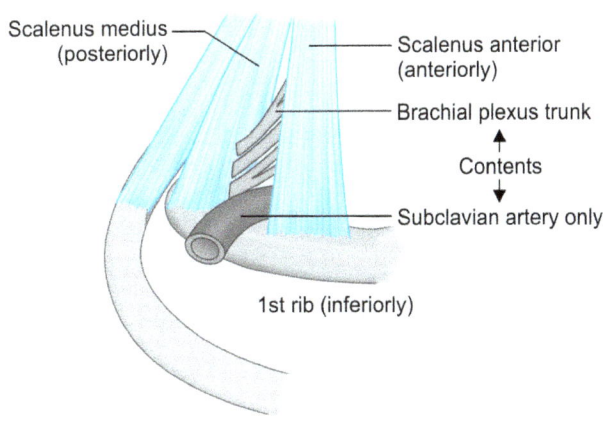

3. Costoclavicular space **(Fig. 23)**
4. Retropectoralis minor space **(Fig. 24)**

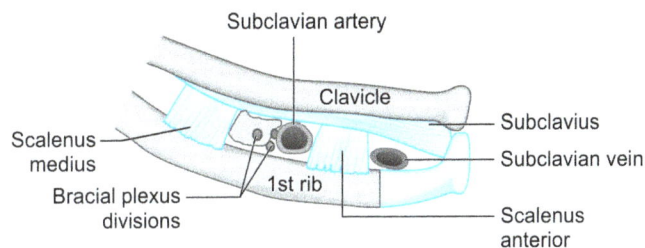

Fig. 23: Costoclavicular space.

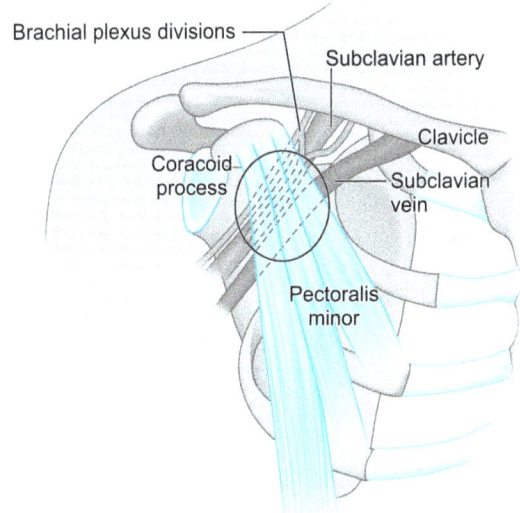

Fig. 24: Retropectoralis minor space

II. ETIOLOGY + PATHOLOGY

Anatomic predisposition + superimposed neck trauma.

A. Soft Tissue (70%)

1. Scalene muscles:
   i. Hypertrophy
   ii. Variable origin and insertion
   iii. Scalenus minimus
2. Abnormal ligament or bands: abnormal insertion of costoclavicular ligament (Paget–Schroetter syndrome)
3. Pancoast tumor

B. Osseous (30%)
  i. Cervical rib
  ii. Prominent C7 transverse process
  iii. AC, SC joint dislocations
  iv. Osseous tumors: Osteoid osteoma, metastasis

III. WILBOURN'S CLASSIFICATION

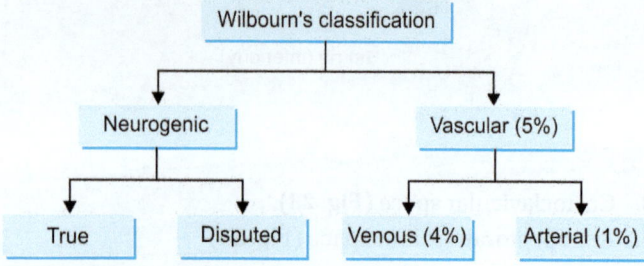

IV. CLINICAL PRESENTATION
F:M = 3:1, Age: 20–60 years

1. Neurogenic
  i. Pain over neck, trapezius, chest, shoulder, arm.
  ii. Upper extremity: weakness, numbness and paresthesia
      ↓
      Non radicular nature and wide anatomic distribution
      ↓   ↓
      Differentiate from   Differentiate from
      cervical nerve   isolated peripheral nerve
      compression   compression
      Root compression nerve root compression.
  iii. True neurogenic: Hypothenar atrophy, decreased grip and sensation.
  iv. Disputed neurogenic: Wide and variable range of complaints.

2. Venous
  i. Episodic cyanotic discoloration
  ii. Swelling of limb
  iii. Distended veins
  iv. Diffuse deep pain in arm and forearm
  v. Upper extremity heaviness.

3. Arterial
Unilateral Raynaud's phenomenon, coolness of hand, claudication, ulceration of finger tips.

4. Special Tests
  i. Adson's
  ii. Roo's
  iii. Halstead
  iv. Hyperabduction

V. RADIOLOGY
1. X-ray: Cervical rib, 7th TP, Pancoast tumor
2. CT: Osseous SOL, malunited fracture of rib and clavicle
3. MRI: Soft tissue abnormality
4. EDS: EMG, NCV
5. Angiography: Thrombosis and embolic aspects

VI. TREATMENT
A. Nonoperative
1. *Activity modification:* Limiting repetitive overhead motion, lifting heavy weight, provocative activities
2. *Pain control:* NSAIDs, muscle relaxants
3. *Physiotherapy:* Shoulder girdle strengthening posture and relaxation, core and back strengthening
4. TENS
5. Anterior scalene blocks

B. Operative
1. *Indications:*
    i. Failure of conservative management (>3–4 months)
    ii. Venous/arterial complications
    iii. Nerve compression (progressive symptoms)
    iv. NCV < 60 m/s
2. *Procedures:*
    i. First rib resection: Lower TOS (transaxillary, supraclavicular, infraclavicular, posterior, VATS)
    ii. Anterior scalenectomy: Upper TOS
    iii. Pectoralis minor tenotomy
    iv. Cervical rib resection
    v. Clavicle malunion: ORIF
    vi. Release of fibromuscular bands and costoclavicular ligaments
    vii. Vascular intervention: Embolism, aneurysm.

VI. COMPLICATIONS
  i. Pneumothorax
  ii. Arterial, venous, nerve injury

CERVICAL RIB

1. Supernumerary rib usually from the seventh cervical vertebra.
2. Usually B/L
3. *Developmental anatomy:*
    i. In embryo → Nerves are larger in proportion to the ribs
       ↓
       Interfere with development of costal process.
    ii. Prefixed plexus → well developed C_4 root and small 1st thoracic root
       ↓
       Formation of C_7 costal process encounters no resistance → cervical rib
4. *Pathoanatomy:*
    i. Hung up neurovascular structures: Brachial plexus and subclavian artery pass over a high barrier
    ii. As age advances → Shoulder girdle droops downward → ↑ tension of NV structures

5. *Classification*:
    i. Complete rib: Articulates with the first rib or manubrium
    ii. Incomplete rib: Free distal bullous tip
    iii. Incomplete rib: Distal attachment via fibrous band
    iv. Short bar of bone extending beyond C_7 transverse process **(Fig. 25)**.

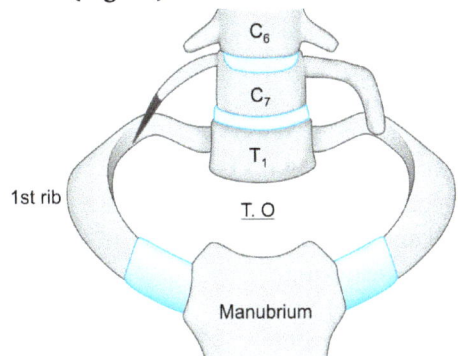

6. Clinical features: Ulnar distribution → Lower trunk
7. Treatment: Non-operative → Same as TOS
8. Surgery: Operative removal of rib

RHEUMATOID ARTHRITIS

I. DEFINITION

Chronic and progressive autoimmune disease leading to destruction of soft tissues, cartilage, and bone along with various systemic manifestations.

II. EPIDEMIOLOGY

1. Most common inflammatory arthritis
2. F > M : 4: 1 Age: 25–45 years

III. ETIOLOGY

1. Multifactorial
2. Genetic → HLADR4
           → HLADW4
3.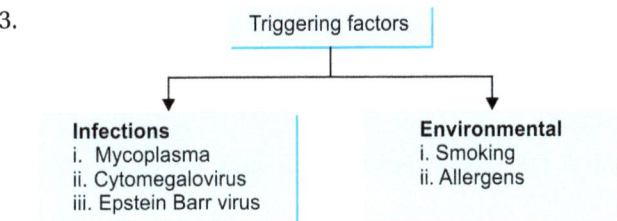

IV. CLASSIFICATION

(Based on Duration of Symptoms)

1. 0–3: Very early RA
2. 3 m–1 y: Early established RA
3. 1–2 y: Late established RA
4. >2 y: Established stable RA

V. PATHOGENESIS

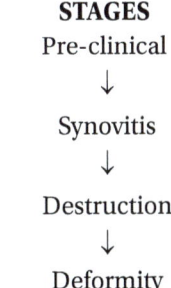

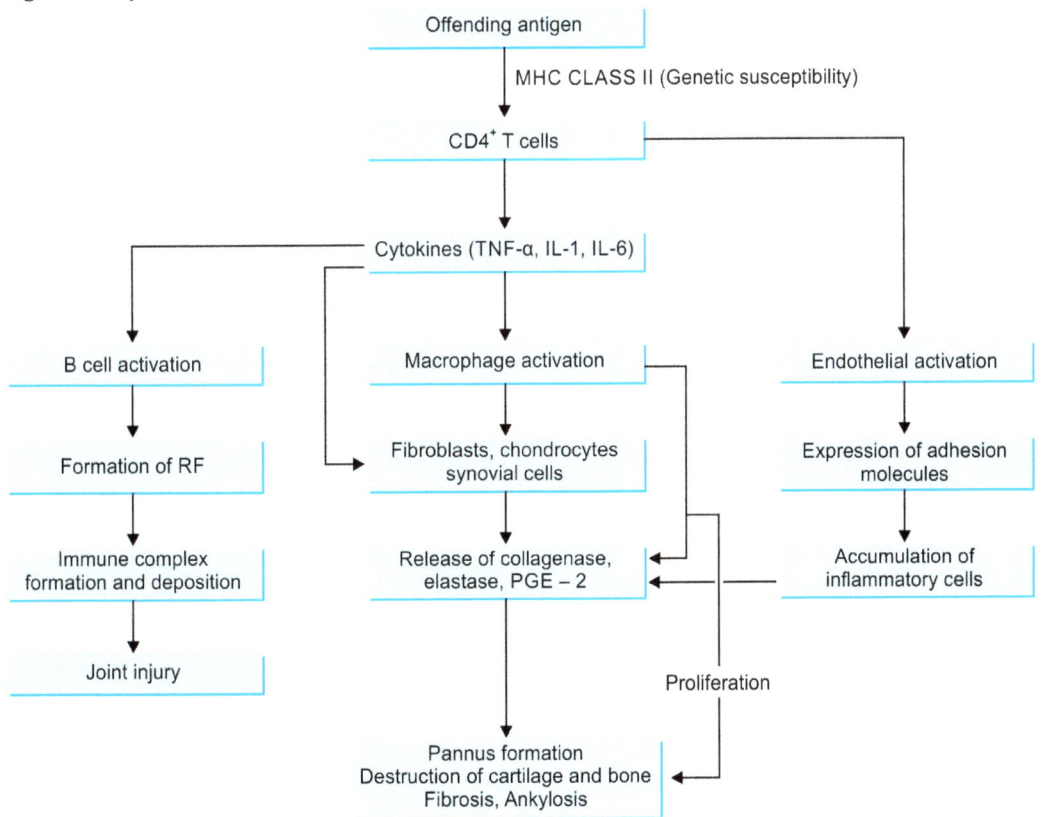

VI. CLINICAL FEATURES
A. Symptoms (Positive Family History)
1. Morning stiffness → Improve with activity.
2. Symmetric polyarticular Joint involvement.
3. Small joints of hand & feet > Large joints
4. Waxing & waning.

B. Signs
1. MCP, PIP, Wrist affected, DIP spared.
2. Tenderness
3. Swelling, stiffness, ↓ROM
4. Subcutaneous nodules (20%) - Olecranon, Achilles.

C. Cervical Spine
1. Atlantoaxial subluxation
2. Basilar invagination
3. Subaxial subluxation
4. Torticollis

D. Fingers
1. Boutonniere deformity
2. Swan neck deformity
3. Arthritis mutilans
4. Ulnar drift at MCP
5. Thumb → Z deformity
   ↓
   Game keepers
6. Triggering
7. Mannerfelt syndrome [FPL ⊗ at the carpal tunnel]
8. Vaughan - Jackson Syndrome
   ↓
   Distal extensor tendon ⊗

E. Wrist
1. Caput ulna syndrome
2. Radiocarpal joint destruction.

F. Toes
1. Hallux valgus
2. Claw toes

G. Hip
1. Protrusio acetabuli
2. Arthritis

H. Knee
1. Valgus deformity
2. **Phemister's triad**: Periarticular osteopenia + peripheral joint erosions + joint space narrowing

I. Extra-articular Manifestations
1. Ocular: Scleritis, Keratoconjunctivitis
2. Pulmonary: Pulmonary fibrosis, Effusion
3. Cardiac: Pericarditis
4. Skin: Vasculitis
5. Renal: GN
6. Fever, malaise, generalized muscle weakness
7. Caplan's syndrome = Pneumoconiosis + RA
8. Felty's syndrome = Triad of RA, Splenomegaly and Neutropenia

VII. RADIOLOGY
A. X-ray
1. Soft tissue shadows
2. Periarticular osteoporosis and synovial cyst
3. Marginal and central joint erosions
4. Joint space narrowing
5. Otto pelvis: B/L protrusion
6. Central glenoid erosion
7. Subluxations
8. Deformity.

B. MRI: Rheumatoid cervical spondylitis

VIII. LAB INVESTIGATIONS
1. WBC ↑ or ↓
2. ESR, CRP ↑
3. RF : IgM against Fc of IgG (80% pts)
4. Anti-cyclic citrullinated peptide
   ↓
   Most sensitive and specific
5. Synovial fluid analysis
   i. Cloudy
   ii. ↓ Viscosity
   iii. 2000 – 50,000 WBCs/mm^3, 50% PMN

IX. DIFFERENTIAL DIAGNOSIS
1. Septic arthritis
2. Gout
3. Pseudogout
4. Ankylosing Spondylitis
5. Psoriatic Arthritis
6. Reactive Arthritis
7. Fibromyalgia
8. SLE
9. Scleroderma
10. TB
11. Self - limiting poly arteritis.

X. ACR/EULAR 200 GUIDELINES (For Diagnosis)
A. Joint Involvement (Swollen or Tender)
1. 1 large joint — 0
2. 2–10 large joints — 1
3. 1–3 small joints with or without ligament inv. — 2
4. 4–10 small joints with or without ligament inv. — 3
5. >10 joints (at least 1 small joint) — 5

B. Serology

1. Negative RF/Anti-CCP — 0
2. Low RF/Anti-CCP — 2
3. High RF/Anti-CCP — 3

C. Acute Phase Reactants

1. Normal ESR/CRP — 0
2. Abnormal ESR/CRP — 1

D. Duration of Symptoms

1. <6 weeks — 0
2. >6 weeks — 1

≥6 Points → RA (Definite)

XI. MANAGEMENT

A. Goals

1. To decrease pain, stiffness.
2. To improve quality of life, achieve disease remission.
3. To prevent joint deformities and loss of function.
4. To treat or cure joint deformities and return to a desirable and productive life.

B.

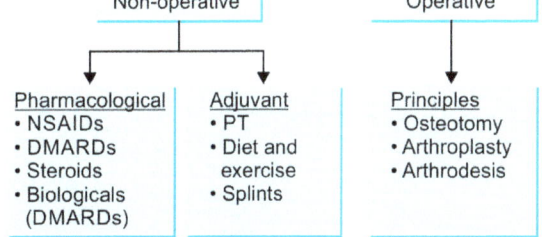

C. Pharmacological: Mainstay of Treatment

1. NSAIDS:
    i. Quick pain relief and onset of action
    ii. Ibuprofen, naproxen, selective COX – 2 inhibitors
2. DMARDS: As per latest guidelines - Add DMARDS as soon as diagnosis is made.

D. Methotrexate (SAQ)

1. Antimetabolite and immune modulator
2. Uses — Inflammatory arthritis → Rheumatoid arthritis (RA)
   — Bone tumors.
3. Mechanism of Action: Analog of folate
    i. RA
        a. Inhibits enzymes of purine metabolism.
        b. ↓ activation of T-cells
        c. Down regulation of B-cells
        d. Inhibits binding of IL-1 to its receptor.
    ii. Bone tumors
        Competitively binds to "Dihydrofolate reductase" → to prevent synthesis of active tetrahydrofolate.
        ↓
        ↓ DNA, ↓ RNA and ↓ Protein synthesis
        ↓
        Tumors cell necrosis.

4. Rheumatoid arthritis: Methotrexate
    i. Backbone of treatment
    ii. Most common used because,
        a. Ease of use (oral/s.c weekly)
        b. Rapid onset of clinical benefit.
        c. Low cost.
        d. Durability.
        e. Well defined toxicities.
        f. Beneficial effect: Combination with other DMARDS.
        g. Ability to retard X-ray changes.
    iii. Dose = 10 mg/week started → Increased by 5 mg/month to max of 25 mg/week.
    iv. Monitoring: CBC, RFT, LFT at initiation and monthly for first 3 months then 2 monthly.
    v. Contraindications
        a. Allergy
        b. Pregnancy
        c. Lactation
        d. Intolerable Side effects
    vi. Side effects
        a. Oral ulcers
        b. Nausea
        c. Diarrhea
        d. Headache
        e. Malaise
        f. Fatigue
        g. Dizziness
        h. Blurred vision
        i. Increased LFTs
        j. Pulmonary fibrosis
        k. Bone marrow suppression
        l. Photosensitivity, rash
        m. Rash
        n. Alopecia.
    vii. Folate administration 1mg/day to reduce side effects.
5. Bone tumors
    i. 1000 times greater doses
    ii. 8–12 g/m^2 dose.
    iii. Needs specialized intensive monitoring.
    iv. Indication: Osteosarcoma

E. Hydroxychloroquine

1. Blocks activation of Toll–like receptors
   ↓
2. Decreased dendritic cell activation.
   ↓
3. Immunomodulation

4. Dose = 200 mg BD (400 mg/day)

F. Sulfasalazine

1. Prodrug → Sulphapyridine + 5–ASA
2. Superoxide radical generation

3. Cytokine inhibition
4. Prostaglandin led inflammation suppressed.
5. Dose = 500 mg–1 g/day

G. Leflunamide

1. Pyrimidine synthesis (Dihydroorotate dehydrogenase) inhibitor : ↓DNA, RNA, ↓T-cell proliferation.
2. 20 mg/day
3. S/E = Hepatotoxicity, weight gain, HTN, pulmonary fibrosis.

H. Old DMARDS

1. Gold
2. Penicillamine
3. Azathioprine.

I. Corticosteroids

1. Used as "Bridge therapy" during high disease activity.
2. Started low dose → Incremented → Tapered off.
3. MPS: 20 mg/day

J. Biologicals (SAQ)

1. Genetically engineered medications from a living organism, virus, or gene to stimulate body's natural response to infection/disease.
2. Reserved for those who are not responding to DMARDS **(Fig. 26)**.

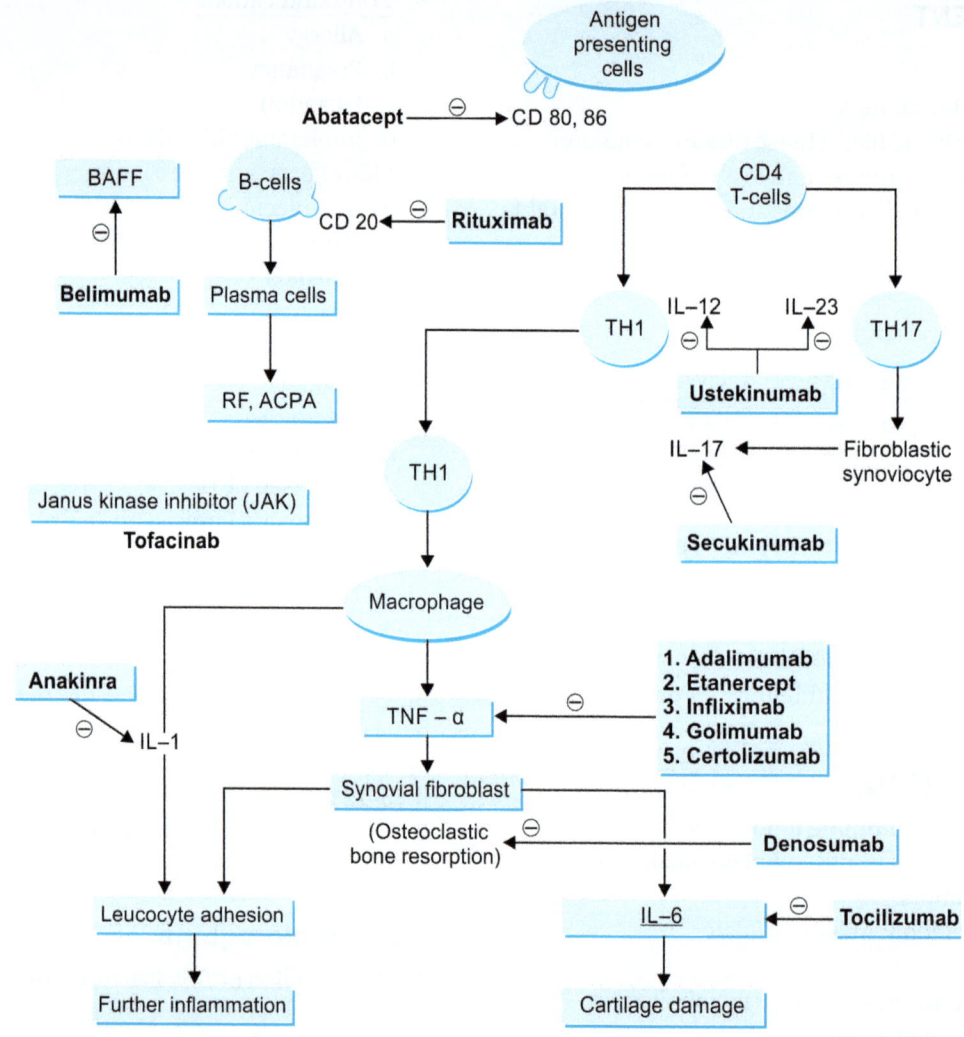

3. Limitation of conventional DMARDS
    i. Onset takes several months.
    ii. Remission induced maybe partial.
    iii. Substantial toxicity
    iv. Loss effectiveness over time
4. Advantages of Biologicals
    i. Very rapid onset of action
    ii. Radiographic efficacy ↑↑
    iii. Well tolerated.
    iv. Well defined and specific M.O.A
5. Disadvantages
    i. Cost
    ii. Adverse Drug Reactions
6. Adverse Drug Reactions
    i. ↑Infections: Skin, Pneumonia, Atypical TB
    ii. Viral reactivation

Orthopedic Diseases

iii. Neutropenia
iv. Severe infusion reactions
v. Hypersensitivity → Anaphylaxis
vi. Malignancy??
7. C/I : Active TB, infections, pregnancy
8. Dosage
    i. SC or IV
    ii. Usually weekly and monthly schedules.

RHEUMATOID HAND

I. DEFINITION (Of Rheumatoid Arthritis from Previous Answer)

II. PATHOPHYSIOLOGY

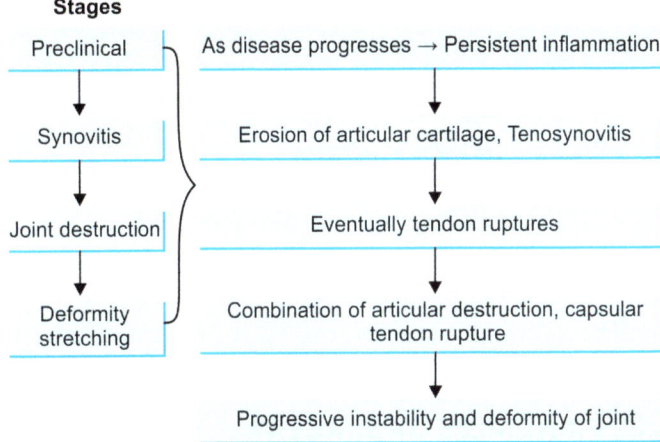

III. DEFORMITIES OF HAND

1. Finger
2. Thumb
3. Wrist
4. Rupture of tendon

MCP and wrist → affected early.
↓
Most significant
Interphalangeal joint → Late

IV. FINGER DEFORMITIES

A. Intrinsic Plus

1. Etiology: Intrinsic muscle contracture.
2. MCP = 90° Flexion
3. IP = Extension
    Test : Bunnel
    ↓
    Flexion of IP joint is more when MCP joint is flexed and less when MCP joint is extended.

B. Swan – Neck (Fig. 27)

1. PIP = Hyperextension
2. DIP = Flexion
3. MCP = Flexed
4. Etiology
    i. Extensor tendon rupture at DIP
    ii. Capsular disruption
    iii. Lateral bands subluxate dorsal to PIP axis of rotation
    iv. Flexor tenosynovitis

5. Classification = Nalebuff

I. Full ROM No intrinsic tightness	Conservative: Splinting, Figure of 8 Surgical: a. Dermodesis of PIP b. PIP flexor tenodesis / Proximal Fowler Tenotomy c. DIP joint fusion d. Retinacular ligament reconstruction
II. PIP ↓ ROM Intrinsic tightness	Lateral band (Intrinsic) release
III. Stiff PIP in all position of MCP	PIP manipulation – Dorsal skin release just distal to PIP & leaving scar to heal.
IV. Severe arthritic Changes	a. PIP Arthrodesis → 2, 3rd finger. b. Arthroplasty – 4, 5th finger.

C. Boutonnière (Fig. 28)

1. MCP = Hyperextension
2. PIP = Flexion
3. DIP = Hyperextension

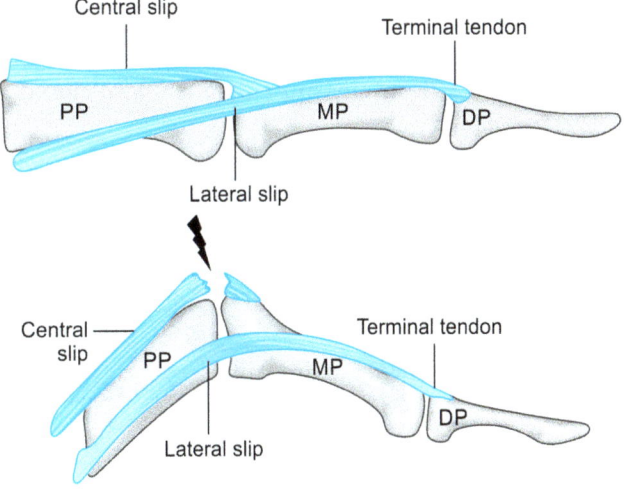

4. Etiology:
   a. PIP synovitis → Central slip and dorsal capsule stretching/weakness.
   b. Lateral bands subluxate volar to PIP axis
5. Grades
   i. Mild: Passively correctable
   Treatment
      a. Splinting
      b. Extensor tenotomy to increase DIP flexion
   ii. Moderate: Not correctable passively, Flexion deformity
   Rx Central slip reconstruction
   iii. Severe: Severe joint destruction - Arthrodesis and Arthroplasty - PIP
6. Elson test: DIP extends when PIP = 90° and blocked. (Normally, DIP remains flaccid.)

D. Ulnar Drift → MCP Joint

1. Volar subluxation + ulnar drifting at MCP
2. Etiology
   i. MCP synovitis → Weakness dorsoradial capsular ligament.
   ii. MCP collateral ligament loosening → ↓ Stability
   iii. Shifting of extensor tendons ulnarly into web space.
3. Treatment
   - Early disease
     • Synovectomy
     • Extensor tendon centralization
     • Intrinsic release
   - Late disease
     • MCP arthroplasty
     • MCP fusion

E. Arthritis Mutilans

1. Gross instability with bone loss = Pencil in cup deformity
2. Treatment: Interposition bone grafting and fusion

F. Rheumatoid Nodules

Treatment: Observe, steroid injection, exercise.

V. THUMB

Nalebuff classification
1. Swan-neck: Z-deformity, most common, MCP flexed, IP Hyperextended
2. Boutonniere deformity
3. Gamekeeper's thumb

VI. WRIST

1. **Caput Ulna syndrome:** Synovitis stretches ulnar carpal ligament.
   i. Dorsal prominence of distal ulna.
   ii. Subluxation of carpus
   iii. Volar subluxation of ECU
   iv. Radial deviation of wrist
   Rx
      a. Darrach's procedure
      b. Sauve-Kapandji
2. **Radio - carpal arthritis:** Zig-zag deformity
   Treatment
      i. Synovectomy
      ii. Radiolunate fusion
      iii. Wrist arthrodesis
      iv. Total wrist arthroplasty.

VII. TENDON

1. **Triggering:**
   Rx - FDS resection
2. **Mannerfelt Syndrome:** FPL ⊗ (MC flexor tendon ⊗), due to scaphoid spur.
   Rx i. FDS4 → FPL
       ii. IP joint fusion
3. **Vaughan - Jackson Syndrome**
   i. Digital extensor tendon ⊗ → ulnar to radial
   ii. DRUJ instability → Dorsal ulna prominence
                                    ↓
                                  Rupture
   Rx
   EIP → EDC + Distal ulna resection.

VIII. PRINCIPLES OF SURGERY

1. Surgery → Proximal joint to distal
2. Alternate fusion with motion sparing surgeries. Wrist fusion, MCP arthroplasty, PIP fusion.
3. MCP/CMC joint → Arthroplasty preferred.
4. Wrist arthrodesis > Arthroplasty
   Wrist arthroplasty: Low demand patient, contralateral wrist arthrodesis.
5. Poor bone and soft tissue quality = Avoid iatrogenic fracture
6. Healing potential in less due to anemia.
7. Multiple staged procedure preferred over single prolonged surgery.

PIGMENTED VILLONODULAR SYNOVITIS (PVNS)

I. INTRODUCTION

1. Idiopathic villus overgrowth and pigmentation of synovial membrane of a joint.
2. Two types
   i. Diffuse villous form
   ii. Localized nodular form

3. PVNS is a slowly progressive, exuberant, benign proliferative process of synovial tissue and is usually monoarticular.
4. It is characterized by Xanthomatous lesions – these are yellow to yellowish brown in color due to cholesterol and hemosiderin deposits.
5. Caused by overexpression of *CSF1* gene.
6. Usual age group → 20-40 years.
7. Knee joint - M/C involved

II. PATHOLOGY

A. Gross

1. Chocolate colored mass with rubbery consistency.
2. Nodular masses (small/large, soft/hard) present on a base of fibrous connective tissue.
3. The synovium is red to brownish in color.
4. It has numerous large, finger-like villi that fuse to form pedunculated nodules (often more than 5 cm).
5. Anterior knee is the most common site of involvement (80%) → most commonly affects the patellofemoral compartment at the infrapatellar fat pad.

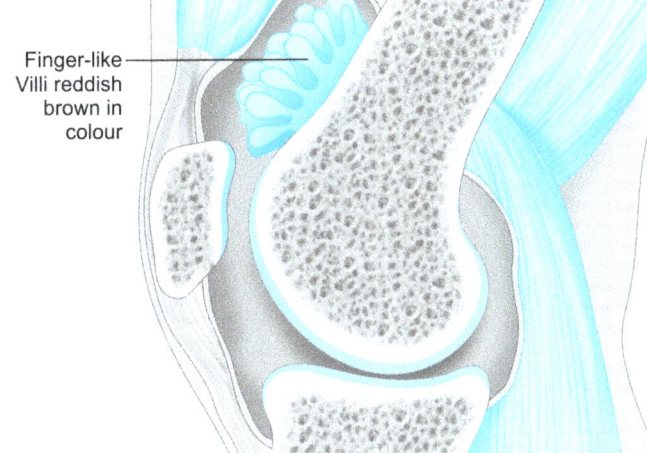

Finger-like Villi reddish brown in colour

B. Microscopy

1. Xanthoma cells or foam cells are present in the nodular masses.

Large oval or polyhedral cells with pyknotic nuclei and foamy cytoplasm
↓
These cells are derived from monocytes or histiocytes which have engulfed lipoid material and hemosiderin and hence the characteristic yellowish brown color.

2. The proliferative synovium invades adjacent cartilage and bone.

III. CLINICAL FEATURES

1. Pain – Gradual in onset, intermittent, starts as discomfort then progresses to mild and moderate.
2. Swollen joint
3. Limp
4. Mechanical block - leading to locking, stiffness, limitation of ROM
5. Symptoms are less pronounced in localized form
6. O/E:
   i. Distended joint due to soft tissue swelling
   ii. Floating patella
   iii. Generalized tenderness
   iv. Examination findings may be less pronounced in the localized form – the mass may not even be palpable
7. On aspiration:
   i. Thick orange brown fluid aspirated – pathognomonic
   ii. In localized form – no abundant effusion, normal synovial fluid may be aspirated

IV. INVESTIGATIONS

1. X-ray
   i. Soft tissue shadows → Hyperdense recurrent effusions
   ii. Smooth cortical saucerized erosions.
   iii. Subchondral cysts
   iv. Joint space initially preserved → progresses to degenerative arthritis.
2. MRI
   i. Mass, either extensive (in diffuse form) or nodular (in localized)
   ii. Hemosiderin (Dark on T1 and T2)
   iii. Thickening of joint lining
   iv. Destructive bone changes
   v. Cartilage damage
   vi. "Blooming artifact" → Signal loss on gradient echo sequences due to iron in hemosiderin.
3. Biopsy
   i. Ultrasound guided
   ii. Percutaneous → Suprapatellar pouch
4. Arthroscopy
   i. IOC
   ii. Direct visualization of the characteristic chocolate colored mass, with synovium thrown into folds → frond-like pattern of papillary projections.

V. MANAGEMENT

1. Observation → Asymptomatic
2. Left untreated, PVNS usually progresses to complete joint destruction.

3. Complete synovectomy is the treatment of choice when joint is preserved.
4. Partial synovectomy
   i. Recurrence rate is very high
   ii. Indicated in localized form
5. Surgical excision → Arthroscopically (preferred) or via open approach.
6. Total knee arthroplasty with excision of the synovium – advanced degenerative changes in the knee.
7. Arthrodesis with synovectomy → Severe ankle PVNS.
8. Radiation therapy:
   i. 30–35 Gy in 15 fractions
   ii. When given postoperatively, it reduces the chances of recurrence.
   iii. Preferred in large masses to reduce them in size → followed by surgical excision.
   iv. Can also be given in patients where surgery is C/I due to medical co-morbidities.
9. Recent advances:
   i. Intra-articular radiation → radioactive fluid is injected into the joint.
   ii. Pexidartinib → CSF-1 receptor antagonist indicated in extensive disease.

SECTION 9

Bone Tumors

INTRODUCTION TO BONE TUMORS—CLASSIFICATION, BENIGN VS MALIGNANT

CLASSIFICATION OF BONE

Based on tissue of origin.

I. Bone

Benign	Malignant
1. Osteoid osteoma 2. Osteoblastoma 3. Osteoma	Osteosarcoma

II. Cartilage

Benign	Malignant
1. Osteochondroma 2. Enchondroma 3. Chondroblastoma 4. Chondromyxoid fibroma	Chondrosarcoma

III. Fibrous

Benign	Malignant
1. Fibrous cortical defect 2. Non-ossifying fibroma 3. Desmoplastic fibroma	Fibrosarcoma

IV. Blood Vessels

Benign	Malignant
Hemangioma	Angiosarcoma

V. Adipose Tissue

Lipoma	Liposarcoma

VI. Marrow

Benign	Malignant
–	1. Multiple myeloma 2. Lymphoma

VII. Notochord

–	Chordoma

VIII. Neural

Neurofibroma	Neurofibrosarcoma

IX. Unknown

Benign	Malignant
1. ABC 2. GCT	1. Ewing's sarcoma 2. Adamantinoma

RADIOLOGICAL DIFFERENCE BETWEEN BENIGN AND MALIGNANT BONE TUMORS

Three most important factors

1. Zone of transition/tumor margin
2. Pattern of bone destruction within lesion
3. Periosteal reaction

1. Zone of transition (ZOT) (Fig. 1)

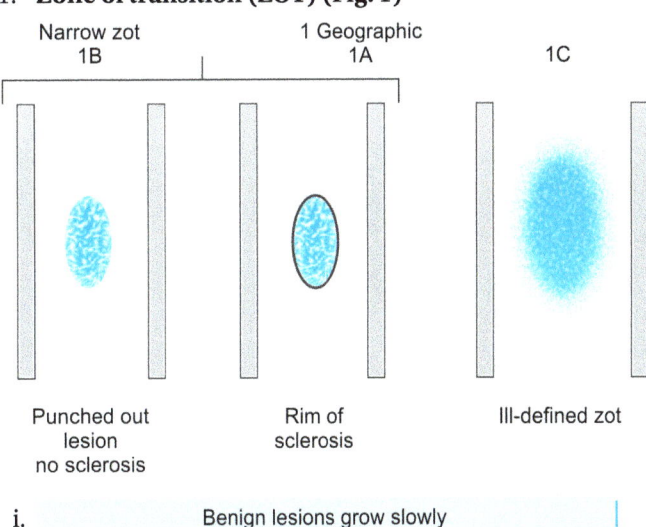

Narrow zot 1B — Punched out lesion no sclerosis
1 Geographic 1A — Rim of sclerosis
1C — Ill-defined zot

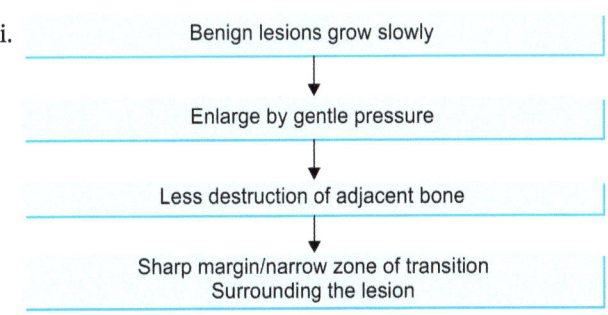

i. Benign lesions grow slowly → Enlarge by gentle pressure → Less destruction of adjacent bone → Sharp margin/narrow zone of transition surrounding the lesion

ii. Malignant lesions grow rapidly → Destroy the adjacent bone area → Wide zone of transition.

iii. Sometimes, fast growing lesions like infection (OM) may also show wide zone of transition.
2. Pattern of bone destruction **(Fig. 2)**

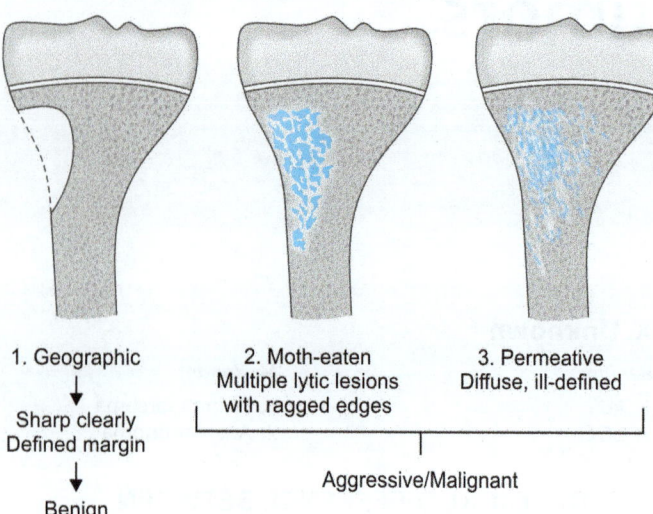

Other differences:

Benign	Malignant
1. Absence of soft tissue mass.	1. Soft tissue mass or extension
2. Metastasis rare	2. Metastasis and skip lesion common
3. Cortical destruction unusual (displaced, remodeled and thin but no cortical destruction)	3. Cortical destruction common
4. Size – variable, often limited	4. Usually, extensive
5. Slow rate of change	5. Rapid rate of change

ENNEKING STAGING SYSTEM

A. Malignant

Stage	Grade	Site	Metastasis
IA	Low G_1	Intracompartmental (T_1)	No
IB	Low G_1	Extracompartmental (T_2)	No
IIA	High G_2	Intracompartmental (T_1)	No
IIB	High G_2	Extracompartmental (T_2)	No
III	Any G	Any T	Regional or distant

B. Benign

Stage:
1. Latent: Remains static or heals spontaneously (e.g., NOF)
2. Active–Progressive growth but limited by natural barriers (e.g., UBC)
3. Locally: Aggressive growth but not limited by natural barriers (e.g., GCT)

MARGINS OF SURGICAL EXCISION (FIG. 4)

3. **Periosteal reaction (Fig. 3)**

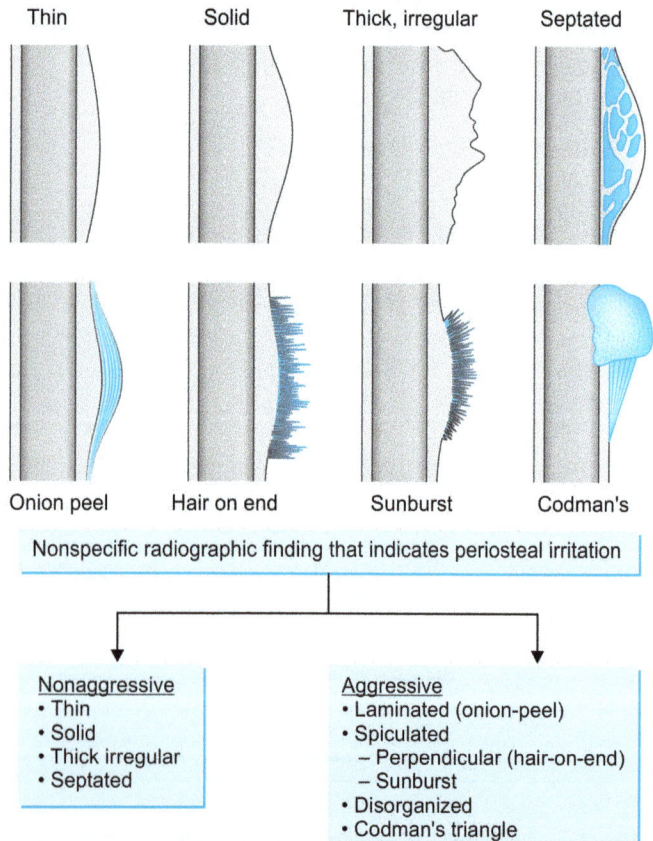

Benign: Low grade chronic irritation allows time for the formation of normal or near normal cortex.
↓
Thick, dense, uniform or wavy.

Malignant: Rapid irritative process does not allow the periosteum time to lay down and consolidate new bone to form normal cortex.

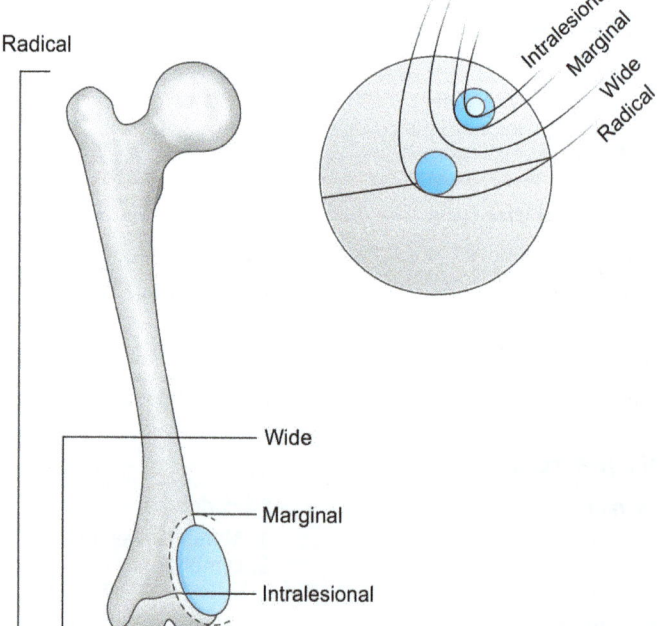

1. *Intralesional:* Piecemeal debulking or curettage, leaves macroscopic disease.
2. *Marginal:* Shell out en bloc through pseudocapsule or reactive zone. May leave satellite or skip lesions.

3. *Wide:* Intracompartmental en bloc with cuff of normal tissue.
4. *Radical:* Extracompartmental en bloc with cuff of normal tissue.

BONE BIOPSY

I. INTRODUCTION
1. Procedure that involves the extraction of sample cells and tissues for diagnostic, grading or therapeutic purposes.
2. Not a substitute for clinical examination and investigation
   ↓
   Purpose: To confirm a suspected Dx.

II. INDICATIONS
1. Aggressive bone/soft tissue lesions.
2. Soft tissue lesions >5 cm, deep to fascia or overlying bone/neurovascular structures.
3. Diagnostic uncertainty in symptomatic patient.
4. Solitary bone lesions in a patient with history of carcinoma.

III. TYPES

1. Fine Needle Aspiration Cytology (FNAC)
i. Cytologic specimen
ii. Needs skilled pathologist → interpretation.

2. Core Biopsy (Tru-cut) (Fig. 5)

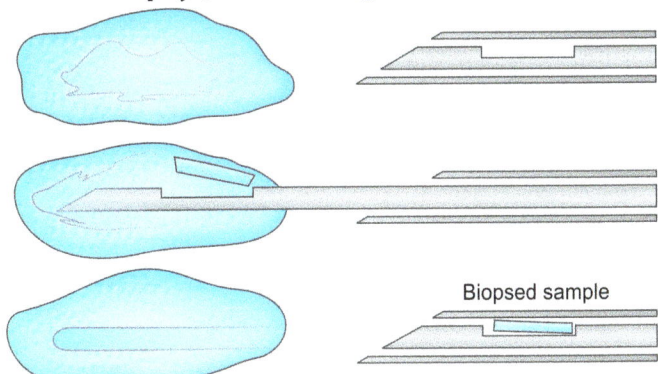

i. Provides cytologic + stromal elements
ii. Used in soft tissue sarcomas.

3. Incisional Biopsy
Small surgical incision.

4. Excisional
Select indications: Small, superficial, soft tissue mass.

IV. PRINCIPLES
1. Who?
   Experienced surgeon who will perform the definite management.
2. Where?
   Center with facilities for diagnosis and oncology experience

3. Incision (Fig. 6)

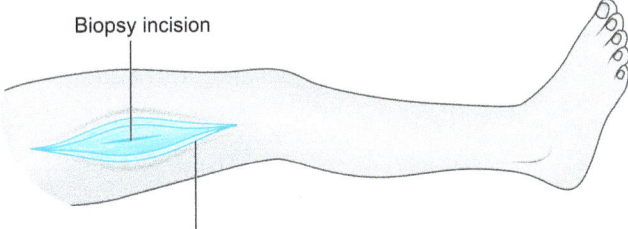

i. Always longitudinal incision in extremities
   ↓
ii. Allows for extension of incision during definitive management.
iii. Never transverse.
4. Approach
   i. All tissues exposed during biopsy considered contaminated → Excised during definitive management.
   ii. ∴ Never expose NVS.
   iii. Maintain meticulous homeostasis.
      ↓
   iv. Release tourniquet prior to wound closure.
      ↓
   v. Since postoperative hematomas considered contaminated.
5. *Compartment:* Through involved compartment. Never violate another.
6. Site
   i. From periphery → Center has high necrotic tissues.
   ii. Sclerosed, ossified, calcified → No yield.
   iii. Lytic areas best.
   iv. Use imaging for help.
   v. No biopsy done through joint or arthroscopic (oncology).
7. *Closure*: If drain is used → bring it out in line with surgical incision.
8. Unclear diagnosis → Repeat.

ANEURYSMAL BONE CYST

I. INTRODUCTION
1. ABCs are locally, destructive, blood-filled, reactive benign lesions.
2. Traditionally, not considered true neoplasms, but recent evidence → Neoplasm
3. MC → Femur and tibia (>60%)
4. 51% → Lower limb
5. 22.5% → Upper limb (commonly proximal humerus)
6. Spine (15%) → posterior elements
7. Calcaneus and metatarsal MC in foot
8. Expansile, intramedullary lesions occurring in the metaphysis of long bones.

II. ETIOPATHOLOGY

ABC	
Primary (70%)	Secondary (30%)
• Recently considered neoplasms • Ubiquitin – specific protease (USP6) gene upregulation • MC translocation = t (16;17) (q22;p13)	• Not considered a neoplasm as no translocation identified • Seen in – Giant cell tumors – Chondroblastoma – Chondromyxoid fibroma – Osteoblastoma – Fibrous dysplasia – Non-ossifying fibroma

Local circulatory disturbance
↓
Increased venous pressure
↓
Hemorrhage and local destruction

III. GROSS

1. Thin osseous shell enclosing honeycombed sponge like mass (cavity) filled with blood.
2. Secondary ABCs have solid areas which represent primary bone lesion.
3. Inside the shell, reddish brown, liver – like fragile mass interspersed with gritty particle of bone.
4. Fibro-osseous septa seen throughout.

IV. MICROSCOPY

1. Anastomosing cavernous areas filled with blood (represent gross honeycombed structure).
2. Cavernous spaces lined by thin fibrous tissue containing fibroblasts, myofibroblasts, <u>osteoid and chondroid tissue (blue zone)</u> and osteoclast like giant cells.
   (Instead of smooth muscle wall or endothelial cells of blood vessels of true cavernous spaces)
3. Solid variant of ABC → <u>Giant cell reparative granuloma</u>.

V. CLINICAL FEATURES

1. *Age*: 75% patients < 20 years
2. *Sex*: Slightly M > F
3. *Pain*: due to ⎡ Bony destruction
              ⎣ Pathological fracture
4. Swelling
5. Limitation of joint movements
6. *Spinal lesion*: ⎡ Backache
                    → Functional spinal deformities
                    → Neurodeficit

VI. RADIOLOGY

A. Radiograph

1. Expansile lytic lesion
2. Eccentrically located in metaphysis
3. Elevates periosteum but remains contained by thin shell of cortex
4. *Margins*: Well-defined > Permeative (mimics malignancy)
5. Honeycombed internal septations

B. Capanna-Morphologic Subgroups (Fig. 7)

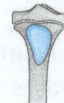 I - Centrally located and well-contained lesion ± slightly expanded outline

 II - Markedly expanded lesions with cortical thinning and involvement of (entire bony segment)

 III - Eccentric lesions in metaphysis involving only one cortex

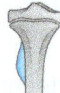 IV - Subperiosteal lesions expanding away from the bone

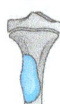 V - Periosteal lesions/meta/diaphyseal/extending into soft tissues/expanding peripherally and penetrating cortical bone

C. MRI

Double density fluid levels, intralesional septations (vs UBC) (Fig. 8)

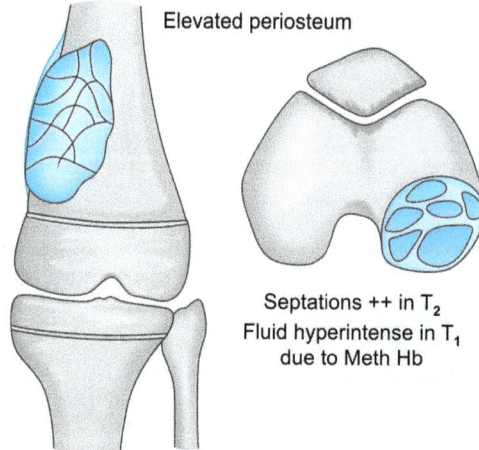

Elevated periosteum

Septations ++ in T_2
Fluid hyperintense in T_1 due to Meth Hb

D. CT Scan

Delineating cyst in areas of bone complex anatomy (spine, pelvis)

E. Bone Scan

Diffuse/peripheral tracer uptake with central area of decreased uptake.

F. Biopsy

Must before planning surgery.

VII. EVOLUTION OF ABC

1. *Incipient*: Small nonexpansile intramedullary lytic lesion
2. *Growth phase*: Rapid growth and lysis of bone, Codman's triangle (±)
3. *Stable*: Expanded bone with shell around and trabeculations within it (bubbly appearance)
4. *Healing*: Self-resolution/post Rx trabeculated bony mass with mineralized matrix.

VIII. TREATMENT

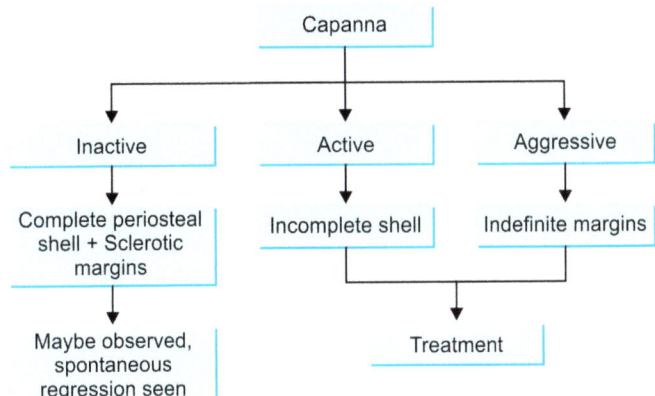

Gold standard: Extended curettage + Bone graft

Extended curettage:

1. High speed burr
2. Adjuvants:
   i. Peroxide
   ii. Phenol
   iii. Zinc chloride
   iv. Cryotherapy
3. Bone cement for central lesions.
4. Use of tourniquet advised, as lesion may produce heavy bleeding.
5. Preoperative embolization = ↓ blood loss
6. Serial embolization → Definitive management in non-resectable tumors (spine, pelvis).
7. Marginal en bloc resection in expandable bones (fibula, clavicle, ribs)
8. Choice of treatment ultimately depends on:
   i. Size
   ii. Extent
   iii. Location
9. In children → Subperiosteal resection + Reconstruction with fibula
10. Recently, percutaneous method for inducing sclerosis (sclerotherapy) and secondary mineralization.
    ↓
11. Alcoholic solution of zein and polidocanol, healing = 6–18 months
12. Demineralized bone particles as paste of allogenic bone powder + autogenous bone marrow
    ↓
    Promote ossification faster than ABC expansion
13. *Contraindications*:
    i. Rapid expansion
    ii. Neurological involvement
    iii. Vascular
    iv. Impending fracture
    v. Allergy to drugs
    vi. Radiation → effective
        = But not used → induces radiation sarcoma

IX. RECURRENCE (20%)

1. Corelated with:
   i. Age < 15 years
   ii. Open physis
   iii. High mitotic index
   iv. More cellular component < Osteoid
2. Least with en bloc resection
3. Rx same as 1° lesion.

GIANT CELL TUMOR

I. INTRODUCTION

1. First described by sir Astley Cooper in 1818, GCT is a benign aggressive tumor.
2. Occurs in skeletally mature individuals
3. F > M (1.5:1), Age: 30–50 years, Peak: 3rd decade.
4. Site = Distal femur > Proximal > distal radius > Sacral ala, phalanges of hand.
5. 50% occur around knee.

II. CLINICAL PICTURE

1. Symptomatic in 97% patients.
2. Pain, maybe associated with mass.
3. Trauma or a pathologic fracture may direct attention to the tumor.

III. PATHOLOGY

A. Gross

1. Epiphysiometaphyseal region
2. Extends up to the adjacent articular cartilage, which usually remains intact.
3. Eccentric
4. The overlying cortex undergoes resorption and the
   ↓
5. Contour of the bone is expanded by the tumor
   ↓
6. Covered by thin shell of subperiosteal new bone.
7. Gray to reddish brown in color.
8. Composed of soft, friable, vascular tissue
9. Firm, gray-yellow areas of fibrosis and collagenization and osteoid production may be found.

B. Microscopy

1. Multinucleated osteoclast – like giant cells in a moderately vascularized network of proliferating round to polygonal mononuclear stromal cells.
2. Giant cells have over 50 nuclei.

3. Uniformly scattered throughout the tumor.
4. Mitoses as well as intravascular extension of tumor do not indicate malignancy in GCT.
5. No correlation between histologic appearance and histological behavior.

IV. RADIOLOGICAL FEATURES

1. Lytic lesion in the epiphysometaphyseal region of long bones.
2. Bulges beyond the confines of the cortex.
3. No periosteal reaction is seen, unless complicated by a pathological fracture.
4. No mineralized tumor matrix
5. Multiple septa traverse the interior and produce characteristic soap – bubble appearance.

MRI

1. T_1W = Low intensity, T_2W = High intensity.
2. Extramedullary tumor best on T_1W.
3. Extraosseous → T_2W.
4. Determines extraosseous extent.
5. Joint involvement.
6. Fluid–fluid levels.

CT

Subtle cortical destruction is better demonstrated on CT.

V. CLASSIFICATION

Campanacci

1. *Grade I*:
   i. Well marginated border of a thin rim of mature bone.
   ii. Cortex intact or slightly thinned but not deformed.
2. *Grade II*:
   i. Relatively well-defined margins, but no radiopaque rim.
   ii. Cortex → Thin, moderately expanded.
   iii. Grade II with fracture.
3. *Grade III*:
   i. Fuzzy borders → Rapid, permeative growth.
   ii. Tumor bulges into soft tissue.
   iii. Not limited by an apparent shell of reactive bone.

VI. DIFFERENTIAL DIAGNOSIS

1. Brown tumor
2. ABC
3. Chondroblastoma
4. Chondromyxoid fibroma
5. OS.

VII. TREATMENT

Aim: Maximize functional preservation, minimizing chance of recurrence (**Fig. 9**)

A.

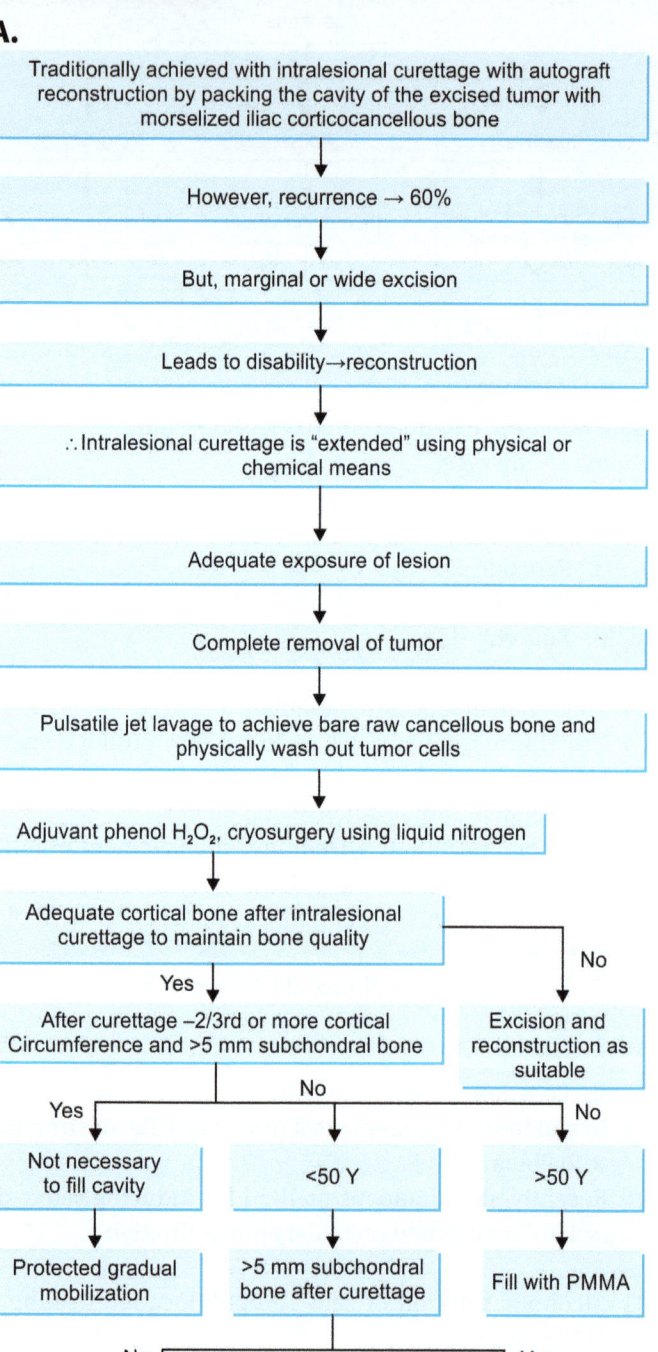

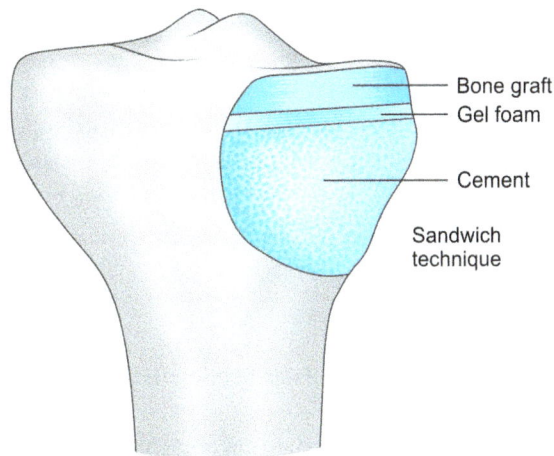

1. Internal fixation as suitable may be used in cases where surgeon feels that stability requires augmentation.
2. Expendable bones (lower end ulna, upper end fibula) → Excision.

B. BG

Advantages	Disadvantages
Remodeling ++, along stress lines	Quantity limited
Reconstruction is permanent	Donor site morbidity
	Expensive → Bone bank
	Recurrence difficult to spot

C. Bone Cement

Advantages	Disadvantages
Cytotoxic → tumor cells ⊗	Not biologically strong
Thermal effect	in compression but weak
Recurrence easy to spot	in shear and torsion → ↑
Immediate structural support, weight bearing	chances of fracture in sites like NOF

D. Reconstruction Options

Megaprosthetic joint replacement
Biological → Autograft arthrodesis
 → Microvascular fibula graft
 → Ilizarov method of bone regeneration.
Recurrence → Total serum acid phosphatase
 ↓
 Usually ≤2 years

OSTEOID OSTEOMA

I. INTRODUCTION

1. Most common true benign bone tumor
2. Small bone forming lesions usually <2 cm ↓
3. Central well-defined hypervascular area of rarefraction → Nidus
4. Vascular fibrous tissue
5. Proliferating fibroblasts
6. Minute spicules of newly formed osteoid
7. Surrounded by zone of normal appearing sclerotic bone
8. 10% of all benign bone tumors.

II. ETIOLOGY

1. Trauma
2. Inflammation
3. Developmental → Altered vascularity in affected area.

III. CLASSIFICATION

1. Subperiosteal
2. Intracortical
3. Endosteal
4. Intramedullary

IV. CLINICAL FEATURES

1. Age: 5–30 years (Peak = 2nd decade)
2. M:F = 2:1
3. Site:
   i. Long bones (MC), Femur + tibia >50% cases
   ii. Proximal femur (MC) site, proximal tibia, posterior elements of spine
4. Dull pain → Progressive, severe
5. Worse at night
6. Pain disappears in response to NSAIDs
7. Reactive sclerosis and pain due to high levels of prostaglandin E_2 and prostacyclin
8. Localized fusiform swelling → Tender
9. LL cases → Limp
10. Intraarticular → Joint effusion, ↓ROM
11. Disuse atrophy of m/s involvement.
12. Spine → m/s spasm, back pain, 2° scoliosis, pelvic tilt
13. Alcohol → ↑ pain due to vasodilatation.

V. RADIOLOGY

1. Small, solitary, rarified lesion, <2 cm, cortical/subcortical/periosteal region.
2. Surrounded by dramatic reactive sclerosis
3. Center of lesion → Osteolytic
 → Partially mineralized
 → Calcified entirely
4. Technetium - 99 bone scan → Intense focus of ↑ uptake in the nidus → "Head light in fog"
5. "Double Density" sign → Focal area of ↑ activity with second smaller area of ↑ uptake is diagnostic.
6. "Bull's eye" → Central nidus surrounded by reactive bone (CT-scan)
 ↓
 Intra-articular, spine, hand, feet
7. MRI: Limited, soft tissue changes, edema

VI. PATHOLOGY (FIG. 10)

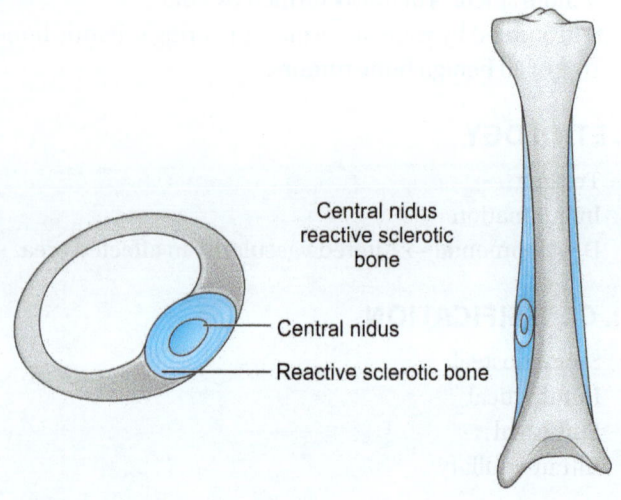

1. Nidus → Red → Due to ↑vascularity → Easily enucleated.
2. Early stages → Soft and granular → Vascularity.
3. Late stages → Dense and gritty → Calcification.
4. Microscopically → Nidus → Immature bone (osteoid) surrounded by osteoblasts and blood-filled capillaries.

VII. DIFFERENTIAL DIAGNOSIS

1. Stress fracture
2. Intracortical abscess
3. Intracortical granuloma
4. Osteoblastoma.

VIII. TREATMENT

1. Self-limiting disease and matures spontaneously over time.
2. Nonoperative → NSAIDs → Prolonged medical treatment
3. Operative: Indications
   i. Severe pain
   ii. Patient not willing to bear pain and long term meds.
   iii. Allergy to NSAIDs.
4. Aim of surgery: To eradicate the pain producing nidus.
5.
```
Percutaneous radiofrequency ablation → Procedure of choice
                    ↓
              Not available
                    ↓
                 Surgery
                ↙        ↘
   En bloc resection    Better → Burr-down technique
                        ↓ removal of bone
                        ↓ pathological fracture
```

CHONDROBLASTOMA

I. INTRODUCTION

1. Rare cartilaginous benign bone tumor arising from immature cartilage forming cells (chondroblasts).
2. Occurs in the epiphysis or apophysis of a long bone
3. Aka Codman's tumor

II. ETIOPATHOLOGY

1. Origin
   i. Secondary centres of ossification in the epiphysis.
   ii. Epiphyseal plate cells
2. Chromosome 5 and 8 structural abnormality
3. Onset is before obliteration of epiphyseal line → 10–20 years
4. Male:Female → 2:1
5. MC sites → Distal and proximal femur, proximal tibia and proximal humerus.

III. CLINICAL FEATURES

1. Pain → Dull, boring, progressive
2. Antalgic gait
3. Joint effusion
4. Muscle wasting
5. Terminal pain and restrict ROM

IV. INVESTIGATIONS

A. Radiograph

1. Site: Epiphyseal and eccentric
2. Radiolucent and well defined with a thin sclerotic border.
3. Geographic pattern of destruction
4. Solid or layered periosteal reaction

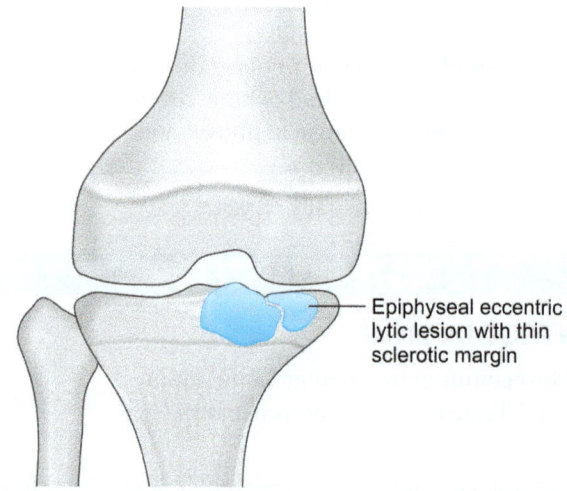

B. MRI

1. T1 → Intermediate signal intensity
2. T2 → Hypointensity
3. These findings are due to chondral matrix and calcification.
4. Reactive joint effusion
5. Periostitis
6. Multiple fluid-fluid levels → Secondary ABC formation

C. Pathology

i. Gross

1. Tan colored or dark red
2. Hemorrhagic
3. Small yellow zones of calcification surrounded by friable tissue.

ii. Microscopy

1. Large sheet of compact polygonal cells with well-defined cytoplasmic borders.
2. Nuclei → Longitudinal grooves
3. Cytoplasm → Clear to eosinophilic
4. Scattered multinucleated giant cells.
5. "Chicken-wire" calcification: Fine, lattice-like matrix pericellular type of calcification

V. DIFFERENTIAL DIAGNOSIS

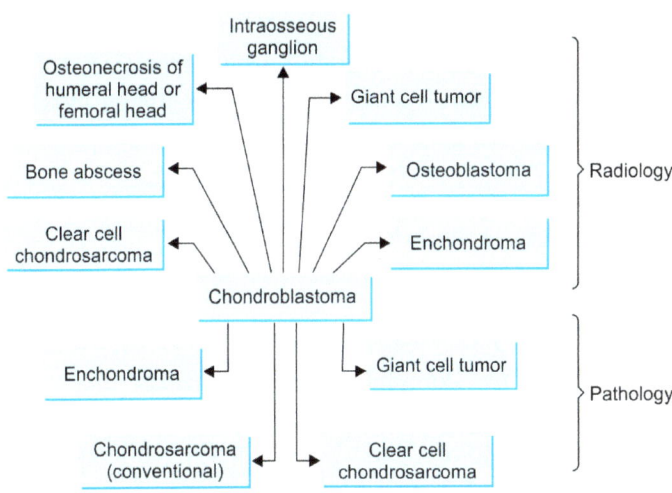

VI. MANAGEMENT

1. Chondroblastoma does not heal spontaneously.
2. Treatment of choice → Intralesional curettage and bone grafting.
3. Radiofrequency ablation
4. Wide excision → may be indicated in tumors arising in the ribs.
5. Rare aggressive forms → Endoprosthetic reconstruction or amputation.

CHONDROSARCOMA

I. INTRODUCTION

1. Malignant tumor of cartilage-producing cells.
2. Third MC primary malignant tumor of the bone.
3. MC sarcoma of bone in patients over 20 years of age.
4. 25% of all sarcomas.

II. CLASSIFICATION

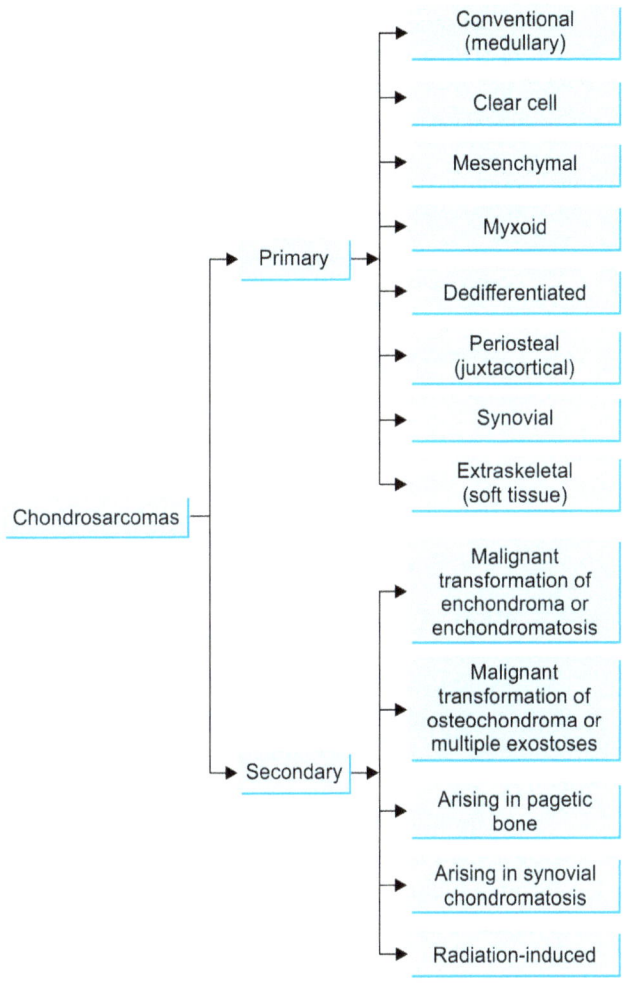

III. CLINICAL FEATURES

1. Pain → most common presentation
2. Slowly growing swelling
3. New onset of pain or rapid increase in swelling → Secondary CS
4. Pathological fracture → H/O of trivial trauma
5. Mass effect in pelvis → Bladder or bowel obstruction

IV. TYPES

A. Conventional (Medullary, Central) CS

1. > 90% of all primary CS.
2. Age → Adulthood and elderly, 5th–7th decade.

3. Male:Female → 3:2
4. MC site → <u>Pelvis (MC Ilium)</u>, proximal femur, proximal humerus, distal femur, ribs.
5. Enchondroma versus low grade CS → Diagnostic dilemma
6. <u>Radiograph</u>
   i. Cortical expansion and thickening
   ii. Expansion of medullary region
   iii. Endosteal scalloping (↑ in aggressive cases)
   iv. Comma-shaped stippled calcification → Rings and arc appearance.
   v. Cortical disruption ±
   vi. Soft tissue mass ±
   vii. Periosteal reaction → usually absent

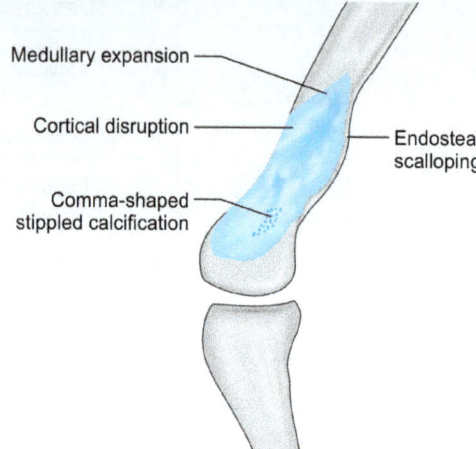

7. <u>CT scan</u>
   i. Assessing the lesions in areas of complex anatomy: Pelvis, sacrum.
   ii. CT chest → Lung is MC site for mets.
8. <u>MRI</u>
   i. T1 → Low intensity, T2 → Very high intensity
   ii. Due to high water content
   iii. Intramedullary extent of lesion
   iv. Soft tissue extension
9. <u>Bone scan</u>
   i. Based on radionucleotide uptake, helps differentiate enchondroma versus chondrosarcoma
   ii. Grade 1 → Uptake < ASIS
   iii. Grade 2 → Uptake = ASIS
   iv. Grade 3 → Uptake > ASIS, (likelihood of CS > enchondroma)
10. Pathology
    i. Gross → Nodular growth with glistening, translucent blue-white colour.
    ii. Microscopy
       a. Irregular lobules of cartilage permeating the host bony trabeculae.
       b. Hyaline cartilaginous matrix
       c. Tumor chondrocytes show nuclear atypia, multinucleation and are present in lacunae.
       d. Mitosis and necrosis

e. HPE grading → based on cellularity and nuclear atypia

Grade 1	Low cellularity, mild nuclear atypia, resembles enchondroma
Grade 2	Increased cellularity, nuclear atypia, plump cartilage cells that are multinucleated
Grade 3	Permeative hypercellular stroma with mitotic figures and pleomorphism

f. HPE of enchondroma and Grade 1 (low grade) CS are same. Therefore, must be differentiated based on clinical and radiological correlation.

B. Dedifferentiated CS

1. Most malignant CS → Very poor prognosis
2. High grade spindle cell component
3. Metastasis + at presentation
4. Large soft tissue mass +
5. 90% patients die with mets within 2 years.

C. Clear Cell CS

1. Low grade CS
2. Epiphyseal end of long bones
3. Bland clear cells along with hyaline cartilage, hence the name.
4. Two-thirds clear CS cases → Femur head and humerus head.

D. Mesenchymal CS

1. Bimorphic pattern → highly undifferentiated, small round cells and islands of well-differentiated hyaline cartilage.
2. Peak incidence → 10–30 years.
3. MC sites → Craniofacial bones, ribs, ilium and vertebrae.
4. MC of extraskeletal site → Meninges.
5. DD → Ewing's sarcoma, small cell OS, synovial sarcoma.

E. Secondary Chondrosarcoma

1. Malignant transformation of a known benign tumor into CS.
2. Histologically indistinguishable from conventional CS.
3. Precursor is → Osteochondroma / Enchondroma
4. Osteochondroma (OC)
   i. >80% of secondary CS.
   ii. Risk of malignant transformation
      a. Solitary OC → <1%
      b. Hereditary multiple exostosis → 5–10%
5. Enchondroma: Risk of malignant transformation
   i. Ollier's disease → 25–30%
   ii. Maffucci's → > 50%
6. Sudden onset or progression of pain and increase in swelling
7. Cartilage cap > 2 cm on MRI

V. MANAGEMENT

1. Percutaneous core needle or open biopsy → must be done compulsorily to confirm diagnosis.
2. Wide surgical excision with clear margins
   i. Most primary CS → Conventional Grade 2 and 3, Grade 1 in pelvis and sacrum
   ii. Clear cell
   iii. Dedifferentiated
   iv. Mesenchymal → Add chemotherapy only in this type.
   v. Secondary CS
3. Intralesional curettage with BG → Grade 1 conventional CS in extremities.
4. No role for chemo and radiotherapy in CS → Tumor is resistant to it.
5. Stabilization → Bone graft, extracorporeal autogenous irradiated bone and fixing with a plate.

OSTEOSARCOMA

I. INTRODUCTION

1. Primary malignant tumor in which the malignant mesenchymal cells produce osteoid and/or immature bone.
2. Most common 1° malignant tumor of bone, excluding those of hematopoietic origin.
3. Most common site → Distal femur > proximal tibia, proximal humerus.
4. Metaphysis (91%), Diaphysis (<9%)

II. CLASSIFICATION

Central (medullary)	Surface (peripheral)
• Conventional (Central) • Telangiectatic • Intraosseous/intramedullary (low grade) • Small cell OS	• Parosteal (low grade) • Periosteal (low to intermediate) • High grade surface OS

1. Conventional intramedullary OS
   ↓
   Most common 80–90% of all OS
2. *Parosteal (juxtacortical or surface OS)*:
   i. Arises directly adjacent to but distinct from the external surface of the bone.
   ii. Most common site → Posterior aspect of distal femur.
   iii. Favorable prognosis, low grade
3. *Periosteal OS*:
   i. Diaphyseal cortex or periosteum.
   ii. Site → proximal tibia
   iii. ↑Cartilaginous component
   iv. Differential diagnosis = Chondrosarcoma.

III. ETIOLOGY

1. Loss of heterozygosity (LOH) at 3q, 13q, 17p, and 18q.
2. Juxtacortical OS → Ring chromosomes.
3. Hereditary retinoblastoma.
4. Germ cell abnormalities: Li Fraumeni syndrome. Mutation of p53 gene.
5. Ionizing radiation/radiation therapy.
6. Paget's disease
7. Werner syndrome, bloom syndrome.

IV. CLINICAL FEATURES

1. 2nd decade, adolescent years second peak → Fifth decade.
2. M:F = 3:2
3. Persistent pain.
4. Pathological fracture – unusual but rare.
5. Deep, firm, fixed mass.
6. Swelling → Near the end of long bones, consistency varies from soft, fluctuant, to firm and indurated to bone hard.
7. Overlying skin → Stretched, thin, glossy. Warmth, erythema
8. The motion of the adjacent joint is unimpaired until the muscle acting on the joint becomes involved by the infiltrating tumor.
9. Telangiectatic OS → Bruits.

V. RADIOLOGY (FIGS. 11A AND B)

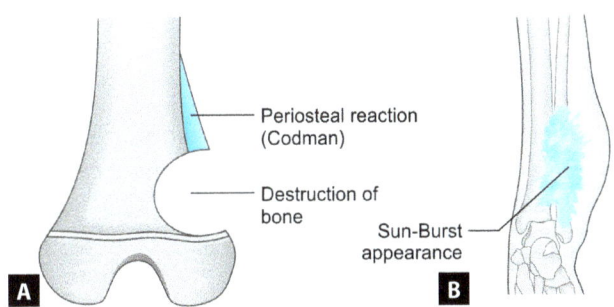

1. Classic high - grade OS → Remarkable osteoblastic lesion.
2. However, radiographic findings variable:
   i. Osteogenesis → Radio-opacity
   ii. Destruction → Radiolucency
3. Metaphyseal portion of long bone outgrows from the medullary canal to extraskeletal region.
4. Permeative growth pattern.
5. Indistinct margins.
6. Cortex erosions
7. Periosteal reaction → Codman's triangle and sunburnt appearance.
8. Telangiectatic and small cell OS → maybe purely lytic
9. CT and MRI → Read from Ewings.

VI. HISTOPATHOLOGY

A. Microscopy

1. Malignant spindle cells produce tumor osteoid.
2. Besides osteoblastic components, OS may also show,

	5 years rate	D. D
Chondroblastic	60%	Chondrosarcoma
Fibroblastic	83%	
Vascular spaces	75%	ABC
Sheets of small round cells		Ewing's

3. High grade OS → Pleomorphic malignant cells with large hyperchromatic nuclei and mitotic figures.
4. OS vs Myositis Ossificans
5. Zonation phenomenon (seen in myositis ossificans) More mature, ossified matrix in periphery.
6. OS → Immature matrix in periphery.

B. Gross

1. Metaphysis of large long bones.
2. During active growth, while the epiphyseal plate is still intact.
↓
Barrier to extension into epiphysis.
3. After physeal closure, tumor may extend to epiphysis, but articular cartilage bars further extension into the joint.
4. Consistency → Stony hard to soft and gritty.
5. Color reflects components:
    i. Fibrous: White
    ii. Osseous: Yellowish white
    iii. Cartilaginous: Bluish white
6. Necrotic foci, cystic degeneration.
7. Most cellular and least differentiated portion of the tumor → Advancing front in the medullary cavity and beneath elevated periosteum.

VII. PROGNOSIS – POOR

1. Trunk and pelvis tumors
2. ↑LDH (>400 IU/L), ↑ALP > 400
3. Secondary OS
4. Pathological fracture
5. Skip lesion
6. Metastasis → Most common site lung.

VIII. TREATMENT

1. High grade osteosarcoma → Surgery excision of primary tumor + Chemotherapy.
Survival rate: Surgery alone = 20%
Surgery + Chemo = 60–70%

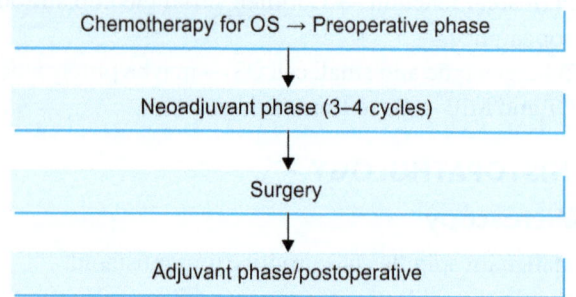

2. *Multiagent chemo treatment is given*:
    i. Doxorubicin
    ii. Cisplatin
    iii. High dose methotrexate [included in most regimens] (8–12 g/m^2)
    iv. Etoposide
    v. Ifosfamide
3. *Preoperative chemo*:
    i. Immediately tackles micrometastatic disease
    ii. Safety margin for resection
    iii. Less resection of normal tissue
    iv. Buys time for surgery planning, manufacture of custom prosthesis
    v. Histological response to chemo
4. *Huvo's system*:
    I: 0–50%
    II: 51–90%
    III: 91–99%
    IV: 100%
    } Necrosis
    ↑ 5Y survival rate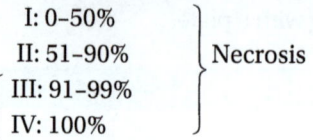
5. *High grade OS*:
    i. Limb salvage
    ii. Amputation
6. Indications of limb – sparing depends on:
    i. Tumor location
    ii. Its relationship with major NVB
7. Adequate local control must not be compromised in attempt to save limb.
8. *Methods of limb – salvage*:
    i. Autografts
    ii. Allografts
    iii. Bone lengthening
    iv. Endoprosthetic replacement
    v. Rotationplasty
    vi. Arthrodesis
9. Low-grade OS → Wide surgical excision + Follow-up (survival >90%)
10. Radiotherapy no longer a part of standard treatment of OS.
11. Very selective group of patients:
    i. Positive or close surgical margins
    ii. Pelvis, thorax, head, neck
    iii. Palliative.

FIBROUS DYSPLASIA

I. INTRODUCTION

1. Developmental disorder in which the body fails to produce normal lamellar bone.
2. Characterized by fibrous replacement of the skeleton.
3. This benign, intramedullary, fibro-osseous lesion is also known as, "Jaffe Lichtenstein syndrome".

II. ETIOPATHOLOGY

1.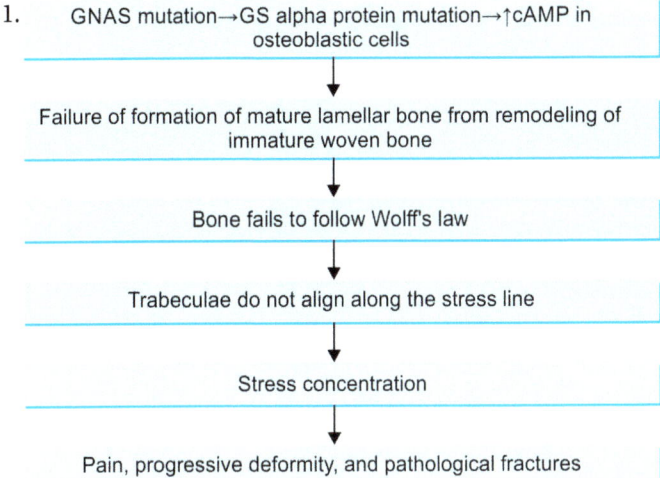

   GNAS mutation → GS alpha protein mutation → ↑cAMP in osteoblastic cells

   ↓

   Failure of formation of mature lamellar bone from remodeling of immature woven bone

   ↓

   Bone fails to follow Wolff's law

   ↓

   Trabeculae do not align along the stress line

   ↓

   Stress concentration

   ↓

   Pain, progressive deformity, and pathological fractures

2. Types — Monostotic (80%)
            — Polyostotic (20%)
3. Associated syndromes
   i. McCune Albright syndrome → Polyostotic fibrous Dysplasia + Precocious puberty + Café-au-lait spots.
   ii. Mazabraud syndrome → Polyostotic fibrous dysplasia + soft-tissue intramuscular myxomas.
   iii. Osteofibrous Dysplasia → Uncommon type affecting only the cortex of tibia.
4. Most common site → Proximal femur f/b ribs, maxilla and tibia.

III. CLINICAL FEATURES

1. F > M
2. Onset → < 30 years in 75% patients
3. Asymptomatic → Incidental finding
4. Bone pain
5. Pathological fractures
6. Shepherd crook deformity → Lateral bow of proximal femur.
7. Scoliosis
8. Limb shortening
9. Limping
10. Tibial bow
11. Protrusio acetabuli
12. Asymmetry of head and face → Hyperostosis at base of skull
13. Café au lait spots → Large, brown, irregular patches of skin.

IV. RADIOLOGY (FIG.12)

1. Radiograph:
   i. Typical localized well-circumscribed central lytic lesions within the medullary canal.
   ii. Cortical thinning
   iii. Sclerotic margins
   iv. Ground glass appearance
   v. Shepherd's crook deformity

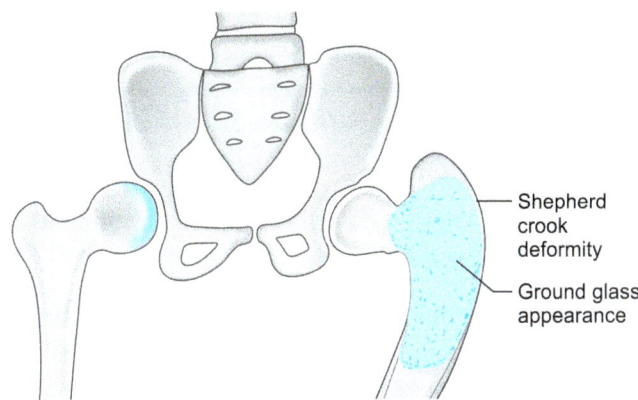

   vi. Most common cause of benign expansile rib lesion
   vii. Harrisons groove following rib fractures
   viii. Vertebral collapse
   ix. Scoliosis
2. CT scan → Cortical discontinuity.
3. MRI → T1 hypointense, T2 hyperintense.

V. GROSS

1. Reddish gray tough fibrous tissue with gritty resistance.
2. Feels like sandpaper in consistency.

VI. MICROSCOPIC APPEARANCE

1. Chinese letter or alphabet soup pattern of trabeculae
2. Islands of woven bone are surrounded by fibroblastic proliferation.

VII. DIFFERENTIAL DIAGNOSIS

1. Paget's disease
2. Neurofibromatosis-1
3. Non-ossifying fibroma
4. Simple bone cyst
5. Enchondromatosis

VIII. TREATMENT

1. Incidental finding → Observation
2. Medical management
   i. Inj. Pamidronate IV (60 mg/day for 3 days) repeated after 6 months
   ii. Zoledronic acid
   iii. Oral risedronate

3. Internal fixation + corticocancellous bone grafting
   i. *Indications*:
      a. Pathological fractures of long bones
      b. Impending fractures in areas of high stresses
   ii. Intramedullary nailing is preferred
4. Subtrochanteric osteotomy → Severe coxa vara deformity

EWING'S SARCOMA

I. INTRODUCTION

1. Malignant, small round cell tumor, most commonly in the diaphysis of long bones.
2. Third most common primary tumor of bone overall.
3. Second most common malignant bone tumor of late childhood and early adulthood, 1% of childhood cancers.
4. It is a small round blue cell tumor
   ↓ORIGIN
   Primitive mesenchymal cells
5. Reciprocal translocation (EWS on chr.22, FLT1 on Chr.11) → t (11:22) (q24;q12)
   ↓
   EWS/FLT1 fusion transcription factor
   ↓
   Fibroblasts → Malignant cells.
6. Prominent neurogenic differentiation
   ↓
   Primitive neuroectodermal tumor
7. Ewings earlier classified it as an endothelial myeloma, as he thought it was a non-osteogenic tumor

II. CLINICAL FEATURES

1. Peak incidence: 1st two decades of life
2. M:F = 1.4:1
3. White population > Asian, African
4. Site: Throughout the skeleton but, most commonly long bones such as femur.
5. Bones of feet > bones of hand → 4 to 1
6. Most common clinical symptom → Pain and Swelling
7. Spontaneously, in association with minor traumatic event
8. May present as pathological fracture
9. Constitutional symptoms of systemic infection
10. In spine, patient may present with symptoms of neurological involvement.
11. Pelvis and other axial sites → diagnosis is delayed and tumor is larger
12. Weight loss and anorexia.

III. RADIOLOGICAL EVALUATION (FIG. 13)

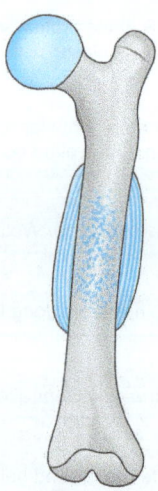

1. Nonmatrix producing destructive lesion in the metaphysis (5%) and diaphysis (50%) of the long bone.
2. Moth eaten appearance.
3. Aggressive periosteal reaction: "Onion peel". Codman's triangle may also be present.
4. In spine, extensive tumor involvement
   ↓
   Fracture and loss of vertebral height (vertebra plana).
5. Chest X-ray → Metastasis
6. *X-ray differential diagnosis*:
   i. Osteomyelitis
   ii. LCH
   iii. Lymphoma
   iv. Small cell osteosarcoma
   v. Metastatic neuroblastoma
7. *CT*:
   i. Extent of cortical destruction
   ii. Distant metastasis in lung
8. *MRI*:
   i. Best modality to assess the degree of intraosseous and extraosseous extension [large soft tissue component] of diseases in bone.
   ii. Initial staging
   iii. Surgery planning
   iv. Assessing response to chemotherapy
   v. Skip lesions
9. *PET–CT*: Staging
   Bone scan→*Very "hot" lesion.*

IV. LAB INVESTIGATIONS

1. Anemia
2. Leukocytosis
3. ↑ LDH (>200 IU/mL)

V. PATHOLOGY

A. Gross

1. Extensive invasion of the medullary bone with destruction of endosteum and cortex.
2. Periosteal new bone formation.
3. Large, firm, often encapsulated by fibrous tissue, grayish - soft white tissue mass.
4. Cysts, hemorrhage and necrosis ±
5. Within the subperiosteal tumor, multiple layers of bone lie parallel with the shaft.

B. Microscopy

1. Sheets of monomorphic small round blue cells with pale and indistinct cytoplasmic border and small, prominent hyperchromatic nuclei.
2. Periodic acid: Schiff → (+) due to intramedullary glycogen
3. Pseudorosettes (circle of cells with necrosis in center) → PNET
4. CD99 (MIC 2) → Immunohistochemical marker (+)
5. EWS translocation → PCR or FISH

V. PROGNOSIS: POOR

1. Male
2. Anemia, fever
3. ↑ LDH
4. Axial tumors
5. C - myc and Ki - 67, p53 expression.
6. Metastasis
7. ↑ Size
8. Poor response to chemo.

VI. TREATMENT

1. Multidisciplinary approach: Surgeon, radiologist, sonologist, pathologist, oncologist.
2. Systemic multiagent chemotherapy and surgery, radiation, a combination of both.
3. Initial chemotherapy: 3-6 cycles after biopsy
  ↓
  Local disease control
  ↓
  6-10 cycles of chemotherapy - 3-week interval
4. Duration of treatment = 10-12 months
5. *Chemotherapeutic agents*:
   i. Vincristine
   ii. Adriamycin/doxorubicin
   iii. Cyclophosphamide
   iv. Ifosfamide
   v. Dactinomycin
   vi. Etoposide
6. Response to chemotherapy → one of the most important prognostic factor.

Histopathology	5Y survival
I – Macroscopic viable tumor	(95%)
II – Microscopic viable tumor	(68%)
III – No viable tumor	(34%)

7. Myeloablative therapy and stem cell transplantation → uncertain value
8. Choice of modality for local disease control depends on:
   i. Age of patient
   ii. Extent of disease at presentation
   iii. Tumor site
   iv. Functional considerations
9. Surgery and radiotherapy → Principle modes of management.
10. Role of RT as 1° means → Reduced due to:
    i. ↓ Survival compared to surgery.
    ii. Secondary malignancy
11. Surgery → Radical or wide resection better outcome than Marginal/Intralesional.
12. Postoperative RT indications when:
    i. Positive or close margins after surgery.
    ii. Widely metastatic disease
    iii. Poor chemotherapy response
13. Appendicular → limb sparing or amputation.
14. Spine → Surgery generally reserved for patients → neurological deficit
15. Decompression and stabilization necessary before initiation of systemic therapy
16. Dose = 5000 cGY.

VII. COMPLICATIONS

1. Secondary neoplasms from Radiotherapy: Bone sarcoma
   Chemotherapy: AML/MDS
2. Recurrence
3. Progression
4. RT → LLD, joint contractures, muscle atrophy, pathological fracture VTE

OSTEOCHONDROMA

I. INTRODUCTION

1. Largest group of cartilage forming benign bone tumor.
2. Also known as "Exostosis"

3. Defined as → "A cartilage capped bony projection arising on the external surface of bone containing a marrow cavity that is continuous with that of the underlying bone"

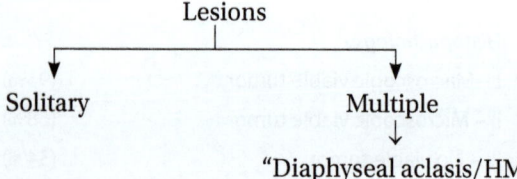

Solitary / Multiple → "Diaphyseal aclasis/HME"

II. ETIOLOGY

1. Traditionally → Developmental disorder, not true tumor. However, recent evidence suggests ↓
2. Mutations in genes encoding "Exostosin 1" (EXT - 1) → ∴ True neoplasm
3. History of prior surgery
4. Salter–Harris fracture
5. Post-radiation
6. Most common radiation induced benign bone tumor in children
7. Most common benign bone tumors
8. Most common bone tumor in children.
9. First 3 decades of life, M > F (2:1)
10. Metaphysis of long tubular bones (Distal femur > proximal tibia)
11. Proximal humerus, ilium, scapula.

III. CLINICAL FEATURES

1. Hard immobile, nontender swelling of long duration
2. Pain due to:
    i. Bursitis
    ii. Fracture
    iii. Mechanical irritation
    iv. Neural irritation
    v. Ischemic necrosis
    vi. Malignant change
3. Limitation of joint movements
4. Deformity
5. Fracture
6. Growth disturbances

IV. IMAGING

A. X-ray (Fig. 14)

Eccentric bony outgrowth from metaphyseal region of long bone, with cortical and medullary portions which are continuous with the cortex and medulla of main bone.

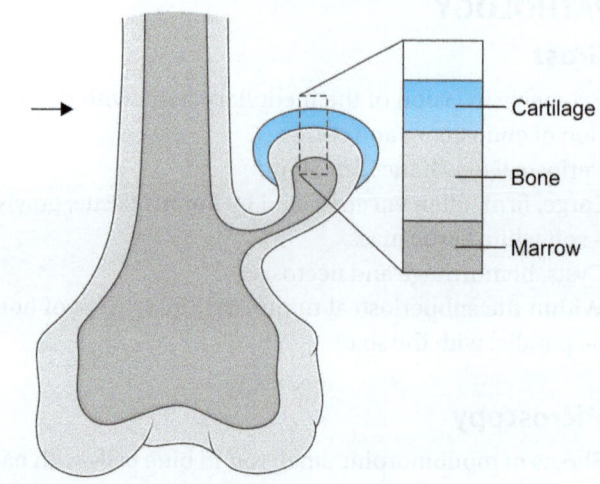

"Lesions are directed away from the growing end of long bones"

B. MRI

1. Medullary continuity
2. Cartilage cap thickness
3. Cartilage cap > 2 cm/more → Higher risk of malignancy

V. GROSS APPEARANCE

Firm, lobulated, pedunculated or sessile varying in size covered by perichondrium.

VI. MICROSCOPY

Three layers:
1. Perichondrium
2. Cartilage
3. Bone

VII. DIFFERENTIAL DIAGNOSIS

1. Parosteal osteomyelitis
2. Parosteal osteochondromatous proliferation (Nora's lesion)
3. Trevor's disease
4. Enchondroma

VIII. TREATMENT

1. Observation → Asymptomatic lesions
2. Surgical excision:
    i. Indications:
        a. Cosmesis
        b. Limitation of joint function
        c. Angular deformity of limbs
        d. Repeated painful bursitis

e. Fracture of lesion
   f. Secondary impingement of tendon or nerve
   g. Suspicion of malignant change
  ii. Complete excision → including perichondrium
  iii. Prevention of recurrence → Removal of tumor from its base.

IX. MALIGNANT TRANSFORMATION

1. Solitary: 1%
2. HME: 20%

AMPUTATION VS LIMB SALVAGE/PRINCIPLES OF SURGERY IN BONE TUMORS

I. INTRODUCTION

1. A set of surgical procedures designed to accomplish removal of a malignant tumor and reconstruction of the limb.
   ↓
   With an acceptable oncologic, functional and cosmetic result.
2. The key principle → Any surgery must first completely resect the tumor and any adjacent involved soft tissues.

II. INDICATION

Every patient with tumor of extremity must be considered for limb salvage.
↓
If the tumor can be excised with an adequate margin and the resulting limb is worth saving.

The decision depends upon factors:
1. Diagnosis
2. Site of tumor
3. Extent of tumor: Especially into soft tissue
4. Response of the tumor to neoadjuvant chemotherapy.
5. Patient's age
6. Financial status of the patient.

A. Barriers to Limb Salvage Surgery (LSS)

1. Poorly placed biopsy incision.
2. Major neurovascular involvement.
   Involvement of main nerve → LSS contraindicated. However, involvement of main vessel not an absolute contraindication → vascular homografts
3. Displaced pathologic fracture.
4. Fungating and infected tumors.
5. Recurrence of malignant tumors.
6. Inability to afford chemotherapy.

B. Three Strike Rule

1. Bone
2. Nerve
3. Vessels
4. Soft tissue envelope

} 3/4th LSS not worth considering.

C. Goal

1. Painless limb
2. Functional and tumor free
3. Good psychological outcome

Proximal the tumor, more likely that LSS will be beneficial to the patient

For example:

Below knee amputation for a tumor around the ankle produces excellent outcome with amputation
↓
Difficult for LSS to match it
and

Proximal femur tumors → LSS significantly better results than achieved with a hip disarticulation or hind quarter amputation.

The risks and benefits of the proposed surgery → must be discussed with the patient → so that they are aware of increased risk of local recurrence and other complications.

In upper limb → Even sacrificing 1 to 2 major nerves → Better results of LSS than amputation

D. Principles

1. Complete resection of tumor
2. Skeletal reconstruction
3. Soft tissue and muscle transfer.

E. Resection

1. Intralesional: Plane of dissection is within tumor
   Indications:
   i. Symptomatic benign tumors
   ii. Palliative in metastatic disease.
2. Marginal:
   Indications:
   i. Most benign lesions
   ii. Few low-grade malignancies.
   iii. Rarely selective high-grade malignancies after preoperative radio and neoadjuvant chemotherapy.
3. *Wide*: Goal of majority of procedures for high grade malignancies
4. *Radical*:
   i. Bone tumors
   ii. Soft tissue sarcomas – removing entire compartment or multiple compartments of any muscle or bone.

III. SKELETAL RECONSTRUCTION

A. Autografts
B. Allografts
C. Endoprosthetic replacement
D. Rotationplasty
E. Bone lengthening
F. Arthrodesis

A. Autografts

1. Bone graft involving transferring a part of bone from the patient himself.
   ↓
   And using it to fill the defect caused by tumor resection.
2. Autograft → vascularized
             → nonvascularized
3. Vascularized fibula graft → Distal radius (fits perfectly)
4. In a skeletally immature, the proximal fibular physis with its blood supply.
   ↓ can replace
   Growth plate of DER and proximal humerus: Epiphysis continues to grow.
5. In the lower limb the vascularized graft needs to be used with other bone grafts.
   ↓
   As singly, it may take up to 18 months or more to get thickened up and hypertrophied.
6. Patient's own tumor bone is sterilized using
   ↓
   Extra-corporeal radiotherapy
   ↓
   Reimplanted at the site of defect
   ↓
   a. Advantages:
      i. Bone fits perfectly at the site of the defect.
      ii. Cheap
      iii. Avoids donor site complications
   b. Disadvantage:
      i. Time consuming.
      ii. Significantly damaged bone may not be able to be used.
7. Dose = 50–300 Gray.

B. Allografts

1. Allografts combined with vascularized fibula graft → Early weight bearing
   ↓
   On allograft
   ↓
   Which gradually becomes redundant
   ↓
   Vascularized fibula graft unites proximally and distally, and then hypertrophies
2. Complications
   i. Nonunion
   ii. Infection
   iii. Delayed fracture
   iv. Disease transmission.

C. Endoprosthetic Replacement

1. Megaprosthesis: Large metallic device designed to replace the excised length of bone and the adjacent joint.
2. Avoids donor site morbidity, risk of nonunion, results as good as grafts
3. Implant material → Usually titanium alloys
   ↓
   Biologically inert, light and strong but cost ↑↑↑
4. Bearing surface → HDPE or XLPE
   ↓
   Wear and loosening (HDPE > XLPE)
5. Fixation → Uncemented
            → Cemented
6. Uncemented → Stress shielding, bone resorption. Requiring time for fixation.
7. Cemented → Immediate strength → Early weight bearing
   ↓
   Aseptic loosening → Long term.
8. Cemented fixation of the prosthesis stem + HA collar on the prosthesis.
   ↓
   Bone ingrowth into the collar
   +
   Advantage of immediate stability of cemented fixation.
9. Bone ingrowth "locks" the prosthesis
   ↓
   Biological "purse – string" to prevent wear debris tracking along the side of the stem.
10. Main complications:
    i. Infection
    ii. Wear
    iii. Breakage and periprosthetic fracture.
    iv. Loosening
    v. Costly ↑↑↑
11. Proximal femur tumors
    ↓
    Resection and proximal femur prosthesis (**Fig. 15**).
12. Main concern → Loss of abductor lever arm attached to GT.
    ↓
    Attached to fascia lata.
13. To prevent dislocation of femur head
    ↓
    Use of large size head
14. Proximal tibia reconstruction (**Fig. 15**)
    i. Main concern → Loss of extensor mechanism attachment on tibial tubercle. Subcutaneous nature of bone
    ii. ↓Rx
        — Gastrocnemius muscle flap —
        Provides soft tissue   Allows attachment
        coverage to prosthesis.   to patellar tendon

15. Distal humerus → Floppy hinge type prosthesis fixed to the ulna.

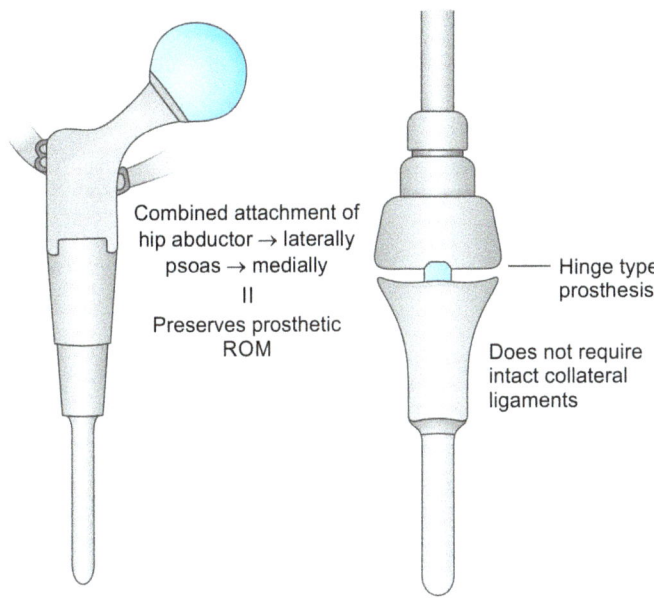

D. Rotationplasty (Fig. 16)

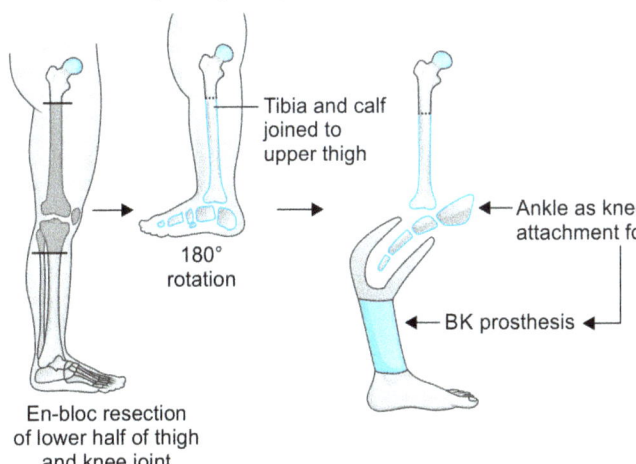

1. Principle = Excision of the diseased part of the limb.
   ↓
   Joining the remaining parts.
   ↓
   Rotating them through 180°
2. Most common site for which it is used → Distal femur.
3. No phantom pain as no amputation.
4. Functions as below knee amputation rather than above knee → Good outcome.

E. Arthrodesis

1. Excision of the diseased bone
   ↓
   Bone graft
   ↓
   Fusion of joint, remaining bone ends.

2. Cost-effective and less time consuming.
3. Ideal for manual laborers needing stability at the cost of movement (ROM).

F. Bone Lengthening

1. Principle → Epiphyseal distraction or cholestasis
2. Bone stabilized using ilizarov fixation
   ↓
   Bone transport → to fill defect
3. Time consuming, intricate
   ↓
4. Length of treatment increases by 2 months for every cm of bone excised.

MULTIPLE MYELOMA

I. INTRODUCTION

1. Neoplastic proliferation of the plasma cells in the bone marrow and other extramedullary sites along with the secreted monoclonal proteins (complete immunoglobulin and/or light chain) resulting in end-organ damage and fatal termination.
2. MC primary bone malignancy.
3. M > F
4. MCC age group involved → 60–70 years

II. ETIOLOGY

1. First degree relatives of patients with multiple myeloma
2. Exposure to radiation
3. Chemical exposure (such as benzene, asbestos, pesticides)
4. Idiopathic

III. PATHOGENESIS

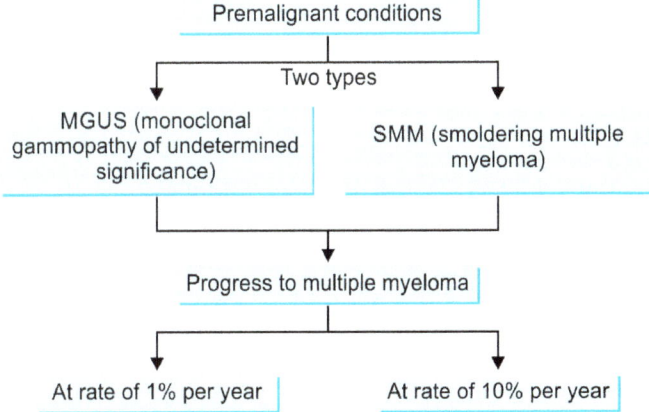

Risk of progression to MM is affected by:
1. Presence of underlying genetic abnormalities
2. Percentage of bone marrow plasma cells

3. Amount of monoclonal protein
4. Involved/Uninvolved free light chain ratio

IV. CLINICAL FEATURES

1. Pre-malignant condition – MGUS and SMM – asymptomatic
2. About 25% patients with MM – asymptomatic, detected incidentally
3. In rest of the patients, symptoms depend on the extent of end organ damage
4. Fatigue, bone pain – M/C symptoms
5. Bone lesions include:
    i. Pathological fractures
    ii. Cord or nerve root compression resulting in backache, radiculopathy, neural deficit with/without bowel/bladder involvement.
6. Renal failure presents as:
    i. Anorexia
    ii. Nausea
    iii. Vomiting   } d/t Uremia
    iv. Decreased urine output
    v. Altered sensorium
7. Hypercalcemia leads to:
    i. Constipation
    ii. Increased thirst
8. Anemia
9. Immune compromise – recurrent infections
10. Secreted M protein – Hyperviscosity syndrome
    i. Headache
    ii. Visual disturbances
    iii. Dyspnea
    iv. Tinnitus
11. Peripheral neuropathy
12. Amyloidosis (cardiomyopathy, proteinuria, neuropathy)
13. POEMS (**P**olyneuropathy, **O**rganomegaly, **E**ndocrinopathy, **M**-protein, **S**kin changes) – seen in osteosclerotic myeloma

V. DIAGNOSIS

1. Careful history taking, thorough examination to look for extent of end organ damage.
2. Lab investigations include:
    i. CBC, ESR
    ii. Metabolic profile (RFT/LFT/serum electrolytes/FBS)
    iii. Serum calcium levels
    iv. Serum LDH
    v. β2-microglobulin levels
    vi. Serum PEP/urine PEP
    vii. Urine for Bence Jones protein
    viii. Serum free light chain assay
3. Bone marrow examination: Aspiration, biopsy, IHC, FISH

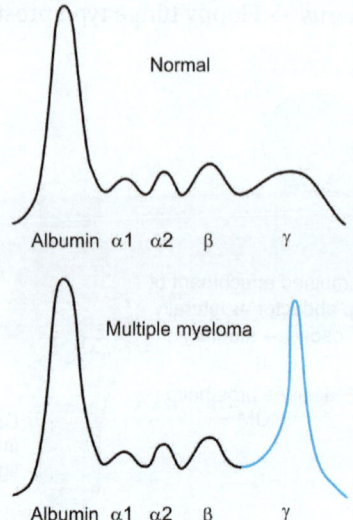

Diagnostic Criteria of MM
i. Presence of >10% clonal plasma cells in bone marrow or biopsy-proven plasmacytoma,
ii. Presence of M protein,
iii. Myeloma defining events, i.e, **CRAB**:
   a. Serum **C**alcium >11 mg/dL
   b. **R**enal dysfunction with serum creatinine >2 mg/dL or creatinine clearance <40 mL/min
   c. **A**nemia with hemoglobin <10 g/dL, and
   d. Lytic **B**one lesion.
4. Radiological imaging done to assess:
   i. Extent of bone involvement
   ii. Extramedullary plasmacytoma
5. Bone lesions include:
   i. Osteopenia
   ii. Multiple, rounded, punched out, lytic lesions seen in skull, vertebrae
   iii. Collapsed vertebral bodies – biconcave vertebral bodies
   iv. Instead a low dose whole body CT can be done rather than skeletal survey to detect extent of bone lesions
6. FDG-PET in nonsecretory myeloma, SMM, extramedullary plasmacytoma

VI. STAGING AND RISK STRATIFICATION

Category	Variable
International staging system (ISS)	
• I	• β2-microglobulin < 3.5 mg/L and serum albumin > 3.5 g/L
• II	• β2-microglobulin 3.5–5.4 mg/L
• III	• β2-microglobulin > 5.5 mg/L
Cytogenetics (FISH)	
• High risk	• Presence of del(17p), t(4;14), t(14;16)
• Standard risk	• No high risk abnormalities
Revised ISS	
• I	• ISS stage I and standard risk cytogenetics and normal LDH
• II	• Neither R-ISS stage I or III
• III	• ISS stage III and either high risk cytogenetics or high LDH

VIII. MANAGEMENT

Annual follow-up and observation → MGUS and asymptomatic myeloma

For MM,
1. Management of hypercalcemia by – Saline hydration, loop diuretics, calcitonin, bisphosphonates, hemodialysis
2. Hydration is essential for patients presenting with hyperviscosity syndrome → may require plasmapheresis
3. Hemodialysis for patients presenting with renal failure
4. Infection, if present – managed with non-nephrotoxic antibiotics
5. Pain – opioid based analgesia
6. Vertebral collapse – vertebroplasty/kyphoplasty
7.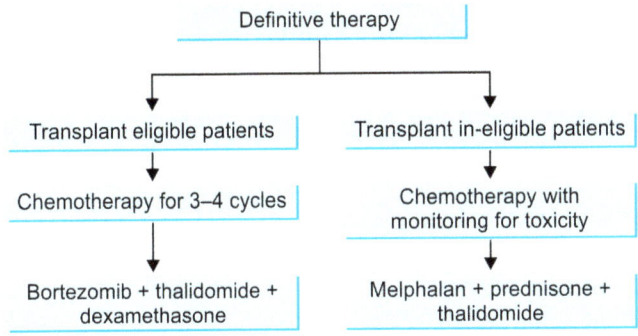
8. Stem cell transplantation → Autologous and allogenic
9. Radiotherapy for solitary plasmacytoma
10. Surgical fixation
    i. Pathological fracture
    ii. Neural deficit due to cord or nerve root compression

METASTATIC BONE DISEASE AND DIFFERENTIALS

I. INTRODUCTION

1. The spread of tumor cells from the primary tumor organ to bones.
2. MC malignant tumor of skeleton
3. Skeleton → 3rd MC site of metastasis
   (1st – lung, 2nd – liver)

II. ETIOLOGY AND PATHOPHYSIOLOGY

1. MC site → Thoracic spine > Ribs > Pelvis > Proximal long bones
2. Breast + Prostate responsible for > 80%.

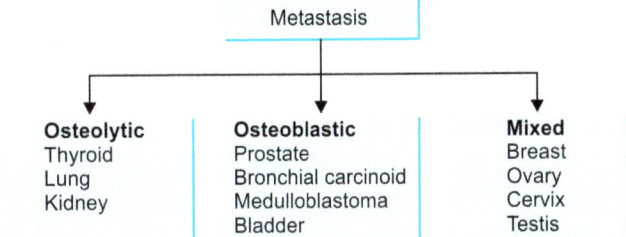

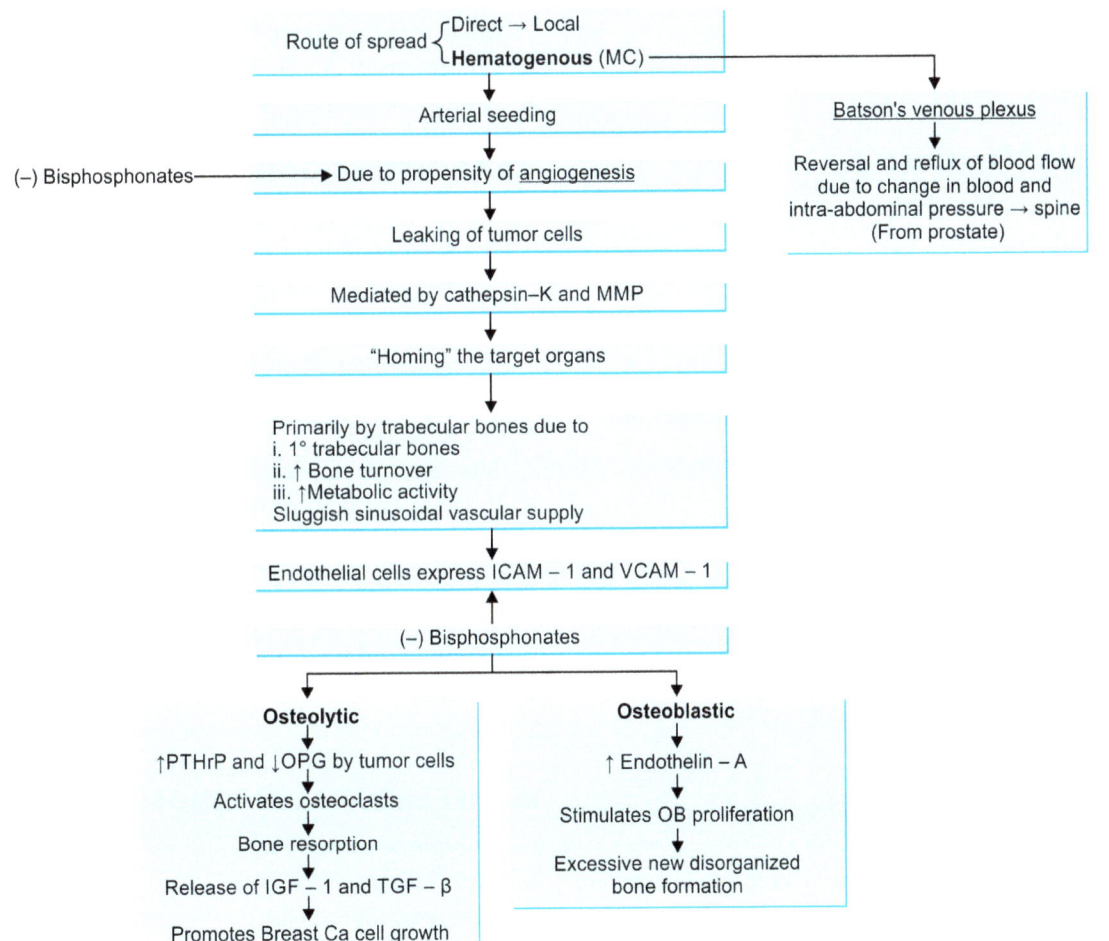

III. CLINICAL PRESENTATION AND ITS PHYSIOLOGY

A. Bone pain
B. Hypercalcemia: Systemic manifestation
C. Pathological fractures
D. Spinal cord involvement
E. Bone marrow infiltration/leukoerythroblastic anemia

A. Bone Pain

1. Continuous deep boring
2. Episodes of stabbing discomfort
3. Worse at night
4. Progressive, unrelenting
5. Leads to decreased quality of life.

Mechanisms

1. Direct pressure and destruction.
2. Release of PG, Histamine, Bradykinin.
3. Hormonal influence
4. Mechanical instability → Backache.

B. Hypercalcemia

1. Most common complication of metabolic bone disease
2. *Dysfunction*:
   - GI
   - Renal
   - CNS
   - Advanced → cardiac arrhythmias
3. Loss of appetite, weight, fatigue.

C. Pathological Fractures

1. Malignancies with long term survival.
   ↓
   Breast and prostate.
   ↓
   Increased chances of pathological fracture.
2. Metabolic destruction of bone → ↓ Load bearing capacities → Trabecular destruction and microfracture
   ↓
   Total loss of bone integrity.
   Bisphosphonates inhibit these effects.

D. Spinal Cord Involvement

1. Neuro deficit
2. Cauda equina syndrome

IV. RADIOLOGICAL INVESTIGATIONS

A. X-ray

1. Osteolytic (visible after >25–50% bone loss → Late), Blastic, mixed.
2. Solitary or multiple → >40 years → multiple lesions are metastasis until proven otherwise

3. Axial > Appendicular
   Distal to elbow → "Acral metastasis"
4. **Mirel's score >9 → fix prophylactically**
   Mneumonic: PISS

	Mild	Moderate	Severe
Pain			
Imaging	Blastic	Mixed	Lytic
Size (Circumference)	<1/3	1/3–2/3rd	>2/3rd
Site	UL	LL	Pertrochanteric
	1	2	3

B. Bone Scan = Tc 99

1. Screening I.O.C →↑ Sensitive
2. Entire skeleton
3. Low cost
4. Identify "easier" site for biopsy
5. "Hot" spots → But false negative in aggressive purely negative scans → FDG-PET

C. CT Scan

1. Chest wall lesions
2. Cortical involvement
3. Intraarticular
4. Planning biopsy

D. MRI

1. Small metastasis not detected on bone scan
2. Low intensity T_1
3. High T_2 → BM edema

V. LAB. INVESTIGATIONS

1. CBC:
   i. Anemia
   ii. Platelets ↓,↑
   iii. Leukocytosis
   iv. Immature and nucleated RBCs
   v. DIC
2. Hypercalcemia
3. Increased alkaline phosphatase
4. Increased acid phosphatase → Ca prostate.
5. BJP, Serum electrophoresis → MM

Tumor Markers

1. Carcinoembryonic antigen (CEA) – GI tumors
2. CA-125 – Female genital tract
3. PSA – Ca Prostate

VI. DIFFERENTIAL DIAGNOSIS

1. Multiple myeloma
2. Paget's disease
3. Hyperparathyroidism

4. Lymphoma
5. Postradiation sarcoma
6. Osteomyelitis

VII. TREATMENT
A. Goals
1. Pain relief
2. Maximize quality of remaining life
3. Functional independence
4. Prevent skeletal related events
5. Biopsy must before commencement of any intervention
6. Multidisciplinary team

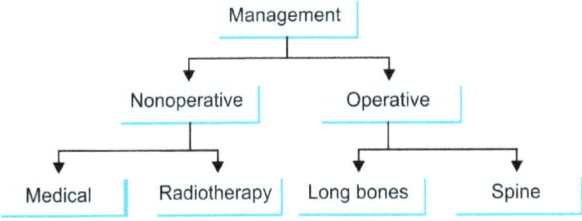

B. Medical
1. Bisphosphonates: Zoledronic acid
   → Inhibits osteoclastic bone resorption
   5 mg IV → yearly
   Adverse drug reactions:
   i. Flu-like illness
   ii. GI distension
   iii. ONJ
   iv. Atypical insufficient fracture
2. Denosumab:
   i. Human monoclonal antibody to RANK-L → ↓ lysis
   ii. 120 mg SC/3 months
   iii. ADR → ONJ, dangerous hypocalcemia: Therefore supplement with calcium

C. Radiotherapy
1. Palliative therapy in multiple metastasis
2. Pain control → destruction of tumor cells
   → ↓ Inflammatory edema
3. External beam radiotherapy (EBRT)
   30 Gray → 10 fractions
4. Stereotactic body radiation therapy (SBRT)
   → Spinal metastasis, low side effects but high cost

D. Radionuclide Therapy
1. Osteoblastic metastasis avidly take up bone seeking radiopharmaceuticals
2. Strontium: 89
3. Phosphorous: 32

E. Others
1. RFA
2. Microwave ablation
3. Cryoablation

F. Operative
Indications
1. Pathologic fracture
2. Impending > 9 Mirels
3. Intractable pain → Not resolved by medical management
4. Estimated survival: Long
5. Spinal instability

Principles
1. Surgery must provide immediate stability
2. Surgeon must assume fracture will not unite and decide management.
3. Fixation must last lifetime of the patient.
   i. Proximal femur (TC) → arthroplasty > Internal fixation.
   ii. Acetabulum involved and good life expectancy → THR
       Acetabulum not involved and lower life expectancy → Bipolar
   iii. Long stem → Prophylactic reinforcement
   iv. Extensive Lesions → Proximal femur megaprosthesis
   v. Subtrochanteric and diaphyseal → IM nailing
   vi. Proximal humerus → Neers/Reverse shoulder
   vii. Use PMMA cement to fill defect.
4. *Spine:*
   i. Stable fracture → for pain management → Vertebroplasty kyphoplasty.
   ii. Unstable fracture → Neural decompression
   iii. Postinstrumentation → spine stabilization after anterior column reconstruction.
5. *Periacetabular*
   i. Palliative → EBRT
   ii. Protusio → Massive allo/autografts, reconstruction cage with screws, cement. Preoperative embolization.

SYNOVIOMA/SYNOVIAL CELL SARCOMA

I. INTRODUCTION
Malignant soft tissue tumor of uncertain histogenesis which usually occurs in proximity to joints and tendon sheaths.
"Synovial" sarcoma: Misnomer

Cell of origin isn't synovium.

II. ETIOPATHOLOGY

1. Chromosomal translocation t(X;18) > 90% cases.
   ↓
2. SYT – SSX$_1$ and SYT – SSX$_2$
   ↓
   Proto-oncogenes and tumor suppressor gene.
3. Epidemiology
   i. MC sarcoma found in young adults (15–40 years)
   ii. M > F: =1.2:1
   iii. MC malignant sarcoma of foot.
   iv. Most commonly occurs in the
       Extremities (70%)
       Trunk (15%)
4. Cell of origin: Controversial → MSC
                                 → Immature myoblasts.
5. Metastasis → Lung (MC)   } Poor prognosis.
               Lymph nodes

III. PRESENTATION

1. Growing mass in proximity to joint
2. Painless/painful
3. ↓ ROM of nearby joints.
4. Regional lymphadenopathy
5. Limp: Lower extremity
6. Constitutional symptoms—weight loss, fatigue, mild fever, loss of appetite.

IV. INVESTIGATIONS

1. *X-ray*:
   i. Soft tissue shadow
   ii. Calcification within (shadow): Focal
   iii. Resembles HO
   iv. Bone involvement rare.
2. *MRI*: Heterogenous mass. Dark on T$_1$. Bright on T$_2$.

V. HISTOPATHOLOGY

1. SS → Biphasic (> common)
      → Monophasic
2.

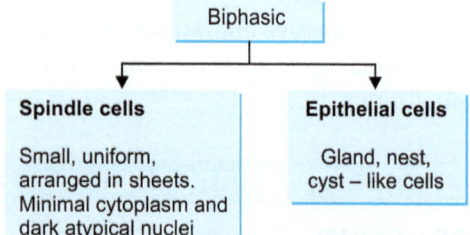

3. Immunohistochemistry → Vimentin (+)
                          S: 100 (+)
                          Cytokeratin (+)
                          (Epithelial cells)

VI. GROSS

1. Well circumscribed: Smooth pseudocapsule.
2. Firm
3. Grayish pink
4. May have necrosis and hemorrhage within.

VII. DIFFERENTIAL DIAGNOSIS

1. Fibrosarcoma
2. Adenocarcinoma
3. Mesothelioma
4. Small round cell tumor.

VIII. TREATMENT

1. Primarily surgical
   ↓
   Wide surgical resection
2. Adjuvant radiotherapy → Pre- or postoperative improved oncological outcome and overall survival.
3. Chemotherapy → High risk patients
   Doxorubicin
   Ifosfamide

MUSCLE BIOPSY

I. INDICATIONS

1. Muscle weakness → Static or progressive
2. Differentiate myogenic versus neurogenic cause
3. Suspected inflammatory myopathies
4. Collagen vascular diseases
5. Muscular dystrophies.

II. PRINCIPLES

1. Moderately affected muscles
2. Avoid severely/minimally affected muscles
3. From muscle belly, not tendon
4. Avoid previously injured sites → Injection and EMG sites
5. Ideal → Quadriceps, biceps
6. Postmortem → Up to 12 hours.

III. CONTRAINDICATIONS

1. Bleeding disorder
2. Endocrine myopathies (relative)
3. Malignant hyperthermia
4. Severely malnourished
5. Bone and Joint Infection

SECTION 10: Bone and Joint Infection

OSTEOMYELITIS–ACUTE AND CHRONIC

I. INTRODUCTION
1. Inflammation of bone and its marrow caused by infecting organism.
2. Acute osteomyelitis → Rapidly destructive pyogenic infection of the bone and its marrow.
   ↓
3. Most commonly in infants and children → usually starting in the metaphysis of an actively growing long bone.

II. CLASSIFICATION
1. Waldvogel and Lew et al.

Duration of symptoms	Source of infection	

• Acute: <2 weeks
• Subacute: 2–6 weeks (less virulent, host has increased immunity)
• Chronic: >6 weeks
	• Hematogenous: Originates from bacteremia
	• Contiguous
	  i. Trauma (external)
	  ii. Surgery (iatrogenic)
	  iii. From nearby tissue
		Presence/absence of generalized vascular disease

2. Cierny-Mader → Chronic osteomyelitis

A. Anatomic Type (Fig. 1)

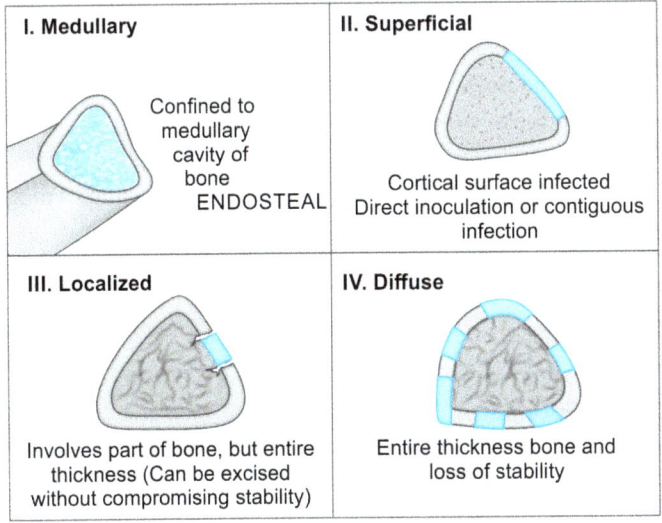

I. Medullary — Confined to medullary cavity of bone ENDOSTEAL
II. Superficial — Cortical surface infected Direct inoculation or contiguous infection
III. Localized — Involves part of bone, but entire thickness (Can be excised without compromising stability)
IV. Diffuse — Entire thickness bone and loss of stability

B. Physiologic Class
A: Host immunocompetent
B: Compromised immunity
Bs: Systemic factors
Bl: Localized factors
C: Severely compromised, unacceptable treatment-risk ratio

III. ETIOLOGY
A. Acute OM
1. *Age:* Infancy and childhood
2. *Sex:* Males > Females = 4:1
3. *Trauma:* History of direct blow frequently there
4. *Location:* Most actively growing end of long bone, metaphysis
5. Malnutrition
6. Remote focus of infection (tonsillitis)
7. *Microbe:* Infant: Most common—*S. aureus, S. Agalactiae, E. coli* >1 year—*S. aureus, S. pyogenes, H. influenzae* Adults most common—*S. aureus*
   Single pathogen → Hematogenous
   Multiple → Direct inoculation

IV. PATHOGENESIS

1. Infective embolus enters the nutrient artery
   ↓
2. Trapped in a vessel of small caliber
   ↓
3. Most of the small end arteries and capillaries are located in the metaphysis adjacent to the epiphyseal plate
   ↓
4. Metaphysis most affected because
   i. Poor phagocytic activity in metaphysis (Hobo's hypothesis)
   ii. U-shaped hair pin bend of small arterioles (Trueta)
   iii. Highly vascularized region
   ↓
Minor trauma
   ↓
Hemorrhage
   ↓
Locus minoris resistentiae
   ↓
Excellent culture medium

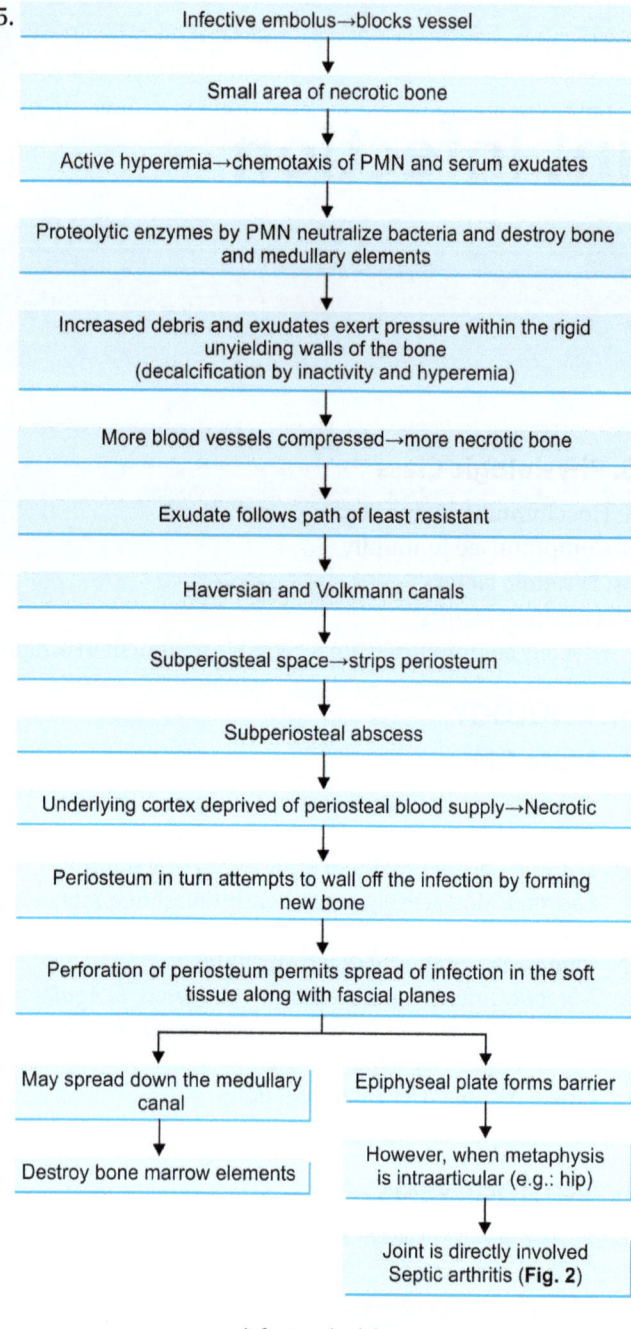

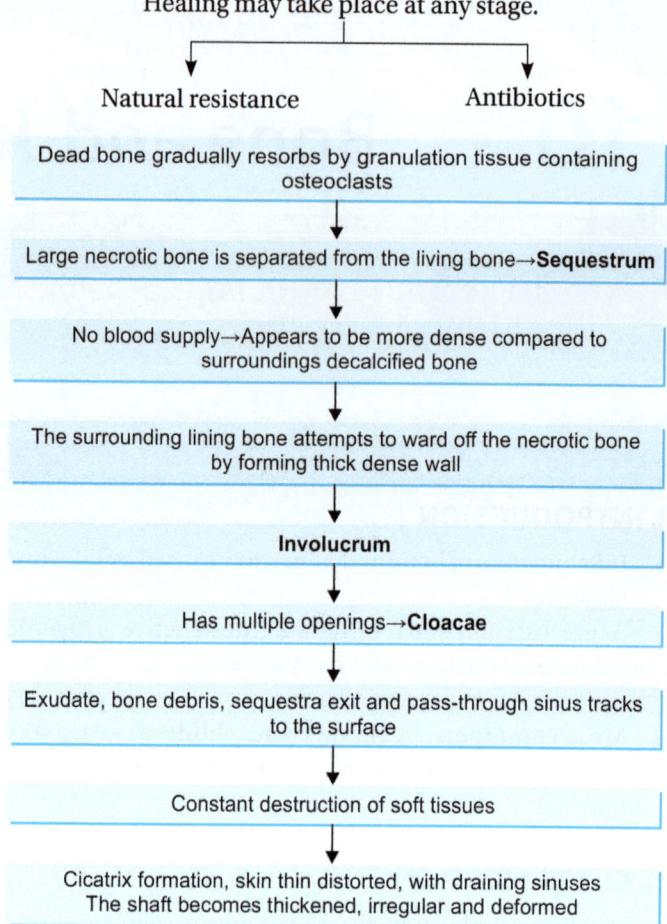

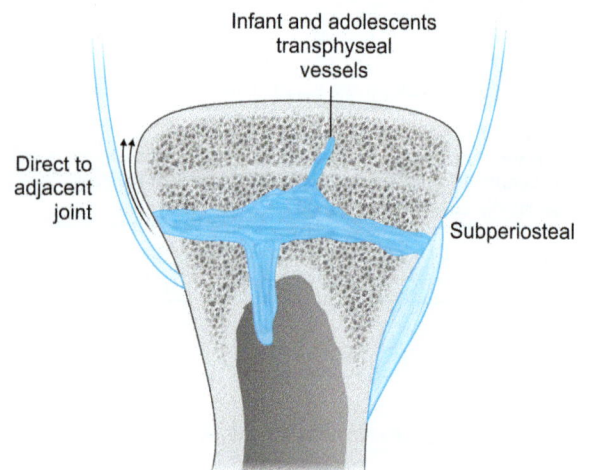

Fig. 2: Spread of infection.

V. CLINICAL PICTURE

A. Acute

1. *History of:*
   i. Pain in the limb
   ii. Recent local infection or trauma
2. *Symptoms:*
   i. Refusal to weight bear, severe pain
   ii. Fever
   iii. Irritable and restless
   iv. Vomiting, convulsions
3. *Signs and examinations:*
   i. Rapid pulse (tachycardia)
   ii. Redness, swelling → evident >few days
   iii. Warmth, tenderness
   iv. Restricted ROM, passive motion resisted due to pain (pseudoparalysis)
   v. Edematous

B. Chronic

1. History of on and off symptoms since childhood acute OM episode
2. During period of inactivity → no symptoms
3. Reactivation of infection → aching pain worse at night
4. Discharging sinus

5. Skin is dusky, thin, scarred, and poorly nourished
6. Break in skin→ ulceration→ allow to heal
7. Bone = Misshapen and thickened
8. Muscles = Scarred, contractures of adjacent joints
9. Overlying tissue = Swollen, edematous, warm, tender and reddened.
10. Sinus may extrude sequestra
11. Recurrent acute flare-ups occur at indefinite intervals over months and years
12. Relapse = Poor health conditions
13. *Walenkamp phenomenon:* Increase in pain over period of time and suddenly decreases with opening up sinus and pus discharge.

VI. DIAGNOSIS

A. Acute OM

1. *X-ray*:
   i. Early radiographs → Normal or loss of soft tissue planes (48-72 hours)
   ii. New periosteal bone formation = 5-7 days
   iii. Osteolysis = 10-14 days (localized osteopenia, trabecular destruction)
   iv. Late films (1-2 weeks) = Metaphyseal rarefaction or abscesses
2. USG = Juxtacortical soft tissue swelling
3. MRI = Gradually becoming the I.O.C → T1 hypointense, T2 hyperintense

   Early marrow and soft tissue edema
   ↓
   Can assist in decision making
4. Technetium 99 bone scan = Sensitive, but not specific
5. CT scan guided pus aspiration

B. Laboratory Findings

1. PMN leukocytosis
2. Elevated ESR, CRP = Increases in <6 hours, in 98% patients, Most sensitive to monitor treatment response. Best indicator of early treatment success. If there is failure in decline within 72 hours → Treatment alter
3. Bone aspiration: 50-70% → Positive cultures
4. Blood culture = 30-50% positive
5. Biopsy and culture = When diagnosis is not clear—rule out malignancy.

C. Chronic OM

1. Moth eaten appearance.
2. Osteoporotic bone and areas of sclerosis.
3. Sequestrum = Dense sclerotic dead bone, surrounded by reactive ring of new bone formation (involucrum)
4. Sequestrum depending on age of patient, pathogen, host response may be → tubular, coke like, cylindrical, ring.
5. The shaft becomes enlarged and misshapen
6. Narrow zone of decreased density between necrotic and living bone → resorption at surface of sequestrum.
7. Sinugram.

VII. TREATMENT

A. Acute OM

1. *Modes of treatment:*
   i. Antibiotic therapy
   ii. Surgical management
   iii. General treatment
   iv. Immobilization
2. **Nades principles** *for acute OM:*
   i. Antibiotic therapy is effective before pus forms (<48 hours)
   ii. Antibiotics cannot sterilize avascular tissue
   iii. Antibiotics prevent formation of pus once evacuated
   iv. Evacuation of pus → Restores blood flow to periosteum
   v. Antibiotics must be continued post-surgery.
2. *Antibiotic therapy:*
   i. Even before the confirmation of diagnosis and culture reports → empirical broad spectrum antibiotics must be started.
   ii. Second generation cephalosporins or penicillin as most common organisms is *S. aureus*
   iii. According to DST once results are obtained
   iv. MRSA suspicion or result = Vancomycin, Clindamycin
   v. 7 days IV followed by oral = 4-6 weeks
3. *Surgery indications:*
   i. Abscess formation (strongest indication)
   ii. Concomitant septic arthritis
   iii. Persistence of symptoms with no improvement for >48 hours of antibiotics
   iv. Slow progression, unsatisfactory clinically >72 hours of antibiotics
   v. Multifocal OM in ill and moribund child
   vi. Delayed presentation >7-10 days (immediate pus evacuation done to preserve as much as bone available
4. *Principles of surgery → Drainage of abscess and debridement*:
   i. Periosteum is incised longitudinally over the point maximally swollen
   ii. Stripped laterally = 1 cm on either side
   iii. Extensive stripping → Contraindicated

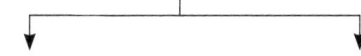

   Decreased blood supply   Allow exudates to spread
   iv. Multiple drill holes away from epiphyseal line
   v. Cortical window is made with help of osteotome → decreased intraosseous pressure and removes pus.
   iv. Postoperative immobilization = slab, cast
5. General treatment:
   i. Maintain hydration
   ii. High protein diet
   iii. Vitamin D, C and calcium

B. Chronic OM

1. *Goal of treatment (similar to orthopedic oncology)*:
   i. Arrest infection—local and systemic chemotherapy
   ii. Radical surgical eradication of infected bone and soft tissue
   iii. Retain functional limb
2. *Timing of intervention*:
   i. Acute phase subsided, no fever
   ii. Discontinue antibiotics 1 week before surgery
   iii. Sequestrum → must be separated from parent bone (2–3 months)
   iv. Involucrum = Strong → 3 cortices on 2 perpendicular views
   v. Klemm's triad → a. Vitality and stability of bone
   　　　　　　　　　　b. Condition of soft tissue envelope
   　　　　　　　　　　c. Virulence of organism
   　　　Identifies chances of providing functional limb
3. *Principles of surgical treatment of OM*:
   i. Bone and soft tissue debridement of infected and necrotic tissue and drainage
   ii. Removal of metal implants, hardware and foreign body
   iii. Stabilization of bone
   iv. Local antibiotic therapy
   v. Dead space management
   vi. *Reconstruction*:
      a. Soft tissue
      b. Bone.

1. TISSUE DEBRIDEMENT

i. *Sequestrectomy and saucerization* (**Fig. 3**):
   All sequestra, scar tissue and surrounding dense bone excised until
   ↓
   Bed of raw bleeding cancellous bone
   ↓
   Paprika skin

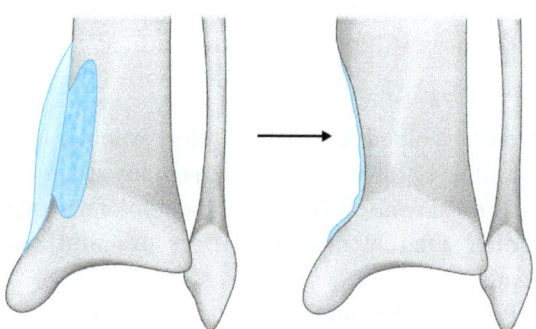

ii. *For closed cavities, Lautenbach method maybe used*:
   Debridement → Reaming → Double lumen catheter (Antibiotic) (**Fig. 4**)

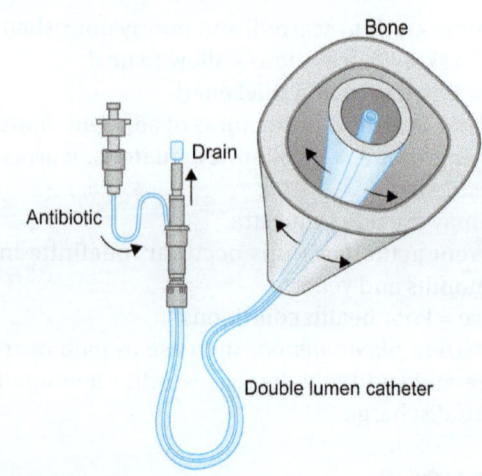

2. BONE STABILIZATION

1. External factors
2. Ilizarov
3. Slabs, splints

3. LOCAL ANTIBIOTIC THERAPY

1. High local levels facilitate delivery of antibiotics to avascular area of bone.
2. Extremely high concentration achieved locally without systemic toxicity.
3. Delivery systems also help in dead space management.
4. Delivery systems

Nonbiodegradable	Biodegradable
a. Bone cement	a. Bone graft substitutes $CaPO_4$
b. PMMA beads	$CaSO_4$, HA, ceramics, polymers

5. Antibiotic impregnated cement

4. DEAD SPACE MANAGEMENT

A. Soft Tissue Defect

i. Local muscle flap → Myoplasty
ii. Myocutaneous flap → Rotational
　　　　　　　　　　　→ Free vascularized
iii. Papineau technique → Open bone grafting technique (**Fig. 5**)

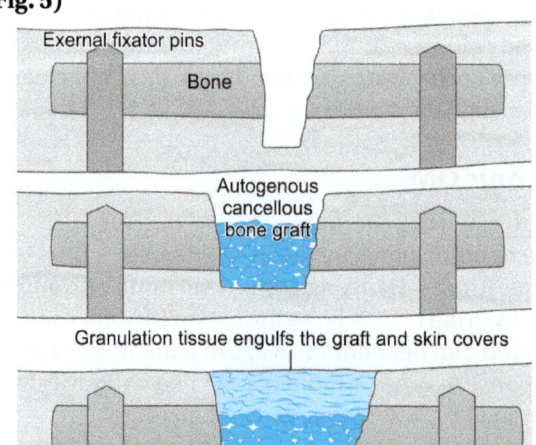

Principles:
a. Granulation tissue markedly resists infection
b. The infected area is completely excised
c. Autogenous cancellous BG rapidly revascularizes and resists infection
d. Adequate drainage
e. Antibiotics
iv. Bead-pouch technique **(Fig. 6)**

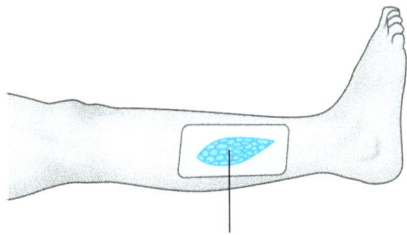

v. Induced membrane technique = Masquelet
vi. Bone transport = Ilizarov ring fixator
vii. Huntington's procedure = Tibialization of fibula **(Fig. 7)**

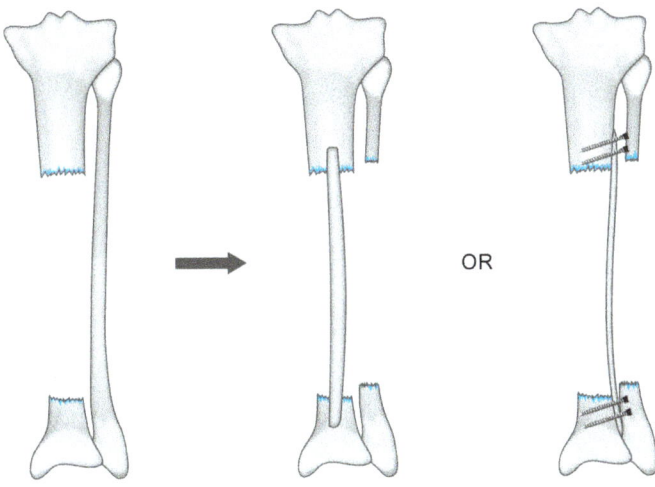

TYPES OF SEQUESTRUM

A piece of devitalized bone that has been separated from its surrounding bone during the process of necrosis.
1. Tubular or diaphyseal sequestrum—acute pyogenic osteomyelitis
2. Ring sequestrum—amputation stump and at Steinmann pins
3. Ivory sequestrum—syphilis
4. Fine sandy—viral osteomyelitis
5. Coarse sandy—out of cavity TB (e.g., central body of vertebra)
6. Flake or feathery sequestrum—in the cavity tuberculosis (for example, TB rib)
7. Kissing sequestrum—peridiscal TB vertebra
8. Button hole sequestrum is seen after radiation
9. Coke sequestrum—cancellous bone
10. Bombay or black—H2S and pollution
11. Black sequestrum—actinomycosis
12. Granular sequestrum—Salmonella osteomyelitis **(Fig. 8)**

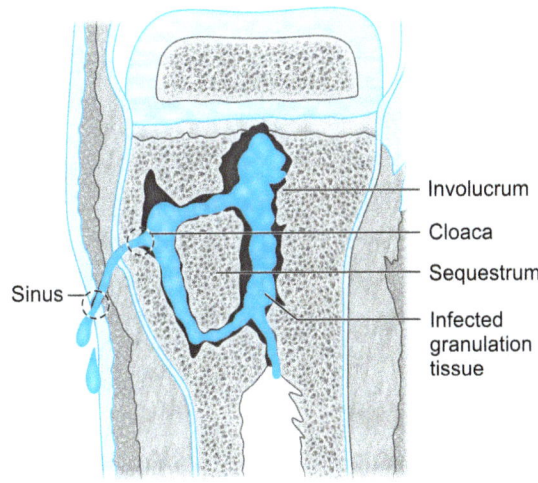

SEPTIC ARTHRITIS

I. INTRODUCTION
Pathological microbial invasion of joint space followed by inflammation.

II. ROUTE OF SPREAD
1. *Hematogenous*: Most common
2. *Direct inoculation*:
   i. Arthrocentesis
   ii. Intra-articular injections
   iii. Animal or human bite
   iv. Trauma
   v. Thorn injury
3. *Contiguous spread in joints with intra-articular epiphysis* **(Figs. 9A and B)**:
   i. Proximal femur
   ii. Distal fibula
   iii. Proximal humerus
   iv. Radial head

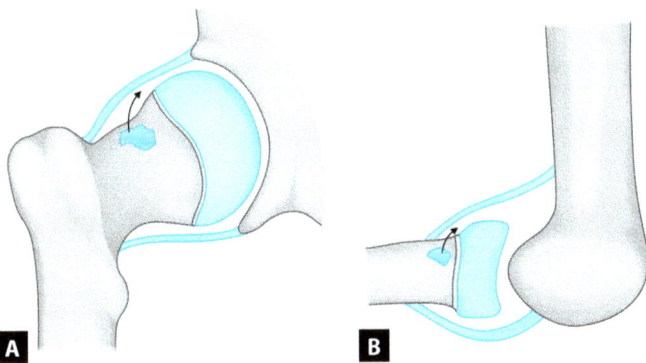

Figs. 9A and B: (A) Proximal femur; (B) Proximal radius.

4. *Metaphyseal extension of infective focus*: Patent transepiphyseal vessel in children < 18 months
5. *Combined*:
   i. Joint arthroplasty
   ii. Tissue allografts

III. RISK FACTORS

1. Age > 80 years
2. DM
3. RA
4. Gout
5. Prosthetic joint
6. Recent joint surgery
7. Skin infection
8. Sickle cell disease
9. End stage renal disease
10. Advance hepatic disease
11. HIV infection
12. Previous septic arthritis
13. IV drug abusers
14. Hemophilia
15. Underlying malignancy
16. Hypogammaglobulinemia
17. Late complement component deficiency

IV. PATHOPHYSIOLOGY

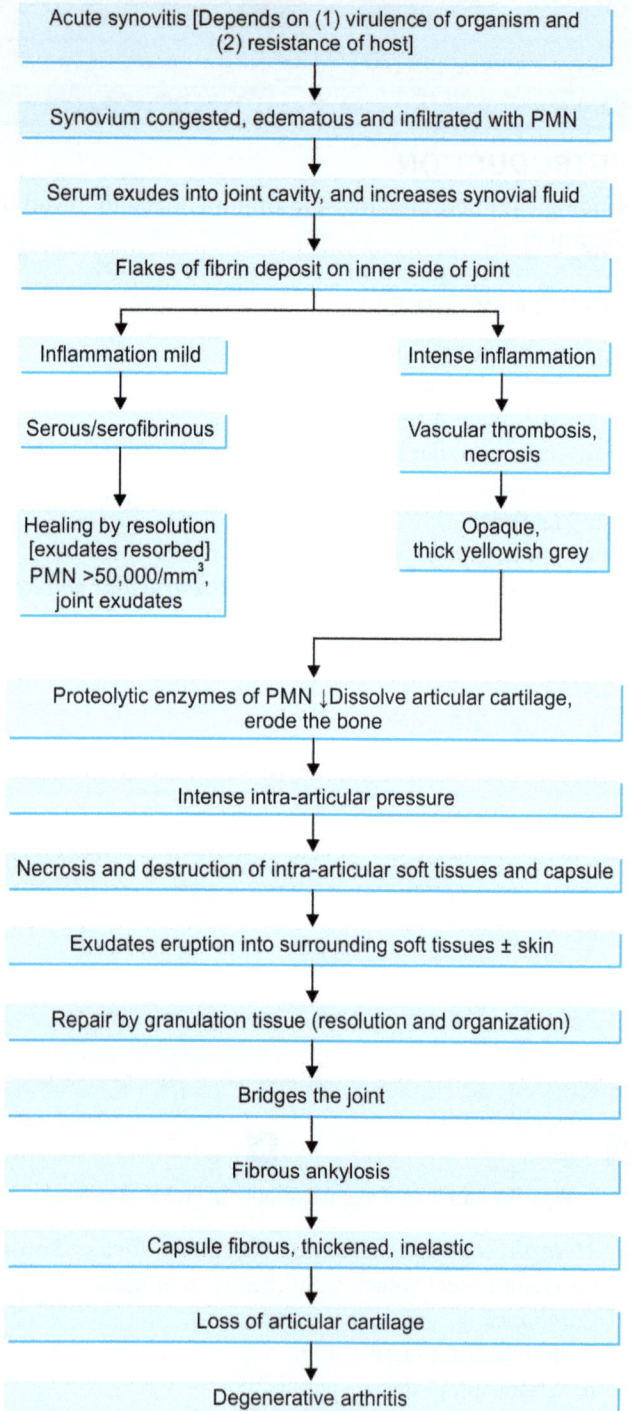

MC → *Staphylococcus aureus*

Microbials common in specific clinical settings.
1. Sexually active young adult—*Neisseria gonorrhoeae*
2. Trauma—Gram-ve bacilli, anaerobes, *S. aureus*
3. Prosthesis: Early—*S. epidermidis*
   Late—Gram-ve cocci, anaerobes
4. IV drug abusers—Pseudomonas
5. RA—*S. aureus*
6. Sickle cell disease and SLE—*Salmonella*
7. Hemophilia—*S. aureus*, Streptococcus
8. Immunosuppression—*S. aureus*, *Mycobacterium*, fungi
9. Neonate—*S. aureus*
10. <2 years—*H. influenzae*, *S. aureus*
11. >2 years—*S. aureus*

V. DIFFERENTIAL DIAGNOSIS (MONOARTICULAR ARTHRITIS)

1. Infection
2. Crystal induced arthritis (Gout, Ca-Pyrophosphate)
3. Trauma
4. Hemarthrosis (Hemophilia, Sickle cell anemia)
5. Osteomyelitis
6. Periarticular syndrome (Bursitis, tendinitis)
7. Ruptured Bakers cyst
8. Deep vein thrombosis
9. Pigmented villonodular synovitis
10. Foreign body
11. OA (acute exacerbation)

VI. CLINICAL FEATURES

1. Fever, rigors ±
2. Warmth
3. Tenderness } of the affected joint
4. Swelling
5. Redness
6. Muscles in protective spasm, Hip → FAbEr, knee → flexion, patella floating
7. Restricted active and passive range of motion
8. Inability to bear weight
9. *In children*:
    i. Fever
    ii. Malaise
    iii. Poor appetite
    iv. Irritability
    v. Reluctance to use affected limb
10. *In neonates*:
    i. Classical signs of fever, malaise, usually absent
    ii. Diagnosis difficult
    iii. Refusal to feed
    iv. Cyanosis during feed
    v. Abdominal distension
    vi. Presence of focus of infection
    vii. Edema of LL/buttocks/genitalia
    viii. Crying on handling

VII. IMAGING

A. Radiograph

1. Joint space widening or effusion
2. Periarticular osteopenia
3. Soft tissue swelling
4. Displacement of fat pad
5. As infection progresses → Joint space narrowing from destruction of cartilage
6. Waldenstrom's sign—increased distance between pelvic teardrop and FH
7. Obturator sign.

B. USG

1. Used to detect small collections of fluid deep in the joints
2. Differentiated between septic arthritis and bursitis, cellulitis by identifying the plane of collection.
3. Non-echo-free effusions from clotted hemorrhagic collections
4. Used to guide initial joint aspiration
5. Inexpensive but heavily operator dependent

C. MRI

Infection extent, abscess formation, status of articular cartilage, viability of FH, adjacent bone involvement → OM.

D. Bone Scan

Increased uptake both in early and "blood pool" images at periarticular region.

VIII. LABORATORY FINDINGS

A. **Kocher's** *criteria (lab + clinical)*   All 4 = 99.6%
   i. Fever > 38.5 °C   3 = 93.1%
   ii. ESR > 40 mm/h   2 = 40%
   iii. Inability to bear weight   1 = 3%
   iv. WBC > 12,000 cells/μL of serum   0 = 0.2%

B. *Septic joint aspirate:*
   i. WBC > 50,000/mm³
   ii. >75% PMN
   iii. Glucose 50 mg/dL < Serum levels
   iv. High lactic acid levels
   v. Appearance → Thick, purulent, yellowish grey
   vi. Crystal analysis
   vii. Gram stain
   viii. Culture

C. *Blood culture:* Maybe +ve when patient is febrile

D. Urine RM and C/S

E. *Lumbar puncture:* Consider in a septic joint by *H. influenzae*, if signs of meningitis present.

IX. TREATMENT

1. Orthopedic emergency
2. *Principles*:
   i. Adequate drainage of joint and resection of infected tissue.
   ii. Antibiotics to diminish the systemic effects of sepsis.
   iii. Resting the joint in stable position.
   iv. Prompt drainage and evaluation of purulent joint fluid is crucial for preservation of articular cartilage and resolution of infection.
3. *Treatment algorithm*:

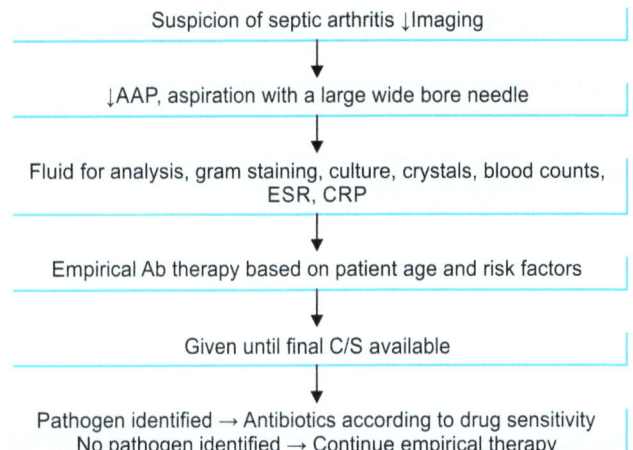

4. *Duration of Ab therapy depends on*:
   i. Type of infecting organism
   ii. Condition of patient
   iii. Response to therapy
   Conventionally—3 weeks of antibiotics (IV) f/b oral antibiotics. (Recent clinical trials → Oral antibiotics as effective as IV)
5. Early drainage of joint → Controversial

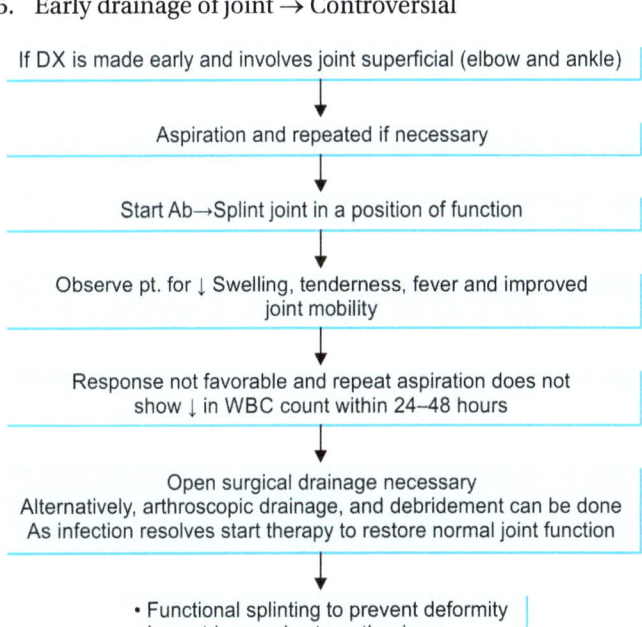

6. For patients with varying degrees of deformity:
    i. Traction
    ii. Dynamic splinting
    iii. Serial casting
    iv. Passive exercises
7. Empirical Ab
    i. Gram +ve cocci (clusters)
        a. MSSA → Third-generation cephalosporin (ceftriaxone)
        b. MRSA → Vancomycin, clindamycin, linezolid
    ii. Gram –ve diplococci → 3rd-generation cephalosporin (*N. gonorrhoeae*) (ceftriaxone) or FQ
    iii. Gram +ve cocci chain (*Streptococcus*) → 3rd-generation cephalosporin (xone)
    iv. Gram –ve bacilli →
        a. Enterobacteriaceae → Piptaz, FQ, third-generation cephalosporin (Ceftazidime)
        b. Pseudomonas → Ceftazidime + AG or meropenem + AG
8. Fluids
9. Blood transfusions
10. Highly nourishing diet

TUBERCULOSIS OF HIP

I. INTRODUCTION

Second most common musculoskeletal region affected after Tb spine.

II. SITE (FIG. 10)

1. Acetabular roof—most common
2. Epiphysis
3. Neck/metaphysis
4. Greater trochanter

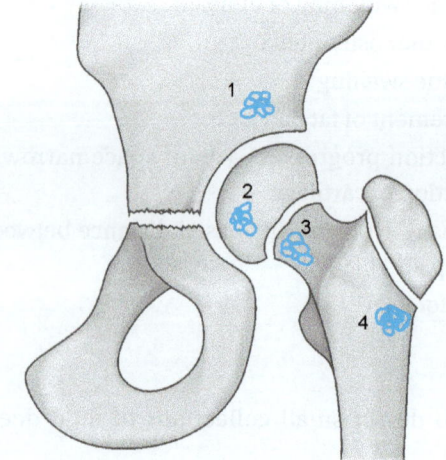

Fig. 10: Sites of infection in TB hip.

III. CLINICAL FEATURES

1. Insidious onset
2. Chronic course
3. Constitutional symptoms
4. Limp → Earliest symptom
5. Antalgic gait
6. Pain
7. Night cries
8. ↓ ROM
9. Fullness around the hip—cold abscess
10. Deformity—depending on the stage
11. Muscle wasting—gluteal and thigh
12. Limb length discrepancy
13. 2° changes (to fixed deformity of hip–Lordosis, scoliosis)

IV. CLINICORADIOLOGICAL STAGING (TULI)

Stages	Clinical findings	LLD	Radiological features
Synovitis	Flexion, abduction, external rotation (FABER)	Apparent lengthening	Haziness of articular margins and rarefaction
Early arthritis	Flexion, adduction, internal rotation (FADIR)	Apparent shortening	Osteopenia, bony erosions in femoral head and acetabulum
Advanced arthritis	FADIR	True shortening	Destruction of articular surface and joint space reduction
Advanced arthritis with subluxation/dislocation	FADIR	Gross shortening	Gross destruction, wandering acetabulum

V. RADIOLOGICAL CLASSIFICATION (SHANMUGASUNDARAM) (FIG. 11)

Type 1	Normal
Type 2	Travelling/wandering acetabulum
Type 3	Dislocating
Type 4	Perthes
Type 5	Protrusio acetabuli
Type 6	Atrophic
Type 7	Mortar and Pestle

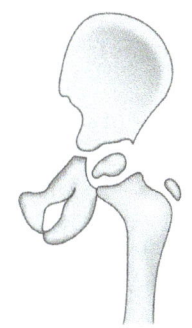
Type 1. Normal
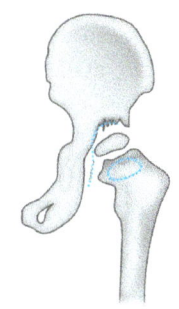
Type 2. Travelling acetabulum
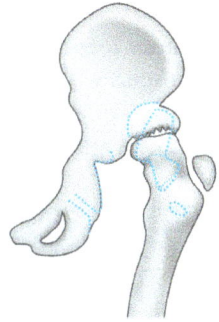
Type 3. Dislocating

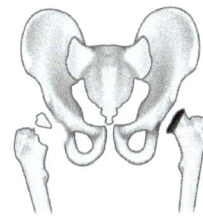
Type 4. Perthes
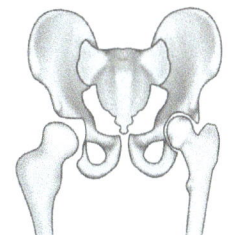
Type 5. Protrusio acetabuli
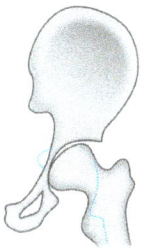
Type 6. Atrophic
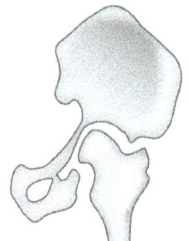
Type 7. Mortar and pestle

VI. INVESTIGATIONS
1. Periarticular osteopenia
2. Soft tissue shadows
3. Minimal periosteal reaction
4. Subchondral cysts and erosions
5. Joint space narrowing.

VII. MANAGEMENT
1. Multidrug antituberculous drug therapy
2. HRZE → 2 months (intensive)
3. HRE → 9-10 months (continuous)
4. Traction
    i. Relieves muscle spasm
    ii. Enforces rest
    iii. Prevents deformity
    iv. Maintains joint space
    v. Prevents pathological dislocation
5. Abduction deformity → Traction more on the well leg. (As ASIS is lower on affected side)
6. Adduction → Traction more on the affected leg
7. Assisted active movement of hip is encouraged during traction
8. Protected weight bearing after 4 months with orthosis
9. Palpable cold abscess → Aspiration
10. *Surgical options*:
    i. Synovectomy/joint debridement
    ii. Excision arthroplasty
    iii. Arthrodesis
    iv. Corrective osteotomies
    v. Total hip arthroplasty
11. *Stage I—synovitis*:
    i. Excellent outcomes on ATT and mobilization
    ii. Synovectomy:
        a. When diagnosis uncertain
        b. Poor clinical response to ATT
    iii. Prognosis → Patients usually have full mobility after treatment
12. *Stage II—Early arthritis*:
    i. Synovectomy—Same as stage I
    ii. Prognosis—70% retained mobility
13. *Stage III and IV—Late arthritis and pathological sub/dislocations*
    i. Initial traction and ATT
    ii. Outcome → Gross fibrous ankylosis
    iii. Girdlestone excisional arthroplasty
        a. Active or painful healed disease in adults
        b. Provides painless, mobile, unstable joint with 3-5 cm shortening
        c. Femoral head-neck and proximal part of the trochanter excised
        d. Postoperatively traction in 30° abduction for 8-12 weeks
        e. Mobilization → Ischial weight-relieving caliper
        f. Severe instability → Pelvic support osteotomy
    iv. *Arthrodesis*:
        a. *Age*: 18 years
        b. *Position*:
            10° adduction (latest consensus)
            5-10° external rotation
            10-30° flexion
        c. *Types*:
            → Intra-articular
            → Extra-articular — Hibbs iliofemoral
                                Brittain ischiofemoral
            → Combined

v. *Total hip arthroplasty*:
   a. Gained popularity leading to ↓ arthrodesis and excisional arthroplasty
   b. Timing: Controversial → However, general consensus 1–3 years after healing of the disease.

TB SPINE

I. MYCOBACTERIUM TUBERCULOSIS— THE *BACILLUS*

1. Properties

Obligate	Aerobe	Acid-fast
Non-motile	Rod-shaped	Non-sporing

2. Does not produce biofilm around implants.
3. Osteoarticular TB–Paucibacillary

II. PATHOGENESIS OF TUBERCULOSIS

1. Pulmonary TB–75%, extrapulmonary–25%
   ↓
   Bone and joint TB 15% of extrapulmonary TB
   ↓
   TB Spine 50% of bone and joint TB (most common)
   TB hip–second most common
2. TB infection
   ↓
   Activation of reticuloendothelial system
   ↓
   Accumulation of PMNs
   ↓
   Rapidly replaced with macrophages and monocytes (phagocytes)
   ↓
   Formation of epithelioid cells → Pale cells with vesicular nucleus with
   (characteristic of TB infection) abundant cytoplasm with indistinct margin
   ↓
   Fusion of large number of epithelioid cells
   ↓
   Langerhan's giant cells (Function-To digest and remove necrosed tissue)
   ↓
   After 1 week, lymphocytes appear and form a ring around peripheral part of lesion.
   ↓
   Tubercle (caseating necrosis)

III. PATHOGENESIS OF SPINAL TUBERCULOSIS (FIG. 12)

1. Secondary to a primary focus of infection via a hematogenous route.
2. Spine highly predisposed due to abundant vascularity of vertebral bodies.
3. Paradiscal (most common): From anterior and posterior spinal arteries → vascular plexus in subchondral region of each vertebra.
4. Central: Valveless paravertebral Batson's venous plexus.
5. Anterior: Begins as destructive lesion in the anterior margins of the vertebral body, usually not involving the disc spaces.
6. Posterior elements: Affects posterior arch, without involvement of the body.

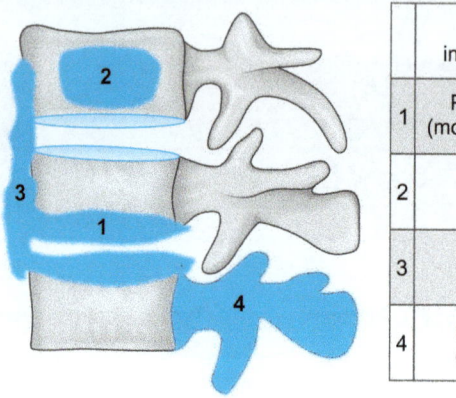

IV. CLINICAL FEATURES

A. Symptoms

1. Malaise
2. Loss of appetite
3. Loss of weight
4. Evening rise of fever
5. Night sweats
6. Night cries → Muscle spasm relaxes during sleep permitting movement between inflamed surfaces causing pain.
7. Weakness, bedridden

B. Examination

Paraspinal muscle spasm
Kyphotic deformity: Knuckle → Single vertebral involvement
                    Gibbus → 2-3 vertebrae
Tenderness → Spinous process
Swelling → Cold abscess
Sinus

C. Neurological Classification (Tuli)

I.	Negligible	Patient unaware of neural deficit. Physician detects extensor plantar response
II.	Mild	Patient aware of deficit but manages to walk without support
III.	Moderate	Non-ambulatory because of paralysis in extension. Sensory loss <50%
IV.	Severe	III + Flexor spasm/Paralysis in flexion/Flaccid/Sensory loss >50%/Sphincters involved

V. CLINICORADIOLOGICAL CLASSIFICATION (KUMAR)

Stage	Clinicoradiological features	Duration
1. Predestructive	• Straightening of curvature • Spasm of paravertebral muscles • Radiolucency • Endplate haziness • Paraspinal soft tissue shadows • MRI (IOC): Marrow edema	<3 months
2. Early destructive	• Diminished disk space + prediscal erosion (K <10°) • MRI: Marrow edema and break in osseous margins • CT: Marginal erosions and cavitations	2–4 months
3, 4, 5 all have vertebral bodies destruction and collapse + appreciable kyphosis		
3. Mild angular kyphosis	2–3 vertebrae involved (K = 10–30°)	3–9 months
4. Moderate angular kyphosis	>3 vertebrae involved (K = 30–60°)	9–24 months
5. Severe kyphosis (humpback)	>3 vertebrae involved (K ≥ 60°)	>2 years

Other Radiological Features

K is the angle of kyphosis measured by technique of Dickson.

Method of measurement of angle of kyphosis (Dickson) **(Fig. 13)**.

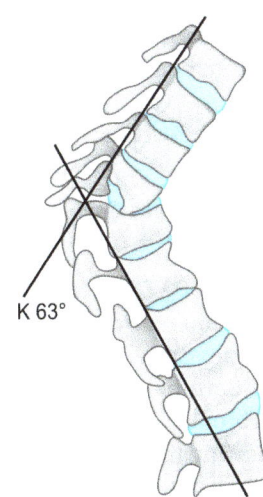

Line drawn along the posterior margins of healthy vertebrae above and below the site of disease.

Angle 'K' increases with increase in degree of kyphosis.

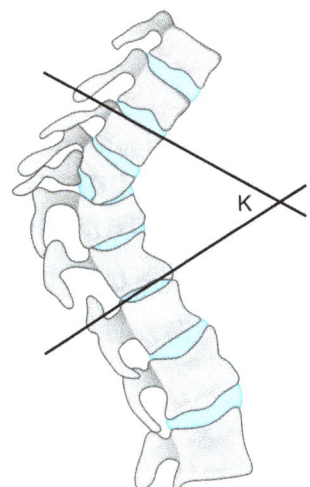

Alternative method for calculating of kyphotic angle.

Angle between the upper end plate of normal vertebrae proximal to affected vertebrae and the lower end plate of the normal vertebra distal to affected vertebrae **(Fig. 14)**.

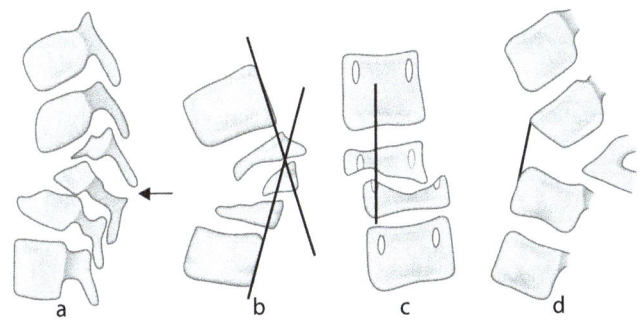

MRI

1. Investigation of choice → Early detection
2. Inflammation → Hypointense T1, hyperintense T2
3. Reduced disc height → due to weakened end plates
4. Scalloping of anterior surface of vertebrae → due to periosteal stripping and devascularization
5. Paravertebral abscess: Mixed signal changes on T1 and T2
6. Post Gadolinium contrast → Thick peripheral rim enhancement: Abscess. Uniform enhancement: Granulation Tissue
7. Cord changes → Myelomalacia: Bright T2 signal within the cord
8. Marrow edema
9. End-plate erosions
10. Subligamentous spread.

VI. SPINE AT RISK SIGNS (RAJASEKARAN) (FIG. 15)

Identifies disease in children with high risk of developing severe deformity.

v. Assists in correction of deformity
   vi. Allows early mobilization and rehabilitation
   vii. MTB does not form biofilms → Safe to use
   viii. Pedicle screws and rod system most commonly used.

D. Surgical Approaches

1. *Posterior*:
   i. Minimal vertebral destruction
   ii. Mild kyphosis and no significant instability
   iii. Cannot be done in patients with severe kyphosis and destruction of 3 or more bodies

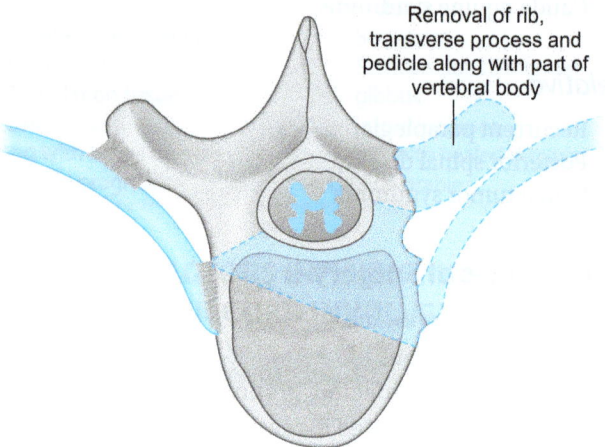

Fig. 16: Costotransversectomy.

2. *Posterolateral*:
   i. Familiarity
   ii. Circumferential exposure of spinal cord
   iii. Simultaneous anterior reconstruction possible
       a. Costotransversectomy **(Fig. 16)**
       b. Transpedicular
       c. Transfacetectomy
   iv. Decreased morbidity compared to anterior
3. *Anterior*:
   i. Adequate neural decompression
   ii. Direct reconstruction of defect
   iii. Rapid healing of lesion
   iv. Technically challenging in upper thoracic and lower lumbar levels
   v. ↑Complications: Major vessel, visceral injury
4. *Combined*:
   i. Staged procedure
   ii. Significant kyphotic deformity
   iii. Junctional lesion–Thoracolumbar
   iv. Three or more vertebral body involvement.

XV. NOTE ON ANTITUBERCULOUS DRUGS

First-line drugs	Dose and property	ADR
Isoniazid	5 mg/kg Most effective bactericidal drug	Hepatitis Peripheral neuropathy CNS toxicity

Contd...

First-line drugs	Dose and property	ADR
Rifampicin	10 mg/kg Kills the persisters	Red colored urine Flu-like symptoms Hepatitis
Ethambutol	15 mg/kg	Color blindness Peripheral neuritis
Pyrazinamide	30 mg/kg	Hepatoxicity Hyperuricemia
Second-line drugs		
Injectables		
Streptomycin		Nephrotoxicity Ototoxicity
Kanamycin	15 mg/kg	
Amikacin		
Capreomycin		
Fluoroquinolones		
Ofloxacin		GI disturbances Tendonitis, tendon rupture Hypersensitivity Muscle and joint pains Headache and insomnia Anxiety and psychosis
Levofloxacin		
Moxifloxacin		
Gatifloxacin	15 mg/kg	
Others		
Ethionamide		Abdominal pain Hepatotoxicity
Prothionamide		
Cycloserine	15 mg/kg	Depression Headache Seizures
Terizidone		Neurologic and psychiatric disturbances
p-aminosalicyclic acid	150 mg/kg	Hypersensitivity
Linezolid	600 mg daily	Myelosuppression Serotonin syndrome
Amoxycillin/clavulanate	875/125 BD	Diarrhea
High dose isoniazid	15 mg/kg	Peripheral neuropathy
New drugs		
Bedaquiline	600 mg weekly	Nausea, vomiting QT prolongation Headaches Hypersensitivity and rash
Delaminid	200 mg daily	Abdominal pain Dizziness Nausea and vomiting

Multidrug Resistant MDR-TB: Isoniazid and Rifampicin resistance

Extensively resistant XDR-TB: Isoniazid + rifampicin + any fluoroquinolone + at least one of the injectables.

Total drug resistant TDR-TB: Resistance to all available ATT drugs.

PSOAS ABSCESS

I. ANATOMY (FIG. 17)

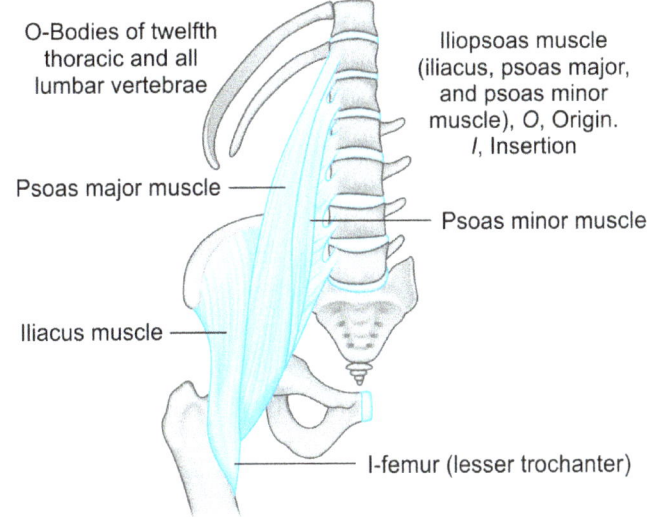

1. *Psoas major muscle*: Supplied by lumbar plexus, origin is from lateral border of T_{12}–L_5
2. *Iliacus muscle*: Origin from upper 2/3rd of iliac fossa, lateral sacrum
3. Both the muscles have common insertion at lesser trochanter
4. Lies in close proximity to organs such as:
   i. Sigmoid colon
   ii. Appendix, jejunum
   iii. Ureters, pancreas
   iv. Kidney, iliac LN
   v. Spine
5. *Nerve supply*: L_1, L_2, L_3, L_4
6. *Function*: Hip flexion

A. PSOAS ABSCESS

Collection of pus in iliopsoas compartment

→ Classification
Psoas abscess

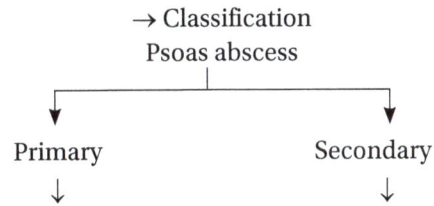

Primary
1. Hematogenous spread from an occult source Source of infection
2. Occurs in patients with immunocompromised
   i. DM
   ii. HIV
   iii. IV drug abusers
   iv. Renal failure
3. *Staph Aureus*

Secondary
1. Due to infection from adjacent organ.
2. Can be
   i. Pyogenic
   ii. Tuberculosis
       ↓
       Pott's spine

II. CLINICAL FEATURES

A. Classical Triad
1. Fever
2. Back ache
3. Limp

B. Other
1. Flank pain
2. Malaise
3. Weight loss
4. Nausea
5. Referred pain to groin or knee
6. Swelling in inguinal region.

C. Tests to Elicit Iliopsoas Inflammation
1. The examiner places his hand just proximal to I/L knee and patient is asked to lift his thigh against examiner's hand.
   ↓
   This will cause contraction of psoas and results in pain → Ludloff's Sign
2. With the patient lying on normal side, hyperextension of affected hip results in pain as psoas muscle is stretched.

D. Differential Diagnosis
1. Hernia
2. Enlarged inguinal LN
3. Iliac artery aneurysm
4. Tumors arising from pelvis or lumbar region

E. Complications
1. Intraperitoneal rupture
2. Septicemia
3. DVT
4. Hydronephrosis

F. Investigations
1. CBC = ↑WBC, ↓Hb
2. ↑ESR
3. ↑CRP
4. Blood culture
5. X-ray = Abdomen → Bulge in psoas
   KUB
   Spine
6. USG
7. CT abdomen = gold standard → low density mass retroperitoneum.
8. MRI-Lumbar spine → Koch's spine
9. Pus → Culture
       → Sensitivity

10. Pus → Gram staining
          → AFB

III. MANAGEMENT
1. Antibiotics → Primary
              → Empirical antistaphylococcal
              → Culture specific
2. Antituberculous therapy
3. Drainage
   i. CT-guided percutaneous drainage
   ii. Open extraperitoneal
      a. Through lateral loin incision
      b. Petits triangle
              ↓
         Boundaries
      c. Medially = Latissimus dorsi
      d. Laterally = EO muscle
      e. Inferiorly = Iliac crest
      f. Floor = Inferior oblique.

MYCETOMA/MADURA FOOT

I. INTRODUCTION
1. Chronic granulomatous infection of exogenous origin often localized to foot.
2. "Madura foot" (term used by Gill in 1842) possibly originates from the modern reporting of disease from Madurai, Tamil Nadu.
3. The infection evolves from multiple nodules beneath the skin followed by formation of cavities within the mass and sinuses (6–12 months) with oozing and colored granules.

II. Risk Factors
1. Minor trauma/thorn prick
2. Walking barefoot
3. Agricultural work and farming, thorny sharp vegetable material
4. Arid hot regions with sunshine, i.e, tropical climate
5. Immunosuppressed patients: HIV infection, postrenal transplant, diabetes

III. ORGANISM

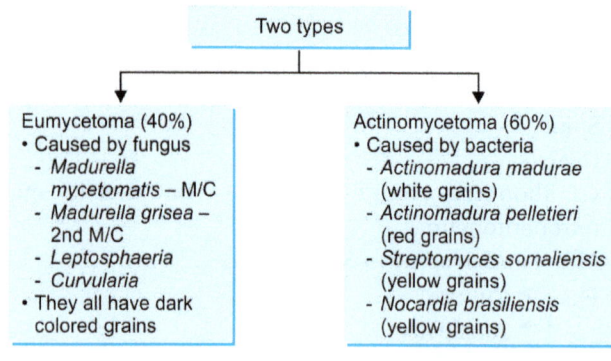

IV. ETIOPATHOGENESIS
1. Initial injury and inoculation of organism
           ↓
   Subcutaneous swelling
           ↓
   Subcutaneous nodule
           ↓
   Sinus formation and pus discharge
2. Host reaction is in the form of granulomatous inflammation.
3. Spread is via following the fascial planes, lymphatic and hematogenous spread are uncommon.

V. CLINICAL FEATURES
1. Painless subcutaneous swelling
           ↓
   Transforms into small, single, painless nodule
           ↓
   The nodule then increases in size, becomes fixed to underlying tissue
           ↓
   Host inflammatory reaction produces cavities and sinuses that discharge typical grains and pus
2. Pus is viscous, translucent yellowish fluid resembling oil.
3. Pain is seen in later stages due to involvement of bone.
4. Scarred skin, discoloration, ulceration.
5. In advanced stage, there is development of deformities and disability.
6. With further progression, regional lymphatic obstruction and fibrosis occurs causing lymphedema and erythema.

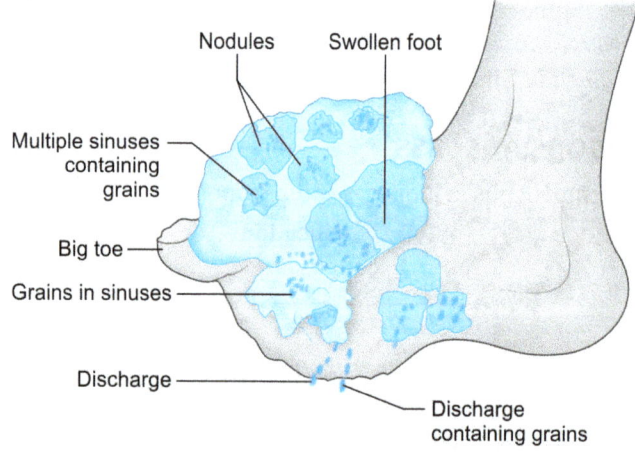

VI. DIAGNOSIS
1. Clinical features of swelling, nodule formation, sinus formation and ultimately pus discharge
2. O/E:
   i. Prolonged duration of the disease
   ii. Absence of pain (especially in early stages of the disease)
   iii. Discharge of grains from the sinus

3. Culture: Gold standard
4. Histopathological examination of the grains
   i. Eumycetoma: Granulomas surrounded by neutrophils and palisading histiocytes. Fungal grains contain short hyphae (branched filaments).
   ii. Actinomycetoma: Chronic abscess surrounded by granulation tissue and fibrosis, lined by neutrophils. Actinomycotic grains contain very fine filaments.
5. Triad:

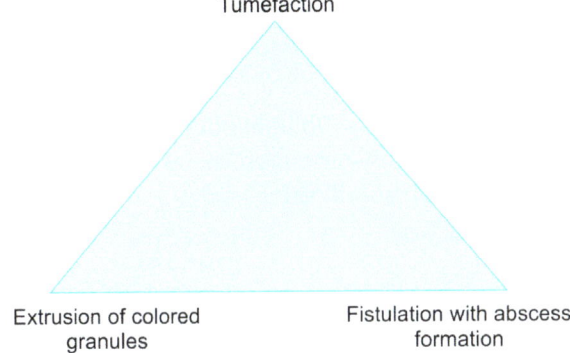

VII. RADIOGRAPHIC FINDINGS

1. Stage 0: Soft tissue swelling (d/t soft tissue granuloma)
2. Stage 1: Pressure effects of swelling on bone (bone scalloping d/t external pressure)
3. Stage 2: Periosteal reaction
4. Stage 3: Cortical erosion and medullary invasion (multiple punched out cavities)
5. Stage 4: Infection spreads along single ray
6. Stage 5: Horizontal spread along other rays
7. Stage 6: Multidirectional and random uncontrolled spread

VIII. TREATMENT

A. Medical Management

1. Actinomycetoma:
   i. Welsh regimen:
      a. Co-trimoxazole + amikacin × 4 weeks
         ↓ f/b
         Co-trimoxazole + doxycycline × 6–8 months
      b. Rifampicin can be added to the above regimen to produce prolonged remission
      c. In resistant cases, streptomycin is the DOC
   ii. Ramam two-step regimen
      a. Intensive phase consisting of gentamicin/amikacin + co-trimoxazole for 5–7 weeks
      b. Maintenance phase consisting of co-trimoxazole + amoxicillin for 2–5 months
2. Eumycetoma: Madurella mycetomatis classically responds to itraconazole 400 mg/day for 3 months f/b 200 mg/day for 9 months

B. Surgical Management

1. Debridement with extended margins
   i. Augments medical treatment
   ii. Reduces the size of the lesion and deformity.
2. Amputation, in cases of extensive infection and deformed limb.

SECTION 11

Trauma

MONTEGGIA FRACTURE–DISLOCATION

Fracture of the proximal ulna + Radio capitellar joint dislocation + Proximal radioulnar joint dislocation.

I. BADO CLASSIFICATION (FIG. 1)

(I) Anterior fracture dislocation
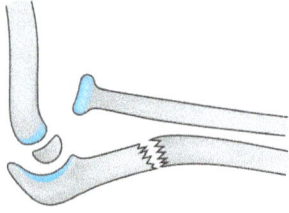

(II) Posterior fracture dislocation
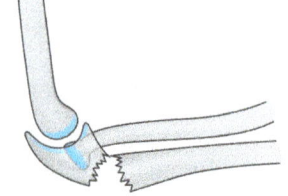

(III) Ulnar metaphysis fracture and lateral dislocation
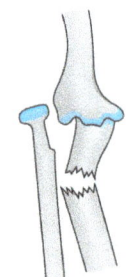

(IV) I + radius fracture at level of ulna
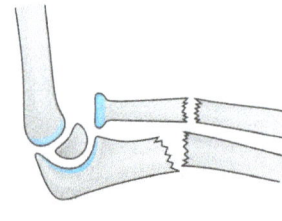

Most common in children and overall → I
2nd most common in children → II
Most common in adults → II

II. MONTEGGIA EQUIVALENTS

Type I = **(Fig. 2)**
1. Isolated radial head dislocation
2. Ulna fracture + Radial neck fracture
3. Isolated radial neck fracture
4. Elbow dislocation

Type II equivalent – Posterior radial head dislocation + fracture radial neck + Ulna fracture.

Type III equivalent – Oblique ulna fracture with varus (lateral angulation) + displaced lateral condyle fracture.
Type IV equivalent → floating elbow

(I) Isolated radial head dislocation
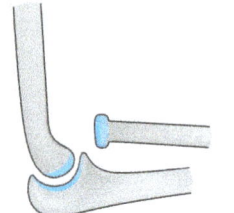

(II) Ulna fracture + Radial neck fracture
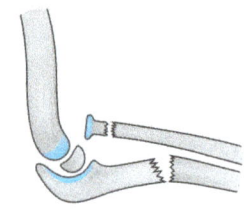

(III) Isolated radial neck fracture
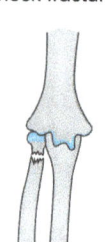

(IV) (Ulnohumeral) elbow dislocation
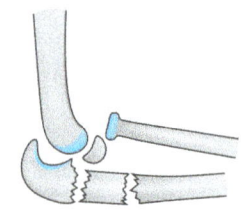

III. MECHANISM OF INJURY

I. Forced pronation of forearm
II. Axial loading of forearm with flexed elbow
III. Forced abduction of elbow
IV. Type I mechanism in which the radial shaft additionally fails.

IV. CLINICAL PRESENTATION

1. Pain
2. Fusiform swelling around elbow
3. Crepitus
4. Deformity
5. Painful and restricted ROM especially supination and pronation
6. Tenting of skin at fracture site
7. Ecchymosis
8. Inability to extend fingers and thumb PIN palsy
9. Wrist drop → Radial nerve palsy

10. Compartment syndrome to be ruled out
    ↓
    Anxiety
    Agitation
    ↑Analgesics
11. Chronic monteggia: Palpation of dislocated RH
12. Age: 4–10 years

V. RADIOLOGY

1. Any disruption of ulna (including plastic deformation)
   ↓
   Proximal R-U joint must be assessed for disruption
2. Radiocapitellar line – A line drawn through the long axis of radial neck and head passes through the capitellum regardless of the degree of flexion or extension on a true lateral.
3. Fracture – dislocation pattern as per classification
4. Chronic: MRI → Congruency of radial head and capitellum

VI. MANAGEMENT

A. Principles

1. Anatomic correction of ulnar deformity.
2. Achieve stable congruent reduction of radiocapitellar joint.
3. Maintenance of ulnar length and fracture stability.
4. Closed reduction and casting should be reserved only for indicated pediatric population.
5. Monteggia is a fracture of necessity and requires operative management.

B.

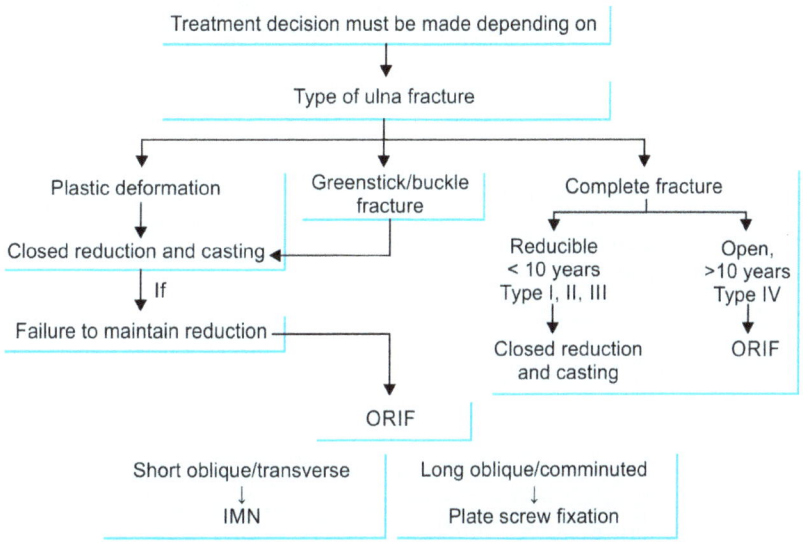

ORIF

1. Closed reduction of RH with ulnar length restoration is the rule
2. Plate application on the tensile (dorsal) surface especially type II
3. After fixation of ulna, RH is usually stable (>90%)
4. Failure of radial head reduction after ulna fracture fixation: Cause inaccurate ulna reduction > Interposed annular ligament

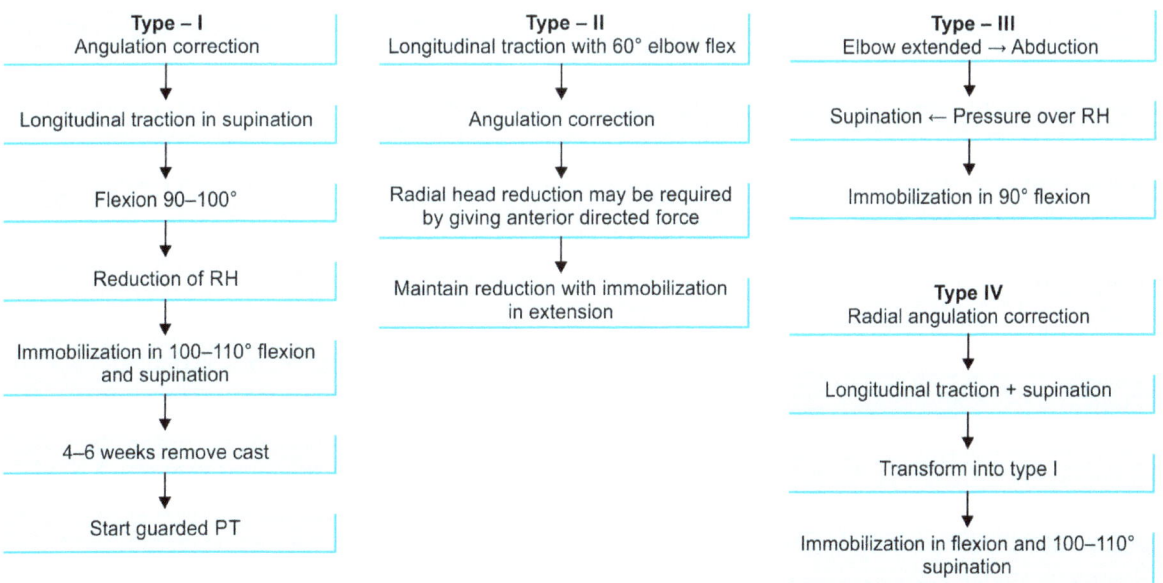

VII. COMPLICATIONS
1. Chronic Monteggia lesions
2. Neurological injury

Acute	Tardy
Radial nerve PIN AIN Median nerve Ulnar nerve	Radial nerve

3. Myositis ossificans
4. Compartment syndrome

VIII. MANAGEMENT OF CHRONIC MONTEGGIA

1. One of the most important criteria for surgical reconstruction.
   ↓
   Preservation of normal concave articular surface of radius and convex capitellum.
2. Appropriate age for RH reduction <10 years
3. Best results when dislocation is <3-6 months
4. Other important indications of surgery:
   i. Pain
   ii. Progressive deformity
   iii. Loss of motion
   iv. Functional disability
5. **Annular ligament reconstruction**
   a. **Kalamchi:** Restoration of stability after open reduction and osteotomy, using the native annular ligament.
   b. **Bell-Tawse:** Central strip of triceps tendon to reconstruct annular ligament. Passing through a single drill hole in ulna and around the radial neck.
   c. *Modified Bell-Tawse*: Lateral strip of triceps + transcapitellar pin.
   d. *Lacertus fibrosis, fascia lata, Palmaris longus tendon*
   e. *Seel and Peterson*: 2 drill holes in ulna for reconstruction of annular ligament
6. **Ulnar osteotomy**
   i. Drill hole ulnar osteotomy
   ii. 1 cm distraction ulnar osteotomy → 5 cm distal to tip of olecranon
   iii. Mehta → Ulnar osteotomy with bone graft.

PELVIS FRACTURES

1. Pelvic fracture typically occurs as result of high energy blunt trauma.
2. Treatment not only includes the orthopedic aspects of fracture fixation but also, effectively manage hemorrhage and other associated injuries.

I. MECHANISM OF INJURY

High energy	Low energy
Pelvic ring disruption, polytrauma ↓ 1. Motor cycle 2. Motor vehicle pedestrian 3. Fall from height 4. Crush injuries	Individual bone fracture ↓ *Elderly patients*: Fall from standing height *Young athletes* → Sudden muscle contraction → Avulsion, straddle type injury from horse

1. Impact injuries occur when moving vehicles strike a stationary victim
2. Direction, magnitude and nature of force → type of fracture
3. Crush injuries: Victim is trapped between injuring force (motor vehicle) and an unyielding environment (ground)
   Duration of crush
   Whether force was direct or a ⎫ Type of fracture
   "rollover" with changing vector ⎭
4. *Anteroposterior force*:
   i. External rotation of hemipelvis
   ii. Pelvis springs open, hinging on the intact posterior ligaments
5. *Lateral compression force*:
   i. Fall on one side "T-bone" in motorcycle crash
   ii. Most common
   iii. Impaction of cancellous bone through the SI joint and sacrum
   iv. Location of application of force:
      a. Posterior ½ of ilium → Classic LC, stable configuration.
      b. Anterior ½ of ilium → Rotates hemipelvis inwards
         ↓
         Disrupts the posterior SI ligamentous complex
         ↓
         If force continues to push the hemipelvis
         ↓
         C/L Hemipelvis external rotation
         ↓
         ∴ LC on ipsilateral side and ER injury on contralateral side
   v. GT region → Transverse acetabular fracture
   vi. ER abduction force → Acts through femoral head and shaft → tears hemipelvis from sacrum.
   vii. Shear force:
        Completely unstable fracture
        ↓
        Triplanar instability due to disruption of sacrospinous, sacrotuberous and SI ligament.

II. CLASSIFICATION
i. Young and Burgess [Based on (MOI)] (Fig. 3)

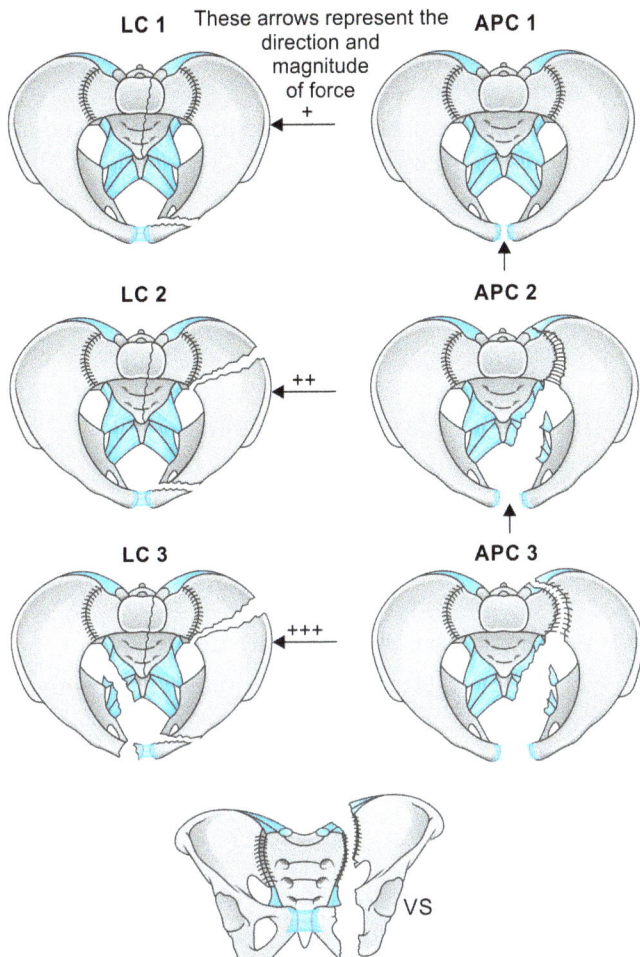

1. *LC* = Lateral compression (MC)
   Anterior injury – Oblique pubic rami fracture
   Further classified based on posterior lesion
   → *LC - I*: Sacral compression on side of impact
   → *LC - II*: Crescent iliac wing fracture on side of impact.
   → *LC - III*: LC I or LC II, with C/L open–book injury (APC) (*windswept pelvis*)
2. *APC*: Anterior posterior compression. Anterior injury- vertical/longitudinal ramii fracture.
   APC I: < 2.5 cm symphysis diastasis.
   Both anterior and posterior ligament intact
   APC II: > 2.5 cm symphysis diastasis. Anterior SI ligament disruption, posterior SI ligament intact.
   APC III: Complete disruption of SI joint. Both anterior and posterior ligaments ⊗
3. *VS*: Vertical shear
   Vertical displacement of hemipelvis
   Anterior → SD/Ramii fracture
   Posterior → Iliac wing, sacral fracture, SIJ disruption
4. *CM*: Combined mechanism: *LC + VS* → *most common*

ii. Tile's Classification
Type A: Pelvic ring stable: *Nonoperative*
   A1: Fracture not involving the ring (Avulsion fracture)
   A2: Minimally displaced pelvic ring fracture
   A3: Sacrum fracture, coccyx
Type B: PR rotationally *unstable*, vertically stable
   B1: Open book
   B2: LC1 → Ipsilateral
   B3: LC → C/L or Bucket-handle
Type C: Pelvic ring rotationally and vertically unstable
   C1 – Unilateral
   C2 – Bilateral
   C3 – Associated with acetabular fracture

III. CLINICAL PRESENTATION
1. Patient may present with polytrauma and be hemodynamically unstable.
   (Groin, buttock, perineum)
2. Traumatic wounds with obvious bleeding
3. Young male patients more common.
4. Symptoms → Pain and inability to bear weight
5. VS → Lower extremity shortening and ER
6. Unstable LC → IR deformity of LL
7. APC → Scrotal oedema in males
8. **Destot sign:** Palpable hematoma over perineum
9. Flank ecchymosis, or **grey turner sign**
   ↓
   Retroperitoneal hemorrhage
10. Palpation of soft tissues to assess for fluctuant areas → Morel – Lavallee lesions
11. Blood at urethral meatus, blood out of vagina
12. Blood in and around rectum
13. Neurological deficit → Lumbosacral plexus
    ↓
    L5 – S1 → Ankle DF, PF, L4 → Knee, S3, 4, 5 → Perineal sensation
14. Leg – length inequality
15. Abnormal pelvic motion on anteroposterior or lateral compression of ASIS and crests.
    → To be performed only once
    → "The first clot is the best clot"
16. High riding prostate on PR exam
17. Associated injuries → Chest, long bone fracture, spine fracture.

IV. RADIOLOGICAL EVALUATION
A. X-ray
1. *AP view of pelvis*:
   i. Anterior lesions → Pubic rami fracture, SD
   ii. SIJ disruption, Sacral fracture
   iii. Iliac fracture
   iv. L5 transverse process fracture → **"Sentinel sign"** → VS injury

2. *Inlet*: Supine patient, Tube 60° caudally
   Anterior/posterior displacement of the SI joint, sacrum, iliac wing.
3. *Outlet*: Tube 45° cephalad
   i. Vertical displacement of hemipelvis
   ii. Widened SI joint
   iii. Disruption of sacral foramina
4. Obturator and iliac oblique views = Acetabular fracture
5. *Radiographic signs of instability*:
   i. Sacroiliac displacement > 5 mm
   ii. Posterior fracture gap
   iii. Avulsion fracture:
      a. 5th transverse process (lumbar)
      b. Lateral border of sacrum (ST Ligament)
      c. Ischial spine (SS Ligament)
6. *Stress views*: Push – pull X-ray, GA → Vertical instability ≥ 0.5 cm mobility

B. CT Scan
1. Better visualization of posterior pelvic injuries
2. Pan CT → Rule out other injuries

C. MRI
1. Genito-urinary injuries
2. Pelvic vascular injuries

V. MANAGEMENT
A. Initial Treatment and Resuscitation
1. Perform ATLS
   ABCDE: Airway, breathing, circulation, disability and exposure.
2. Identification of all injuries to pelvis and extremity
3. Bleeding sources:
   i. Intra-abdominal (MC)
   ii. Intrathoracic
   iii. Extremity
   iv. Pelvic
   Source of hemorrhage:
   → Venous 80% Retroperitoneal hematoma (up to 4 litres of blood)
   → Arterial (20%)
   i. Superior gluteal artery (MC): Posterior pelvic ring injury, APC
   ii. Internal pudendal (anterior pelvic ring, LC)
4. Transfusion PCV: FFP: Platelets = 1:1:1 → ↓Mortality
5. *Pelvic binder*:
   i. Initial management of unstable pelvic injury
   ii. Centered over GT
6. *External fixation*:
   i. Indications:
      a. PR injuries with an external rotation component (APC, VS, CM)
      b. Unstable PR with ongoing blood loss
      c. Must be applied before emergency laparotomy.
   ii. Contraindications:
      a. Ilium fracture that prevents application
      b. Acetabular fracture
   iii. Works by ↓ pelvic volume.
   iv. ↑Stability of bleeding bone surfaces and venous plexus → Clot formation
7. *Angiography/embolization*:
   i. CT angiography has NPV (98-100%) to determine ongoing arterial hemorrhage.
   ii. Selective embolization in patients with uncontrolled bleeding.

B. Definitive Rx (Based on Classification)
LC – I = Nonoperative
LC – II = ORIF–Ilium
LC – III = Posterior stabilization with plate and SI screws
APC – I = Nonoperative
APC – II = Anterior symphyseal plate (ASP)/Ex. Fix.
APC – III = ASP/Ex. Fix and Posterior stabilization with SIJ Screws

VS – Posterior Stabilization.

C. Nonoperative
1. Mechanically stable pelvic injuries (LC, APC –I)
2. Bed rest → Protected weight bearing with walker or crutches
3. Serial X-ray → Check displacement.

D. Operative
a. *Absolute indications*:
   1. Open pelvic fracture
   2. Fracture associated with visceral perforation requiring surgery.
   3. Open book fracture ⎫
   4. Vertically unstable fracture ⎭ with HD unstable patient
b. *Relative indications*:
   1. SD > 2.5 cm
   2. LLD > 1.5 cm
   3. Rotational deformity
   4. Sacral displacement > 1 cm
   5. Intractable pain

E. ORIF
a. *Anterior ring stabilization*:
   Single superior plate → Rectus splitting. Pfannenstiel approach

b. *Posterior ring stabilization*:
   i. Anterior S1 plating: risk of L4–5 injury
   ii. Iliosacral screws
       Safe zone in S1 vertebral body
c. Anterior + posterior stabilization = VS

ACETABULAR FRACTURES

I. INTRODUCTION
1. 3/100,000 population per year
2. *Epidemiology*: Bimodal distribution
   i. Young patients: High energy trauma (MVA)
   ii. Old patients: Low energy (fall from standing height)

II. PATHOANATOMY
1. Innominate osseous structural support to acetabulum → 2 column construct → Inverted Y **(Fig. 4)**

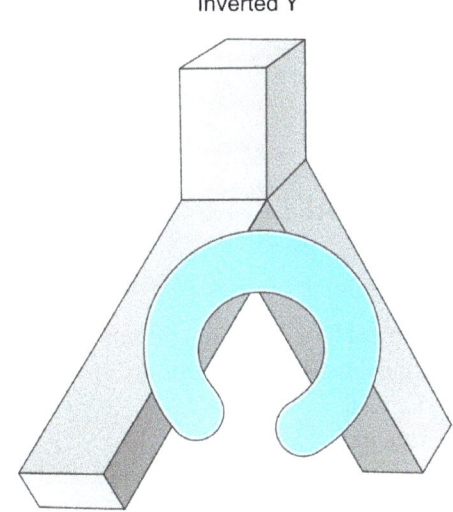

   i. Anterior column (iliopubic component)
      Iliac crest → Symphysis pubis with anterior wall of acetabulum.
   ii. Posterior column (Ilioischial component)
       Superior gluteal notch → Ischial tuberosity with posterior wall of acetabulum
   iii. Acetabular dome → Superior weight-bearing portion of the acetabulum at junction of anterior and posterior column.
2. *Fracture pattern*: Depends on:
   - Force vector
   - Bone quality
   - Position of FH at time of injury

III. MECHANISM OF ACTION
1. Direct impact on GT
   Hip abducted   Hip adducted
   ↓   ↓
   Low transverse fracture High transverse fracture

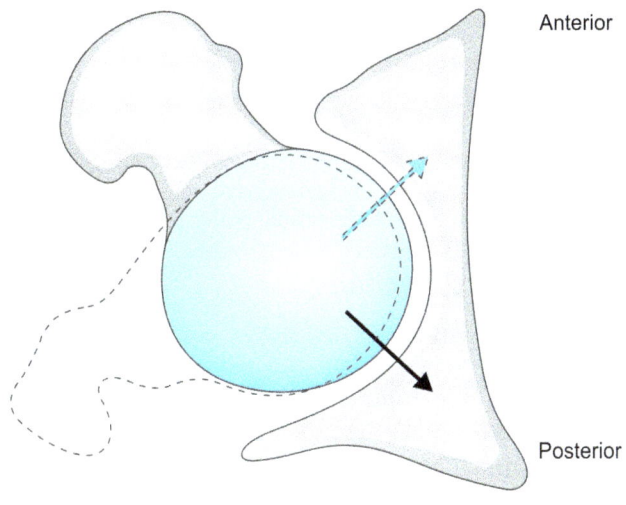

2. ER hip → Anterior column injury **(Fig. 5)**
3. IR hip → Posterior column injury
4. Indirect trauma (dashboard injury to flexed knee)
   ↓
5. As degree of hip flexion ↑ → Posterior wall is fractured in increasingly inferior position
6. As hip flexion decreases, superior portion of the posterior wall fracture.

IV. CLASSIFICATION
Judet–Letournel: 10 fracture patterns **(Fig. 6)**

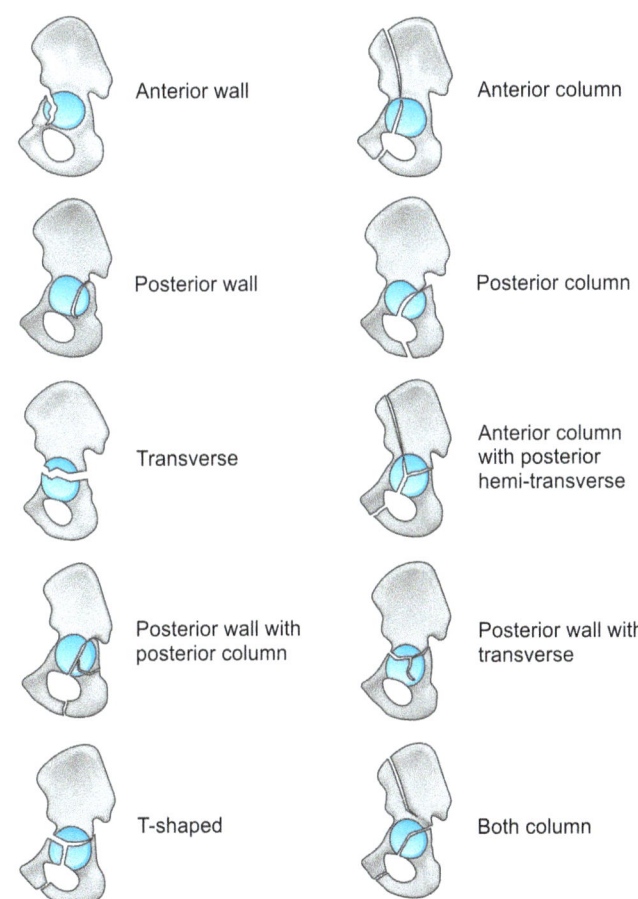

Elementary	Associated
1. Posterior wall	1. T-shaped
2. Posterior column	2. Posterior column and posterior wall
3. Anterior wall	3. Transverse and posterior wall
4. Anterior column	4. Anterior column/posterior hemitransverse
5. Transverse	5. Associated both column

A. Elementary Fracture

1. *Posterior wall*:
   i. Separation of posterior articular space
   ii. Posterior column not disturbed (ilioischial line normal)
   iii. "Marginal impaction" present in posterior fracture dislocation
       Articular cartilage impacted in underlying cancellous bone
   iv. **Gull sign:** Dome impaction in osteoporotic fractures
2. *Posterior column*:
   i. Ilioischial line broken
   ii. Fracture line originates at greater sciatic notch, travels across the retroacetabular surface and exits at obturator foramen
   iii. Ischiopubic ramus fracture
3. *Anterior wall fracture*:
   i. Least common
   ii. Teardrop displaced medially
4. *Anterior column*:
   i. Disruption of iliopectineal line
   ii. Classified according to the level at which the superior margin at the fracture line divides the innominate bone
       Low +
       Intermediate ++   Greater involvement of weight bearing surface.
       High +++
5. *Transverse*:
   i. Innominate bone separated into 2 fragments as per fracture line
       a. Transtectal: Through acetabular dome
       b. Juxtatectal: Through junction of dome and fossa acetabuli
       c. Infratectal: Through fossa acetabuli
   ii. Both iliopectineal and ilioischial lines broken

B. Associated Fracture

1. *PW + PC*: Only associated fracture that does not involve both columns
2. Transverse + PW: 2/3rd – Femoral head dislocation posteriorly, 1/3rd – Centrally. Most common associated fracture
3. Anterior column + Posterior hemitransverse: Hemi-transverse because the transverse component involves only 1 column.
4. *Both column*:
   i. "Central acetabular fracture"
   ii. Most complex
   iii. Floating acetabulum
   iv. "Spur sign" → Distal most portion of the fractured ilium that is still attached to the axial skeleton.

V. CLINICAL PRESENTATION

1. Patient may present with polytrauma and be hemodynamically unstable
2. Pain and inability to move involved extremity
3. Morel–Lavallee lesion: Closed soft tissue degloving injury
4. Neurological deficit
   Sciatic nerve → Peroneal division
                    ↓
              Foot drop
5. Shortening of limb → Hip dislocation
                         ↓
                   FADIR → Posterior
6. *Associated injuries*:
   i. Long bone fracture.   iv. Chest injury
   ii. Spinal injury   v. Abdomen injury
   iii. Head injury   vi. Genitourinary

VI. RADIOLOGICAL EVALUATION

A. X-ray

i. *AP view*:
   1. Iliopectineal line: Anterior column
   2. Ilioischial line: Posterior column
   3. Anterior wall
   4. Posterior wall
   5. Superior weight bearing surface of acetabulum
   6. Teardrop
   7. Shenton's line
   8. Roof arc angle: Angle between vertical line through femoral head and line through fracture.
      i. Defines fracture pattern stability
      ii. Considered stable if fracture line exits outside the weight bearing dome of acetabular >45° on AP, obturator and iliac views
      iii. Not applicable for both column and posterior wall fracture as no intact portion of acetabulum to measure.
   9. Gull sign: Impaction of superomedial roof on iliac oblique view, pathognomonic for posterior wall fracture
   10. Spur sign:
ii. Judet views
   1. Obturator oblique
   2. Iliac oblique
   3. Inlet/outlet views
iii. Obturator oblique: Anterior column and posterior wall
iv. Iliac oblique: Posterior column and anterior wall
v. Inlet/outlet views → PR involvement.

B. CT Scan
1. Fracture pattern orientation
2. Defines fragment size and orientation
3. Identifies marginal impaction
4. Identifies loose bodies–postreduction
5. Articular gap/step off.

VII. TREATMENT
A. Goals of Treatment
1. Anatomic restoration of articular surface
2. Achieve join stability
3. Prevent post-traumatic arthritis

B. Treatment Algorithm

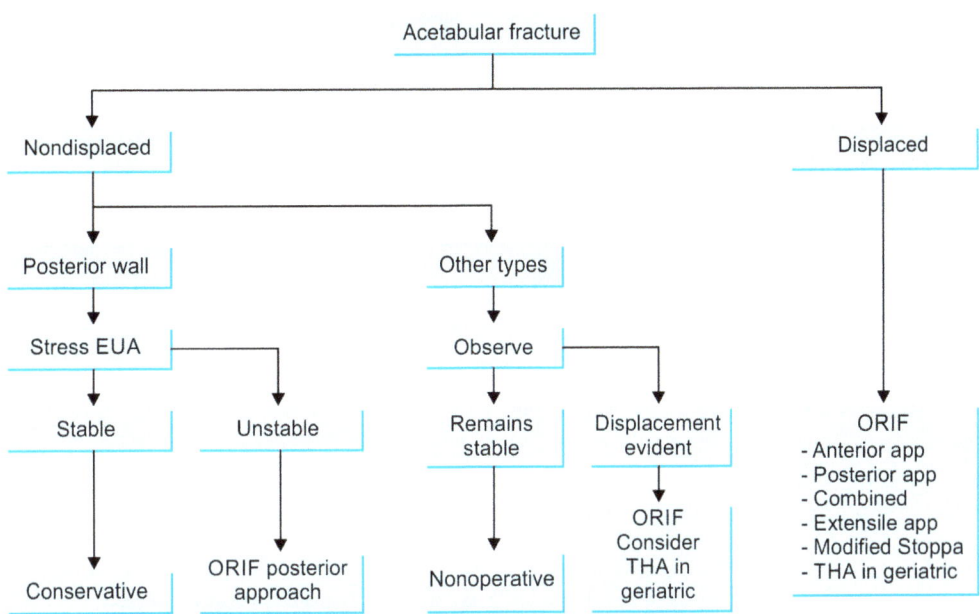

C. Fracture Pattern Dictates Approach
1. Anterior–ilioinguinal
    i. Anterior wall and anterior column
    ii. Transverse with minimal posterior displacement
    iii. Posterior hemitransverse
    iv. Most both column fractures
    v. Select T-shaped transtectal
   Risks:
    i. Femoral nerve
    ii. LCFN
    iii. Femoral vessel thrombosis
    iv. Laceration of corona mortis
        ↓
        Anatomical variant with anastomosis between
        External iliac (epigastric) and internal iliac (obturator)
        ↓
        Lateral dissection over superior pubic ramus
2. Posterior: Kocher-Langenbeck
    i. Posterior wall and posterior column
    ii. Most transverse fractures
    iii. T-shaped → Infratectal
                 → Juxtatectal
   Risks:
    i. ↑Heterotopic ossification compared to anterior approach
    ii. Sciatic nerve injury
    iii. Damage to FH blood supply: MCFA
3. Extensive approach: Extended iliofemoral
    i. Only single approach that allows direct visualization of both columns
    ii. Both columns needing direct reduction of posterior column
        Risk → Post. Gluteal muscle necrosis
             → Massive Heterotopic ossification
4. Modified Stoppa approach
    i. Access to quadrilateral plate to buttress comminuted medial wall fracture
    ii. Risk: Coronal Mortis

D. Initial Management–Skeletal Traction
i. Minimizes further soft tissue damage
ii. Allow associated injuries to be addressed
iii. Maintain length of limb
iv. Maintain femoral head reduction within the acetabulum

E. Nonoperative
Indications
1. Undisplaced fracture without hip instability.
2. Maintenance of medial, anterior and posterior roof arcs >45°

3. Posterior wall fracture fragment
   <20% → Nonoperative
   >50% → Operative
   20–50% → Stress examination ↓ C-Arm
4. Elderly low-demand patients

VIII. COMPLICATION

1. Post-traumatic degenerative joint disease (most common complication)
2. Heterotrophic ossification = Indomethacin X 5 weeks
3. Osteonecrosis
4. DVT and PE
5. Infection, bleeding, NV injury
6. Abductor muscle weakness
7. Intra-articular hardware placement.

HIP DISLOCATION

I. INTRODUCTION

1. Hip is an inherently stable joint due to the bony anatomy and soft tissue constraints involving the capsule and the ligaments.
2. Hip dislocations are traumatic hip injuries that result in femoral head dislocation from the acetabular socket.

II. ETIOLOGY

1. High energy trauma → ↑ incidence of associated injuries.
2. The position of the hip, the force vector applied, and the individual's anatomy all affect the direction of the dislocation and whether a fracture dislocation or pure dislocation occurs.

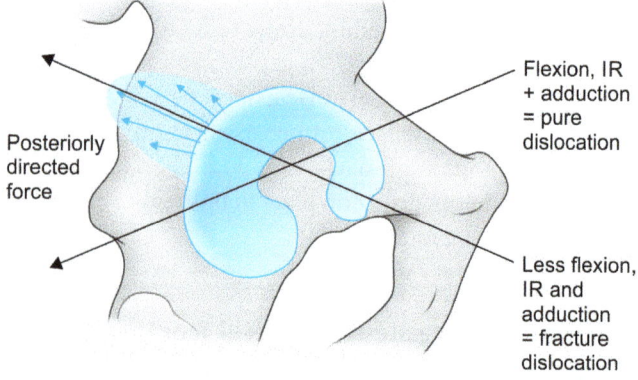

Direction of hip versus injury pattern	
Flexion, adduction, IR	Pure posterior dislocation
Partial flexion, less adduction, IR	Posterior fracture dislocation
Hyperabduction, extension, ER	Anterior dislocation
(IR: internal rotation of the hip; ER: external rotation of the hip)	

3. Posterior dislocation (PD): Anterior dislocation (AD) → 9:1

III. CLASSIFICATIONS
A. Anterior Hip Dislocation

Epstein classification of anterior hip dislocations
Type I: Superior dislocations, including pubic and subspinous
IA: No associated fractures
IB: Associated fracture or impaction of the femoral head
IC: Associated fracture of the acetabulum
Type II: Inferior dislocations, including obturator, and perineal
IIA: No associated fractures
IIB: Associated fracture or impaction of the femoral head
IIC: Associated fracture of the acetabulum

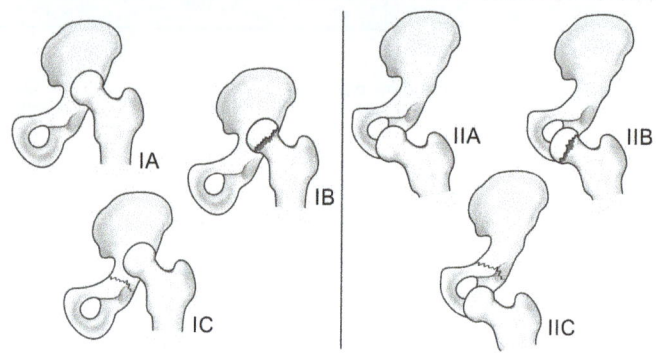

B. Posterior Hip Dislocation

Thompson and Epstein's classification of posterior hip dislocations	
Type	Description
I	With or without minor fracture of the acetabulum
II	With a large, single fracture off the posterior acetabular rim
III	With comminuted fractures of the acetabular rim (with or without a major fragment)
IV	With fracture of the acetabular rim and floor
V	With fracture of the femoral head

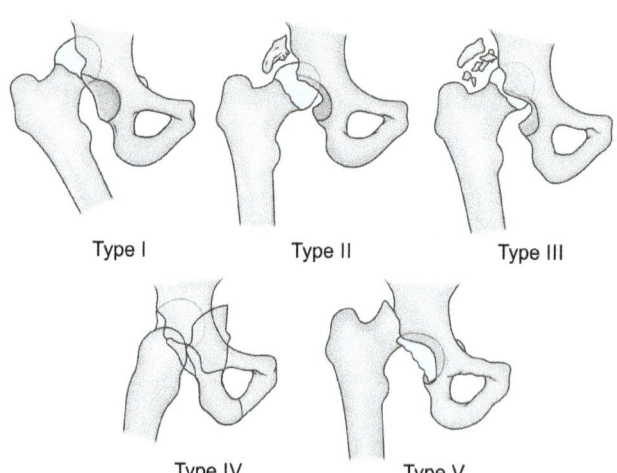

C. Femur Head Fracture with Hip Dislocation

Femur head fracture occurs almost always with hip dislocation.

Pipkin classification

Type I	Posterior dislocation with femoral head fracture caudad to the fovea
Type II	Posterior dislocation with femoral head fracture cephalad to the fovea
Type III	Femoral head fracture with associated femoral neck fracture
Type IV	Type I, II, or III with associated acetabular fracture

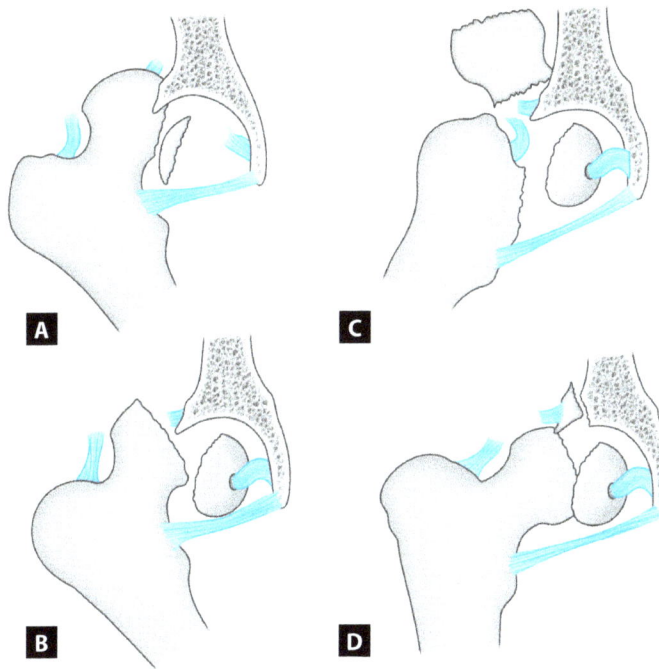

IV. CLINICAL FEATURES

1. Severe pain, tenderness, inability to bear weight
2. Limb appears shortened.
3. Large ecchymosis around thigh and gluteal region.
4. Anterior dislocation (AD)
    i. Superior (pubic) = Extension + ER + Abduction
    ii. Inferior (obturator) = Flexion + ER + Abduction
    iii. Femur head may be felt over pubic bone or the perineum.
    iv. Femoral nerve injury ±
5. Posterior dislocation (PD)
    i. Flexion + IR + Adduction
    ii. Head of the femur is felt as a hard mass in the gluteal region and it moves along with the femur.
    iii. Sciatic nerve injury ±
    iv. Vascular sign of Narath → Negative

V. INVESTIGATIONS

A. Radiograph

1. Views → AP, cross-table lateral, inlet, outlet and Judet views (before and after reduction)
2. Congruence of femur head with acetabulum is lost.
3. Shenton's line disrupted.
4. Anterior dislocation
    i. Femoral head (FH) appears larger than contralateral FH.
    ii. FH is medial or inferior to the acetabulum.
5. Posterior dislocation
    i. FH → appears smaller than contralateral FH.
    ii. FH superimposes the roof of acetabulum.
    iii. ↓ visualization of lesser trochanter due to IR of femur.

B. CT Scan

1. Direction of dislocation
2. Presence of loose bodies
3. Associated fractures

C. MRI

1. Not routinely indicated in acute cases.
2. Determines status of labrum, cartilage and FH vascularity.

VI. TREATMENT

A. Emergency Closed Reduction within 12 Hours

1. Hip dislocations are emergencies and must be reduced to prevent complications like osteonecrosis and post-traumatic arthritis.
2. C/I → Ipsilateral femur neck fracture
3. Reduction maneuvers (for details read the review article "Waddell et al. *Orthopedic reviews 2016*")
    i. Allis method
    ii. Bigelow method
    iii. Classical Watson-Jones method
    iv. Stimson's gravity method
    v. Whistler's technique
    vi. Captain Morgan's method

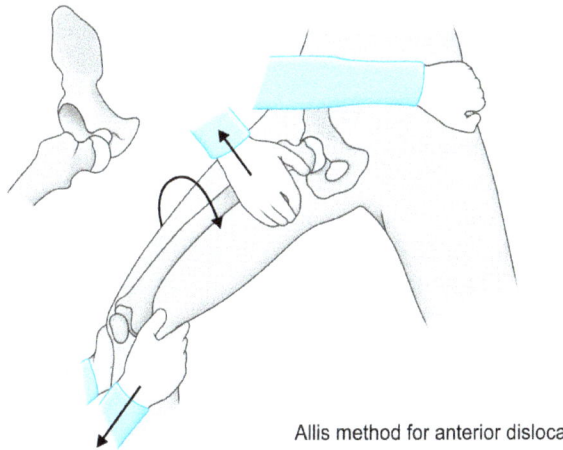

Allis method for anterior dislocation

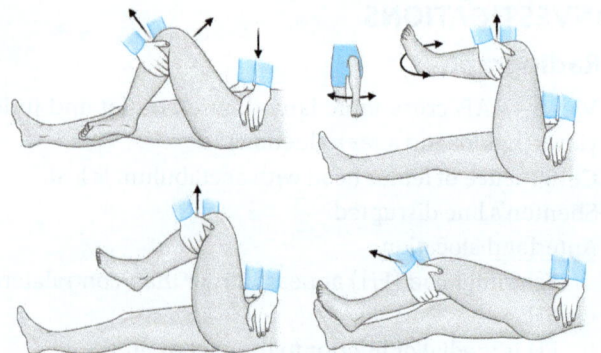

Allis method for posterior dislocation

4. In general, patient is supine, traction is applied in line of the deformity to reduce the hip joint.

B. Open Reduction

1. Indications
   i. Irreducible dislocation
   ii. Incarcerated fracture fragment
   iii. Delayed presentation
   iv. Nonconcentric reduction
   v. Acetabular fracture + Sciatic nerve injury (exploration)
2. Approach
   i. PD → Kocher-Langenbeck
   ii. AD → Smith-Peterson
3. Internal fixation is needed along with open reduction in cases having associated fractures → Femur head, neck and acetabulum.

C. Hip Arthroscopy

1. Removal of loose bodies
2. Chondral injuries
3. Labral tears

D. Hip Dislocation and Femur Head Fracture Management Algorithm

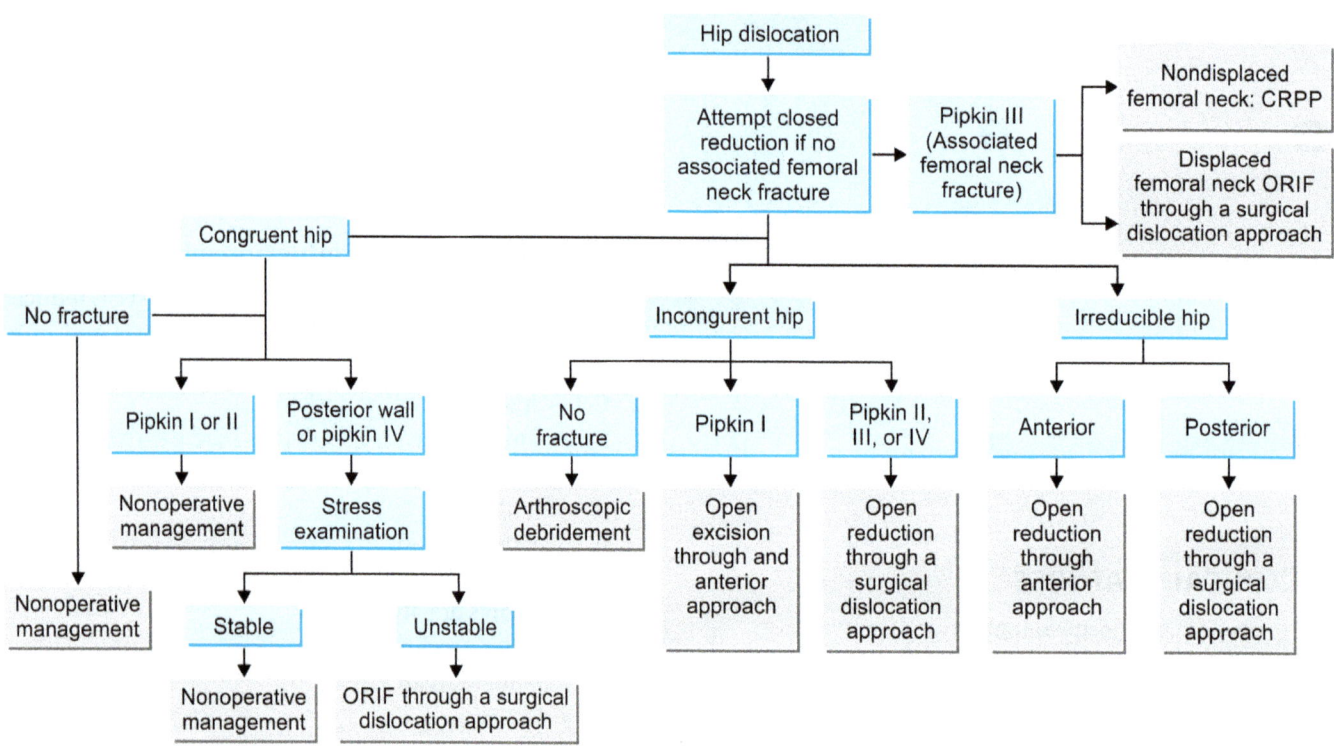

VII. COMPLICATIONS

1. Myositis ossificans
2. Post-traumatic arthritis
3. Femur head osteonecrosis
4. Sciatic nerve injury → PD
5. Femoral nerve injury → AD
6. Recurrent dislocations

SPINAL CORD INJURIES

I. ETIOLOGY

1. RTA
2. Falls
3. Building collapse
4. Gunshot wounds
5. Improper immobilization and transport after initial traumatic event

II. PATHOPHYSIOLOGY

- Primary injury → damage to neural tissue due to direct trauma → irreversible
  i. Compression
  ii. Stretch
  iii. Laceration
  iv. Contusion
- Secondary injury → additional neural tissue damage from the biologic response initiated by physical tissue disruption.
  i. Decreased perfusion
  ii. Tissue edema
  iii. Lipid peroxidation
  iv. Free radical and cytokines
  v. Cell apoptosis

III. CLASSIFICATION

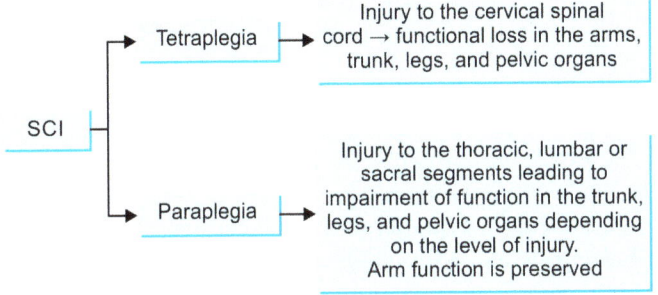

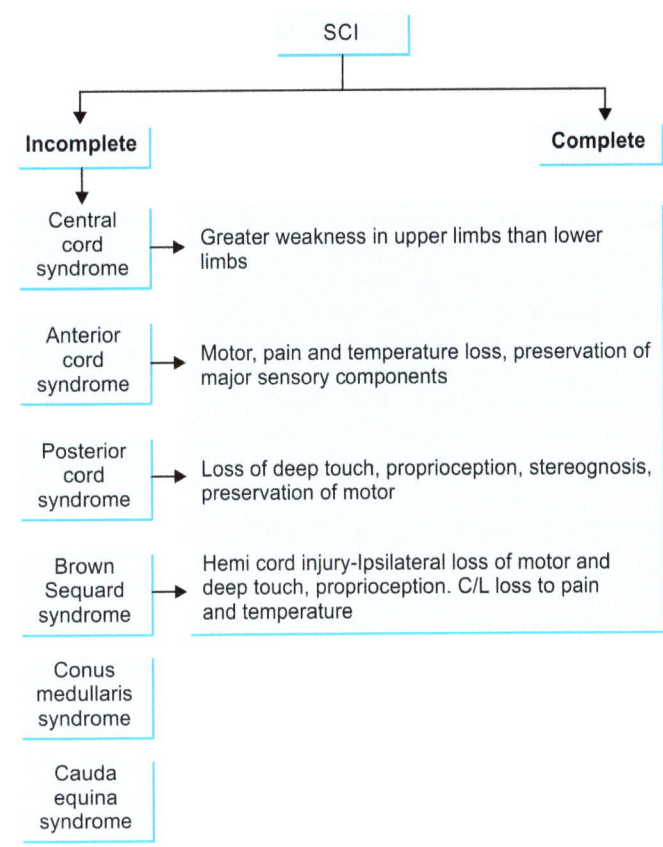

	Conus medullaris syndrome	Cauda equina syndrome
Vertebral level	L1–L2	L2-sacrum
Spinal level	Sacral cord segment and roots	Lumbosacral nerve roots
Presentation	Sudden and bilateral	Gradual and unilateral
Radicular pain	Less severe	More severe
Low back pain	More	Less
Motor strength	Symmetrical, less marked hyperreflexic distal paresis of LL, fasciculation	More marked asymmetric areflexic paraplegia, atrophy more common
Reflexes	Ankle jerks affected	Both knee and ankle jerks affected
Sensory	Localized numbness to perianal area, symmetrical and bilateral	Localized numbness at saddle area, asymmetrical, unilateral
Sphincter dysfunction	Early urinary and fecal incontinence	Tend to present late
Impotence	Frequent	Less frequent

ASIA impairment scale		
	Motor	Sensory
A. Complete	No motor function	Complete deficit
B. Incomplete	No motor function	Incomplete deficit
C. Incomplete	Motor function partially preserved; more than half of key muscles below the neurological level have a muscle grade less than 3	Incomplete deficit
D. Incomplete	Motor function is partially preserved at least half of key muscles below the neurological level have a muscle grade of 3 or more	Incomplete deficit
E. Normal	Normal motor	Normal sensory

IV. ACUTE PHASE CONDITIONS

i. Spinal Shock

Temporary loss of spinal cord function and reflex activity below the level of a spinal cord injury.
1. Flaccid areflexic paralysis
2. Bradycardia and hypotension due to loss of sympathetic tone
3. Absent bulbocavernosus reflex.

Bulbocavernosus Reflex "Osinski Reflex" (Fig. 7)

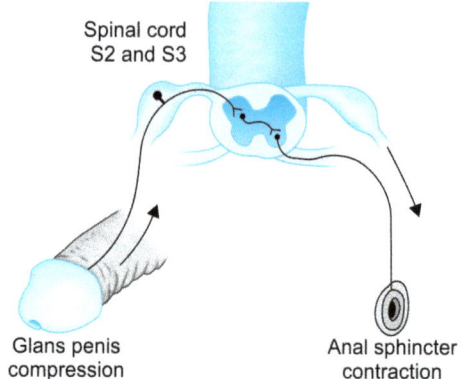

1. Oligosynaptic sacral reflex used to assess integrity of sacral sensory and motor fibers as well as sacral spinal cord segments S2–S4
2. Used for testing spinal shock and understanding the nature of the SCIs.
3. Contraction of the anal sphincter in response to a squeeze on the glans penis in a male, the clitoris or the mons pubis in a female, or a pull on the urethral catheter.
4. Absence of this reflex indicates spinal shock.
5. Return of the bulbocavernosus reflex heralds the end of spinal shock and generally occurs within 48 hours of the initial injury.
6. The presence of a complete lesion after spinal shock has resolved virtually nonexistent chance of neurologic recovery.
7. The bulbocavernosus reflex is not prognostic for lesions involving the conus medullaris or the cauda equina.
8. Delayed BCR is seen in diabetics.

Mechanism → Neurophysiologic in nature → Neurons become hyperpolarized and unresponsive to stimuli from brain.
Timing: May occur up to several hours after injury time
More severe the anatomic and physiologic nature of injury → Profound spinal shock
Usually resolves by 48 hours → Spasticity, hyperreflexia and clonus develops
Evaluation: One cannot evaluate neurologic deficit until spinal shock phase has resolved
End of spinal shock indicated by return of the bulbocavernosus reflex.
Conus or cauda equina injuries may lead to permanent loss of the bulbocavernosus reflex.

Phases

1. Hyporeflexic: 0–48 hours
2. Initial reflex return:
   i. 1–2 days
   ii. Polysynaptic reflexes return (bulbocavernosus reflex)
   iii. Monosynaptic (patellar) remain absent
3. Initial hyperreflexia: 1–4 weeks
4. Spasticity: 1–12 months:
   Characterized by altered skeletal performance

Characteristics of Spinal Shock
Motor effect → Paraplegia, quadriplegia
Loss of tone → flaccidity
Areflexia → All superficial and deep reflexes lost
Sensory → All sensations are lost below the level
Complete lesion → Above T1
↓
All sympathetic outlow is lost
↓
Between T1–T6 lesion → Preserves sympathetic tone in upper limb but lost to LL and adrenals

Prognostic Factor for Neurological Recovery

- **Good prognostic factor**
  1. Spinal shock of < 24 hours
  2. Early appearance of DTR
- **Poor prognostic factor**
  1. Complete lesion
  2. Spinal shock for >1 week
  3. Flexion spasm within 3 weeks
  4. Persistence DTR beyond 7 days
- During recovery optimized conditions must be provided for new synapse growth
  1. Nutrition
  2. Optimized general health
  3. Co-ordinating active exercise and functional training
  4. Controlling interfering spasticity
  5. Electrical stimulation

- **Intervention to enhance synapse formation**
    1. Medications to increase excitability of spinal neurosis
        i. 5 HTP
        ii. Clonidine
        iii. Theophylline
        iv. TRH
    2. Stimulates axonal growth
        i. Inosine
        ii. Clenbuterol
    3. Inhibition of glutamate toxicity
       Dizocilpine
    4. Cell replacement strategies
       Stem cell therapy

ii. Neurogenic Shock

Characterized by hypotension and relative bradycardia in patient with an acute spinal cord injury—potentially fatal.

Mechanism: Circulatory collapse from loss of sympathetic tone

Disruption of autonomic pathway within the spinal cord leads to:
- Decreased systemic vascular resistance
- Pooling of blood in extremities

V. EVALUATION

1. *Primary Survey* → ABCDE:
    i. Avoid head chin lift maneuver
    ii. Severe SCI above C5 → require intubation
    iii. Seat belt sign (abdominal ecchymoses) → flexion distraction injuries of thoracolumbar spine.
2. *Secondary survey*:
    i. Inspection: Rotational deformity of head → U/L facet dislocation
    ii. Palpate: Tenderness along posterior midline cervical spine.
    iii. Log rolling of patient for entire spine exam
    iv. Neurology
    v. Sacral Sparing

VI. RADIOLOGICAL EVALUATION

1. *X-ray*: AP, lateral, open mouth for C1–C2. Fracture, Dislocation, Fracture-Dislocation.
2. *CT scan*: Posterior element bony involvement, Facet dislocations, Posterior wall involvement.
3. *MRI*: Spinal cord edema hemorrhage, ligamentous complex injuries, spinal compression by disc or osseous material.

VII. MANAGEMENT: INITIAL MANAGEMENT

1. Philadelphia collar
2. *Intubation*: If breathing absent.
3. *Hemodynamic monitoring and stabilization*: Avoid hypotension
4. *Steroids*: High dose MPS → Controversial but recommended within 8 hours of injury by NASCIS III trials.
    i. Loading 30 mg/kg over 1st hour
    ii. Maintenance 5.4 mg/kg/h
        a. For 23 hours if started < 3 hours after injury
        b. For 47 hours if started 3–8 hours after injury
5. *ADR*: GI hemorrhage, wound infection, sepsis, and pneumonia
6. *Newer drugs*: GM-1 ganglioside, Riluzole
7. *Reduction*: Acute closed reduction with axial traction
    i. Indications: Alert and oriented patient with neurologic deficits and compression due to fracture/dislocation
    ii. Bilateral facet dislocation with spinal cord injury in alert and oriented patient is most common reason to perform acute reduction with axial traction
    iii. When to stop:
        a. Overdistraction
        b. Worsening neurologic examination
        c. Failure to obtain reduction

Operative: **Surgical decompression and stabilization**

Indications

1. *Most incomplete SCI (except GSW)*:
    i. Decompress when patient hits neurologic plateau or if worsening neurologically
    ii. Decompression may facilitate nerve root function return at level of injury (may recover 1–2 levels)
2. *Most complete SCI (except GSW)*:
    i. Stabilize spine to facilitate rehab and minimize need for halo or orthosis
    ii. Decompression may facilitate nerve root function return at level of injury (may recover 1–2 levels)

A. THORACOLUMBAR INJURIES (FIG. 8)

I. Pathoanatomy

1. Thoracic spine from T2 to T10 has increased stiffness → Less fractures
    i. Increased rigidity by articulation with ribs
    ii. Ribs articulate with sternum, adding secondary stability
    iii. Facet joints oriented in coronal plane
    iv. Discs are thin increasing stiffness and rotational stability
    v. Kyphosis concentrates axial load on anterior column
2. Thoracolumbar region (T11 to L2): More commonly affected by spine trauma due to fulcrum of motion (intersection between stiff thoracic spine and increased motion of lumbar spine)
3. Blood supply: "Watershed area" in middle thoracic spine → Artery of Adamkiewicz → Cord Ischemia
4. Spinal cord ends at lower border of L1 - Cord/Conus/Cauda equina affected.

II. Algorithm for Morphological Classification

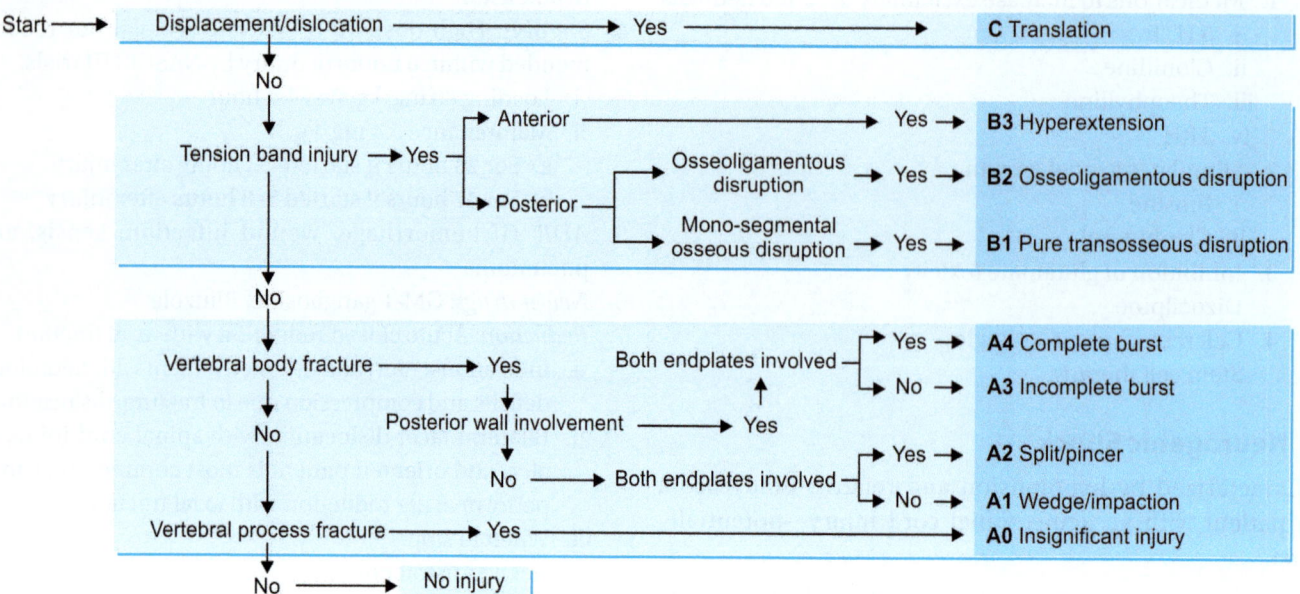

Compression (A)	Tension band (B)	
A0: Minor fractures that don't compromise integrity of spine (e.g., spinous or transverse process)	B1: Posterior distraction injury only involving bony structures	B2: Posterior distraction injury involving ligaments +/-bony structures
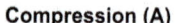	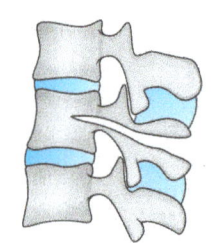	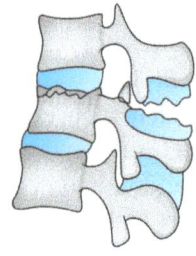
A1: Single end-plate fracture without involving posterior wall	A3: Incomplete burst fracture involving single end-plate and posterior wall	B3: Anterior distraction injury involving bony and/or soft tissues
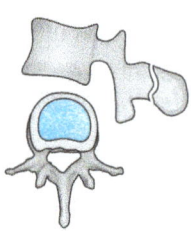	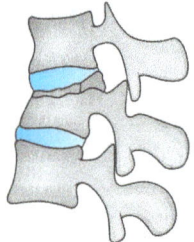	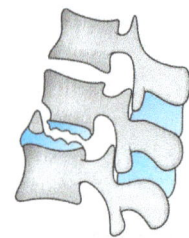
A2: Fractures involving both endplates without involving posterior wall	A4: Complete burst fracture involving both end-plates and posterior wall	Translation (C) C: In axis displacement of one vertebral body in any direction relative to another
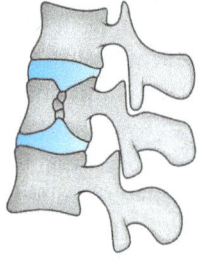	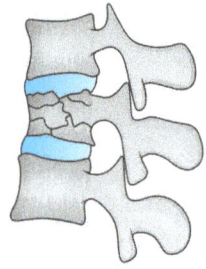	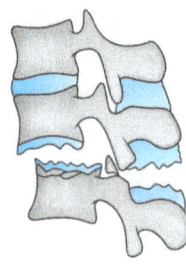

Classifications

Dennis and McAfee → Magerl → AO → New AO classification and also TLICS.

Thoracolumbar injury classification and severity (TLICS) score

Category	Parameter	Description	Points
1	Injury morphology	Compression	1
		Burst	2
		Translation/rotation	3
		Distraction	4
2	PLC integrity	Intact	0
		Suspected disruption	2
		Disruption	3
3	Neurological status	Intact	0
		Nerve root injury	2
		Complete cord injury	2
		Incomplete cord injury	3
		Cauda equina injury	3

PLC = posterior ligamentous complex

Total points	Management
1–3	Non-surgical
4	Surgical or non-surgical
5–10	Surgical

III. **Spinal stability**: "The ability of the spine under physiologic loads to maintain relationships between vertebrae in such a way that there is neither **initial damage** nor **subsequent irritation** to the spinal cord or nerve roots and, in addition, there is no development of incapacitating **deformity or pain** due to the structural changes."
Instability – 5 or more
Instability usually based on middle column integrity.

White and Punjabi's checklist for thoracic instability:
1. Anterior elements destroyed or unable to function : 2
2. Posterior elements destroyed or unable to function: 2
3. Relative sagittal plane translation >2.5 mm : 2
4. Relative sagittal plane rotation > 5° : 2
5. Spinal cord/cauda equine damage : 2
6. Disruption of costovertebral articulations : 1
7. Dangerous lading anticipated :1
   Thoracolumbar spine – 90% of vertebral body fractures

IV. TREATMENT

Treatment is based on:
 i. Degree of neurologic deficits
 ii. Degree of spinal cord compression and imaging evidence of myelomalacia
 iii. Spinal stability.

A. Compression Fractures
1. Usually stable. No neurodeficit
2. Rx → ASH brace/Jewett/Thoracolumbar orthosis with early ambulation.

B. Chance Fracture

Flexion–distraction injury → compression failure of the anterior column and tension failure of the posterior and middle columns.

Type A: One-level bony injury → Bony chance → Hyperextension brace

Type B: One-level ligamentous injury ⎫
Type C: Two-level injury through bony middle column ⎬ Posterior fusion and instrumentation
Type D: Two-level injury through ligamentous middle column ⎭

Increased interspinous distance on the AP and lateral views.

C. Burst

Compression failure of the anterior and middle columns under an axial load.

Dennis Classification
1. Type A: Fracture of both endplates 2nd MC
2. Type B: Fracture of superior endplate MC
3. Type C: Fracture of inferior endplate
4. Type D: Burst rotation
5. Type E: Burst lateral flexion
   Most can be treated with - ASH brace/Jewett/Thoracolumbar orthosis with early ambulation.

D. Indications of Surgery
1. Neurologic deficits
2. Loss of vertebral body height >50%
3. Angulation >20 to 30 degrees
4. Canal compromise of >50%
5. Scoliosis >10 degrees
6. Instability.

E. Goals
1. Decompression
2. Achieving normal spinal alignment
3. Anterior column reconstruction
4. Spinal stabilization

F. Approaches
1. Anterior
2. Posterior
3. Combined
  i. *Posterior surgery:*
   1. Indirect decompression via ligamentotaxis
   2. Avoids the morbidity of anterior exposure
   3. Shorter operative times
   4. Decreased blood loss
   5. Easier to perform
  ii. *Anterior approaches:*
   1. Direct decompression
   2. Direct anterior column reconstruction → kyphosis >30 degrees.

G. Thoracic

1. Midline transverse
2. Costotransverse: Open or arthroscopic
3. Transthoracic → Lateral thoracotomy
4. Fusion → BG → Iliac crest, ribs, fibula
5. Instrumentation → Pedicle Screw and rods posteriorly
6. Anterior → Cage.

V. COMPLICATIONS

1. Neurological injury
2. Dural tear
3. Cauda equina syndrome
4. DVT
5. Non-union after spinal fusion
6. Pseudoarthrosis
7. Post-traumatic pain
8. Scoliosis
9. Progressive kyphosis
10. Flat back
11. Depression

B. CERVICAL SPINE INJURIES (FIG. 9)

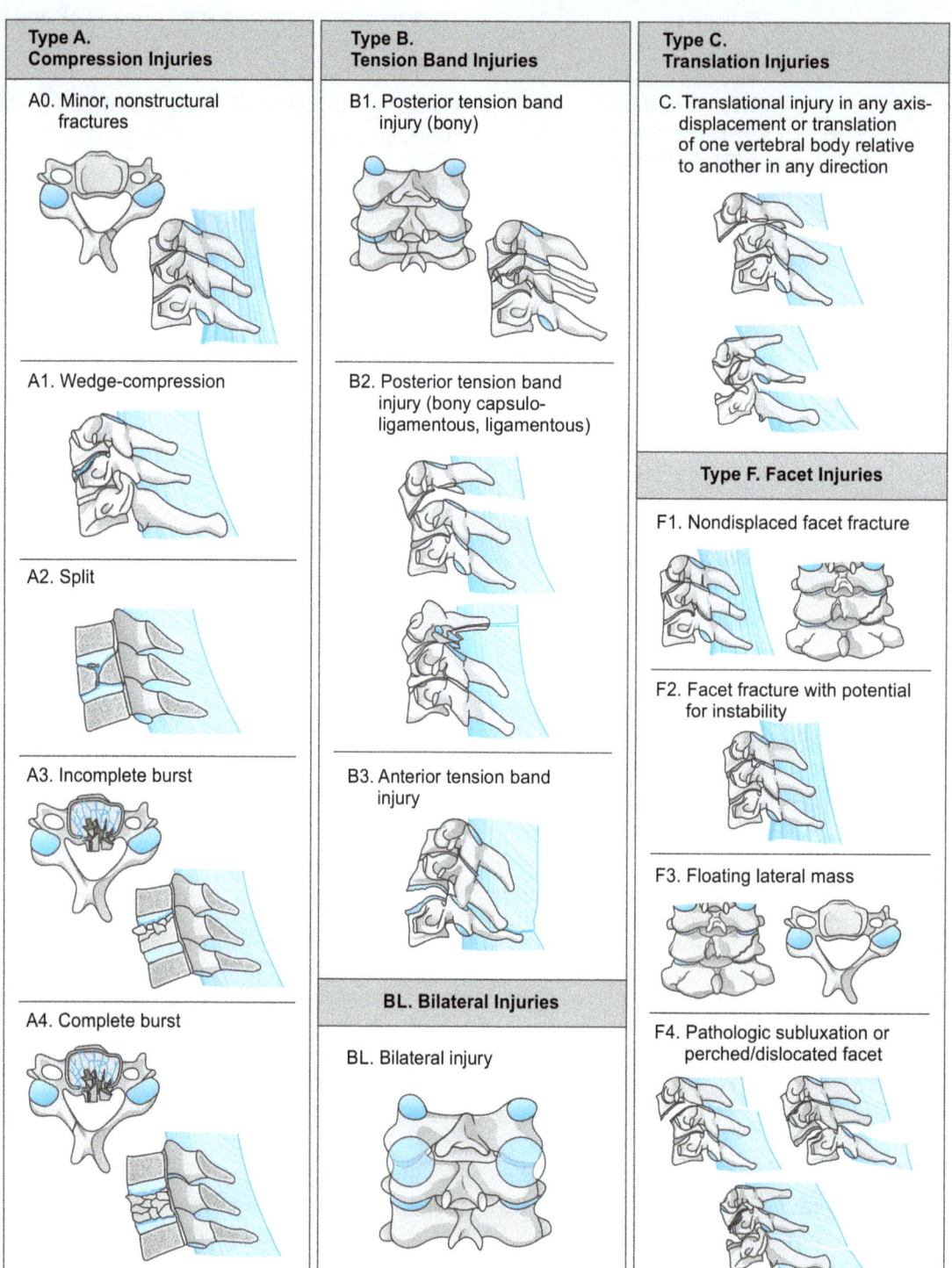

Type A. Compression Injuries
- A0. Minor, nonstructural fractures
- A1. Wedge-compression
- A2. Split
- A3. Incomplete burst
- A4. Complete burst

Type B. Tension Band Injuries
- B1. Posterior tension band injury (bony)
- B2. Posterior tension band injury (bony capsulo-ligamentous, ligamentous)
- B3. Anterior tension band injury

BL. Bilateral Injuries
- BL. Bilateral injury

Type C. Translation Injuries
- C. Translational injury in any axis-displacement or translation of one vertebral body relative to another in any direction

Type F. Facet Injuries
- F1. Nondisplaced facet fracture
- F2. Facet fracture with potential for instability
- F3. Floating lateral mass
- F4. Pathologic subluxation or perched/dislocated facet

I. Etiology

1. High energy → Young
2. Low energy → Old
3. Pathoanatomy → Spectrum of osteoligamentous pathology
4. Facet fractures → More frequently involves superior facet → unilateral or bilateral.
5. Decreases the threshold for facet dislocation
6. Unilateral facet dislocation → Most frequently missed cervical spine injury on plain X-rays
    i. Leads to ~25% subluxation on X-ray
    ii. Associated with monoradiculopathy that improves with traction → Inferior facet of the cephalad vertebrae encroaches the neuroforamina
7. Bilateral facet dislocation → leads to ~50% subluxation on X-ray → associated with significant spinal cord injury (~80% of cases)

II. Mechanism

Flexion and distraction forces +/- an element of rotation. Rotational moment associated with unilateral facet dislocation.

Allen and Ferguson classification (of sub-axial cervical spine injuries)
Typically used for research and not in a clinical setting based solely on static radiographs and mechanisms of injury

1. Flexion-compression
2. Vertical compression
3. Flexion-distraction
4. Extension compression
5. Extension-distraction
6. Lateral flexion

Flexion-distraction injuries
Stage 1: Facet sprain with slight subluxation, focal kyphosis <10°
Stage 2: Unilateral facet dislocation
Stage 3: Bilateral facet dislocation with 50% displacement (perched facets)
Stage 4: Complete dislocation (100% displacement)

III. Symptoms

1. Pain → neck pain in setting of flexion-distraction mechanism
2. Unilateral dislocation → numbness and tingling radiating down a single arm
    i. C5/6 presents with numbness in thumb
    ii. C6/7 presents with numbness in index and middle finger
3. Bilateral dislocation:
    i. Subjective weakness in b/l upper and lower extremities
    ii. Paresthesias and sensory changes in b/l lower extremities
4. Physical examination:
    i. Inspection:
       Gross spinal alignment → angular deformity may suggest a unilateral facet dislocation
    ii. Monoradiculopathy → seen in patients with unilateral dislocations
        a. C5/6 unilateral dislocation:
            1. Presents with a C6 radiculopathy
            2. Weakness to wrist extension
            3. Numbness and tingling in the thumb
        b. C6/7 unilateral dislocation:
            1. Presents with a C7 radiculopathy
            2. Weakness to triceps and wrist flexion
            3. Numbness in index and middle finger
    iii. Spinal cord injury symptoms → seen with bilateral dislocations
        a. Motor and sensory status
        b. Neurologic reflexes
        c. ASIA scoring

IV. Treatment

Nonoperative

1. Stable facet fracture, no spinal cord compression
2. Philadelphia collar, PT, NSAIDs

Operative

1. Single level instrumented stabilization:
   Indications:
   a. Unstable facet fracture
   b. Bilateral facet fracture
   c. Unilateral fracture involving >40% of the lateral mass or an absolute height >1 cm
   d. If no anterior disc herniation can be performed from anterior or posterior approach

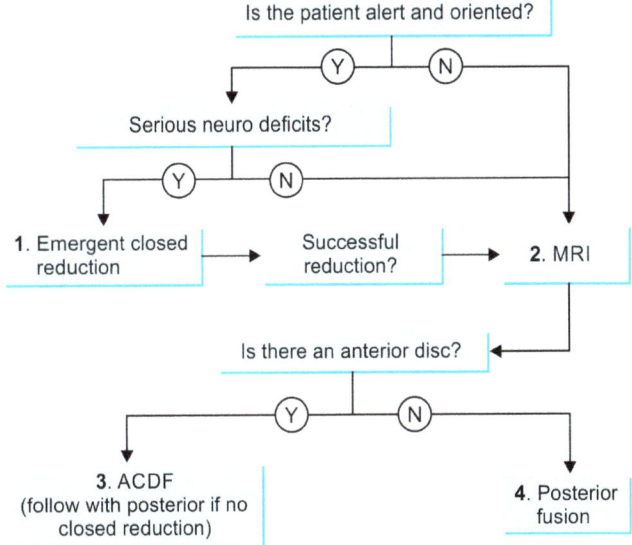

2. Anterior cervical discectomy and fusion (single level) → Smith Robinson approach:
   Indications:
   a. Large disc herniation → compression on the spinal cord or nerve roots
   b. Failed CR → open reduction from anterior approach by distracting across Casper pins with simultaneous rotation.
   c. 1-level interbody arthrodesis with anterior plating

3. Posterior reduction and instrumented stabilization:
   Indications:
   a. No anterior disc present
   b. bilateral or unilateral facet dislocations that are not reducible from the front or through closed reduction
4. Combined anterior decompression and posterior reduction/stabilization:
   When disc herniation present that requires decompression in patient that cannot be reduced through closed or open anterior technique.

HANGMAN'S FRACTURE

Traumatic anterior spondylolisthesis of the axis
   ↓(d/t)
Bilateral fracture of the pars inter-articularis

ETIOLOGY

1. Motor vehicle accident: MC
2. Falls
3. Dives
4. The term "hangman's fracture" is not accurate for majority of the cases as it lacks the massive traction force present in judicial hangings.

MECHANISM

1. Forcible Hyperextension + Axial loading → Pars fracture
2. Secondary flexion → tears PLL and disc, allowing subluxation.

CLASSIFICATION (FIG. 10)

Effendi (Levine and Edwards)

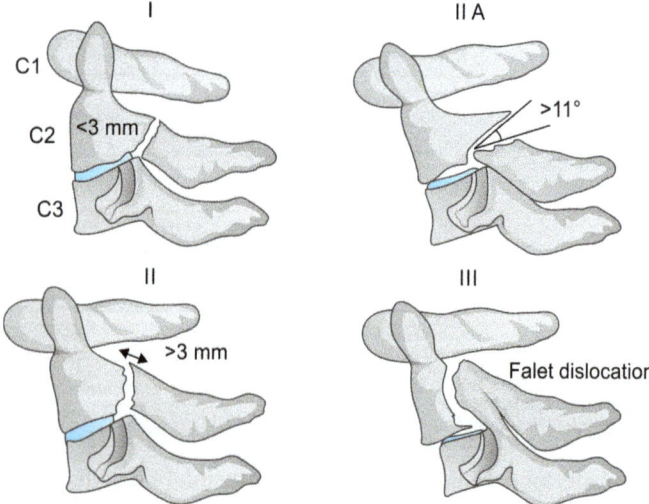

Type I

1. MOA → Hyperextension
2. Minimally displaced (0–2 mm)
3. No angulation
4. C_2 - C_3 disc intact
5. Stable fracture pattern

Type II

1. Hyperextension + Axial load f/b rebound flexion.
2. 3 mm horizontal translation.
3. Vertical fracture line
4. C_2 - C_3 disc and PLL disrupted
5. Unstable fracture pattern.

Type IIA

1. Flexion - Distraction.
2. No horizontal displacement.
3. Horizontal fracture line.
4. Significant angulation (>11°)

Type III

1. Flexion compression.
2. Severe angulation and displacement
                        +
   Unilateral or B/L facet dislocation C_2 - C_3

   Variant to type III → Fracture extends posteriorly into the axis → associated with ↑ Neurological deficit.

CLINICAL FEATURES

1. MC symptom → Neck pain
2. Patients are usually neurologically intact.
3. However, if involved → Sensory loss
                          Weakness
                          Paralysis
                          Death

INVESTIGATIONS

1. X-ray → Flexion and Extension radiograph (under strict supervision)
      ↓
   Subluxation
2. CT → Delineates fracture pattern
3. MRI → Ligament injuries
4. MRA → Suspected injury to vertebral artery.

TREATMENT

1. Type I: Rigid cervical collar for 6–8 weeks
2. Type II → <5 mm displacement
            ↓
         Reduction with traction
            ↓f/b
         Halo immobilization × 8–12 weeks
       >5 mm displacement
            ↓
         Prolonged traction or surgical fixation
3. IIA: Traction Contraindicated
   Reduced immediately with gentle axial load + extension, and then compression in halo immobilization × 10–12 weeks.
   Type III: Surgical reduction and stabilization

4. *Surgery*:
   i. Fusion at C_2 - C_3 with C_2 pedicle and C_3 lateral mass screw root system (Posterior) (posterior > anterior)
   ii. C_1 - C_3 fusion
   iii. Anterior C_2 - C_3 stabilization → but exposure difficult.

ODONTOID FRACTURE

1. MC fracture of axis (50-60%) (2nd MC Hangman)
2. MC cervical spine fracture in elderly.
3.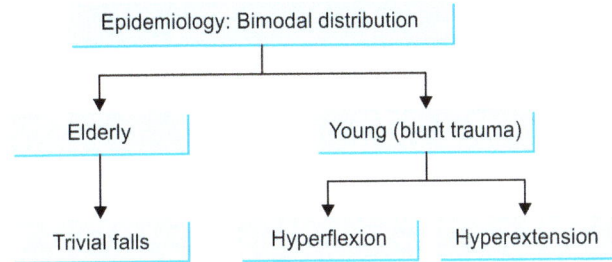

I. PATHOPHYSIOLOGY

1. Displacement

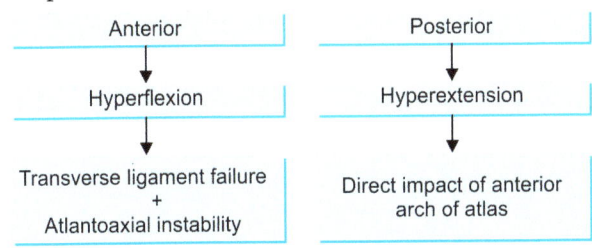

2. Fracture through base of odontoid
   ↓
   Severely compromises the stability of the upper cervical spine.
3. Os odontoideum → Failure of fusion at base of odontoid. DD of type II
4. Blood supply → Base → Vertebral artery
   Apex → Internal carotid
   Junction of apex and base → Watershed area
   ↓
   ↑Nonunion in type II

II. CLASSIFICATION (FIG. 11)

A. Anderson D'Alonso

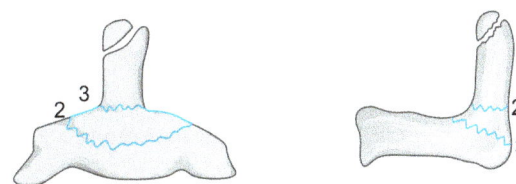

1. Oblique avulsion fracture through tip
2. Through base of dens.
3. Through body of C_2.

B. Grauer Classification of Type 2 Odontoid Fractures (Fig. 12)

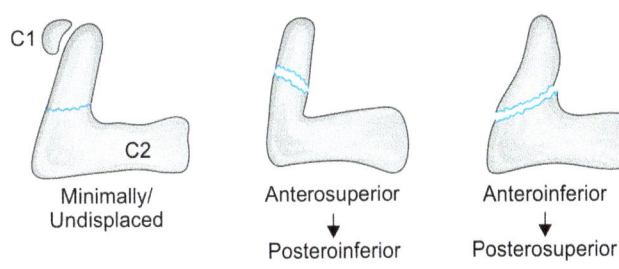

Minimally/Undisplaced | Anterosuperior ↓ Posteroinferior | Anteroinferior ↓ Posterosuperior

III. CLINICAL FEATURES

1. Neck pain → Worse with motion → Especially rotation
2. Dysphagia → Maybe present due to large retropharyngeal hematoma.
3. Neurological deficit → Rare due to large cross section area of spinal canal.

IV. INVESTIGATIONS

1. X-ray: AP, lateral, open - mouth odontoid view → Best to see fracture pattern.
2. Flexion - Extension: For occipitocervical instability in type 1 and os odontoideum.
3. Instability: Atlanto–Dens interval (ADI) >10 mm <13 mm space available for cord
4. CT angiogram → To determine location of vertebral artery prior to posterior instrumentation.
5. MRI → If neurological deficit.

V. TREATMENT

Type 1: Rigid cervical collar for 6 weeks
Type 2: Less than 40 years: Halo Vest for 8-12 weeks
   40-80 years: Surgical management
   More than 80 years = Rigid cervical collar
Type 3: Rigid cervical collar } 8-12 weeks

Surgery

A. Posterior C_1 - C_2 fusion
   1. Indications:
      i. Type IIC fractures with risk of nonunion (40-80 years)
      ii. IIC/III nonunions
B. Anterior odontoid screw: IIB
   ↓
   Screw trajectory must be perpendicular to fracture
C. Transoral odontoidectomy
   ↓
   Severe displacement of dens with spinal cord compression
   ↓
   But rarely performed due to ↑ complications

CANADIAN C-SPINE RULE

Assessment decision making tool utilized by clinicians to determine when radiography should be done following cervical spine trauma.

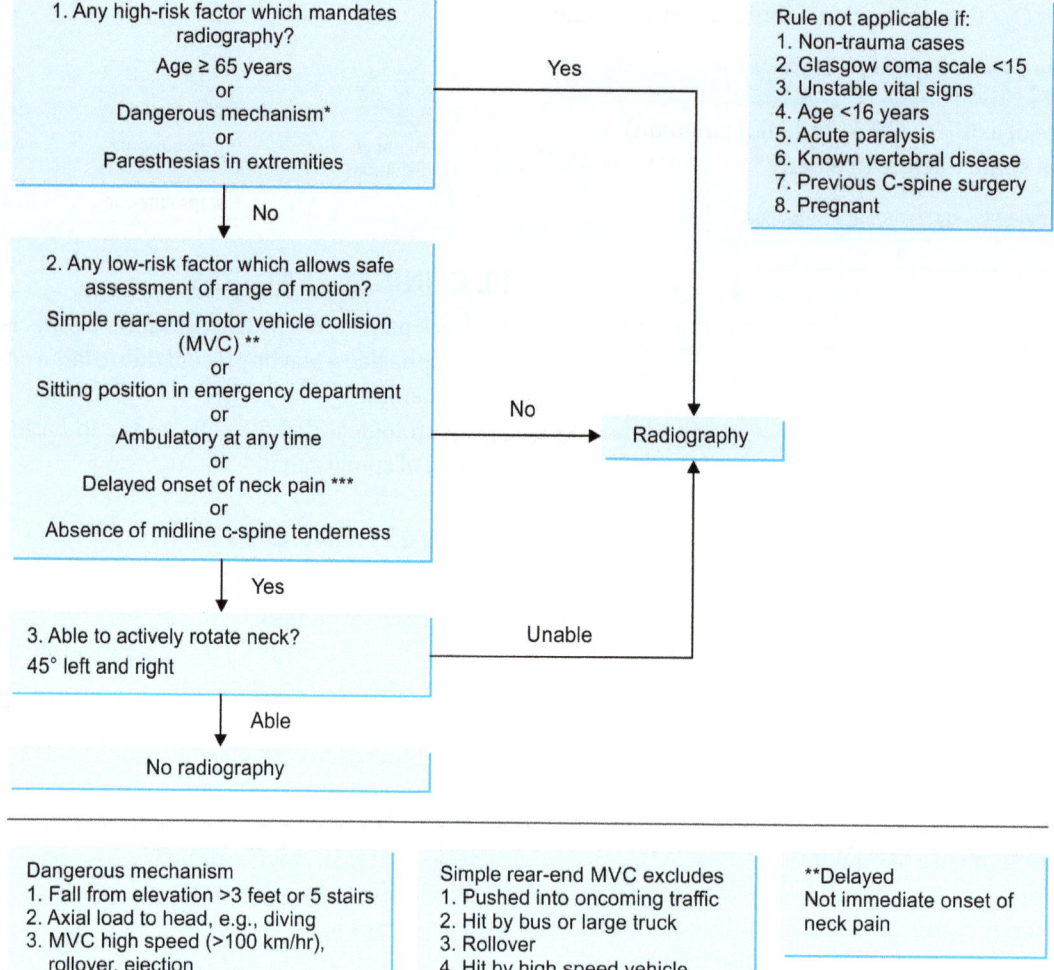

NEXUS

1. National Emergency X-radiography Utilization Study Criteria
2. Decision making tool to help doctors risk-stratify cervical spine trauma patients to determine if they need imaging to rule out clinically relevant C. spine injury.

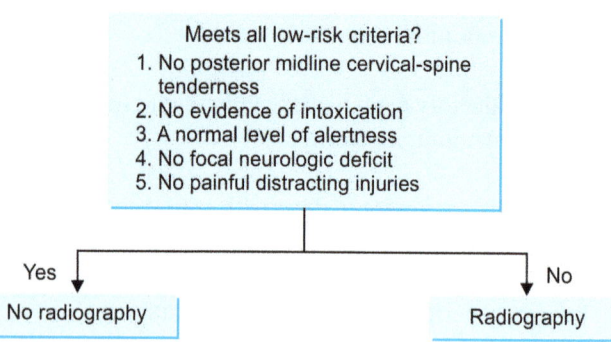

MOREL LAVALLEE LESION

I. INTRODUCTION

1. A closed traumatic soft tissue degloving injury characterized by separation of the skin and superficial fascia from the underlying deep fascia due to a shearing force.
2. *Anatomic location*:
    i. Greater trochanter
    ii. Gluteal
    iii. Lumbosacral
    iv. Abdominal areas
3. *Risk factors*:
    i. Motor vehicle accidents (Most common)
    ii. Blunt Trauma – High energy fall, sports
4. *Associated orthopedic conditions*:
    i. Pelvic and acetabular fractures
    ii. Proximal femur fractures
5. Bacterial colonization is seen in 50% cases.

II. PATHOPHYSIOLOGY

It has four stages:
1. Shearing forces to soft-tissue envelope → separation of the dermis from the underlying fascia
2. Injured lymphatics and vasculature from the subdermal plexus → Blood and Lymph
3. These components are then replaced by serosanguinous fluid as the lesion enlarges
4. Local inflammation leads to pseudocapsule formation and lesion maturation as the body attempts to sequester the space **(Fig. 13)**.

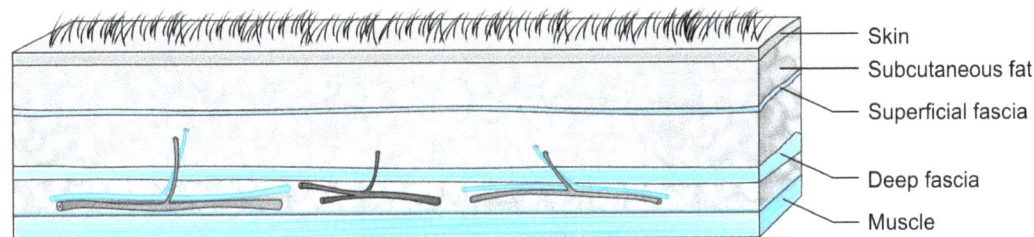
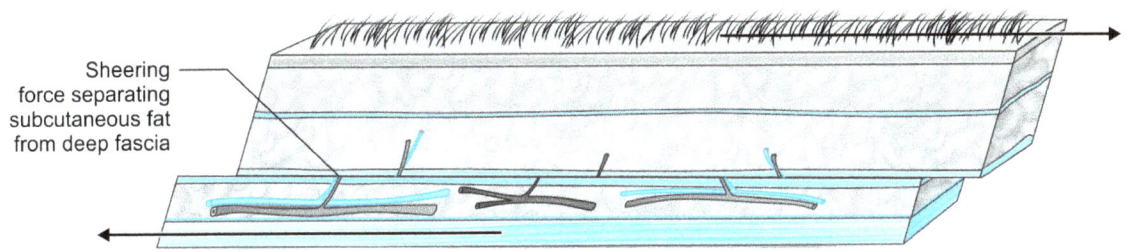
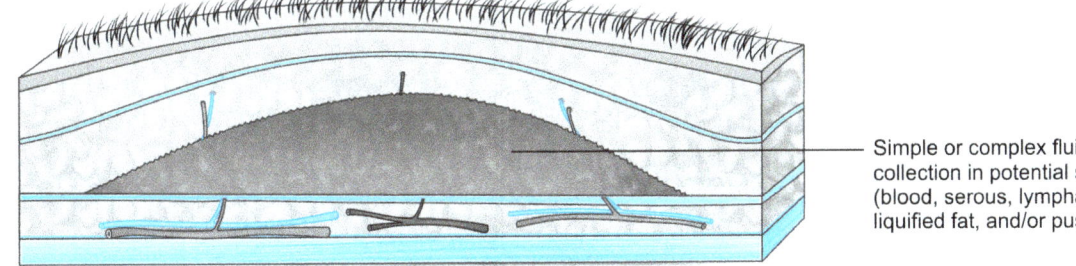

III. CLINICAL FEATURES

1. History: Polytrauma patient with high energy pelvic injury.
2. Presentation → Early or Late (months).
3. Swelling: Compressible, fluctuant, non-illuminant
4. Paraesthesia over skin: Disruption of subdermal vessels.
5. Ecchymosis
6. Other signs of fracture
7. Secondary changes in skin → Drying, discoloration, necrosis.

IV. INVESTIGATIONS

1. *Radiographs*:
   i. Evaluate underlying proximal femur, acetabulum or pelvis fractures
   ii. May show soft tissue swelling
2. *USG*:
   i. Rapid, readily available, inexpensive.
   ii. Hypoechoic space superficial to fascial layer
3. MRI
   i. Imaging modality of choice
   ii. Classification → Acute or chronic based on presence of pseudocapsule.

V. DIFFERENTIAL DIAGNOSIS

1. Bursitis
2. Neoplasm
3. Seroma
4. Subcutaneous hematoma.

VI. MANAGEMENT

A. Conservative

1. Compressive therapy → < 50 cc
2. NSAIDs, bed rest.

B. Surgical
1. Percutaneous drainage with drain placement → USG, CT based
2. Open irrigation and debridement:
    i. Larger lesions: >50 cc
    ii. Failed non-operative management
    iii. Lesion overlies surgical approach for fracture management.
3. Resection of fibrous capsule → Chronic MLL
4. Aggressive debridement of cavity performed with scrub brush and cobbs.
5. Placement of a drain exiting away from lesion (consider using 15 Fr or larger drain) → Recommend leaving drain until minimal output (<20–30 cc/day)

VII. COMPLICATIONS
1. Recurrence: Most common complication
2. Pseudocyst formation
3. Skin necrosis
4. Perioperative infection: Presence of a MLL has been cited as an independent risk factor for postoperative surgical site infection following pelvic and acetabular surgery.

SCAPHOID NON-UNION

I. INTRODUCTION
1. MC carpal bone fracture (62–87% of all carpal #)
2. "Unsolved fracture" due to high rates of NU and AVN.
3. Diagnosis missed in emergency → treated as sprain → Inadequate splint
4. Union time → Waist fracture: 6–8 weeks
     → Proximal pole fracture: 10–12 weeks
5. Incidence: Fracture Waist = 65%
     Distal 1/3 = 10%
     Proximal 1/3 = 25%

II. ANATOMY
1. Twisted, peanut or boat shaped
2. Surface covered 80% by cartilage
     ↓
3. ↓ Area for ligamentous attachment and entry for blood vessels.
4. Largest bone in proximal carpal row.
5. The radioscaphocapitate (RSC) ligament (volar) → Fulcrum on which scaphoid flexes.

III. BLOOD SUPPLY (FIG. 14)
1. Retrograde blood flow.
2. Supplied by the dorsal and volar branches of radial artery.

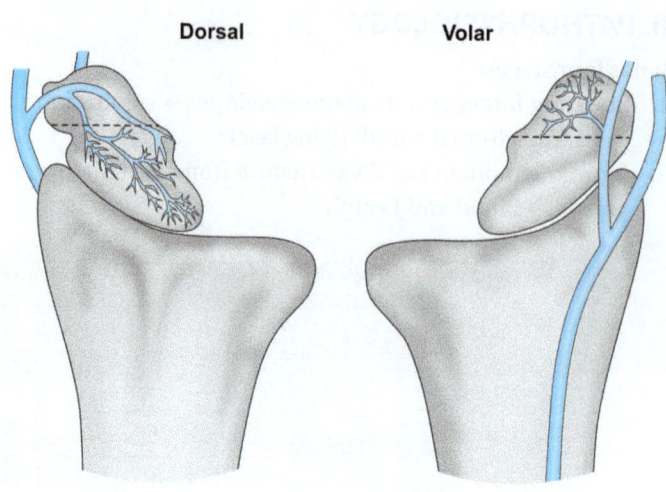

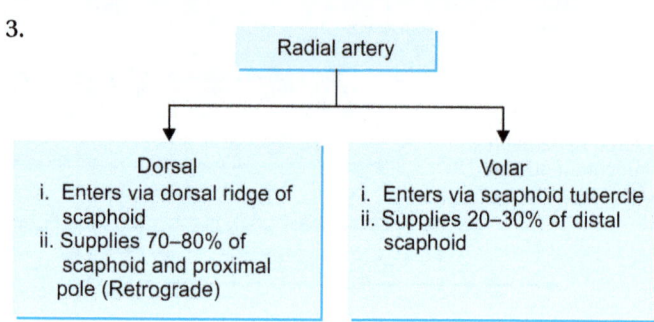

3.

4. Waist of the scaphoid → minimal and no perforating vasculature.
5. Creates a vascular watershed and poor fracture healing environment.
6. No vessel perforates the proximal dorsal cartilaginous area.

IV. ETIOPATHOGENESIS
1. Retrograde blood supply
2. Limited cancellous bone
3. Limited soft tissue attachments
4. Lack of periosteum
5. Intra-articular nature of fracture
6. Improper diagnosis and inadequate immobilization
7. Instability of carpus
8. Improper fixation
9. *Risk factors*:
    i. Vertical oblique fracture pattern
    ii. Displacement > 1 mm
    iii. Advancing age
    iv. Nicotine use

V. CLINICAL FEATURES
1. Pain: Radial side of wrist, ↑ on activity, difficulty in grip.
2. Tenderness over the anatomical snuff box.
3. Swelling over the radial dorsal side of wrist.

4. ROM affected in later stages.
5. History of FOOSH/past immobilization for wrist pain.
   ↓
   (Axial load→ hyperextended wrist + ulnar deviation)
6. M:F = 2:1, 3rd decade peak.
7. Site = Proximal pole (Most common).
8. In later stages, features of wrist arthritis.
9. **Watson's** test: Scapholunate interosseous ligament insufficiency.

VI. IMAGING
A. X-ray
1. *Views*:
   a. Neutral rotation PA views
   b. True lateral view
   c. Semi-pronated oblique view (45%)
   d. "Scaphoid view": PA in ulnar deviation with tube 20–30° angulated forward
2. Cysts, sclerosis, bone resorption at fracture site.
3. Hardware failure/loosening.
4. Humpback deformity **(Fig. 15)**

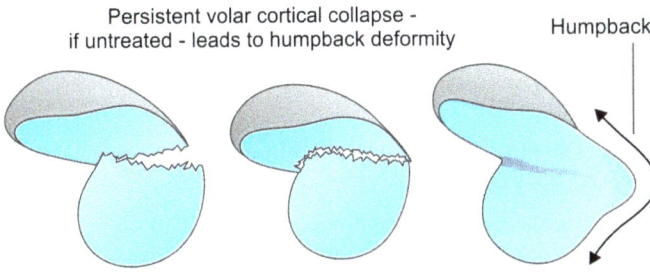

5. SNAC (Scaphoid NU advanced collapse)
6. Intrascaphoid angle→ Anteroposterior (normal=40°) and Lateral (normal = 30°). Perpendicular from plane of proximal and distal poles. Decreased in volar collapse.
7. Scapholunate (normal = 45°)
   Capitolunate
   Radiolunate   } 0° (DTS) } lateral view
   ↓
   All Increase in DISI (Dorsal intercalated instability.)

B. CT Scan
1. Best modality to evaluate NU
2. Surgery planning
3. CT scan must be oriented in plan of scaphoid without 1 mm cuts.
4. "Height-to-length" ratio → Degree of deformity (> 0.65 = Collapse)

C. MRI
1. Evaluation of osteonecrosis.
2. Gadolinium diffusion MRI
3. Bone marrow edema of avascular necrosis.

VII. CLASSIFICATION
1. Herbert
2. Slade and Geissler
3. Lichtman

i. Slade and Geissler
1. Delayed presentation = 4–12 weeks
2. Stable fibrous union → (minimal fracture line) appearing healed on X-ray, but CT scan shows gap
3. Minimal Sclerosis <1 mm
4. Cyst formation 1–5 mm
5. Humpback Deformity + cyst > 5 mm ± pseudoarthrosis
6. Wrist arthrosis

VIII. TREATMENT
A. Principles
1. Make on early diagnosis
2. Perform complete resection of NU
3. Correct the deformity 2° to carpal collapse

B. Surgical Options
1. *Compression screw fixation* → Headless screw.
   i. Acute fracture > 4 weeks
   ii. Fibrous Union
   iii. Early NU without minimal gap (SGI, II, III)
2. *Fixation with bone grafting*:
   i. Russe inlay non-vascularized cortico-cancellous bone graft: Indicated when there is no adjacent carpal collapse **(Fig. 16)**.

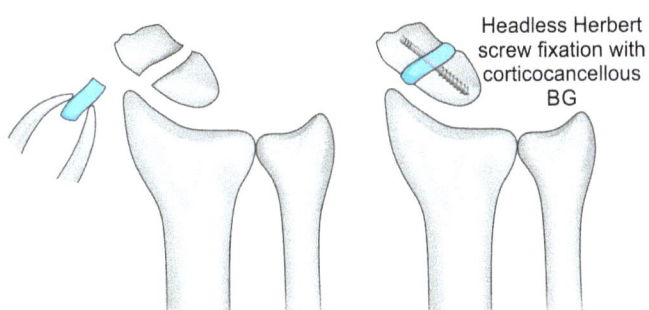

   ii. Fisk interposition non-vascularized corticocancellous bone graft. When adjacent cortical collapse and humpback deformity are present.
3. *Vascularized bone grafting*:
   A. Indications:
      i. Proximal pole NU
      ii. AVN
   B. Options:
      i. Pronator quadratus muscle pedicle graft
      ii. Free vascularized → Iliac crest graft
                           → Medial femoral condyle
4. Wrist arthrodesis → Arthritis, SNAC.

TERRIBLE TRIAD OF ELBOW

Traumatic injury of the elbow characterized by elbow dislocation, radial head fracture, and coronoid process fracture.

I. PATHOANATOMY
1. *Radial head*:
   i. A primary restraint to posterolateral rotatory instability (PLRI)
   ii. Secondary valgus stabilizer
   iii. Forearm in neutral rotation, lateral portion of articular margin devoid of cartilage → roughly between radial styloid and listers tubercle
2. *Coronoid process*:
   i. Provides an anterior and varus buttress to ulnohumeral joint.
   ii. Resists posterior subluxation beyond 30° of flexion
   iii. Fracture fragment typically has some anterior capsule attached → useful in repair
3. *Medial collateral ligament*—3 components:
   i. Anterior bundle: Most important to stability, restraint to valgus and posteromedial rotatory instability. Inserts on sublime tubercle (anteromedial facet of coronoid)
   ii. Posterior bundle
   iii. Transverse ligament **(Fig. 17)**.

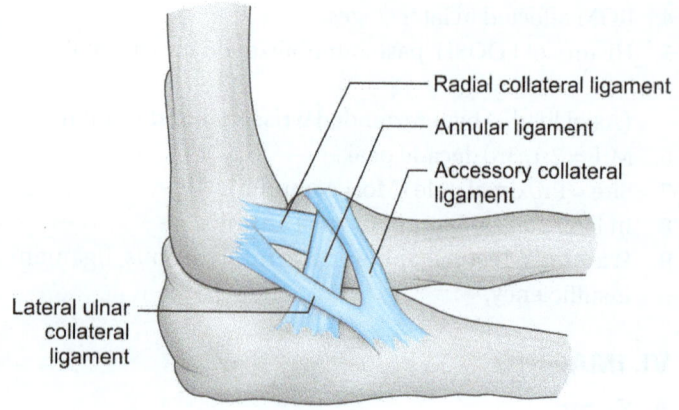

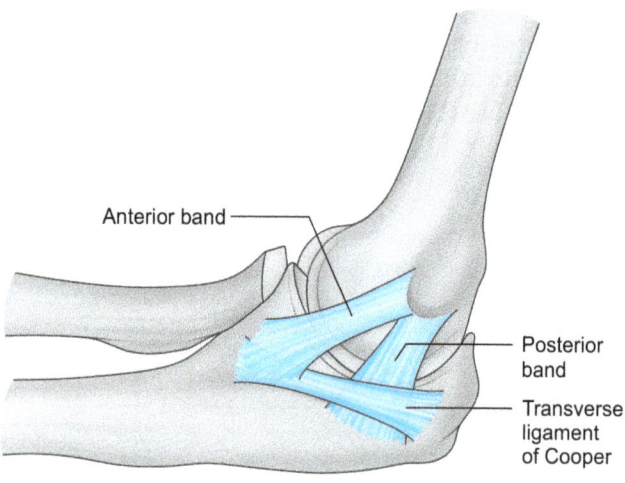

4. *Lateral collateral ligament*:
   i. Inserts on supinator crest distal to lesser sigmoid notch
   ii. The primary restraint to posterolateral rotatory instability
   iii. 4 components: When injured usually avulsed off of the lateral epicondyle
      a. **Lateral ulnar collateral ligament** (most important for stability)
      b. Radial collateral ligament
      c. Annular ligament
      d. Accessory collateral ligament **(Fig. 18)**

II. PATHOPHYSIOLOGY
1. Fall on extended arm → a combination of valgus, axial, and posterolateral rotatory forces → produces posterolateral dislocation.
2. Structures of elbow fail from lateral to medial:
   i. LCL disrupted first
   ii. Anterior capsule injured next
   iii. MCL disruption ±

III. CLINICAL FEATURES
A. *Symptoms*:
   1. Pain
   2. Clicking and locking with elbow in extension
B. *Examination*:
   1. Varus/valgus instability ±
   2. Posterolateral pivot shift instability test +
   3. Distal radioulnar joint (DRUJ) injury → Essex-Lopresti injury

IV. RADIOLOGY
A. *Radiograph*:
   1. Concentricity of ulnohumeral and radiocapitellar joints
   2. Line drawn through center of radial neck should intersect the center of the capitellum regardless of radiographic projection
   3. Lateral radiograph → coronoid fracture
   4. Prereduction and postreduction films
   5. Films of wrist and forearm → DRUJ, Essex-Lopresti injury
B. *CT*: Better evaluation of coronoid fracture. 3D imaging for determining fracture line propagation.
C. *MRI*: Ligament disruptions

V. MANAGEMENT
Usually managed operatively: High Instability
A. *Open reduction and Internal fixation of radial head fracture*:
   1. Non-comminuted fractures that involve <40% articular surface.

2. 1.5, 2.0, or 2.4 mm countersunk screws
3. Plate if indicated → position should be posterolateral.
4. Safe zone: 90-110° arc from radial styloid to Lister's tubercle with arm in neutral rotation.

B. *Radial head arthroplasty*:
  1. Comminuted radial head fractures → >3 pieces
  2. Implant should articulate 2 mm distal to the tip of the coronoid process.
  3. Radial head resection without replacement is contraindicated in presence of Essex-Lopresti lesion or in ligamentously injured elbows.

C. *Coronoid fracture fixation*:
  1. Type 1 → Do not need fixation as they don't disrupt stability.
  2. Type 2 and 3 → Fracture fixed using sutures, suture anchors or screws.

D. *LCL repair*:
  1. Usually avulsed from origin on lateral epicondyle.
  2. Reattached with suture anchors or transosseous sutures → must be reattached at center of capitellar curvature on lateral epicondyle
  3. If MCL is intact → LCL is repaired with forearm in pronation
  4. If MCL injured, LCL is repaired with forearm in supination to avoid medial gapping due to overtightening.

E. *MCL repair*: Indicated if instability on exam after LCL and fracture fixation, especially with extension beyond 30 degrees.

F. *Posterior skin incision advantageous*:
  1. Allows access to both medial and lateral aspect of elbow
  2. Lower risk of injury to cutaneous nerves
  3. More cosmetic.

VI. COMPLICATIONS

1. Instability
2. Failure of internal fixation: Most common following repair of radial neck fractures → poor vascularity leading to osteonecrosis and nonunion
3. Post-traumatic stiffness
4. Heterotopic ossification
5. Post-traumatic arthritis.

TFCC INJURY

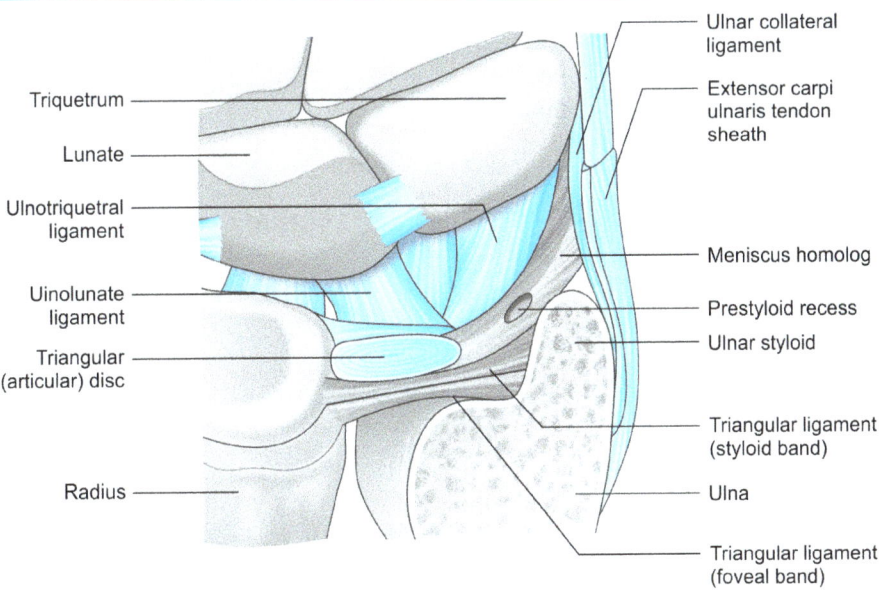

I. PATHOANATOMY (FIG. 19)

1. *Components*:
   i. Dorsal and volar radioulnar ligaments
   ii. Central articular disc
   iii. Meniscus homolog
   iv. Ulnar collateral ligament
   v. ECU subsheath
   vi. Ulnocarpal ligaments:
      a. Ulnolunate
      b. Ulnotriquetral ligaments
2. *Blood supply*:
   i. Periphery → well vascularized
   ii. Central portion → avascular

II. FUNCTION

1. Stabilizes DRUJ during rotator movements
2. Cushions forces that are transmitted through ulnocarpal axis
3. Connects ulna to volar carpus.

III. ETIOLOGY

1. Traumatic:
   i. Fall on outstretched hand
   ii. Acute rotational injury
2. Degenerative lesions:
   i. Repetitive movements
   ii. Anatomical variation (+) ulnar variance

IV. CLASSIFICATION

Class 1: Traumatic TFCC injuries
1A Central perforation or tear
1B Ulnar avulsion (without ulnar styloid fx)
1C Distal avulsion (origin of UL and UT ligaments)
1D Radial avulsion

Class 2: Degenerative TFCC injuries
2A TFCC wear and thinning
2B 2A + Lunate and/or ulnar chondromalacia
2C 2B + TFCC perforation
2D 2C + Ligament disruption
2E 2D + Ulnocarpal and DRUJ arthritis

V. CLINICAL FEATURES

A. *Symptoms*:
   1. Ulnar sided wrist pain
   2. Popping, clicking with rotational movements
   3. ↓ ROM
   4. ↓ Grip strength
   5. Turning door key → painful
B. *Examination*:
   1. Positive "fovea" sign → tenderness in the soft spot between the ulnar styloid and FCU tendon, between the volar surface of the ulnar head and the pisiform
   2. Pain elicited with ulnar deviation (TFCC compression) or radial deviation (TFCC tension)
   3. DRUJ instability: Piano key test
   4. Press test 100% sensitivity: Asked to get up from chair.

VI. INVESTIGATIONS

A. Radiograph → Positive ulnar variance
B. Arthrography → Joint injection shows extravasation
C. MRI → Tear at ulnar part of lunate indicates ulnocarpal impaction
D. Arthroscopy → Most accurate method of diagnosis.

VII. MANAGEMENT

A. Immobilization, NSAIDs, steroid injections
   1. All acute type I injuries
   2. First line of treatment for type 2 injuries
B. **Arthroscopic debridement**
   1. Type 1A
   2. diagnostic gold standard
C. **Arthroscopic repair: Inside out, outside in – Peripheral tears only**
   1. Type 1B, 1C, 1D
   2. Best for ulnar tears
   3. Acute, athletic injuries more amenable to repair than chronic injuries
D. **Ulnar diaphyseal shortening** → Type II with ulnar positive variance is >2 mm
E. **Wafer procedure: Central articular disc and ulnar pole debrided, cortex not disrupted.**
   1. Type II with ulnar positive variance is < 2 mm
   2. Type 2A-C
F. **Limited ulnar head resection** → Type 2D
G. **Darrach procedure**

BENNET AND ROLANDO FRACTURES

I. INTRODUCTION

1. Base of thumb metacarpal fractures
   i. Extra-articular fractures (most common)
   ii. Bennett fractures (partial intra-articular)
   iii. Rolando fractures (complete intra-articular)
2. 80% of thumb fractures involve the metacarpal base
3. Mechanism of injury: Axial force applied to the thumb in flexion.

II. CLASSIFICATION

Classification of fractures of the first metacarpal	
Extra-articular oblique	Oblique fracture line not involving the articular surface
Extra-articular transverse	Pure transverse fracture line not involving the articular surface
Intra-articular Bennett	Intra-articular fracture with a palmar radial fragment
Intra-articular Rolando	Y or T shaped complete intra-articular fracture
Intra-articular comminuted	Severely comminuted complete intra-articular fracture (**Fig. 20**)

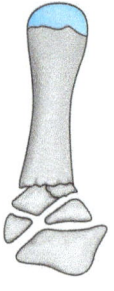
Intra-articular comminuted

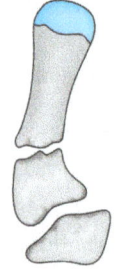
Extra-articular transverse

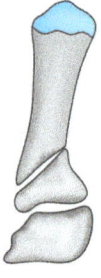
Extra-articular oblique

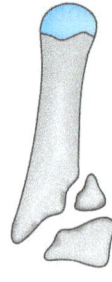
Intra-articular Bennett

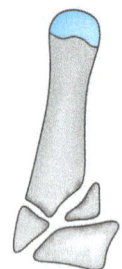
Intra-articular Rolando

III. CLINICAL FEATURES

1. Acute pain at the base of thumb with
2. Swelling
3. Ecchymosis
4. Tenderness → CMC joint
5. Range of motion → Painful, restricted

IV. RADIOLOGY

A. *X-ray*:
   1. Views:
      i. Robert's view – True AP of thumb – arm in full pronation with dorsum of thumb on cassette
      ii. True lateral of thumb – hand pronated 30° and beam angled 15° distally
      iii. Oblique
      iv. Traction view → fracture pattern in Rolando and severely comminuted fractures.
   2. Findings:
      i. Bennett fractures: A small fragment of 1st metacarpal base articulating with trapezium
      ii. Rolando fractures: Y sign → Splitting of the 1st metacarpal base into volar and dorsal fragments.
   3. Criteria dictating treatment:
      i. Extra-articular fracture
         → <30 degrees angulation
      ii. Bennett's fracture
         → <1 mm articular step-off
      iii. Rolando
         → comminution dictates operative strategy
B. *CT*: Complex fracture patterns.

V. MANAGEMENT

A. Conservative

Closed reduction and thumb spica casting:
   i. Extra-articular fractures → <u><30° angulation</u> after closed reduction
   ii. Bennett fractures → <u>< 1 mm displacement</u>
   iii. Fractures > 3 weeks old only thumb spica cast
   iv. Reduction is achieved with longitudinal traction, palmar abduction, and pronation.

B. Surgical

1. *Closed reduction and percutaneous k-wire fixation*:
   i. Extra-articular fractures → >30° angulation after closed reduction
   ii. Inability to maintain reduction < 30° with thumb spica
   iii. Rolando fracture <1 mm displacement
   iv. Small fracture fragments not amenable to screw fixation
2. *Open reduction internal fixation*:
   i. Bennett, Rolando, and severely comminuted fractures → >1 mm displacement + large fracture fragments amenable to fixation
3. *Distraction and external fixation*:
   i. Rolando fracture with >1 mm displacement + major soft tissue injury
   ii. Severely comminuted fractures + major soft tissue injury or impacted articular fragments
   iii. Bennett, Rolando, or severely comminuted fractures fragments too small for ORIF

VI. COMPLICATIONS

1. Stiffness
2. Instability
3. Post traumatic arthritis
4. Malunion.

CARPAL INSTABILITY

Carpal instability is a term that comprises of a spectrum of injuries within or around the carpus, leading to loss of congruity or abnormal loading between the carpal bones.

I. CARPAL BIOMECHANICS

1. The lunate is the "keystone" of the carpus.
2. Lies at the center of the proximal carpal row (linking the scaphoid and the triquetrum), and also at the center of the longitudinal chain (linking the radius with the capitate) → termed the intercalated segment.
3. In the proximal row, the scaphoid has an inherent tendency to flex, while the triquetrum has an inherent tendency to extend.
4. The lunate, placed between the two, is in dynamic equilibrium and maintains the alignment of the proximal row.

II. OVERVIEW

Overview of carpal instability	
Carpal instability dissociative (CID) **Intracarpal row instability**	
DISI	Scapholunate (SL) ligament
VISI	Lunotriquetral (LT) ligament
Carpal instability nondissociated (CIND) **Intercarpal row instability**	
Midcarpal instability	
Radiocarpal (ulnar translation, distal radius malunion)	Rupture of extrinsic ligaments
Carpal instability combined (CIC) Intercarpal and intracarpal row instability	
Perilunate dislocation	SL, CL, and/or LT deficiency
Scaphocapitate	
Carpal instability adaptive (CIA) Instability in response to malalignment of skeleton extrinsic to wrist	

III. SCAPHOLUNATE DISSOCIATION

1. Most common dissociative carpal injury (CID).
2. Rupture of the scapholunate ligament disconnects the scaphoid and lunate, widening the interval between them.
3. The scaphoid flexes while the lunate (which is still connected to the triquetrum) extends
4. Acute injury → 10–30% of intra-articular distal radius fractures or carpal fractures
5. Degenerative injury → Degenerative tears in >50% of people over the age of 80 years old

IV. PATHOPHYSIOLOGY

1. Mechanism of injury → sudden impact force → Wrist → extension, ulnar deviation and carpal supination.
2. If left untreated the DISI deformity can progress into a SLAC wrist.

V. CLINICAL FEATURES

A. Symptoms
1. Dorsal and radial-sided wrist pain
2. ↑ Pain with loading across the wrist (e.g., push ups)
3. Clicking or catching in the wrist
4. Wrist instability or weakness ±

B. Physical Examination
1. Inspection → Swelling over the dorsal aspect of the wrist ±
2. Palpation → Tenderness in the anatomical snuffbox or over the dorsal scapholunate interval (just distal to Lister's tubercle)
3. Motion → ↑ Pain with extreme wrist extension and radial deviation
4. Provocative tests → Watson test
   a. When deviating from ulnar to radial → pressure over volar aspect of scaphoid subluxates the scaphoid dorsally out of the scaphoid fossa of the distal radius → and a clunk is palpated when pressure is released as the scaphoid reduces back over the dorsal rim of the radius.

VI. RADIOLOGY

A. AP X-rays
1. Terry Thomas sign: SL gap >3 mm with clenched fist view
2. Cortical ring sign due to scaphoid malalignment
3. Humpback deformity with DISI associated with an unstable scaphoid fracture
4. Scaphoid shortening.

B. Lateral X-rays
1. Dorsal tilt of lunate leads to SL angle >70° on neutral rotation lateral
2. Capitolunate angle > 20°.

VII. MANAGEMENT

A. Conservative
1. Rest
2. Immobilization
3. Indications:
   i. Acute, undisplaced SLIL injuries
   ii. Chronic, asymptomatic tears

B. Surgical
1. SLL repair and reconstruction:
   a. Acute SLL injury without carpal malalignment
   b. Chronic but reducible SLL injuries <18 months
2. **Brunelli Reconstruction**: FCR sling to keep scaphoid in place.
3. Scaphoid ORIF → If associated#
4. Wrist fusion – Rigid, unreducible and DJD
5. Scapho-Trapezo-Trapezoid or Scapho-Luno-Capitate fusion

VIII. COMPLICATIONS

1. Disease progression (e.g., SLAC wrist)
2. Arthritis
3. Post-operative pain, stiffness, fatigue
4. Reduced grip strength.

LUNATE DISLOCATION (PERILUNATE DISSOCIATION)

I. INTRODUCTION

1. Lunate/perilunate dislocations are high energy injuries to the wrist associated with neurological injury and poor functional outcomes.
2. Lunate → "carpal keystone."
3. Commonly missed (~25%) on initial presentation
4. Mechanism of injury → Traumatic, high energy
5. Position: Wrist extended and ulnarly deviated → leads to intercarpal supination

II. CLASSIFICATION

Mayfield Progression and Classification

1. Sequence of injuries **(Fig. 21)**

Stage I	Scapholunate dissociation
Stage II	+ lunocapitate disruption
Stage III	+ lunotriquetral disruption, "perilunate"
Stage IV	Lunate dislocated from lunate fossa (usually volar) associated with median nerve compression

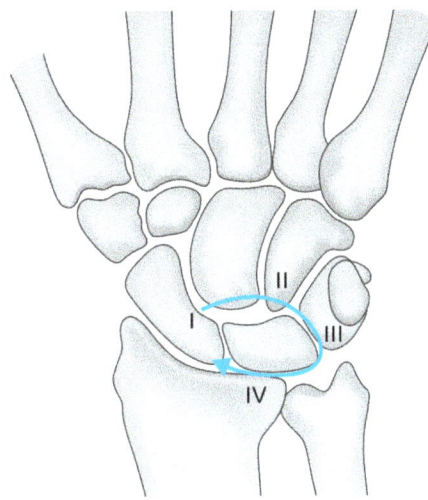

2. Dislocation can course through:
   i. Greater arc → Ligamentous disruptions with associated fractures of the radius, ulna, or carpal bones
   ii. Lesser arc → purely ligamentous **(Fig. 22)**

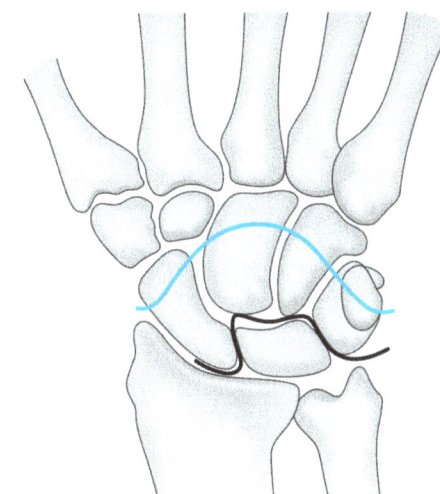

III. CLINICAL FEATURES
1. Pain and swelling at the wrist
2. Tenderness
3. Numbness and paraesthesia in the hand
4. Chronic injuries → Median nerve involvement: Motor + Sensory.

IV. RADIOLOGY
A. PA View
1. Break in Gilula's arc
2. Lunate and capitate overlap
3. "Piece-of-pie sign":
   i. Triangular appearance of lunate
   ii. Abnormal widening of the scapholunate interval >3 mm
4. Other associated fractures.

B. Lateral
1. Loss of collinearity of radius, lunate, and capitate
2. SL angle >70 degrees
3. Spilled teacup sign.

V. MANAGEMENT
1. Closed reduction should be performed with adequate sedation.
2. Emergency closed reduction → ↓↓ risk of median nerve and cartilage injuries
3. Technique of closed reduction by Tavernier:
   i. Longitudinal traction → 5 to 10 minutes for muscle relaxation
   ii. For dorsal perilunate injuries, the wrist is hyperextended and volar pressure is applied to the lunate to rotate the lunate into extension
   iii. Wrist palmar flexion and traction then reduces the capitate into the concavity of the lunate
4. Closed reduction of lunate dislocations are frequently unsuccessful.
5. Early surgical reconstruction is performed if swelling allows.
6. Indications: All acute injuries less than 8 weeks.
7. Immediate surgery: Open reduction and pinning + Scapholunate ligament repair
8. Open carpal tunnel release if → Progressive signs of median nerve compromise.
9. The lunate is reduced and pinned to the radius in neutral alignment.
10. The triquetrum and scaphoid can then be pinned to the lunate with additional pins from scaphoid to capitate if required to achieve stability.
11. **Proximal row carpectomy** → Chronic injury (defined as >8 weeks after initial injury)
12. **Total wrist arthrodesis** → Chronic injuries with degenerative changes.

VI. COMPLICATIONS
1. Median neuropathy
2. Posttraumatic arthritis
3. Chronic perilunate injury
4. CRPS.

FLEXOR TENDON INJURIES – HAND

I. INTRODUCTION
1. Traumatic injuries to the flexor digitorum superficialis and flexor digitorum profundus tendons
2. Mechanism: Volar lacerations
   i. Industrial accidents
   ii. Suicidal injury
   iii. Assault
   iv. Household injury
   v. Farming injury.

II. PATHOPHYSIOLOGY

1.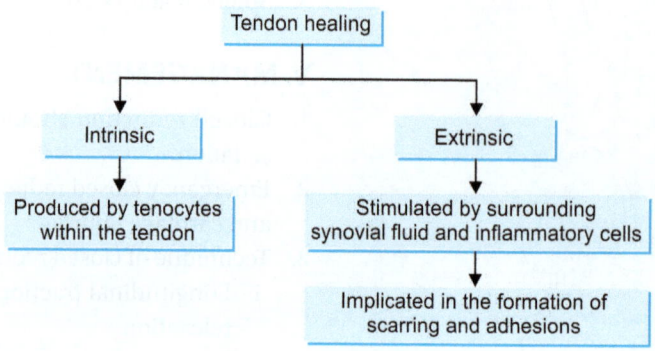

2. 3 phases of healing:

Phases of Tendon healing			
Phase	Days	Histology	Strength
Inflammatory	0–5	Cellular proliferation	None
Fibroblastic	5–28	Fibroblastic proliferation with disorganized collagen	Increasing
Remodeling	>28 days	Linear collagen organization	Will tolerate active range of motion

III. PATHOANATOMY

1. Camper chiasm → At the level of the proximal phalanx where FDP splits FDS
2. Pulley system 2nd–5th fingers contain,

5 annular pulleys (A1 to A5)	3 cruciate pulleys (C1 to C3)
• Thicker and stiffer than cruciate pulleys • A2 and A4 arise from the periosteum → Most important pulleys to prevent flexor tendon bowstringing • A1, A3, and A5 arise from the volar plate	• Collapsible and flexible • Allows the annular pulleys to approximate each other during digital flexion (**Fig. 23**)

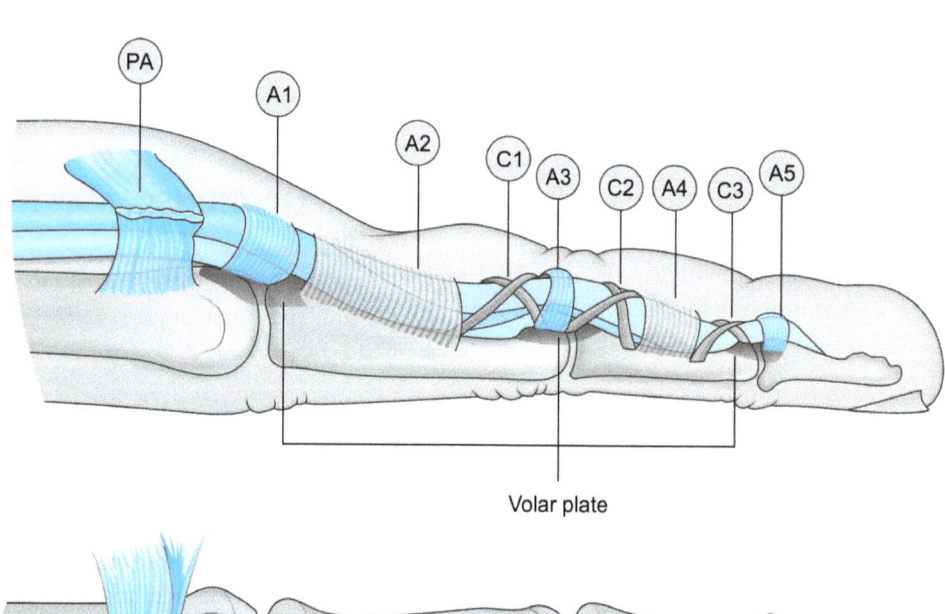

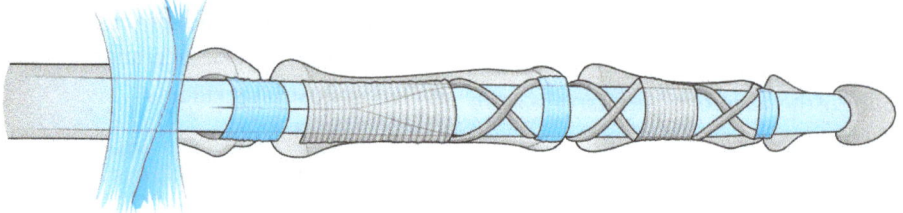

IV. ZONES (FIG. 24)

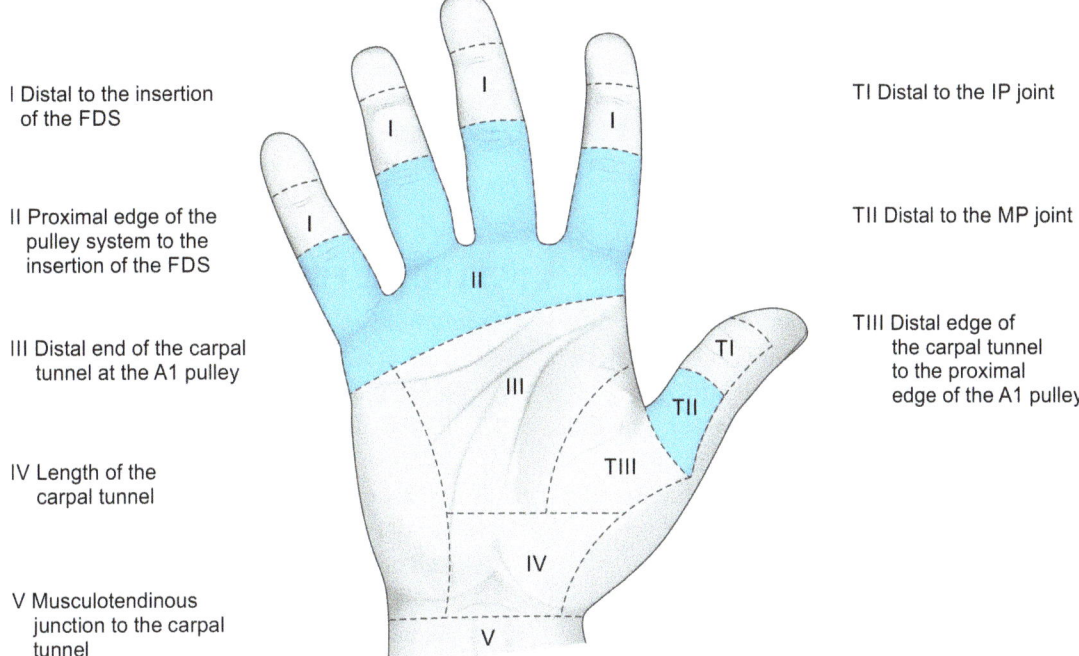

- I Distal to the insertion of the FDS
- II Proximal edge of the pulley system to the insertion of the FDS
- III Distal end of the carpal tunnel at the A1 pulley
- IV Length of the carpal tunnel
- V Musculotendinous junction to the carpal tunnel
- TI Distal to the IP joint
- TII Distal to the MP joint
- TIII Distal edge of the carpal tunnel to the proximal edge of the A1 pulley

V. CLINICAL FEATURES

A. *Symptoms*:
   1. Loss of active flexion strength or motion
   2. Lacerated wound
B. *Examination*:
   1. Assessment of the digital cascade → Malalignment or malrotation → fracture
   2. Skin integrity to help localize potential sites of tendon injury
   3. Evidence of traumatic arthrotomy
   4. Passive wrist flexion and extension → tenodesis effect
      i. Normally wrist extension causes passive flexion of the digits at the MCP, PIP, and DIP joints
      ii. Maintenance of extension at the PIP or DIP joints with wrist extension indicates flexor tendon discontinuity
   5. Active PIP and DIP flexion is tested in isolation for each digit
   6. Digital neurovascular bundle assessment.

VI. MANAGEMENT

A. **Wound care and early range of motion** → partial lacerations < 60% of tendon width
B. **Flexor tendon repair and controlled mobilization**
   1. Indications:
      i. Lacerations > 60% of tendon width with triggering
      ii. Lacerations >75%
   2. Epitendinous suture at the laceration site
   3. Fundamentals of repair:
      i. Easy placement of sutures in the tendon
      ii. Secure suture knots
      iii. Smooth juncture of the tendon ends
      iv. Minimal gapping at the repair site
      v. Minimal interference with tendon vascularity
      vi. Sufficient strength throughout healing to permit application of early motion stress to the tendon
   4. Repair must be done within 2 weeks of injury.
   5. Incisions → must cross flexion creases transversely or obliquely to avoid contractures (never longitudinal)
   6. Meticulous atraumatic tendon handling minimizes adhesions
C. **Flexor tendon reconstruction and intensive postoperative rehabilitation**
   1. Failed primary repair
   2. Chronic untreated injuries
   3. Graft selection:
      i. Palmaris longus: Most common
      ii. Plantaris: If longer graft is needed
      iii. Extensor digitorum longus
      iv. Extensor indicis proprius
      v. FDS
D. **FDS4 transfer to thumb**
   1. Single stage procedure
   2. Indicated in → chronic FPL rupture

VII. COMPLICATIONS

1. *Tendon adhesions*:
   i. Most common complication following flexor tendon repair
   ii. Higher risk with zone 2 injuries
   iii. Rx - physical therapy, tenolysis
2. Re-rupture

3. Joint contracture
4. Swan-neck deformity
5. Trigger finger
6. Lumbrical plus finger

GAME KEEPER'S THUMB

I. INTRODUCTION

1. Thumb Collateral Ligament Injuries [most commonly ulnar collateral (UCL)], are athletic injuries that lead to a decrease in effective thumb pinch and grasp.
2. Ulnar collateral ligament (UCL) injury is 10 times more common than radial collateral ligament (RCL) injuries.
3. UCL injuries → 86% of all athletic thumb injuries.
4. Acute injuries → Skier's thumb: Football, soccer, downhill skiing
5. Chronic injuries due to weakening of the ligament under repeated stress → Gamekeeper's thumb

II. PATHOANATOMY

Both UCL and RCL composed of:
1. Proper collateral ligament resists load with thumb in flexion.
2. Accessory collateral ligament and volar plate → resists load with thumb in extension.
3. Both ligaments run in dorsal to volar direction from proximal to distal.
4. Valgus laxity in both flexion and extension is indicative of a complete collateral rupture.

III. PATHOPHYSIOLOGY

1. Mechanism → Radially-directed force causing hyperabduction moment at the thumb MCP
2. **Stener lesion** → Avulsed ligament with or without bony attachment is displaced dorsal and superficial to the adductor aponeurosis → the interposed adductor does not allow healing without surgical repair **(Fig. 25)**

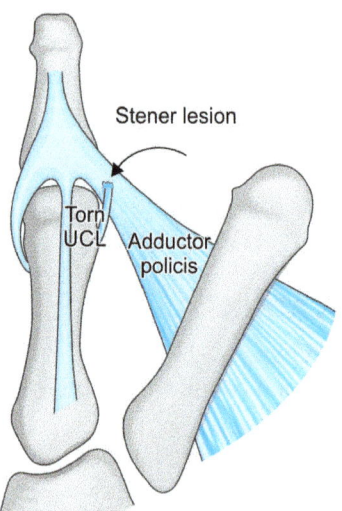

3. Grading

UCL/RCL instability grading	
Grade 1	Sprain with no joint instability (incomplete tear)
Grade 2	Asymmetric joint laxity but endpoint present (incomplete tear)
Grade 3	Joint instability without endpoint and 30–35 degrees of joint space opening or 10–15 degrees more than contralateral thumb (complete tear)

IV. CLINICAL FEATURES

A. *Symptoms*:
   1. Pain at ulnar aspect of MCP joint worse with pinch or grasp most common for UCL tear
   2. Radial-sided MCP pain most common complaint for RCL tear
B. *Examination*:
   1. Tenderness at site of ligament injury (distal for UCL and proximal for RCL)
   2. Tender mass signifying Stener lesion
   3. Radial instability in 30° of flexion → Proper UCL injury
   4. Radial instability in extension → Accessory and proper UCL and/or volar plate injury
   5. Weakness with resisted pinch.

V. RADIOLOGY

1. Avulsion or condylar fracture
2. Sag sign → supination of proximal phalanx relative to the metacarpal
3. Volar subluxation of proximal phalanx (lateral view)
4. Ultrasound: Operator-dependent
5. MRI: 100% sensitivity and specificity

VI. MANAGEMENT

A. **Thumb spice splint/cast immobilization for 4 to 6 weeks**
   1. Grade 1 and 2 partial UCL and RCL tears
   2. <15° side to side variation of varus/valgus instability
B. **RCL/UCL repair**
   1. Acute Grade 3 injuries with
      i. >15° side to side variation of varus/valgus instability
      ii. >30–35° of opening
   2. Stener lesion
   3. Chevron Incision over MCP joint.
   4. Transosseous sutures, suture anchors used
C. **Ligament reconstruction using Palmaris longus tendon graft**
   1. Chronic injury (older than 3–8 weeks)
   2. Incompetent ligament tissues
D. **Adductor advancement**
   For acute UCL rupture → in conjunction with UCL repair
E. **MCP fusion – 15 degrees of flexion**
   1. Chronic injuries
   2. Salvage procedure for failed repairs or reconstructions

PAEDIATRIC FRACTURES – PRINCIPLES AND MANAGEMENT

I. INTRODUCTION
1. Younger the patient → greater the remodeling potential. Therefore → Absolute anatomic reduction in a child is less important than in a comparable injury in an adult.
2. Approximately 50% of all children will fracture at least one bone during childhood.
3. Boy: Girl = 2.7:1
4. Peak incidence a boys 16 years, girls 12 years.

II. ANATOMY
1. ↑Water content and ↓ mineral content per unit volume than adult bone → lower modulus of elasticity (less brittle) and a higher ultimate strain-to-failure than adult bone → stronger in tension than compression compared to adult bone.
2. Physis varies in thickness depending on age and location. Weaker than bone in torsion, shear and bending → injury.
3. Divided into zones: Reserve (resting/germinal), proliferative, hypertrophic, and provisional calcification **(Fig. 26)**

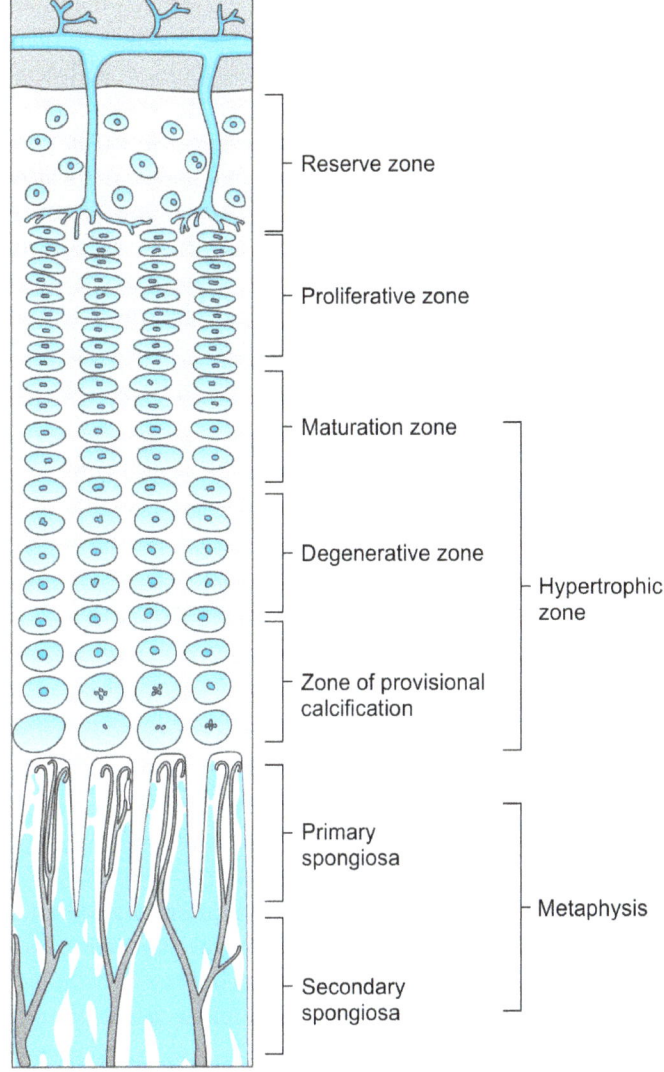

Zone	Property	Pathology
Reserve zone	• Cells store lipids, glycogen, and proteoglycan • Low oxygen tension	Gaucher's
Proliferative zone (C)	• Proliferation of chondrocytes with longitudinal growth and stacking of chondrocytes • Highest rate of extracellular matrix production • Increased oxygen tension in surroundings inhibits calcification	• Achondroplasia • Gigantism • HME
Hypertrophic zone	• Zone of chondrocyte maturation, chondrocyte hypertrophy, and chondrocyte calcification • Three phases occur in the hypertrophic zone • **Maturation zone:** Preparation of matrix for calcification, chondrocyte growth • **Degenerative zone:** Further preparation of matrix for calcification, further chondrocyte growth in size (5x) • **Provisional calcification zone:** Chondrocyte death allows calcium release, allowing calcification of matrix	• SCFE • Rickets (provisional calcification zone) • Enchondromas • Mucopolysaccharide disease • Fractures most commonly occur through zone of provisional calcification
Primary spongiosa (metaphysis)	• Vascular invasion and resorption of transverse septa • Osteoblasts align on cartilage bars produced by physeal expansion. • Primary spongiosa mineralized to form woven bone	• Metaphyseal "corner fracture" in child abuse • Scurvy
Secondary spongiosa (metaphysis)	• Internal remodelling (removal of cartilage bars, replacement of fiber bone with lamellar bone) • External remodelling (funnelization)	Renal SCFE

4. Periosteum → thick fibrous structure → encompasses the entire bone except the articular ends. It thickens and is continuous with the physis at the perichondral ring (ring of LaCroix), additional resistance to shear force.
5. Ligaments in children are functionally stronger than the physis. Therefore, a higher proportion of injuries that produce sprains in adults result in physeal fractures in children.
6. Rich metaphyseal circulation with fine capillary loops ending at the physis (in the neonate, small vessels may traverse the physis, ending in the epiphysis).

III. MECHANISM OF INJURY
1. Pediatric fractures occur at lower energy than adult fractures
2. Compression fractures → MC at the metaphyseal diaphyseal junction and are referred to as "Buckle/torus fractures" → impacted and stable → Rx. Manipulative reduction.
3. Torsional injuries → 2 patterns of fracture based on maturity of the physis.

a. Young child → thick periosteum → diaphyseal bone fails before the physis → long spiral fracture. Toddlers # - Tibia.
b. In the older child, similar torsional injury → physeal fracture.
4. Bending moments → "greenstick fractures" → incompletely fractured, resulting in a plastic deformity on the concave side of the fracture. The fracture may need to be completed to obtain an adequate reduction.
5. Bending moments can also result in microscopic fractures that create plastic deformation of the bone with no visible fracture lines on plain radiographs; permanent deformity can result.
6. In the older child, bending moments result in transverse or short oblique fractures.

IV. CLINICAL EVALUATION

1. Pediatric trauma patients → full trauma evaluation → ABCDE
2. Children → unreliable history. Parents may not be present at the time of injury and cannot always provide an accurate history.
3. Evaluate the entire extremity → Young children cannot always localize the site of injury.
4. Neurovascular evaluation mandatory → both before and after manipulation.
5. Periodic evaluation for compartment syndrome. Particularly in a nonverbal patient who is irritable and who has a crush-type mechanism of injury.
6. A high index of suspicion should be followed by compartment pressure monitoring.
7. Anxiety, ↑ analgesia requirement, agitation – 3A's of compartment syndrome in children.

8. Intracompartmental blood loss from long bone # of the lower limbs → serious complications.
9. *Child abuse suspicion*:
    i. Transverse femur fracture in <1 year old
    ii. Transverse humerus fracture in <3 years old
    iii. Metaphyseal corner fractures (caused by a traction/rotation mechanism)
    iv. History → inconsistent with the fracture pattern
    v. An unwitnessed injury that results in fracture
    vi. Multiple fractures in various stages of healing
10. *Skin stigmata of abuse*:
    i. Multiple bruises in various stages of resolution, cigarette burns
    ii. If abuse → child should be admitted to the hospital and social services notified.

V. RADIOGRAPHIC EVALUATION

1. Radiographs → Orthogonal views of the involved bone as well as the joint proximal and distal to the suspected area of injury.
2. Comparison views of the opposite extremity to confirm if in doubt of normal ossification pattern.
3. "Soft signs", such as the posterior fat pad sign in the elbow.
4. Skeletal survey → suspected child abuse or multiple traumas.
5. CT → Complicated intra-articular fractures in the older child.
6. MRI → evaluate a fracture not clearly identifiable on plain films due to lack of ossification.
7. Arthrogram → Intraoperative assessment of intra-articular fractures → Radiolucent cartilaginous structures will not be apparent on fluoroscopy.
8. Bone scans → Osteomyelitis or tumor.
9. Ultrasound → Epiphyseal separation in infants.

VI. CLASSIFICATION–SALTER HARRIS (FIG. 27)

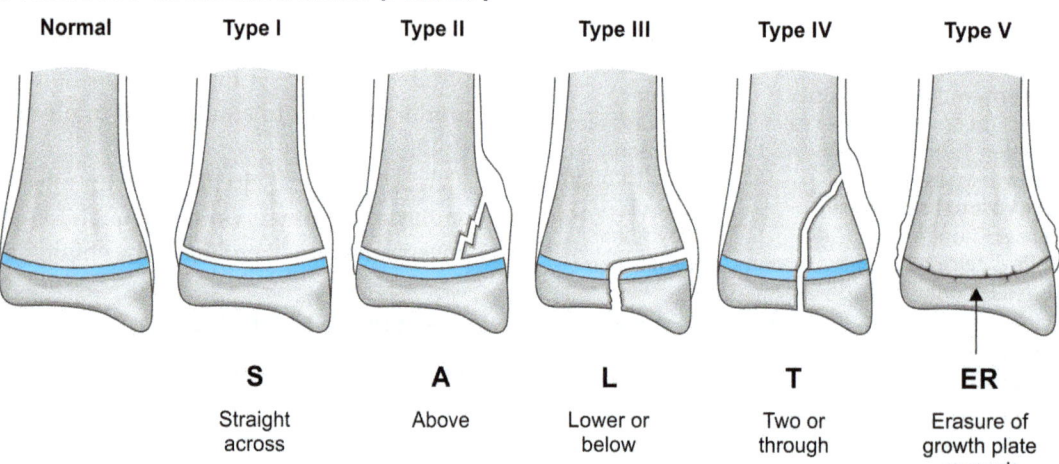

VI. Perichondral ring
VII. Epiphysis only
VIII. Metaphyseal fracture
IX. Diaphyseal fracture

VII. TREATMENT

1. Fracture management in the child differs from that in an adult → presence of a thick periosteum in diaphyseal fracture or open physis → metaphyseal fractures.
2. Periosteum → aid to reduction → usually intact on the concave side of the deformity → hinge preventing overreduction. Longitudinal traction will not reliably unlock the fragments when the periosteum is intact.
3. Controlled recreation and exaggeration of the fracture deformity are effective means of disengaging the fragments to obtain reduction.
4. Unlike in the adult, considerable fracture deformity may be permitted because the remodeling potential of the young child is great.
5. In general, the closer the fracture is to the joint (physis), the better the deformity is tolerated (e.g., 45–60° of angulation in a proximal humeral fracture in a young child is permissible, whereas the midshaft fracture of the radius or tibia → within 10 degrees of normal alignment).
6. Rotational deformity does not spontaneously correct or remodel – Avoid.
7. Severely comminuted or shortened fractures may need skin or skeletal traction. Traction pins proximal to the nearest distal physis (e.g., Distal femur). Traction pin not through the physis.
8. Fracture reduction should be performed under conscious sedation, followed by immobilization in either a splint or bivalved cast.
9. In children, casts or splints should encompass the joint proximal and distal to the site of injury, because post immobilization stiffness is not a common problem for children.
10. All fractures → elevated at above the heart level, iced, and frequently monitored → warmth, color, capillary refill, and sensation.
11. Pronounced swelling → admitted to the hospital for observation.
12. Reduction not achieved → splinted → child prepared for GA → complete relaxation.
13. Intra-articular fractures, SH III and IV → anatomic reduction (<1 to 2 mm of displacement both vertically and horizontally) to restore articular congruity and to minimize physeal bar formation.
14. Pathological fractures → Management of Malignancy.
15. Indications for operative management: SCII, III, IV, NOF, forearm both bone, femur with no acceptable reduction
16. Indications for open reduction include:
    i. Most open fractures
    ii. Displaced intra-articular fractures (Salter-Harris types III and IV)
    iii. Fractures with vascular injury
    iv. Fractures with an associated compartment syndrome
    v. Unstable fractures that require abnormal positioning to maintain closed reduction

VIII. COMPLICATIONS

1. Complete growth arrest
2. Overgrowth
3. Progressive angular or rotational deformities
4. Nonunion: NOF #, lateral condyle
5. Osteonecrosis

LATERAL CONDYLE OF HUMERUS FRACTURE – PAEDIATRICS

I. INTRODUCTION

1. 2nd most common fractures of the pediatric elbow.
2. Notorious for having an ↑↑ risk of non-union, malunion and AVN.
3. Typically occurs in patients aged ~ 6 years
4. Most commonly → Salter-Harris IV fracture patterns of the lateral condyle.

II. PATHOANATOMY

1. Fractures originate proximally at the posterior aspect of the distal humerus metaphysis and extend distally and anteriorly across the physis and epiphysis into the elbow joint
2. Fractures can extend medially into the trochlear groove → making the elbow unstable and prone to dislocation.
3. 180 degree displacement in coronal plane and 90 degree in vertical.
4. **CRITOE + CTE + DH + I**

Ossification centers in elbow	Appearance
i. **C**apitellum	1
ii. **R**adial head	3
iii. **I**nternal epicondyle	5
iv. **T**rochlea	7
v. **O**lecranon	9
vi. **E**xternal epicondyle	11
	Fusion
i. C+T+E	13
ii. CTE→ Distal humerus metaphysis	15
iii. I → Metaphysis	17

5. "Fracture of necessity"

   Factors leading to nonunion:
   i. Displaced by extensor tendon origin
   ii. Bath by synovial fluid
   iii. Precarious blood supply
   iv. Articular cartilage distal surface facing the proximal fragment

III. CLASSIFICATION

Milch classification	
Type I	Fracture line is lateral to trochlear groove (less common, elbow is stable as fracture does NOT enter trochlear groove)
Type II	Fracture line extends medially into trochlear groove (more common, more unstable)

Fracture displacement classification-Weiss		
	Characteristics	Treatment
Type 1	<2 mm, indicating intact cartilaginous hinge	Casting
Type 2	>2 mm <4 displacement, intact articular cartilage on arthrogram	Closed reduction and fixation
Type 3	>4 mm, articular surface disrupted on arthrogram	Open reduction and fixation

IV. CLINICAL FEATURES

A. Symptoms
1. Lateral elbow pain and swelling
2. Refusal to move elbow joint

B. Examination
1. Lacks the obvious deformity often seen with supracondylar fractures
2. Swelling and tenderness → limited to the lateral side
3. Lateral ecchymosis → tear in the aponeurosis of the brachioradialis → unstable fracture
4. Crepitus at the fracture site.

V. RADIOLOGY

A. Radiographs
1. Internal oblique view most accurately shows fracture displacement as the fracture is posterolateral.
2. Comparison X-rays of the contralateral elbow when ossification is not completed.
3. Capitellum is laterally displaced in relation to radial head.
4. **Thurston-Holland fragment** seen posteriorly on the lateral view.

B. Arthrogram
1. Minimally displaced fractures
2. Incomplete epiphyseal ossification → to assess cartilage surface
3. Permits dynamic assessment

C. MRI
1. Assessment of cartilaginous integrity of the trochlea
2. Surgical planning of delayed or nonunions

VI. MANAGEMENT
1. Closed reduction + Percutaneous pinning → 2–4 mm of displacement with intact articular cartilage.
2. *Open reduction and pinning*:
   i. >4 mm of displacement
   ii. Open reduction may be necessary most times to align the joint surface
   iii. Avoid dissection of the posterior aspect of lateral condyle (compromises blood supply)
3. Supracondylar osteotomy → Deformity correction in late-presenting cubitus valgus – rarely needed
4. Immobilization in an above elbow cast for 3–6 weeks

VII. COMPLICATIONS
1. Stiffness: Most common complication:
   i. Early sign of a non-union or delayed union ±
   ii. Usually self-resolving by 24–40 weeks.
2. Delayed Union → fractures that do not heal with 6 weeks of immobilization
3. Non-union treatment:
   i. Rx Goal → Achieve metaphyseal fragment union, not restoration of joint surface
   ii. ORIF with screw + Bone graft
4. Cubitus Valgus ± tardy ulnar nerve palsy:
   Rx → Supracondylar osteotomy after skeletal maturity and ulnar nerve transposition
5. AVN
6. Fishtail deformity
7. Lateral overgrowth/prominence
8. Growth arrest

SUPRACONDYLAR FRACTURE HUMERUS – PAEDIATRICS

One of the most common pediatric traumatic fractures resulting from a fall on an outstretched hand.

I. PATHOPHYSIOLOGY
1. *Age group*: 5–7 years
2. M = F
3. *Mechanism*:
   i. Fall on outstretched extremity
   ii. Thin cross section of bone in that region
4. *Associated injuries*:
   a. Neuropraxia:
      i. Anterior interosseous nerve (AIN): Most common
      ii. Radial nerve palsy → second most common
      iii. Ulnar nerve palsy → seen with flexion-type injury patterns
      iv. Most cases of neurapraxia in supracondylar humerus fractures resolve spontaneously
   b. Vascular compromise (10%) → Abundant collateral blood supply can maintain circulation despite vascular injury.
   c. Ipsilateral distal radius fractures.

II. CLINICAL FEATURES

A. Symptoms
1. Pain
2. Swelling
3. Refusal to move the elbow

B. Examination
1. Gross deformity
2. Swelling
3. Ecchymosis in antecubital fossa
4. Puckering sign: Brachialis → indicates proximal fragment buttonholed through brachialis
5. Limited active elbow motion
6. Neurovascular examination must before any reduction maneuver to be certain nerve or vascular injury is not iatrogenic.
7. Evaluate for:
   i. AIN neurapraxia (Kiloh-Nevin sign)
      a. FPL ⊗ → Unable to flex the interphalangeal joint of the thumb
      b. FDP ⊗ → Distal interphalangeal joint of the index finger
   ii. Median nerve injury: Loss of sensation over volar index finger
   iii. Radial nerve neurapraxia → inability to extend wrist, MCP joints, thumb IP joint
   iv. Pulse
   v. Assess vascular perfusion:
      a. Well perfused:
         1. Warm
         2. Pink
      b. Poorly perfused:
         1. Cold
         2. Pale
         3. Arterial capillary refill >2 seconds

III. CLASSIFICATION

Extension type most common (95–98%)
Flexion type less common (<5%)

Gartland classification (may be extension or flexion type)	
	Characteristics
Type I	• Undisplaced • Beware of subtle medial comminution leading to cubitus varus which technically means it is not a Type I fracture
Type II	• Displaced, in 1 plane • Posterior cortex and posterior periosteal hinge intact • Deformity is in the sagittal plane only
Type III	• Displaced, in 2 or 3 planes
Type IV	• Complete periosteal disruption with instability in flexion and extension • Diagnosed with examination under anesthesia during surgery
Flexion type	• Mechanism of injury is usually a fall on the olecranon

IIIA – Posteromedial more common than IIIB – Posterolateral

IV. RADIOLOGY
1. Posterior fat pad sign
2. Displacement of the anterior humeral line:
   i. Normally, the anterior humeral line intersects the middle third of the capitellum.
   ii. Capitellum moves posteriorly to this reference line in extension type fractures and anteriorly in flexion type fractures
3. Abnormal Baumann angle:
   Baumann's angle → a line parallel to the longitudinal axis of the humeral shaft and a line along the lateral condylar physis (AP view). Normal: ~ 75° **(Fig. 28)**

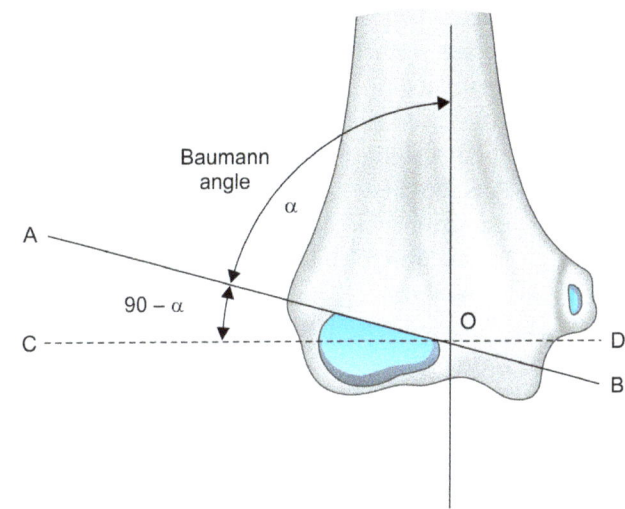

V. MANAGEMENT

A. Above elbow slab after closed reduction (elbow flexion less than 90°) → converted to a cast after swelling subsides
   1. Indications:
      i. Type I (nondisplaced) fractures
      ii. Type II fractures when:
         a. Anterior humeral line intersects the capitellum
         b. Minimal swelling present
         c. No medial comminution
   2. Hand must be warm perfused without neurological deficits
   3. Immobilization in pronation for posteromedial displacement and supination for posterolateral → for 3 weeks
   4. Repeat radiographs at 1 week to assess for interval displacement

B. Closed reduction and percutaneous pinning (CRPP):
   1. Indications:
      i. Type II and III supracondylar fractures
      ii. Flexion type
      iii. Medial column collapse
   2. Timing:
      i. Non-urgent (can wait overnight) → warm perfused hand without neuro deficits

ii. Urgent (same day - do not wait overnight)
     a. Pulseless, well-perfused hand
     b. Sensory nerve deficits
     c. Excessive swelling
     d. "Brachialis sign" → ↑ chances of arterial injury
     e. Floating elbow → to decrease the risk of compartment syndrome from swelling
  iii. Emergent (within hours) → pulseless, poorly perfused hand sos vascular exploration
 3. Technique:
    i. **2 lateral pins** → usually sufficient in type II fractures
       a. Maximize separation of pins at fracture site (50% of width of supracondylar region)
       b. Engage both medial and lateral columns
       c. Engage sufficient bone in proximal and distal segments.
       d. Low threshold for 3rd lateral pin if concern about stability with first 2 pins
       e. Pins should be inserted with elbow in flexion for extension-type injury and elbow in extension for flexion-type injury
    ii. **3 lateral pins:** Biomechanically stronger in bending and torsion than 2-pin constructs
       a. Comminution
       b. Type III and type IV (free floating distal fragment)
    iii. Crossed pins:
       a. Biomechanically strongest to torsional stress
       b. ↑ risk of ulnar nerve injury
       c. ↑↑ risk if placed with elbow in hyperflexion as ulnar nerve subluxates anteriorly over medial epicondyle in some children
       d. Reduce the risk of ulnar nerve injury by → placing medial pin with elbow in extension → use small medial incision (rather than percutaneous pinning)
  C. Open reduction and pinning: Closed reduction fails

VI. COMPLICATIONS

1. Pin migration: Most common complication
2. Infection
3. Cubitus varus (gunstock deformity)
4. Recurvatum
5. Cubitus valgus
6. Neuropraxia
7. Vascular Injury
8. Volkmann ischemic contracture → Results from elbow hyperflexion casting

PAEDIATRIC DIAPHYSEAL FOREARM FRACTURES

I. INTRODUCTION

1. Both bone forearm fractures are one of the most common pediatric fractures, estimated around 40% of all pediatric fractures.
2. *Greenstick fracture:* Incomplete fracture resulting from failure along tension (convex) side
3. *Torus Latin (tori): A swelling or protuberance*:
   i. Failure of cortex on compression side usually 2-3 cm proximal to physis
   ii. Torus (buckle) fracture of distal metaphysis of radius and ulna is most common lower forearm fracture in young children.
4. *Anatomic location*:
   i. 14% distal physis
   ii. 60% distal metaphysis
   iii. 20% midshaft
   iv. 4% proximal third

II. PATHOPHYSIOLOGY

1. *Mechanism of injury*:
   i. Fall from a height, on outstretched hand
   ii. Sports, or playground equipment injury
2. Nerve injury – Rare (<2%), most common – Median nerve
3. *Osteology: Normal*:
   i. Radius: Apex lateral bowing
   ii. Ulna: Apex posterior bowing
4. *Muscles*:
   i. Biceps and supinator flex and supinate the proximal fragment
   ii. Pronator teres and pronator quadratus pronate the distal fragment
   iii. Brachioradialis dorsiflexes and radially deviates the distal fragment

III. CLASSIFICATION

1.

```
                    Fracture type
                    /          \
            Incomplete         Complete
            i. Greenstick fractures
            ii. Torus fracture
            iii. Plastic deformation
```

Plastic deformation: Deforming force overtime resulting in shape change of bone without clear fracture line.
Due to a large number of microfractures resulting from a relatively lower force over longer time compared to mechanism for complete fractures.

2. *Fracture location and pattern*:
   i. Proximal-third, middle-third, distal-third
   ii. Apex volar or apex dorsal pattern.

IV. CLINICAL FEATURES

1. M > F
2. Pain and swelling
3. Child refuses to use arm
4. Gross deformity ±

5. Ecchymosis and swelling
6. Puncture wounds
7. Compartment syndrome and neurovascular injury evaluation in all forearm fractures.
8. *Rule out child abuse*:
   i. Mechanism or history appears inconsistent with injury
   ii. Multiple injuries, especially different ages
   iii. Child's affect
   iv. Grip marks/ecchymosis

V. RADIOLOGY

1. Fracture of both radius and ulna
2. Fracture of a single bone with plastic deformation of the other bone
3. No fracture with atypical bowing patterns suggesting plastic deformation
4. *Rotational malalignment*:
   i. Bicipital tuberosity and radial styloid should be 180° apart on the AP view
   ii. Ulnar styloid and coronoid are 180° apart on the lateral view
   iii. The diameter of proximal and distal fragments should match
   iv. Thickness of cortices should match on proximal and distal fragments.
5. *Evaluation for associated injuries*:
   i. Scapholunate interval
   ii. DRUJ (distal radioulnar joint)
   iii. Ulnar styloid
   iv. Elbow injuries.

VI. MANAGEMENT

A. General Principles

1. Deformities in the plane of joint motion are more acceptable.
2. Distal deformity (closer to distal physis) more acceptable than mid shaft.
3. The radius and ulna function as a single rotational unit. Therefore a final angulation of 10° in the diaphysis can block 20–30° of rotation.
4. Rotational deformities do not remodel and are increasingly being considered as not acceptable.

Acceptable closed reduction criteria in pediatric forearm fractures

Age	Shaft/both bone fx		Distal radius/ulna	
	Acceptable bayonetting	Acceptable angulations	Malrotation	Dorsal angulation
<10 years	<1 cm	15–20°	45°	30 degrees
>10 years	None	10°	30°	20 degrees

B. Conservative

1. *Closed reduction and immobilization*:
   i. Most pediatric forearm fractures → when an adequate reduction is maintained.
   ii. Greenstick injuries
   iii. Plastic deformation of over 20 degrees
2. *Closed reduction*:
   i. Plastic deformation:
      a. Steady three-point bending to counteract bending deformity
      b. Complication → A fracture may occur with abrupt force rather than a slow gradual increase in force.
   ii. Greenstick fracture:
      a. Reduction → a combination of traction, direct pressure with thumb, rotation, and three-point bending.
      b. Apex volar fractures are treated with pronation and apex dorsal fractures are treated with supination.
      c. Casting maintains reduction through three-point molding and interosseous mold.
      d. Compartment syndrome due to excessive swelling and tight circumferential casting
         Rx. → Bivalve cast to mitigate this risk.

C. Surgical

1. Intramedullary nailing
2. Percutaneous, sos open reduction
   Indications:
   i. Unacceptable alignment following closed reduction
   ii. Both bone forearm fractures in children >13 years
   iii. Open fractures
   iv. Refractures
   v. Segmental
   vi. Highly comminuted

VII. COMPLICATIONS

1. Re-fracture
2. Malunion
3. Compartment syndrome: Multiple attempts at reduction
4. Synostosis

PEDIATRIC NECK OF FEMUR FRACTURES

I. INTRODUCTION

1. *Bimodal distribution*:
   i. Children < 2–3 years → non-accidental trauma
   ii. Adolescents → motor vehicle accidents
2. M:F = 2.5:1
3.

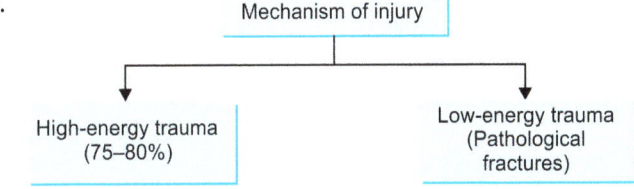

4. Commonly associated with polytrauma in children (approximately 50%)

II. BLOOD SUPPLY (FIG. 29)

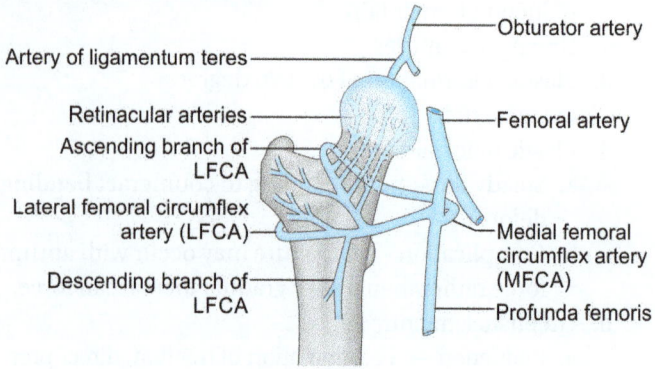

1. *Medial femoral circumflex artery (MFCA)*:
   a. Via the retinacular branches
   b. Supplies the femoral head with the LFCA and artery of ligamentum teres at birth
   c. Primary blood supply → at 4 years after regression of the LFCA and artery of ligamentum teres
2. Lateral femoral circumflex artery (LFCA)
3. Artery of the ligamentum teres
4. *Metaphyseal vessels*:
   a. Supply the head < 3 years old and after 14–16 years
   b. Between 3 and 14–16 years → Physis blocks metaphyseal supply
   c. After 14–16 years → anastomoses between metaphyseal-epiphyseal vessels.

III. CLINICAL FEATURES

1. *Symptoms*:
   i. Severe pain in affected hip
   ii. Inability to bear weight
2. *Physical examination*:
   i. Swelling and ecchymosis
   ii. Tenderness
   iii. Shortened, externally rotated lower extremity
   iv. Crepitus
   v. Neurovascular examination: Sciatic nerve

IV. CLASSIFICATION

Delbet classification				
	Description	Incidence	AVN	Nonunion
Type I	Transphyseal (with or without epiphyseal dislocation)	<10%	38–100%	
Type II	Transcervical	40–50%	28%	15%
Type III	Cervicotrochanteric (or basicervical)	30–35%	18%	15–20%
Type IV	Intertrochanteric	10–20%	5%	5%

V. INVESTIGATIONS

A. *Radiographs*:
   1. AP and cross-table lateral
   2. Bone survey if suspected non-accidental trauma
   3. Break or offset of bony trabeculae near Wards triangle → undisplaced or impacted fracture
B. *CT*: Undisplaced suspected fractures
C. *MRI*:
   1. Undisplaced fractures and stress fractures (preferred over CT)
   2. Pathologic fractures
   3. Well-defined hypointense line and surrounding hyperintense bone edema on T2- images
D. *Ultrasound*:
   1. Infants → Undisplaced fractures
   2. Hemarthrosis difficult to differentiate from effusion due to inflammation or infection
   3. Subtle epiphyseal mobility.

VI. DIFFERENTIAL DIAGNOSIS

1. Legg-Calve-Perthes disease
2. Toxic synovitis
3. Spontaneous hemarthrosis
4. Infection

VII. MANAGEMENT

A. **Closed reduction percutaneous pinning or screws – Rx of choice**
   1. Indicated in almost all pediatric neck fractures when closed reduction is successful
   2. Fixation → Smooth pins adequate in very small children.
      → 2 cannulated cancellous screws in older children and adolescents
   3. Pin or screw placement:
      Short of the physis → Patients < 4 years
      → Type III and IV fractures
   4. Transphyseal:
      i. Indications:
         a. Children close to skeletal maturity (>12 years)
         b. Crossing the physis is necessary to achieve stable fixation
      ii. Management of LLD from premature physeal closure is simpler than treating nonunion.
      iii. Must be within 5 mm of subchondral bone
      iv. Prevent injury to vasculature by avoiding anterolateral epiphyseal quadrant and posterior perforation of femoral neck.
   5. Postoperative → Hip Spica cast
B. **Open reduction** → inability to achieve closed anatomic reduction
C. **Open reduction with pediatric dynamic hip system (DHS)** → Displaced type IV or > 4 years old
D. **Open reduction capsulotomy: Smith-Peterson anterior approach**
   1. Epiphyseal dislocation

2. Open fractures
3. Vascular injury

E. **Conservative** → Closed reduction and spica abduction casting: Rarely indicated in undisplaced fractures in less than 4 years old children.

VIII. COMPLICATIONS

1. *Osteonecrosis – most common complication:*
   i. Pathophysiology:
      a. Kinking or laceration of vessels
      b. Tamponade by intracapsular hematoma
   ii. Risk factors:
      a. ↑ with ↑ age
      b. fracture type → > type I and II
      c. Delayed reduction > 24 hours
      d. Inadequate or unstable reduction
   iii. **Ratliff classification:**
      Type I: Entire head involved
      Type II: Partial head affected
      Type III: Necrosis in femur neck from fracture line to physis
   iv. Treatment:
      a. Core decompression
      b. Vascularized fibular graft
2. Coxa vara (neck-shaft angle <120°): 2nd most common complication
3. Coxa valga: Type IV fractures → due to premature GT apophysis closure
4. *Nonunion*:
   i. Etiology:
      a. Conservative treatment of type II or III fractures
      b. Occult infection at fracture site
      c. Incorrect reduction
   ii. Treatment:
      a. ORIF and hip spica cast
      b. Subtrochanteric valgus osteotomy
      c. Bone grafting
5. Physeal arrest
6. Limb length discrepancy (LLD)
7. Chondrolysis
8. Infection.

COMPLICATIONS OF COLLES' FRACTURE

Defined as: Extra-articular fracture of the distal end of radius (corticocancellous junction) with dorsal displacement.

1. MALUNION

i. Inadequate fracture reduction or stabilization.
ii. Common in elderly → Collapse
   ↓
   However functional disturbance is minimal
iii. Definition of malunion in Colles' **(Fig. 30)**:
   a. Radial inclination (RI) <10°
   b. Volar or dorsal tilt (VT) > 20°
   c. Radial height (RH) < 10 mm
   d. Ulnar variance > 2 + mm
   e. Intra-articular incongruity > 2 mm

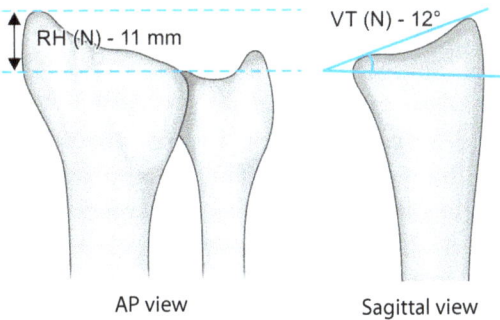
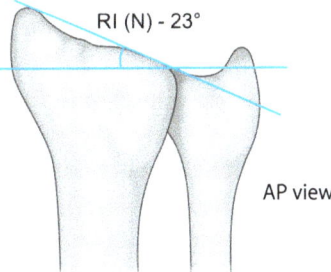

AP view

Mnemonic for normal measurements: 11 + 12 = 23
RH = 11 mm
Volar tilt = 12 degrees
RI = 23 degrees

v. However, malunion may be better defined based on loss of functional outcome rather than radiographic app.
vi. Symptoms →
   Decreased grip strength
   ↓ROM, pain
   Cosmetic deformity (unacceptable)
vii. Rx = Corrective osteotomy → Principle: Restore normal RC and RU alignment.

2. CARPAL TUNNEL SYNDROME

i. Median nerve dysfunction
ii. Acute, subacute, delayed
iii. Median nerve contusion
   ↓
   Nonprogressive → Improves over time.

Indications for Surgery

a. Median nerve dysfunction – developed after reduction → Remove splint wrist neutral. Still no improvement → Surgery
b. Complete/Incomplete lesion in a fracture requiring Surgery → relative indication
c. Complete lesion → No improvement

3. TENDON INJURY
i. MC: EPL. Rx EIP transfer → EPL
ii. Tendonitis, irritation (hardware), rupture
iii. *Prevention*:
   a. Plate proximal to watershed line
   b. Avoid prominent screws

4. FINGER AND WRIST STIFFNESS
i. Etiopathogenesis → Prolonged immobilization in cast or External Fixator
ii. Rx → Aggressive PT/OT of fingers and wrist while cast is present and after cast removal wrist too.

5. POST-TRAUMATIC ARTHRITIS
Due to:
i. Radiocarpal and radioulnar articular injury
ii. Screw penetration
Rx → Adequate reduction

6. CRPS
1. Mid-carpal instability (DISI and VISI) (Dorsal and volar intercalated segmental instability)
2. Ex Fix → Pin tract infection
3. Nonunion = Rare
4. Osteoporosis → Future marker of ↑ risk of frailty fracture

ANKLE SPRAIN

I. INTRODUCTION
1. Ankle sprain is one of the most common injuries, 1 inversion injury per 10,000 people per day.
2. A sprain is defined as a partial or complete rupture of the fibers of a ligament.
3. Any ligament about the ankle may be torn by a force that exerts traction in the direction of the fibers.
4. When the ligament is strong, a fragment of bone is avulsed from the point of insertion of the ligament.

II. PATHOANATOMY
Three ligaments:
1. *Anterior talofibular ligament*:
   i. Most commonly injured ligament in low ankle sprains
   ii. Plantar flexion and inversion injury
2. *Calcaneofibular ligament*:
   i. 2nd most common ligament injury in lateral ankle sprains
   ii. Dorsiflexion and inversion injury
3. *Posterior talofibular ligament*:
   i. Very strong → only torn in severe trauma
   ii. May lead to complete dislocation

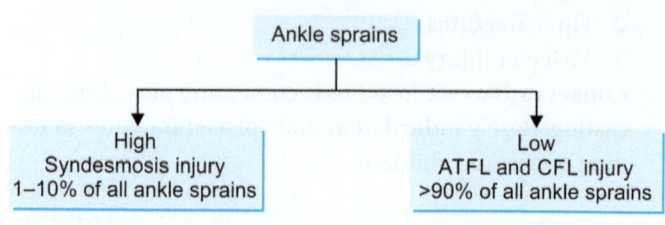

III. CLASSIFICATION
Ankle sprain types: The American Medical Association
Grade 1: Ligament stretched
Grade 2: Ligament partially torn
Grade 3: Ligament completely torn.

IV. CLINICAL FEATURES
A. Symptoms
1. Pain with weight bearing
2. Recurrent instability
3. Catching or popping sensation.

B. Physical Examination
1. Ecchymosis
2. Focal tenderness and swelling
3. Anterior drawer test: Excessive anterior displacement of talus relative to tibia
   ATFL tested in plantarflexion, CFL in dorsiflexion
4. Talar tilt test: ↑ ankle inversion (>15°) compared to C/L side → injury to ATFL and CFL.

V. RADIOLOGY
1. Ottawa ankle rules → indications for radiographs with an ankle injury
   i. inability to bear weight or walk >4 steps
   ii. medial or lateral malleolus point tenderness
   iii. 5th Metatarsal base tenderness
   iv. Navicular tenderness
   v. 96-99% sensitive in ruling out ankle fracture
2. When the ligament is strong, a fragment of bone is avulsed from the point of insertion of the ligament.
3. MRI → Pain persists for 6-8 weeks following sprain
   i. Peroneal tendon pathology
   ii. Osteochondral injury
   iii. Syndesmotic injury

VI. MANAGEMENT
A. Conservative
1. Rest
2. Ice fomentation
3. Compression - crepe bandage to minimize swelling
4. Limb elevation
5. Aircast or walking boot for 3 weeks.

B. Surgical

1. *Arthroscopy: Debridement of impinging tissue*:
   i. Indicated in recurrent ankle sprains and chronic pain caused by impingement lesions.
2. *Ligament repair and reconstruction*:
   i. **Gould modification of Brostrom anatomic reconstruction**
      a. Anatomic shortening and reinsertion of the ATFL and CFL
      b. Gould modification is the reinforcement with inferior extensor retinaculum and distal fibular periosteum.
   ii. **Tendon transfer and tenodesis (Watson-Jones, Chrisman-Snook):** Non-anatomic reconstruction using peroneus brevis tendon.

VII. COMPLICATIONS

1. Chronic pain
2. Instability
3. Stress neuropraxia

ANKLE INJURIES

I. INTRODUCTION

1. 2nd MC lower limb fracture after hip fractures
2. Mean age: 45 years
3. Mode → High energy, Sports → Young, low energy → Old

II. RISK FACTORS

1. Osteoporosis
2. Obesity
3. Smoking
4. Alcohol
5. Previous ankle sprains.

III. PATHOANATOMY

1. Distal tibia (Plafond) + MM + LM is called Mortise
2. *Ligament complex*:
   i. Syndesmotic –4:
      1. Anterior inferior tibiofibular ligament
      2. Posterior inferior tibiofibular ligament
      3. Inferior transverse tibiofibular ligament
      4. Interosseous ligament
   ii. **Medial:** Deltoid ligament → Superficial + Deep
      A. Superficial – from anterior colliculus
         1. Naviculotibial ligament
         2. Tibiocalcaneal ligament
         3. Talotibial Ligament → Most prominent
      B. Deep: Intraarticular deep tibiotalar → Medial stabilizer against lateral displacement of talus.
   iii. Fibular collateral ligament complex:
      1. Anterior talofibular ligament → weakest
      2. Posterior talofibular ligament → strongest
      3. Calcaneofibular ligament.

IV. MECHANISM OF INJURY AND CLASSIFICATION

i. **Lauge-Hansen:** 1st word: Position of foot at the time of trauma
2nd word: Direction of injuring force
Fibular # above syndesmosis: Pronation
Fibular # below syndesmosis: Supination **(Figs. 31A and B)**

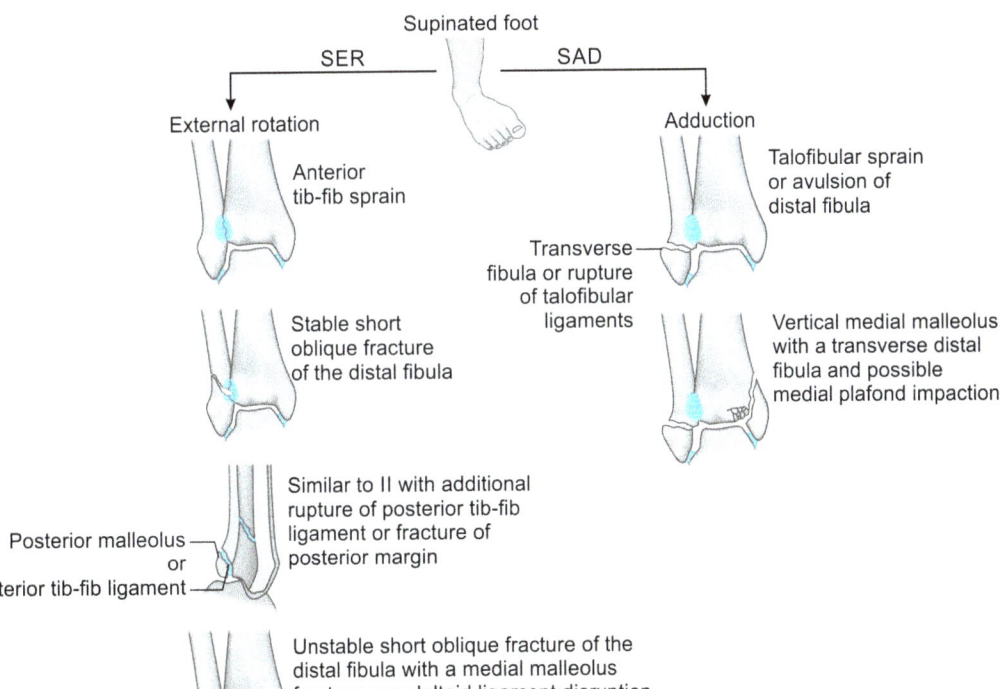

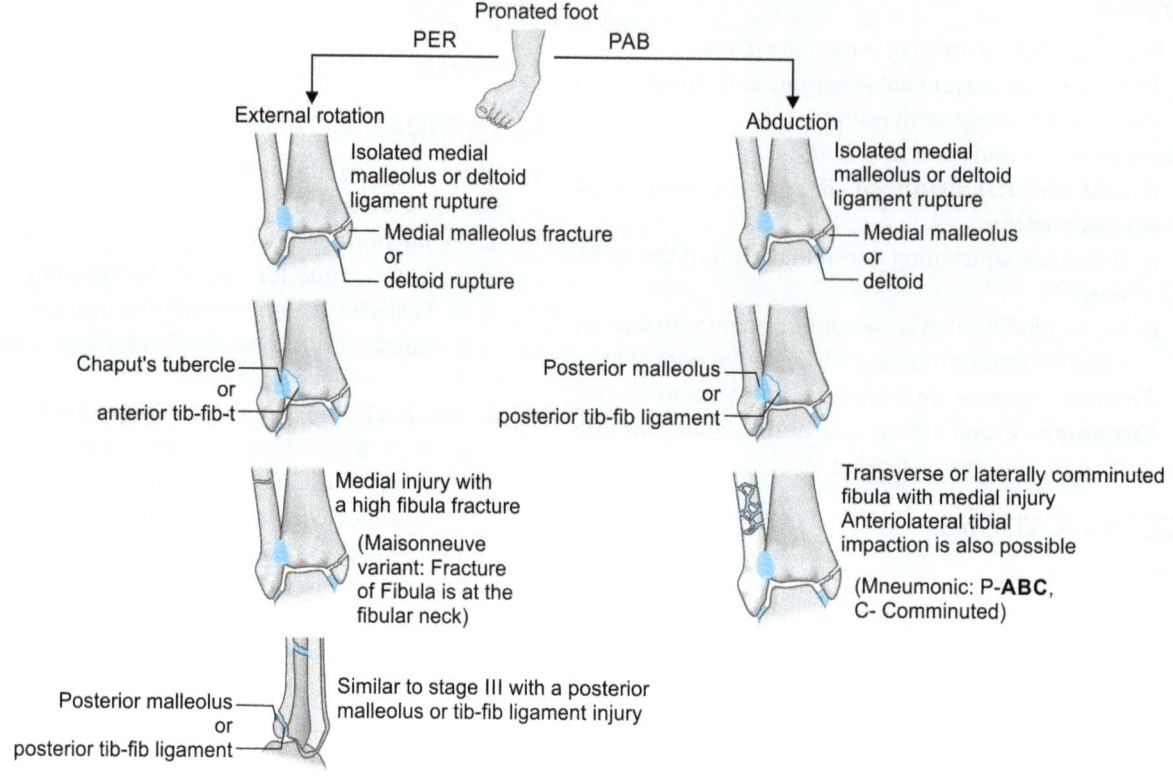

ii. **Weber classification**
   A. Infra-syndesmotic
   B. Trans-syndesmotic
   C. Supra-syndesmotic.

V. CLINICAL FEATURES

1. History of mechanism of trauma
2. Symptoms: Ottawa ankle rules
3. Examination: Swelling, tenderness, crepitus, ↓ ROM, neurovascular status.

VI. RADIOLOGY

1. AP, lateral, mortise
2. External rotation stress - most appropriate stress X-ray → competency of deltoid ligament
3. Full-length tibia → to rule out Maisonneuve-type fracture
4. *Syndesmotic injury*:
   i. Decreased tibiofibular overlap:
      - Measure at point of maximum overlap → normal >1 mm on mortise view
   ii. Increased medial clear space:
      - Normal ≤4 mm on mortise or stress view
      - >5 mm with ER stress to a DF ankle → deep deltoid disruption
   iii. Increased tibiofibular clear space → measure clear space 1 cm above joint
      - Normal <6 mm on mortise views.
5. *Lateral malleolus fractures*:
   i. Increased talocrural angle → measured by bisection of line through tibial anatomical axis and another line through the tips of the malleoli
   ii. Ball sign: Short mal reduced fibula – ball broken
6. Posterior malleolus fractures: Volkmanns fragment
   i. Double contour sign
   ii. Misty mountains sign
   iii. Spur sign.

VII. MANAGEMENT

A. Conservative
1. Rest, Nil weight bearing
2. Ice fomentation
3. Limb elevation
4. *Below knee cast*:
   i. Isolated undisplaced medial malleolus fracture or tip avulsions
   ii. Isolated lateral malleolus fracture → <3 mm displacement and no talar shift
   iii. Bimalleolar fracture → elderly or unfit for surgery.
   iv. Posterior malleolar fracture → <25% joint involvement or <2 mm step-off

B. Surgical
1. *Open reduction internal fixation*:
    i. Any talar displacement
    ii. Displaced isolated medial malleolar fracture
    iii. Displaced isolated lateral malleolar fracture
    iv. Bimalleolar fracture and bimalleolar-equivalent fracture
    v. Posterior malleolar fracture with >25% or >2 mm step-off
    vi. Bosworth fracture-dislocations → Posterior dislocation of fibula
    vii. Open fractures
    viii. Malleolar nonunion
2. Goal of treatment is stable anatomic reduction of talus in the ankle mortise →1 mm shift of talus leads to 42% decrease in tibiotalar contact area
3. *Modalities*:
    i. Lag screw fixation → stronger if placed perpendicular to fracture line
    ii. Anti-glide plate with lag screw → best for vertical shear fractures
    iii. Tension band fixation
    iv. Fibula locking plate
4. Soft tissue poor, open fracture: Delta external fixator
5. Syndesmotic injury → Syndesmotic screw.

VIII. COMPLICATIONS
1. Wound problems
2. Deep infections
3. Malunion
4. Postoperative stiffness
5. Post-traumatic arthritis.

LISFRANC INJURY

I. INTRODUCTION
A Lisfranc injury is a tarsometatarsal fracture dislocation characterized by traumatic disruption between the articulation of the medial cuneiform and base of the second metatarsal.

II. PATHOANATOMY
1. *Lisfranc joint consists of three articulations*:
    i. Tarsometatarsal (TMT) articulation
    ii. Intermetatarsal articulation
    iii. Intertarsal or intercuneiform articulations
2. *Columns of the midfoot*:
    i. Medial column → 1st TMT joint
    ii. Middle column → 2nd and 3rd TMT joints
    iii. Lateral column → 4th and 5th TMT joints (most mobile)
3. 2nd MT "Keystone" of the transverse arch.
4. Lisfranc ligament → A planter interosseous ligament from medial cuneiform to base of 2nd metatarsal → Stabilizes the 1st and 2nd TMT joints and maintenance of the midfoot arch
5. Dorsal TMT ligaments are weak → ∴ Dislocation dorsal
6. Intermetatarsal ligaments → 2nd to 5th. No ligament between 1st and 2nd.

III. PATHOPHYSIOLOGY
1. Mechanism of injury →
    i. Road traffic accidents
    ii. Fall from height
    iii. Sports injuries
2. Indirect rotational forces and axial load through hyper-plantarflexed forefoot
    ↓
    Metatarsals displaced in dorsal/lateral direction
3. Lisfranc equivalent injuries can present in the form of contiguous proximal metatarsal fractures or tarsal fractures.

IV. CLASSIFICATION (FIGS. 32A TO C)

Hardcastle and Myerson classification	
Type A	Complete homolateral dislocation
Type B1	Partial injury, medial column dislocation
Type B2	Partial injury, lateral column dislocation
Type C1	Partial injury, divergent dislocation
Type C2	Complete injury, divergent dislocation

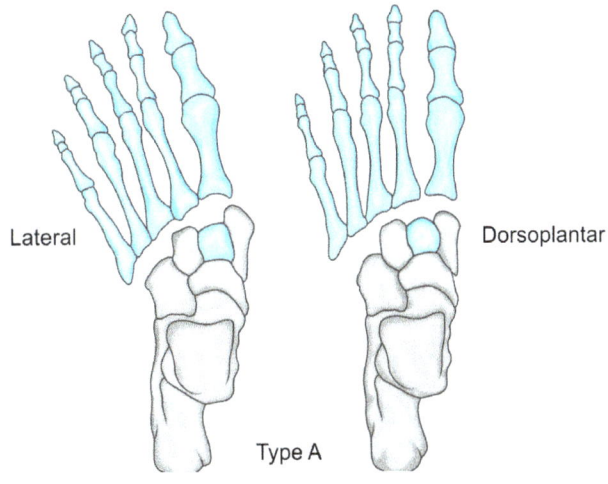

Fig. 32A: Total incongruity

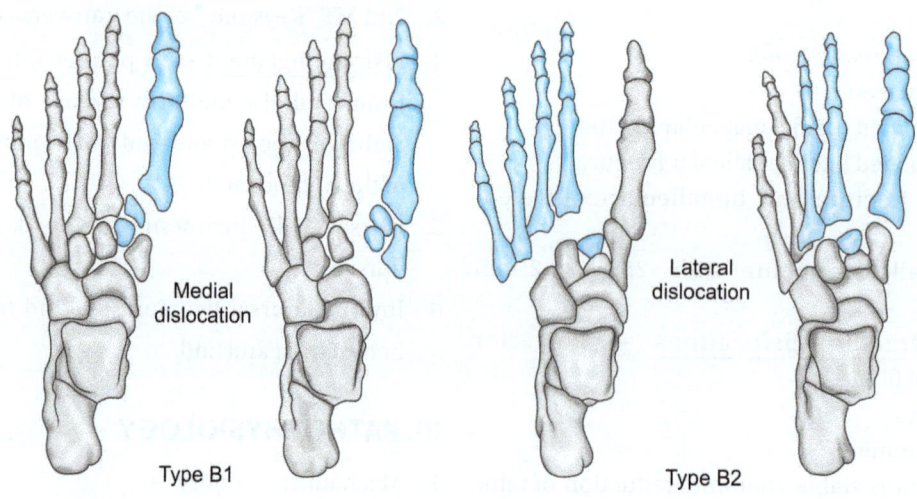

Fig. 32B: Partial incongruity

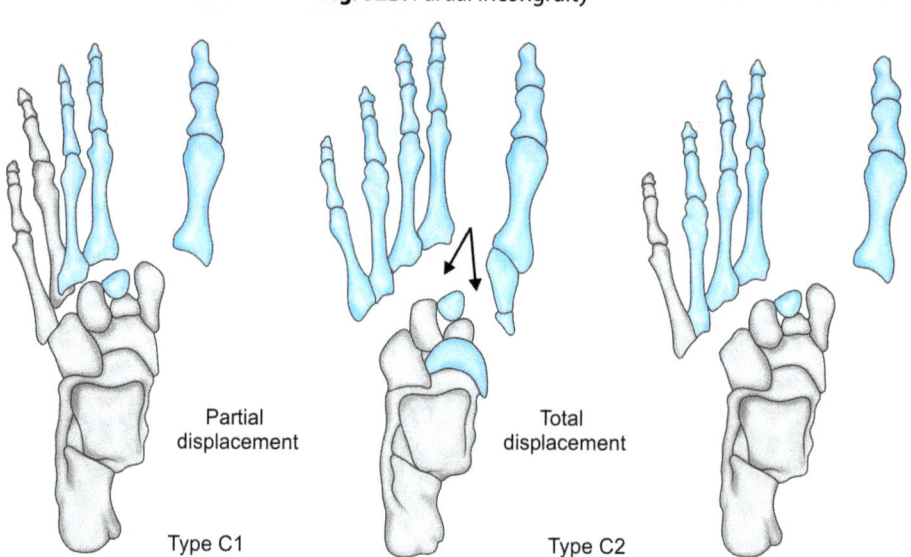

Fig. 32C: Divergent

V. CLINICAL PRESENTATION

1. Males > females
2. MC → 3rd decade
3. Variable foot deformity, pain, swelling, and tenderness on the dorsum of the foot.
4. Medial plantar ecchymosis is pathognomonic for a Lisfranc injury.
5. Neurovascular examination: Dorsalis pedis artery
6. Rule out compartment syndrome
7. Stress test: Passive forefoot abduction and pronation
8. Instability test: Grasp metatarsal heads and apply dorsal force to forefoot while other hand palpates the TMT joints → dorsal subluxation suggests instability

VI. RADIOLOGY

1. *X-ray*:
    i. Discontinuity of a line drawn from the medial base of the 2nd metatarsal to the medial side of the middle cuneiform (AP view)
    ii. 1st and 2nd ray interval widening (AP view)
    iii. Bony fragment (*fleck sign*) in 1st intermetatarsal space → represents avulsion of Lisfranc ligament from base of 2nd metatarsal (diagnostic of Lisfranc injury)
    iv. Dorsal displacement of the proximal base of the 1st or 2nd metatarsal (Lateral)
2. CT: Preoperative planning → comminuted bony injuries, subtle injuries
3. MRI: Presence of purely ligamentous injury.

VII. MANAGEMENT

1. *Conservative* → Below knee cast immobilization for 8 weeks
    i. Non-displaced injuries that are stable with weight bearing
    ii. Non-operative candidates
        a. Non-ambulatory patients
        b. Presence of serious vascular disease
        c. Severe peripheral neuropathy

2. *Surgical*:
   i. Open reduction and rigid internal fixation
      a. Instability > 2 mm shift
      b. Anatomic reduction required for a good result
      c. 2 long incisions: 1st – between 1st and 2nd MT → NVB
      d. 2nd → over 4th MT
      e. The key to reduction is correction of the fracture-dislocation of the second metatarsal base.
      f. Fixation → Cancellous screws, Headless screws, K wires.
   ii. Temporary percutaneous pinning and delayed ORIF or arthrodesis significant soft tissue swelling
   iii. Primary arthrodesis of the 1st, 2nd and 3rd TMT joints
      a. Delayed treatment
      b. Chronic deformity
      c. Complete Lisfranc fracture dislocations (Type A or C2)
   iv. Midfoot arthrodesis
      a. Destabilization of the midfoot's architecture with progressive arch collapse and forefoot abduction
      b. Chronic Lisfranc injuries → advanced midfoot arthrosis and have failed conservative therapy

VIII. COMPLICATIONS

1. Post-traumatic arthritis: MC complication
2. Malunion
3. Nonunion
4. Hardware removal
5. Deep infection
6. Planovalgus foot deformity
7. Compartment syndrome
8. Neurovascular injury
9. CRPS.

TALUS NECK FRACTURES

I. INTRODUCTION

1. High energy injuries to the hindfoot that are associated with a high incidence of talus avascular necrosis
2. Neck: Most common fracture of talus (50%)
3. Mechanism → Forced dorsiflexion with axial load

II. CLASSIFICATION

	Hawkins classification	
Type	Description	AVN risk
Hawkins I	Nondisplaced	0–13%
Hawkins II	Subtalar dislocation	20–50%
Hawkins III	Subtalar and tibiotalar dislocation	20–100%
Hawkins IV	Subtalar, tibiotalar, and talonavicular dislocation	70–100%

III. RADIOLOGY

1. Radiographs → Mortise, lateral, Canale view
2. Canale view → Best view to demonstrate talar neck fractures
   Maximum equinus, 15 degrees pronated, X-ray beam 75 degrees cephalad from horizontal.
3. CT scan → best study for degree of displacement, comminution and articular congruity.
   Assesses ipsilateral foot injuries as well (up to 89% incidence)

IV. MANAGEMENT

A. Conservative

1. **Emergent reduction in ER** → all cases require emergent closed reduction in ER
2. **Short leg cast for 8–12 weeks (NWB for initial 6 weeks)**
   i. Nondisplaced fractures (Hawkins I) → CT to confirm an undisplaced fracture without articular step off.

B. Surgical

1. *Indications*:
   i. All displaced fractures (Hawkins II-IV)
   ii. Talus extrusion
2. *Open reduction and internal fixation*:
   i. Approach → two approaches recommended
      a. Visualize medial and lateral neck to assess reduction
      b. Typical areas of comminution are dorsal and medial
   ii. Anteromedial: Between tibialis anterior and posterior tibialis
      a. Preserve soft tissue attachments, especially deep deltoid ligament (blood supply)
      b. Medial malleolar osteotomy to preserve deltoid ligament
   iii. Antero-lateral:
      a. Between tibia and fibula proximally, in line with 4th ray
      b. Elevate extensor digitorum brevis and remove debris from subtalar joint
3. Anatomic reduction essential
4. Mini and small fragment screws, cannulated screws and mini fragment plates
5. Medial and lateral lag screws → simple fracture patterns
6. Mini fragment plates in comminuted fractures to buttress against varus collapse
7. Postoperative Nil weight-bearing for 10–12 weeks

V. COMPLICATIONS

1. Osteonecrosis
2. Post-traumatic arthritis
3. Varus malunion
4. Non-union
5. Infection
6. Wound dehiscence

CALCANEAL FRACTURES

I. INTRODUCTION
1. Calcaneum (Os Calcis) → Most commonly fractured tarsal bone.
2. Mechanism of injury → Traumatic axial loading
   i. Fall from height
   ii. Motor vehicle accidents

II. PATHOANATOMY

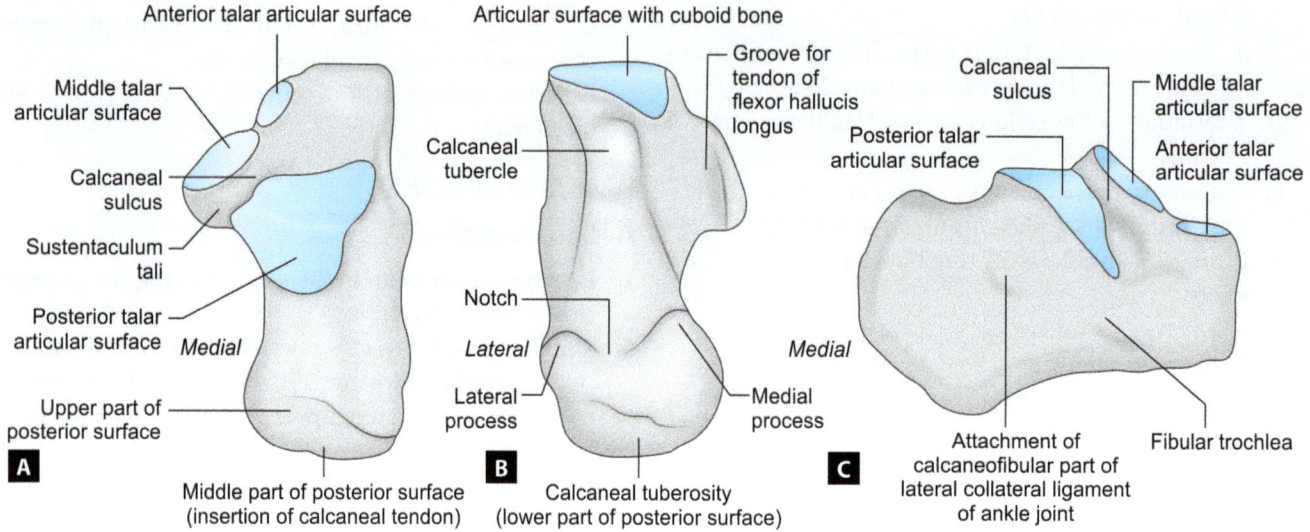

1. Three facets articulate with the talus:
   i. Posterior facet → largest and constitutes the major weight-bearing surface.
   ii. Middle facet → located anteromedially on the sustentaculum tali.
   iii. Anterior facet → confluent with the middle facet.
2. Between the middle and posterior facets → lies the interosseous sulcus (calcaneal groove), which, with the talar sulcus, forms the sinus tarsi.
3. Sustentaculum tali
   i. Supports the neck of the talus medially
   ii. Attached to the talus by the interosseous talocalcaneal and deltoid ligaments → "Constant fragment"
   iii. FHL tendon passes beneath the sustentaculum tali medially.
4. The peroneal tendons pass laterally between the calcaneus and the lateral malleolus.
5. The Achilles tendon attaches to the posterior tuberosity.

III. CLINICAL FEATURES
A. Symptoms
1. Pain
2. Swelling
3. Inability to bear weight
4. Gross deformity
5. Open wound with fracture visible

B. Examination
1. Ecchymosis
2. Skin blisters
3. Short and widened heel
4. Diffuse tenderness
5. Compartment syndrome
6. Posterior heel skin necrosis → d/t displaced tongue type fracture
7. Neurovascular exam to rule out compromise.

IV. INVESTIGATIONS
A. Radiograph
1. Views → Foot AP, lateral, oblique, broden, harris heel.
2. **Bohler's (tuber) angle** (normal 20–40°) → Decreased
   i. Angle between line from highest point of anterior process to highest point of posterior facet + line tangential to superior edge of tuberosity.
   ii. Represents collapse of the posterior facet

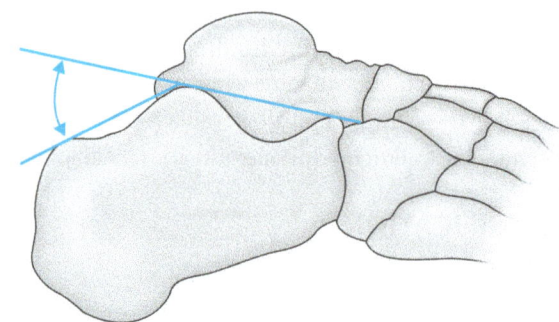

3. Crucial/Critical angle of Gissane (normal 120–145°) → Increased
   i. Angle between line along lateral margin of posterior facet + line anterior to beak of calcaneus.

ii. This also represents collapse of the posterior facet

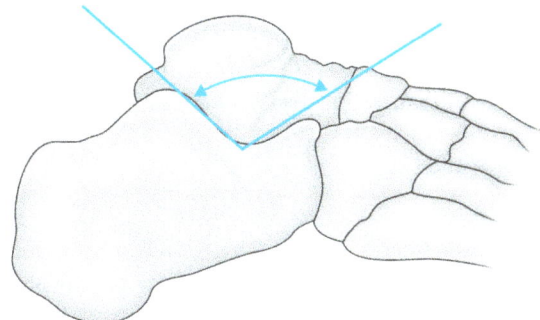

4. Double-density sign → represents subtalar incongruity indicates partial separation of facet from sustentaculum.
5. Calcaneal shortening
6. Varus tuberosity deformity
7. Broden's view:
   i. Visualization of posterior facet → Intraoperatively
   ii. With ankle in neutral dorsiflexion and ~45° internal rotation, X-rays at 40, 30, 20, and 10° cephalad from neutral.
8. Harris heel view
   i. Visualizes tuberosity fragment widening, shortening, and varus positioning
   ii. Foot in maximal dorsiflexion and X-ray beam at 45°

B. CT Scan → Gold Standard

V. CLASSIFICATION

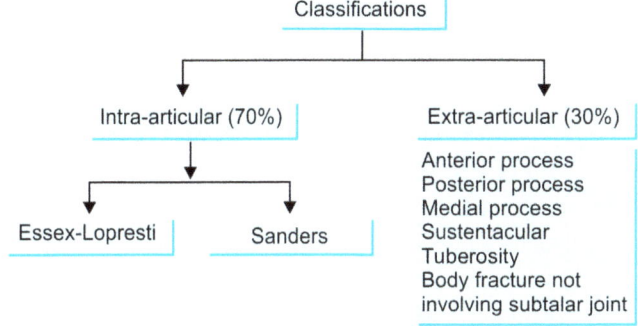

A. Essex-Lopresti

1. Primary fracture line runs obliquely through the posterior facet forming two fragments.
2. Secondary fracture line runs in one of two planes, leading to →
   i. Tongue type: Exits posteriorly, the superolateral fragment and posterior facet remain attached to the tuberosity posteriorly
   ii. Joint depression type: Exits inferiorly and depresses the subtalar joint.

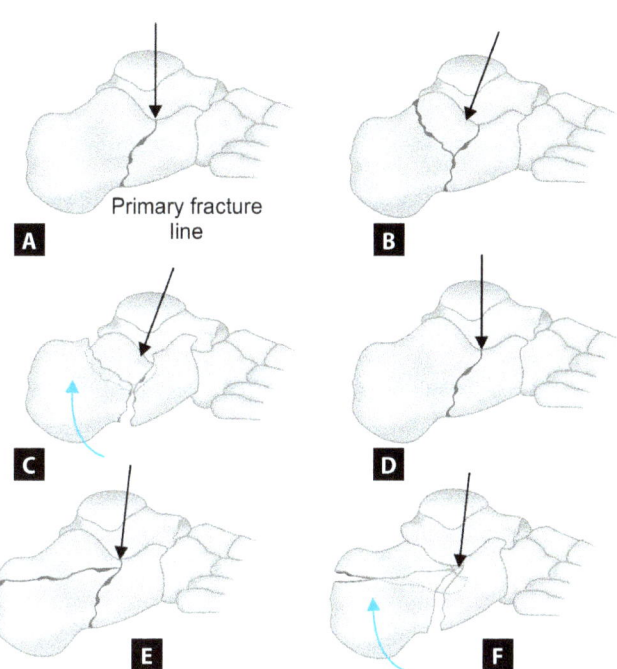

[Mechanism of injury according to Essex-Lopresti. (A to C) Force of Talus (A) creates the primary facture line, involving the posterior facet (B) and leading to depression of the facet fragments (C). (D to F) Primary fracture line again created by axial force of talus (D), secondary fracture line exists posteriorly (E) and pull of the Achilles displaces the tuberosity fragment (F)]

3. Sanders (CT based)
   i. Based on the number and location of articular fragments
   ii. Utilizes coronal sections → which shows the widest surface of the posterior facet of the talus.
   iii. The posterior facet of the calcaneus is divided into three fracture lines (A, B, and C), corresponding to lateral, middle, and medial fracture lines.
   iv. Four potential pieces → lateral, central, medial, sustentaculum tali.

Type I	All nondisplaced fractures regardless of the number of fracture lines
Type II	Fractures of the posterior facet; subtypes IIA, IIB, IIC, based on the location of the primary fracture line
Type III	Three-part fractures with a centrally depressed fragment; subtypes IIIAB, IIIAC, IIIBC
Type IV	Four-part articular fractures; highly comminuted

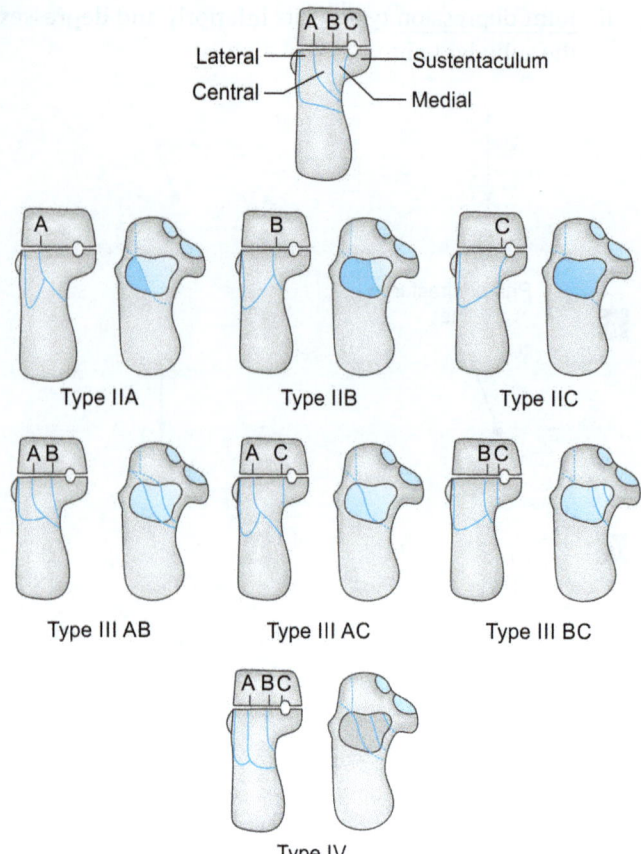

VI. MANAGEMENT

A. Conservative

1. Below knee cast immobilization
2. Nonweight bearing × 6–8 weeks
3. Indications
   i. Minimally displaced extra-articular fractures
   ii. Sanders type I
   iii. Comorbidities leading to poor outcomes (DM, smoking, PVD) → High wound complication rates after surgery.

B. Operative

1. Goals of surgery are to restore
   i. Congruity of subtalar joint
   ii. Böhler's angle and calcaneal height
   iii. Width
   iv. Correct varus malalignment
2. Closed reduction with percutaneous pinning
   i. Minimally displaced tongue type
   ii. Large extra-articular
3. Open reduction and internal fixation
   i. Displaced tongue-type fractures (>1 cm)
   ii. Threatened soft tissue → urgent reduction and fixation to avoid skin necrosis
   iii. Open fractures → thorough debridement of contaminated tissue.
   iv. Large extra-articular (> 2 mm displacement)
   v. Sanders Type II and III
4. Primary subtalar arthrodesis → Sander IV

C. Approaches

1. Extensile lateral
   i. Extensile lateral L-shaped incision is most common
   ii. Vertical part of incision → between posterior fibula and Achilles tendon.
   iii. Horizontal part → in line with 5th metatarsal base
   iv. Also provides access to the calcaneocuboid and subtalar joints
   v. Full-thickness skin, soft tissue, and periosteal flaps are developed → to preserve blood supply to the flap which is supplied by lateral calcaneal branch of peroneal artery.
   vi. Sural nerve and peroneal tendons are retracted superiorly
   vii. Lateral calcaneal wall visualized
   viii. Fracture is opened and medial wall is reduced going medial to lateral → reduction confirmed via fluoroscopy
   ix. Tuberosity reduction is done under direct visualization using manual traction, Schanz pins, and mini distractors.
   x. Provisional fixation with K-wires and definitive with plates and screws.
2. Sinus tarsi
   i. Minimally invasive incision → minimizes soft tissue dissection
   ii. Reduces wound complications associated with extensile lateral incision
   iii. Allows direct visualization of the posterior facet, anterolateral fragment, and lateral wall.
   iv. Decreased surgical time.
   v. Lateral decubitus position
   vi. Incision → In line with the tip of the fibula and the base of the 4th MT (2–4 cm)
   vii. Extensor digitorum brevis retracted cephalad to expose sinus tarsi and posterior facet
   viii. Peroneal tendons retracted posteriorly
   ix. Schanz pin inserted percutaneously in posteroinferior tuberosity going from lateral to medial → provides distraction and aids with reduction.
   x. Fibrous debris and fat removed from sinus tarsi.
   xi. Elevator or lamina spreader placed under posterior facet fragment to aid in reduction
   xii. K-wires inserted for provisional fixation aimed toward the sustentaculum

xiii. Two screw are placed lateral-to-medial to engage sustentaculum and support facet.
xiv. Large fully threaded screw from posterior-to-anterior to support axial length of calcaneum
xv. Low-profile plate is applied underneath a well-developed soft tissue cover.

VII. COMPLICATIONS

1. Chronic heel pain
2. Subtalar arthritis
3. Malunion
4. Wound complications
5. Sural nerve neuroma
6. FHL injury
7. Compartment syndrome → Claw toes

JONES FRACTURE/5TH METATARSAL BASE

I. INTRODUCTION

1. One of the most common fractures of the foot and are predisposed to poor healing due to precarious blood supply to the specific areas of the 5th metatarsal base.
2. Account for 25% of all metatarsal fractures → 90% are zone 1 fractures
3. Common in athletes, military recruits, and manual laborers
4. *Mechanism of injury*:
    i. Zone 1: Plantarflexion and hindfoot inversion
    ii. Zone 2: Forefoot adduction
    iii. Zone 3: Repetitive microtrauma

II. PATHOANATOMY

1. *Parts of the metatarsal*:
    → Head, neck, diaphysis, metadiaphysis, base and tuberosity.
    i. Base and tuberosity:
        a. Highly vascularized cancellous bone
        b. Tuberosity → Peroneus brevis insertion
        c. Open apophysis or Os vesalianum → confused for fracture. Comparison radiographs must be taken when in doubt.
    ii. Metadiaphyseal region → No tendinous attachments and is vascular watershed
    iii. Diaphysis → Peroneus tertius inserts on dorsal diaphysis
2. *Blood supply*:
    i. Metaphyseal vessels and diaphyseal nutrient artery
    ii. Zone 2 (Jones fracture) represents a vascular watershed area → prone to nonunion

III. CLASSIFICATION

Zone 1
1. Pseudo-Jones fracture
2. Proximal tubercle avulsion
3. Contraction of the peroneus brevis

Zone 2
1. Jones fracture
2. Metaphyseal-diaphyseal junction
3. Involves the 4th-5th metatarsal articulation
4. Vascular watershed area
5. Acute injury
6. Increased risk of non-union (15–30%)

Zone 3
1. Proximal diaphyseal fracture
2. Distal to the 4th-5th metatarsal articulation
3. Stress fracture in athletes
4. Associated with cavovarus foot deformities or sensory neuropathies **(Fig. 33)**

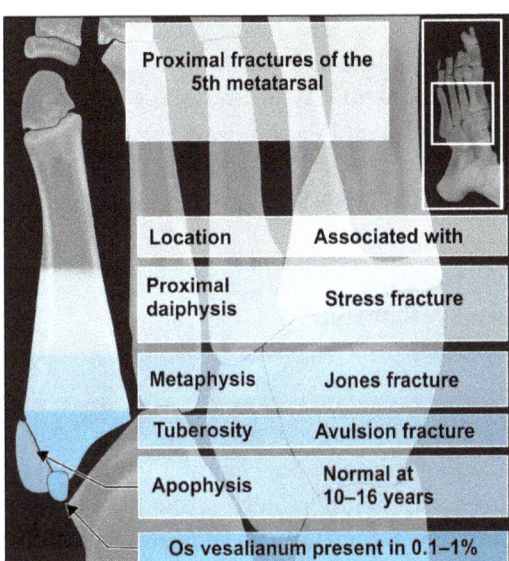

IV. CLINICAL FEATURES

1. Pain over lateral border of foot, ↑ with weight bearing
2. Swelling
3. Tenderness to palpation along bone at fracture site
4. Varus hindfoot on weight-bearing
5. Cavus foot deformity
6. Fifth metatarsal head callosity
7. Pain with resisted foot eversion → peroneal tendon weakness.

V. RADIOLOGY

1. *X-rays*:
    i. Narrow fracture line without intramedullary sclerosis → Acute fracture
    ii. Widened fracture line with intramedullary sclerosis → Delayed Union
    iii. Widened intramedullary canal with no callus → Non-union

2. Bone scan → IOC for bilateral stress fractures
3. CT → Nonunion/delayed union following surgical fixation
4. MRI → Unilateral stress fractures.

VI. MANAGEMENT
1. *Conservative*:
   i. Below knee cast or Air cast for 6 weeks → Nil weight bearing for 4 weeks
   ii. Partial Weight bearing → after 4 weeks.
   iii. Union → 8 weeks
2. *Surgical* → Very high rates of union:
   i. Indications:
      a. Pseudo-Jones fracture → Rotational displacement or skin tenting
      b. Jones, stress fractures → Athletes
   ii. Intramedullary screw fixation
   iii. ORIF with miniplate and screws → Salvage for nonunion after IM screw fixation.

VII. COMPLICATIONS
1. Re-fracture
2. Painful hardware
3. Sural nerve injury
4. Chronic pain.

TENDOACHILLES TENDON RUPTURE

Achilles tendon ruptures are common tendon injuries that occur due to sudden dorsiflexion of a plantarflexed foot, most commonly associated with sporting events.

I. PATHOANATOMY
1. Largest tendon in body
2. Formed by the tendons of soleus and gastrocnemius
3. Blood supply → posterior tibial artery
4. *Rupture site*:
   i. 4–6 cm proximal to the calcaneal insertion: Most common → Hypovascular area
   ii. Myotendinous junction
   iii. Insertion.

II. ETIOPATHOLOGY
1. M > F
2. Most common in ages 30–40 years
3. *Risk factors*:
   i. Episodic athletes, "weekend warrior"
   ii. Fluoroquinolones antibiotics
   iii. Steroid injections
4. Mechanism → usually traumatic injury during a sporting event
   i. Sudden forced plantar flexion
   ii. Violent dorsiflexion in a plantar flexed foot.

III. KUWADA CLASSIFICATION
According to severity of the tear and degree of retraction it is classified into four types:
1. *Type I*: Partial ruptures ≤50% → Conservative management
2. *Type II*: Complete rupture with tendinous gap ≤3 cm → End-end anastomosis
3. *Type III*: Complete rupture with tendinous gap 3 to 6 cm → often requires tendon/synthetic graft
4. *Type IV*: Complete rupture with a defect of >6 cm (neglected ruptures) → Requires tendon/synthetic graft and gastrocnemius recession

IV. CLINICAL FEATURES
1. Symptoms
1. A "pop" at the time of injury.
2. Weakness and difficulty walking
3. Acute onset swelling
4. Pain in heel

2. Examination
1. ↑ Resting ankle dorsiflexion in prone position with knees bent
2. Calf atrophy may be apparent in chronic cases
3. Palpable gap
4. Weakness to ankle plantar flexion
5. Increased passive dorsiflexion
6. **Thompson test** → lack of plantar flexion when calf is squeezed
7. Knee flexion test: Prone position, patient flexes knee to 90°, neutral position or dorsiflexion of ankle suggests torn tendon.

V. RADIOLOGY
1. *X-ray*:
   i. Used to rule out other pathology
   ii. Loss of posterior border of **Kager's triangle** (K). (Fat-filled triangular space in front of tendoachilles)
   iii. Toygar's sign (T) – ↓ in the **Toygar's angle**. Measured on the posterior skin surface on lateral X-ray. **(Fig. 34)**

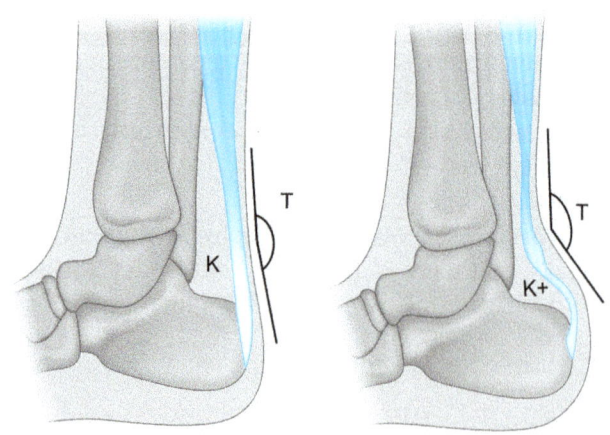

2. Ultrasound: To determine complete vs. partial ruptures
3. MRI: When equivocal physical examination findings, chronic ruptures, acute rupture with retracted tendon edges

VI. MANAGEMENT

1. Functional Cast in resting plantar flexion for 8 weeks
    i. Kuwada 1 acute injuries
    ii. Sedentary patient
    iii. Medically frail patients
2. Open end-to-end Achilles tendon repair → acute ruptures (<6 weeks) **Kessler, Krackow or Bunnel** methods
3. Percutaneous Achilles tendon repair
    i. Lesser wound complications, better cosmesis
    ii. ↑ Sural nerve damage
4. Reconstruction with VY advancement → chronic ruptures with defect <3 cm **(Fig. 35)**

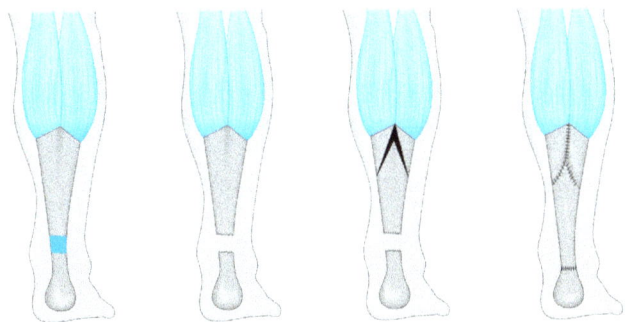

5. Flexor hallucis longus transfer ± VY advancement of gastrocnemius → chronic ruptures with defect > 3 cm

VII. COMPLICATIONS

1. Re-rupture: Higher with nonsurgical management
2. Wound healing complications: Smoking (most common), female, steroids.
3. Sural nerve injury.

CHEST INJURIES

1. Injuries to the chest may affect one or more of:
    i. Ribs
    ii. Lungs and the pleura
    iii. Cardiovascular → Heart and the aorta
    iv. Trachea
    v. Esophagus
2. 25% of all trauma deaths → Chest trauma
3.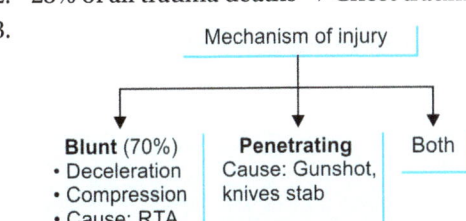

4. "Deadly dozen" threats to life from chest injuries

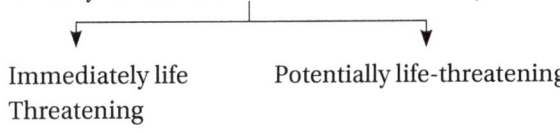

Immediately life   Potentially life-threatening
Threatening

1. IMMEDIATELY LIFE-THREATENING

i. Airway obstruction
ii. Tension pneumothorax
iii. Pericardial tamponade
iv. Open pneumothorax
v. Massive hemothorax
vi. Flail chest.

2. POTENTIALLY LIFE-THREATENING

i. Aortic injuries
ii. Tracheobronchial injuries
iii. Myocardial contusion
iv. Rupture of diaphragm
v. Esophageal injuries
vi. Pulmonary contusion.

3. CLINICAL EXAMINATION

i. Respiratory rate and depth: Tachypnea, bradypnea
ii. Chest wall asymmetry
iii. Paradoxical movement
iv. Bruising, seat belt, steering wheel wounds
v. Penetrating wounds
vi. Tracheal deviation
vii. Adequacy and equal chest wall movement
viii. Chest wall tenderness
ix. Crepitus
x. Pulse and blood pressure
xi. Respiratory effort → Labored
                     → Retractions
                     → Progressive respiratory distress.
xii. Breath sounds → Absent or decreased
                   → Unilateral or bilateral
                   → Bowel sounds in chest?
xiii. Percussion → Hyperresonance: Pneumothorax
                → Hyporesonance: Hemothorax
xiv. Subcutaneous emphysema
xv. JVD: Jugular venous distention.

4. INVESTIGATIONS

i. *Chest X-ray:* First investigation
ii. *USG*:
    a. Differentiates between contusion and the actual presence of blood
    b. USG eFAST → Extended focused assessment with sonography in trauma

iii. *CT scan (HRCT Chest)*:
   a. Principle and most reliable
   b. With contrast → 3D reconstruction of chest with bony skeleton
   c. Track or presence of missile → proper planning of surgery.
iv. *Chest tube insertion* – Diagnostic as well as therapeutic
v. Angiography
vi. ABG

5. MANAGEMENT IN GENERAL

i. Follow the ATLS protocol
ii. A: Airway
    B: Breathing
    C: Circulation
    D: Disability
    E: Exposure
iii. Early assessment and primary survey
iv. Simultaneous aggressive resuscitation
v. Secondary survey with full examination
         ↓
vi. Transfer to definitive care

6. MANAGEMENT OF SPECIFIC INJURIES

i. Airway Obstruction

1. Early intubation is essential, particularly in neck hematoma or possible airway oedema
2. Airway distortion → Insidious
              ↓
   Delayed intubation very difficult

ii. Pneumothorax

Abnormal collection of air in the pleural space between the lungs and the chest wall.

1. CLASSIFICATION/TYPES

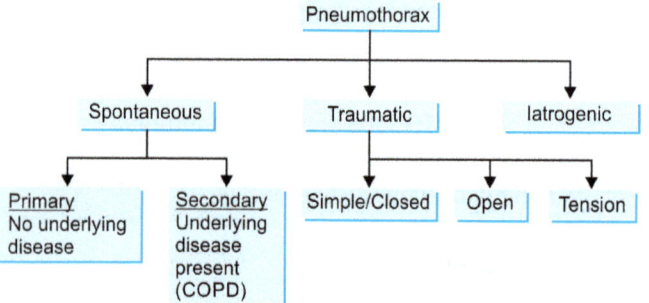

A. Closed (Fig. 36)

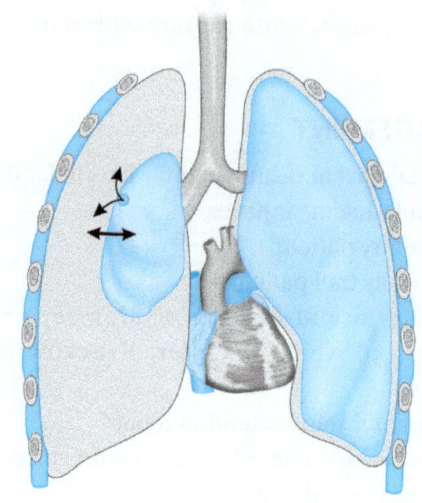

1. Chest wall is intact
2. Air enters the pleural space from the lung surface
         ↓
   Rupture of alveoli
3. Atmospheric pressure > Pleural cavity pressure
4. Pleural cavity pressure = Pulmonary pressure

B. Open (Sucking Chest Wound) (Fig. 37)

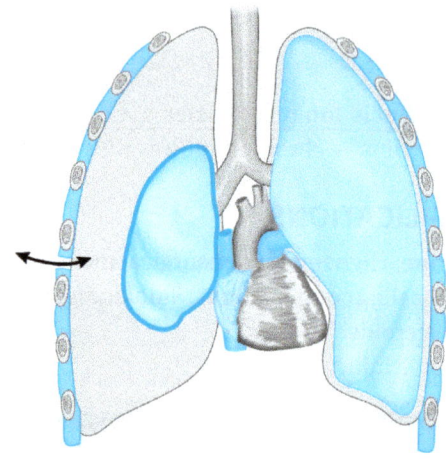

1. Chest wall integrity compromised (large open defect in chest = 3 cm)
         ↓
2. Communication between the pleural cavity and outside atmosphere.
3. Air enters during inspiration and exits during expiration, there is "no tension"
4. Pleural pressure = Atmospheric pressure

C. Tension (Fig. 38)

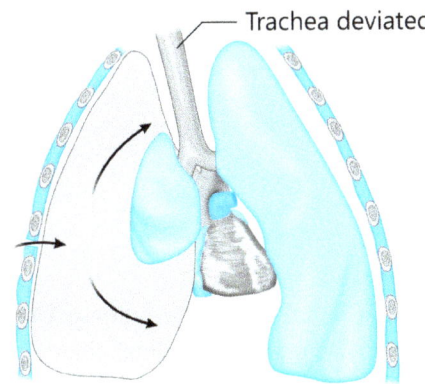

1. Communication between pleural cavity and outside atmosphere is through a **one-way valve**
2. Air enters the pleural cavity during inspiration
   ↓
   Unable to exit → further accumulation of air during inspiration.
   ↓
   "tension"
   ↓
3. Pleural cavity pressure > Atmospheric pressure
   ↓
   Compresses the lungs and mediastinal structures → Tracheal deviation
   ↓
   Progressive cardiopulmonary compromise
   ↓
   Life-threatening emergency

2. CLINICAL FEATURES

1. Dyspnea
2. Pleuritic chest pain
3. ↓ Breath sounds or absent
4. Tactile vocal fremitus absent
5. Hyperresonant percussion note
6. Closed → Relatively mild symptoms
7. Tension pneumothorax → <u>Dramatic presentation</u>
   a. Displacement of trachea to opposite side
   b. Jugular venous distention
   c. Decreased BP
   d. Respiratory failure
   e. Open → Red bubbles on exhalation from wound → "Sucking chest wound"
   f. Cyanosis
8. <u>Open</u>: Red bubbles from the wound on exhalation

3. INVESTIGATIONS

a. Hyperlucency between lung and thoracic cage (loss of lung mark)
b. Razor sharp border of collapsed lung
c. Shift of mediastinum → opposite side

4. TREATMENT

1. General treatment (discussed earlier)
2. Simple pneumothorax → Supplemental O_2 → to facilitate resorption of pleural air and accelerate resolution.
   i. Small <20% (lung edge < 2 cm from chest wall) → observation if symptom free (clinically stable) and Repeat CXR
   If patient must receive positive pressure ventilation or has evidence of multisystem trauma.
   ↓
   Chest tube
   ↑
   ii. Moderate/Large Pneumothorax (>20% or lung edge > 2 cm from chest wall)
   iii. Small to moderate → aspiration may be tried

   Simple   Catheter

3. *Open (Fig. 39)*:

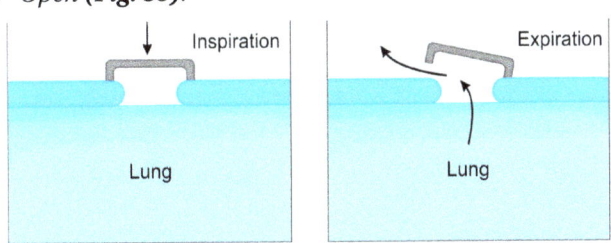

   i. Occlusive dressing → Taped on 3 sides → acting as a one-way valve
   ↓
   Followed by chest intubation.

4. *Tension*:
   i. Surgical emergency
   ii. Emergency needle decompression **(Fig. 40)**

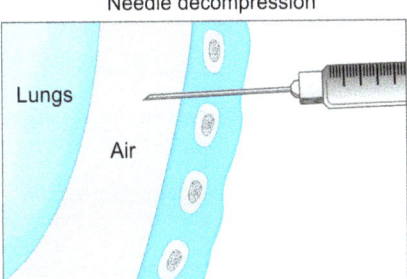

Adults	Paediatric
5th IC space mid-axillary line	2nd IC space, mid-clavicular line

   iii. Followed by chest intubation.
5. Chest tube is connected to a water seal device with/without suction until pneumothorax resolves.

6. *Chemical pleurodesis*:
   A. Goals:
      i. Prevent PT recurrence
      ii. To produce inflammation of pleura and adhesions
   B. Indications:
      i. Persistent air leak
      ii. Repeated PT
      iii. Complicated with bullae
      iv. B/L PT
   C. Sclerosing agents:
      i. Tetracycline/doxy/mino
      ii. Erythromycin
7. Mechanical pleurodesis → VATS: Video-assisted thoracic surgery
8. No flights for 4 weeks → ↓ air pressure → Pneumothorax.

iii. Flail Chest (Fig. 41)

≥ 3 consecutive ribs with segmental fractures
↓
Segment of chest wall does not have bony continuity with the rest of the thoracic cage.

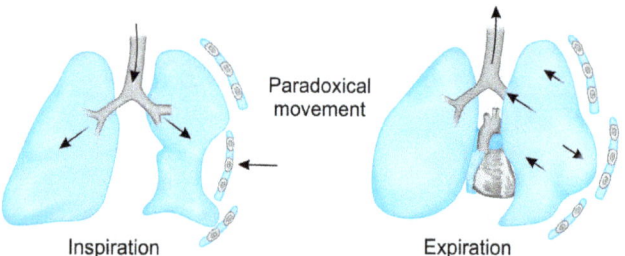

I. Etiology

1. MCC → RTA
2. Fall from height
3. Industrial accidents.
4. Assault
5. Old patients → osteoporosis
   ∴ Bimodal distribution

II. Pathophysiology

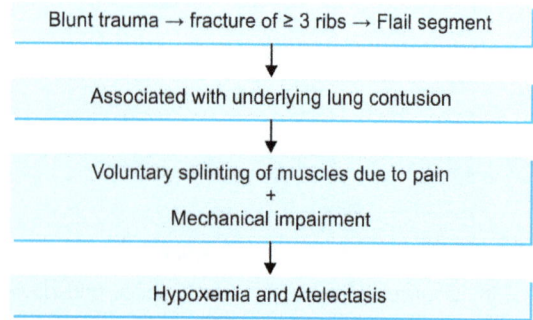

III. Clinical Features

1. Clinical diagnosis, Not radiological
   ↓
2. Paradoxical chest movement
3. Tenderness
4. Crepitus
5. Shallow breathing
6. Chest wall deformity.

IV. Investigations

X-ray (CXR), CT scan - ↑ accuracy.

V. Treatment

1. *Conservative*:
   i. O_2 administration → Positive pressure ventilation
   ii. Adequate analgesia → Including opiates
   iii. Physiotherapy
2. *Operative*:
   i. Indications:
      a. Displaced rib fracture → intractable pain
      b. Rib fracture associated with failure to wean off from ventilator
      c. Open rib fractures
      d. Displaced fracture with flail chest segment
   ii. Approach:
      a. Full thoracotomy
      b. Limited exposure
   iii. Open reduction and internal fixation

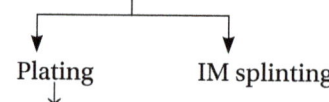

   a. 3.5 recon
   b. Anatomical plate
   iv. Postoperative: Early shoulder and scapular ROM

VI. Complications

1. Intercostals neuralgia
2. Periscapular muscle weakness
3. Pneumonia
4. Restrictive pulmonary dysfunction.

iv. Pericardial Tamponade (Fig. 42)

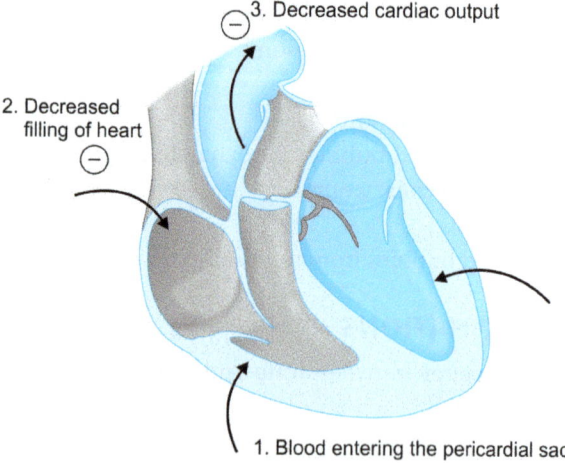

I. Pathophysiology

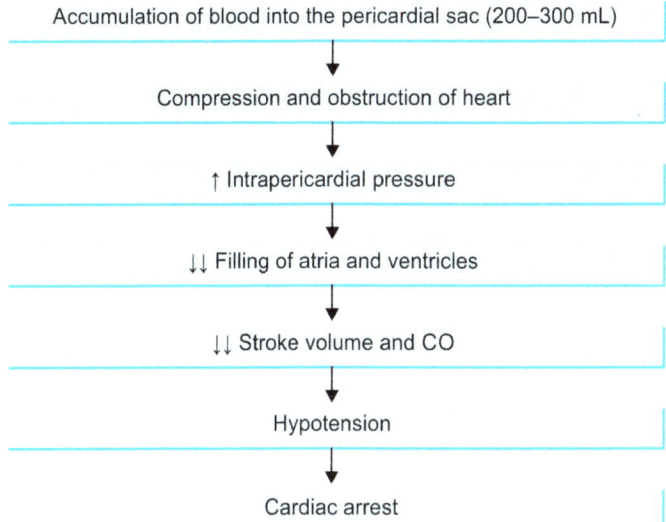

II. Clinical Features

1. **Beck's triad:** Hypotension
   Distended neck veins
   Muffled heart sounds
2. Kussmauls sign → ↓ JVP during inspiration
3. Pulsus paradoxus
4. Shock
   D/D → Tension pneumothorax

III. Investigations

1. USG = Pericardial effusions + RV collapse
2. CXR → Globular heart shadow
3. ECG → Electrical alternans

IV. Treatment

1. Initial resuscitation and general Rx
2. Volume expansion via crystalloids with 2 large bore iv lines
3. Pericardiocentesis → Temporary measure. Dramatic improvement
   High complication rates → Injury to heart
4. Emergency left thoracotomy is the definite surgical repair technique.

v. Hemothorax

Accumulation of blood in pleural space after blunt or penetrating injury.
   X-ray → 200 mL fluid
   Rx → chest tube
Indication for emergency thoracotomy:
1. >1,500 mL of blood initially itself
2. >300 cc blood/h over 2-3 hours
3. Need for persistent blood transfusion.

THORACIC AORTIC DISRUPTION

1. Control arterial BP
2. Endovascular intra-aortic stent
3. Direct repair.
4. Excision and grafting (dacron graft).

POLYTRAUMA

INTRODUCTION

1. *New Berlin definition*:
   Injury to ≥ 2 body regions/systems with abbreviated injury score (AIS) of ≥3 along, with ≥1 of following conditions.
   i. Hypotension (SBP < 90 mmHg)
   ii. Unconsciousness (GCS ≤ 8)
   iii. Acidosis (Base excess ≤ −6.0)
   iv. Coagulopathy (INR ≥ 1.4)
   v. Age (>70 years)

AIS	Body region
1. Mild	1. Head
2. Moderate	2. Face
3. Serious	3. Neck
4. Severe	4. Thorax
5. Critical	5. Abdomen
6. Unsurvivable	6. Spine
	7. UL
	8. LL
	9. External

2. Simply put, 2 major organ system + 1 bony injury
   or
   2 bony injuries + 1 major organ system.
3. Polytrauma → MCC death (18-45 years) worldwide.
4. ISS ≥ 18 → Polytrauma.

II. PATHOPHYSIOLOGY

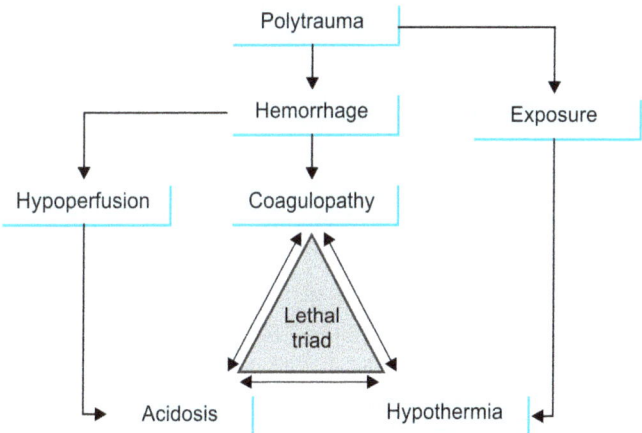

III. DEATH IN POLYTRAUMA

1. *Immediate (50% deaths)*:
   i. Severe head injury, brain stem
   ii. Disruption of heart, aorta

iii. Most deaths in polytrauma in this phase
iv. Amenable to public health measures
   ↓
   Safety helmets, seatbelts
2. *Early (30%)*:
   i. Few hours after injury
   ii. Intracranial bleeding.
   iii. Chest, abdominal, pelvis injury
   iv. Most common cause of death in this period → Hypovolemic shock
3. *Late (20%)*:
   i. Several days or weeks
   ii. Sepsis, organ failure

IV. GOLDEN HOUR

1. The first 60 minutes following trauma
   ↓
   Critical period for getting patients to trauma center for definitive care
   ↓
   After which morbidity and mortality increase

V. MANAGEMENT
A. ATLS Guidelines

1. *A – Airway*:
   i. Ensure patency of airway
      ↓
   ii. Remove foreign body, endotracheal intubation, tracheostomy.
   iii. Cervical spine protection (if injury)
2. *B – Breathing*:
   i. Ventilation and oxygenation
   ii. Rule out chest injury → Pneumothorax
                               Flail chest
                               Hemothorax
   iii. Chest tube insertion
   iv. Respiratory O_2 support
3. *C – Circulation*:
   i. Hemorrhage control and resuscitation
   ii. 2 – Large bore IV lines
   iii. Blood pressure, pulse, urine output monitoring
   iv. Classification of hemorrhage:
       I – <15% blood loss
           No change in BP
           Rx → Crystalloid
       II – 15–30%
           Tachycardia with normal BP
           Rx – Crystalloid.
       III – 30–40%
           Tachycardia, tachypnea, hypotension
           Rapid crystalloid, then blood
       IV – >40% life-threatening
           Marked tachycardia and ↓BP
           Immediate blood replacement
   v. Indicators of adequate resuscitation:
      a. Urine output 1mg/kg/h
      b. Serum lactate < 2.5 mmol/L
         Most sensitive indicator
      c. Base deficit – normal –2 to +2
   vi. Fractures:
      a. Thomas splint → Femur fracture
      b. Pelvic binder → Pelvis
      c. Direct pressure over bleeding vessel
   vii. DD shock
        Types of shock
        1. Cardiogenic
        2. Neurogenic shock
        3. Septic shock

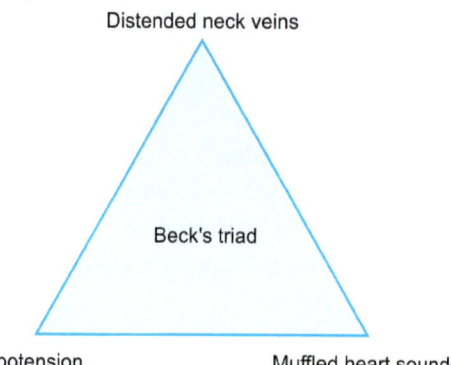

   →Cardiogenic: Beck's
   →Neurogenic (Head/spine): Hypotension + Bradycardia
   →Septic shock: Hypotension + Tachycardia + Fever.
   Multiorgan failure, ↓ Systemic vascular resistance
4. *D – Disability*
   Neurologic assessment, Glasgow Coma Scale
5. *E – Exposure:* Uncover the patient to examine entire body → Unmask hidden injuries

B. Radiological Evaluation

1. CXR – Chest injuries
2. X-ray – Limb fracture, PBH, spine
3. USG FAST → Internal bleeding
4. CT Scan → Intra-abdominal and pelvic injury

C. Damage Control Orthopedics
   ↓
i. Contains and stabilizes orthopedic injuries to allow patients overall physiology to improve.
ii. 4 phases:
    1. Acute: Life saving procedures
    2. Second: Control hemorrhage
               Temporary stabilization of major Skeletal fractures
    3. Third: Monitoring in ICU
    4. Last: Definitive fixation

iii. Spectrum of physiological status:

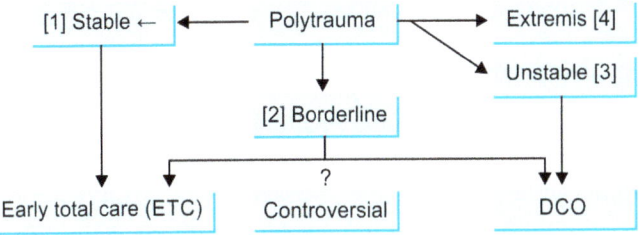

iv. Timing of surgery (**Fig. 43**)

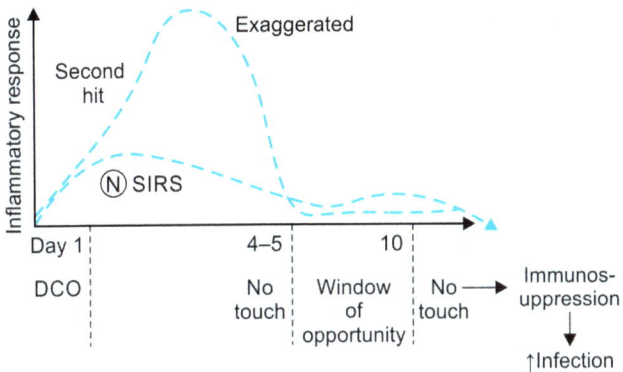

v. **Second hit concept:**

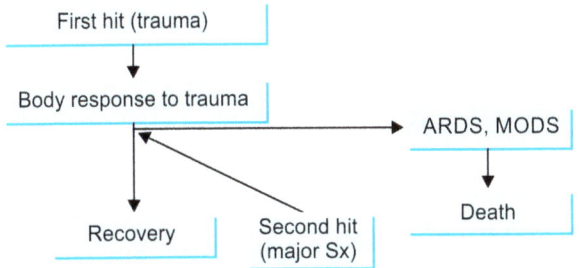

GAS GANGRENE

I. INTRODUCTION
1. Highly lethal soft tissue infection caused by *Clostridium* species.
2. Characterized by rapidly progressive gangrene of the injured tissue along with the production of foul-smelling gas.
3. Aka myonecrosis with *Clostridium perfringens* being the most common.

II. RISK FACTORS
1. *Post-traumatic*:
   i. Car accidents (most common)
   ii. Crush injuries
   iii. Gunshot wounds with foreign bodies
   iv. Burns and frostbite
   v. IV drug abuse
2. Postoperative: Very rare in orthopedic surgeries. Seen in abdominal surgeries.

III. PATHOPHYSIOLOGY
1. **Clostridium perfringens (most common)**, *Clostridium Novyi, Clostridium Septicum*
2. Found in soil and gut flora
3. Gram-positive obligate anaerobic spore-forming rods that produce exotoxins
4. C. perfringens → Alpha toxin
   i. causes muscle necrosis and vessel thrombosis
   ii. can cause hemolysis and shock
5. Incubation period <24 hours
6. Gas produced by fermentation of glucose → main component is nitrogen

IV. CLINICAL FEATURES
A. Symptoms
1. Sudden progressive pain out of proportion to injury from thrombotic occlusion of large vessels
2. Tachycardia not explained by fever
3. Feeling of impending doom

⎫ Triad

B. Examination
1. Swelling, edema
2. Discoloration and ecchymosis
3. Blebs and hemorrhagic bullae
4. **"Dishwater pus" discharge**
5. Crepitus
6. Sweet smelling odor
7. Altered mental status
8. Low urine output

V. RADIOGRAPH
1. Linear streaks of gas in soft tissues
2. Associated fractures

VI. LABORATORY FINDINGS
1. Gram stain reveals gram-positive bacilli with spore formation
2. Elevated LDH
3. Elevated WBC
4. Absence of neutrophils → lack of acute inflammatory response is hallmark of gas gangrene
5. Myoglobinuria
6. Metabolic acidosis and renal failure
7. Raised LFTs

VII. DIFFERENTIALS
1. Necrotizing fasciitis
2. Septic shock
3. Toxic shock syndrome

VIII. TREATMENT
1. True orthopedic emergency
2. Radical surgical debridement with fasciotomies
3. Amputation of the limb
4. *High dose IV antibiotics*:
    i. 1st line is penicillin G and clindamycin
    ii. Alternative treatment is erythromycin, tetracycline or ceftriaxone
    iii. Clindamycin and tetracycline inhibit toxin synthesis
5. Adjuvant hyperbaric O_2

IX. PREVENTION
1. Thorough cleaning and wound wash of open fractures and trauma → 9 liters
2. Debridement of all necrotic tissue during primary management
3. Early antibiotics

X. COMPLICATIONS
1. Shock
2. Renal failure } TNF alpha, IL-1, IL-6

XI. PROGNOSIS
1. Overall mortality → 25%
2. Bacteremia mortality → 50%
3. Delay in treatment → 100% mortality
4. Poorer prognosis for older patients with comorbidities.

DYNAMIZATION OF FRACTURES

The methods of altering the fixation of fractures to improve the bone healing process → "Weaken stability"

I. TYPES
1. Primary: Dynamic locking of axially and rotationally stable fractures at the time of initial fracture fixation.
2. Secondary: Removing the interlocking screws from the longer fragment, control maintained over shorter fragment.

II. PHYSIOLOGY
1. Telescopic movement between the nail and tubular bone
    ↓
    Closes gaps in bony continuity
    ↓
    Potentially compresses the fracture fragments.
2. The favorable results of axial dynamization are attributed to repeat cyclic loading of bony ends due to free axial movement and closure of the osseous gap at the fracture or nonunion site.

III. EFFECTS
1. Induces new bone formation
2. Callus maturation
3. Faster callus remodeling.

IV. RATIONALE
Interlocking intramedullary nailing (IMN) → gold-standard for long bones → "static nailing" → in essence prevents appreciable axial loading at the fracture site, raising concerns of a potential adverse impact on the timely evolution of the healing process → Axial loading across the fracture is believed to stimulate an osteogenic response.

An alternative dynamization method involves decreasing the stiffness of the fracture fixation during the healing process.

This method is used mainly with external fixation → Stabilizing elements of the fixator are removed at some time during the treatment leading to greater flexibility of the fixation.

V. INDICATIONS
1. Delayed Union
2. Fracture gap → Prolonged time to heal
3. Established pseudoarthrosis
4. Nonunion along with BMAC

VI. TIMING
10–16 weeks after nailing.

VII. CONTRAINDICATIONS
Unstable construct.

VIII. COMPLICATIONS
1. Loss of reduction
2. Leg-length inequality
3. Nonunion: Early dynamization.

STRESS FRACTURE

I. INTRODUCTION
1. Stress fracture: Normal bone exposed to abnormal stress → Summation of stress any of which by itself wouldn't have caused a fracture.
2. Insufficiency: Abnormal bone exposed to normal stress.

II. ETIOLOGY
Risk factors
1. Athletes and military recruits
2. "Female athlete triad" → amenorrhea, eating disorder, and osteoporosis
3. Weight bearing. LL>UL → Tibia 50% MC
4. Nutritional deficiency → Ca and vitamin D
5. NSAID intake
6. Smoking

Extrinsic	Intrinsic
• Excessive load on the body • Training errors • Unsuitable training environment • Poor training equipment • Ineffective training rules	• Mal-alignments (e.g., tibia vara) • Leg length discrepancy • Tarsal coalition • Previous surgery • Overweight • Muscle weakness or imbalance

Stages in Development
- Crack initiation
- Crack propagation
- Rapid failure of bone

III. PATHOPHYSIOLOGY

1. Excessive, repetitive, submaximal loads on bones that cause an imbalance between bone resorption and formation
2. An abrupt increase in the duration, intensity, or frequency of physical activity without adequate periods of rest may lead to an escalation in osteoclast activity
3. During periods of intense exercise, bone formation lags behind bone resorption
4. When bone subjected to hyper physiological loads, its ultimate strength decreases→ susceptible to microfractures
5. Continuous loading → microcracks coalesce to stress fracture.

Low risk	High risk
Compression side	Tension side
Conservative	Operative

IV. CLASSIFICATION

Kaeding-Miller stress fracture classification system

Grade	Pain	Radiographic findings (CT, MRI, bone scan, or X-ray)
I	–	Imaging evidence of stress fracture No fracture line
II	+	Imaging evidence of stress fracture No fracture line
III	+	Nondisplaced fracture line
IV	+	Displaced fracture (>2 mm)
V	+	Nonunion

V. RADIOLOGY

1. Radiograph:
   i. 1st 2–3 weeks → Normal
   ii. Periosteal response → 2 months after onset
   iii. Periosteal reaction, endosteal callus, frank fracture line
   iv. Tibia → lateral X-ray → "dreaded black line" anteriorly indicating tension fracture from posterior muscle force
2. MRI: Most sensitive – IOC – Unilateral stress fracture
3. Bone scan: IOC – B/L stress fractures
4. CT: Navicular bone, Pars and sacral stress fracture

VI. DIFFERENTIALS

1. Stress reaction
2. Periostitis, infection
3. Avulsion injuries, muscle strain
4. Bursitis, neoplasm
5. Exertional compartment syndrome, and nerve entrapment.

VII. MANAGEMENT

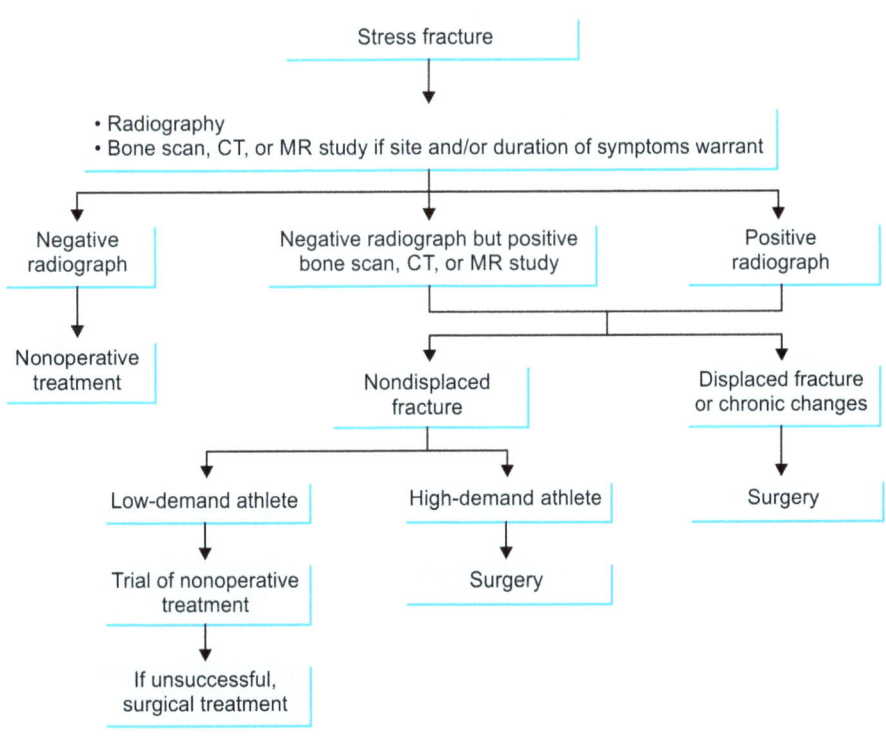

Fundamental Principles

1. Rest → allow bone remodeling
2. Identify and correct predisposing factors
3. Low risk fracture: Trial of conservative
4. High risk fracture: Treated as acute fractures

1. *Proximal Femur*

i. Tensile lateral surface → 3 screw
ii. Compressive medial surface: Rest

2. *Tibia*

i. Posteromedial → Compression side → MC → Conserve
ii. Anterior cortex of middle 1/3rd shaft → Tensile → IMN

3. *Navicular*

i. Sprinting and jumping sports
ii. Insidious onset vague medial arch pain
iii. Avascular central third of bone → Predisposed to fracture
iv. Acute fracture → Initial 6 week → NWB cast mobilization
v. Delayed Dx/union: Compression screw stabilization
vi. Displaced fracture or Established sclerotic NU : ORIF + BG

4. *Metatarsal*

i. 5th MC followed by 2nd
ii. Acute fracture → Initial 6 week → NWB cast mobilization
iii. Delayed Union → IM compression screw
iv. Displaced fracture or Established sclerotic NU – ORIF + BG.

5. *Great Toe Sesamoids*

i. Medial Sesamoid
ii. Acute: Initial 6 week → NWB cast mobilization
iii. Sx: Sesamoidectomy.

SECTION 12

Orthopedic Radiology

IMAGE INTENSIFIER

I. INTRODUCTION

1. A *C-arm* is an image scanning intensifier
2. Name derived from the C-shaped arm connecting the X-ray source and the detector at the other end.
3. The image intensifiers convert low intensity X-rays → visible light output.

II. PARTS (FIG. 1)

1. Monitor
2. C-arm
3. Image intensifier
4. Flat panel detector
5. Collimator.

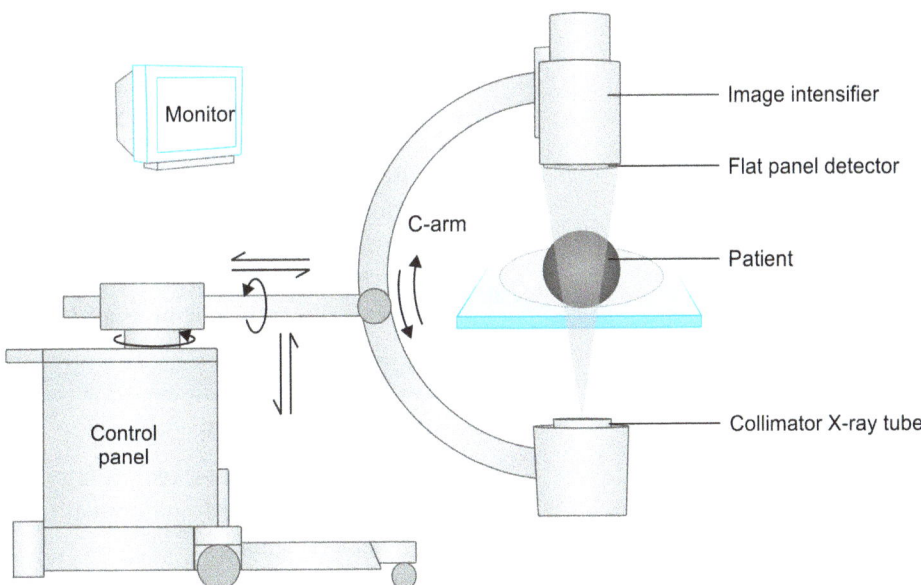

III. PRINCIPLE OF IMAGE INTENSIFIER (FIG. 2)

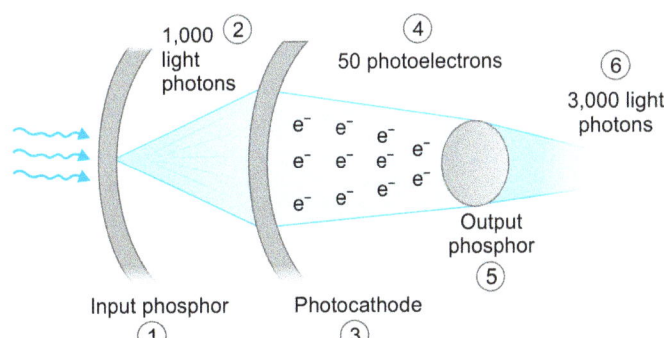

X-ray beam → from patient → enters image intensifier → through input phosphorous window → light photons created → these hit the Photocathode
                ↓Photoelectric effect
Photoelectrons → output phosphor
                ↓
Large number of light photons
∴ Image intensifier significantly reduces radiation.

IV. USE

1. Closed reduction of fractures f/b cast → Colles fracture, etc.
2. Foreign body removal: Glass, metal

3. *Before surgery:*
   i. Closed reduction on operating table → TC, IT, femur
   ii. Confirmation of spinal level for incision
4. *Intraoperatively:*
   i. Fracture reduction and fixation
   ii. Rule out intraarticular screws
   iii. Fluoroscopy for locking of IM nails
   iv. Correct placement of pedicular and lateral mass screws
   v. Angle of osteotomy (HTO and VITO)
   vi. Vertebroplasty and kyphoplasty
   vii. Nerve root blocks
   viii. Reduction of dislocated joints, not managed in the emergency room
   ix. Revision arthroplasties.
   x. Confirm position of endobutton → ACL reconstruction
   xi. Scoliosis curve corrections
   xii. Malrotation of fractured fragments intraoperatively **(Fig. 3)**.

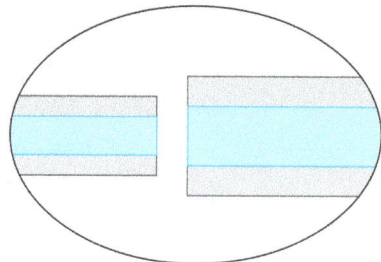

Fig. 3: Malrotation assessed by different dimensions of the proximal and distal fragment cortices.

V. PROTECTIVE EQUIPMENT

1. Wrap around lead apron (0.5 mm lead)
   ↓
   16-fold ↓ in scattered radiation
2. Thyroid shield → 2.5 fold
3. Eye protective glasses (0.25 mm lead) 70% ↓ radio beam
4. Gloves: Use if hand in beam zone.

VI. RADIATION REDUCTION

1. X-ray tube under the patient → ↓ scattered radiation **(Fig. 4)**

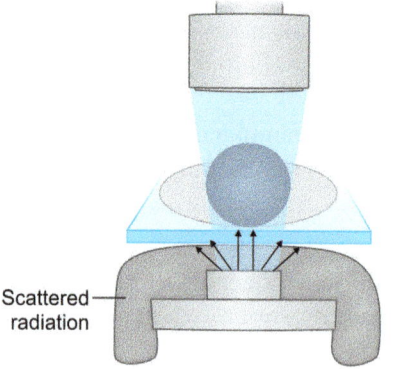

2. Integrated lasers on image intensifiers for positioning
3. Maintain distance from C-arm and patient
4. Rely on stored images when possible
5. Radiation dosimeter
   ↓
   <20 mSV/year averaged over 5 years
   150 mSV → thyroid and eyes, 500 mSV hands
6. Lead aprons on racks → Hanging
   No folding and bending → Cracks

VII. RECENT ADVANCES

1. O-arm
2. 3D image intensifier

VIII. RADIATION HAZARDS

Types

⇒ Stochastic—unrelated to dose → leukemia → no threshold
⇒ Deterministic—dose related → erythema, loss of hair, cataract formation, ↓fertility

⇒ Somatic—self → affect somatic cells
⇒ Genetic—next generation → affect germ cells

1. Skin—Nails → brittle, blunting of finger ridges, dryness, skin atrophy, progressive pigmenting keratosis, telangiectasia, indolent ulcers.
2. Thyroid—papillary carcinoma
3. Eye—cataract
4. Mouth—mucositis, xerostomia
5. Acute radiation syndrome—rare
   i. BM → ↓granulocytes, platelets, ↓ erythrocytes
   ii. GIT → nausea, vomiting, diarrhea

MRI

I. INTRODUCTION

Noninvasive imaging technology that produces three dimensional detailed anatomical images using magnetic resonance imaging.

II. PRINCIPLE (FIG. 5)

1. The protons (H^+) in the body spin in a random arrangement.
2. MRI uses superconducting magnets and radiofrequency (RF) coils to manipulate these hydrogen protons.
3. A powerful magnet (field strength 1.5 to 3T).
   ↓
   Aligns these H^+ protons with its magnetic field.

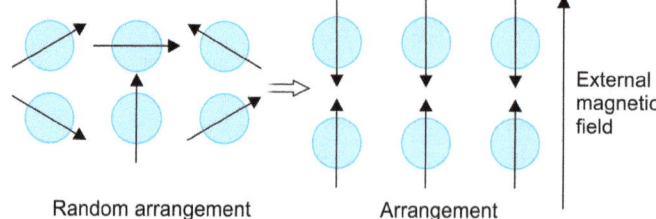

4. RF pulse applied → atoms absorb energy.
5. RF turned off → atoms release energy at different rates.
6. Decides T_1 and T_2 time.
7. T_1 time takes the protons to realign themselves with the magnetic field.
8. T_2 time taken for the synchronized proton spinning to lose its coherence.
9. RF receiver or coil → used to detect emitted energy → "signal".
10. Converted to detailed, high contrast image by the computer.

III. SPECIAL TYPES

1. *Gradient echo (GRE):* Fast MR scan for cartilage imaging.
2. *Short tau inversion recovery (STIR):* Suppression of fat signal → detects edema in soft tissue and marrow (trauma and neoplasia)
3. *Contrast MRI:*
    i. MC IV contrast: Gadolinium
    ii. Use: Inflammation, blood vessels, tumors
4. *Dynamic MRI:* In flexion and extension → cervical myelopathy.

IV. INDICATIONS

A. Knee (Figs. 6A and B)

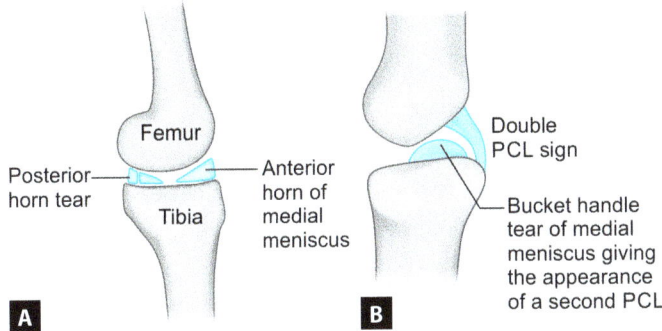

Figs. 6A and B: Double PCL sign seen in Bucket handle tear of meniscus. (Usually medial meniscus).

1. Meniscal tears
2. ACL, PCL, collateral ligament tears
3. Patellar and quadriceps tendon tears
4. Cysts → Para, peri, synovial
5. SPONK
6. Physeal injuries in children
7. Osteochondritis dissecans
8. Chondromalacia patellae
9. Evaluation of articular cartilage
10. Occult fractures
    Chosen plane for scanning (sagittal) is 15° IR → Parallel to ACL

B. Hip

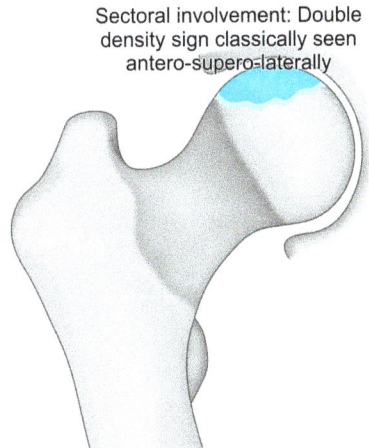

1. Osteonecrosis (modified Ficat-Arlet) of hip: Double density sign **(Fig. 7)**
2. Evaluation of acetabular labrum
3. Septic arthritis of hip
4. Transient osteoporosis of hip
5. Inflammatory arthritis: RA and AS
6. Perthes disease
7. DDH

C. Spine (Fig. 8)

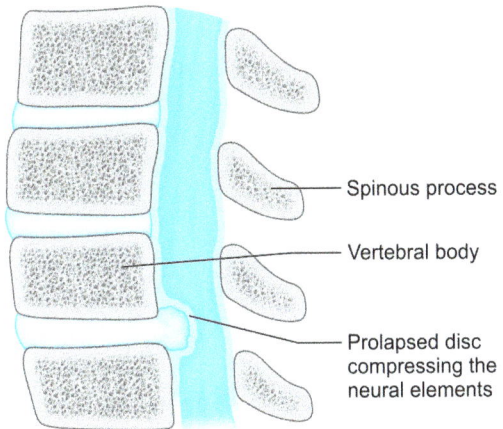

Fig. 8: Sagittal section of MRI.

1. Intervertebral disc disease:
    i. Prolapsed
    ii. Extrusion
    iii. Sequestration
    iv. Nerve root compression
2. Spinal trauma → Spinal cord compression
                   → Ligament injury
3. Lumbar canal stenosis
4. Tuberculous and pyogenic infections
5. Epidural hematoma or abscess
6. Developmental deformities of the vertebral column
7. Intradural and extradural spinal cord tumors

D. Shoulder

1. Rotator cuff tear **(Fig. 9)**
2. Impingement syndromes
3. *Instability*: Bankart, Hill Sach's
4. Long head of biceps tendon—rupture, tendinitis.
5. Osteonecrosis
6. Acromioclavicular joint

E. Wrist

1. Triangular fibrocartilage complex injuries
2. Intrinsic carpal ligament injuries
3. ON—scaphoid, lunate (Kienbock's disease)
4. Edema, swelling of median nerve—carpal tunnel syndrome.

F. Foot and Ankle

1. Tendinopathy—Achilles
2. Ligament tears—Deltoid
3. Articular disorders
4. Osteochondral injuries
5. ON—Talus
6. Osteomyelitis—Marrow edema.

V. MRI IN TUMORS

1. MR uses the principle of resonance of hydrogen protons with static magnetic field
   ↓
   Excellent soft tissue and bone contrast
2. Radiograph primary investigation followed by MRI
3. *Tumor MR application*:
   i. Narrows down differential diagnosis when lesion indeterminate or shows aggressiveness
   ii. Demonstrates several tissue components - muscles, bone, joints, subcutaneous
   iii. Tumor extent
   iv. Skip lesions, satellite lesions
   v. Detects bone marrow lesions
   vi. Contrast enhanced MRI → Most vascularized part of the tumors
      ↓
      Helps guide biopsy site
   vii. Local staging of tumor
   viii. Surgical planning.
   ix. *Invasion of adjacent*:
      a. Physeal plates
      b. Joints
      c. Compartments
      d. Neurovascular bundles
   x. Response to neoadjuvant chemotherapy
   xi. Post therapeutic follow-up
   xii. Intratumoral necrosis and hemorrhage
   xiii. *Dynamic contrast enhanced MRI*:
      a. Differentiates reactive edema around tumor from viable tumor
      b. Viable tumor enhances in early phase
      c. Reactive edema → late phase
   xiv. Faint lytic/sclerotic bone lesions = MRI superior
   xv. Differentiates between OM and Ewings → soft tissue extension
4. *Specific tumors*:
   i. *Osteosarcoma*: Hypointense (dark) on both T_1 and T_2 → due to osseous matrix
   ii. *Chondrosarcoma*: High water content of chondroid matrix → cartilaginous tumors hyperintense of T_2.
   iii. *Osteochondroma*: Cartilage cap hyperintense on T_2 → Size ↑ = ↑ Malignancy.
   iv. *Fibrosarcoma*: Tumors with fibrous matrix are dark on both T_1 and T_2
   v. *Lymphoma*: Multiple osteolytic lesions → Dark on T_1 and bright on T_2 as other round cell tumors.
   vi. *Fluid-fluid levels*: GCT and ABC
      ↓
      CE–MRI → Solid components-Biopsy
5. Planes:
   i. *Axial*: Extraosseous involved best seen. Anatomy of various compartments.
   ii. *Sagittal and coronal*: Proximal and distal extent of lesion.

VI. CONTRAINDICATIONS

A. Absolute

1. Intracerebral aneurysm clips
2. Cardiac pacemakers and automatic defibrillators
3. Implanted infusion devices and interval hearing aids
4. Metallic orbital foreign bodies
5. Metallic external fixators.
6. Cochlear implants
7. Ferromagnetic foreign bodies like shell shrapnel

B. Relative
1. First trimester pregnancy
2. Middle ear prosthesis

CT SCAN

I. PRINCIPLE (FIG. 10)

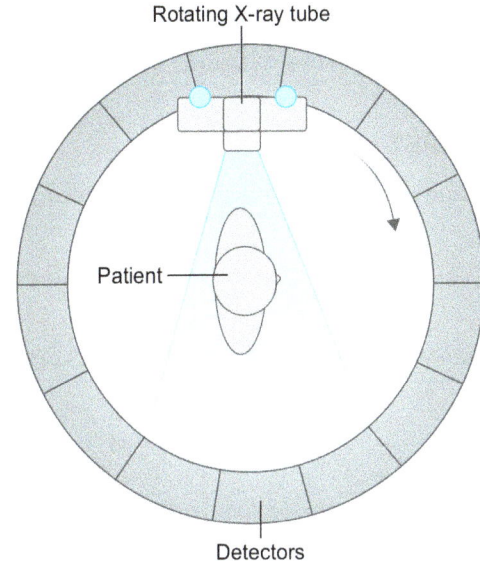

1. "The internal structure of an object can be reconstructed from multiple projections of the object"
2. CT scan collimates the X-ray beams and transmits them only through small cross-sections of the body.
3. Rotating X-ray tube and a row of detectors in the gantry to measure X-ray attenuations by different tissues in the body.
4. Numerical data → Gray scale representing different tissue densities → Visual image.

II. INDICATION
1. *Complex fractures*:
   i. Intra-articular extension (proximal tibia, distal femur)
   ii. Surgical planning (lag screws, plate, approach)
   iii. Decision making regarding (IT → [THR, fixation]) management options.
   iv. Bony Bankart—Glenoid bone loss (Bankart, Latarjet)
   v. Spinal fractures—Posterior wall fracture
      Posterior element—fracture-dislocation
2. Union → Suspected nonunion
3. CT angiography—Vertebral artery course for cervical spine surgeries
4. Deformity correction (CT scanogram)—Planning the osteotomy angles
5. Bone loss—Revision hip and knee arthroplasties
6. Spine:
   i. CT-guided biopsies
   ii. Intact pedicles for screw fixation in TB, pyogenic spondylodiscitis
   iii. OPLL
   iv. OLL
   v. Facetal arthritis
   vi. Spinal stenosis (central, lateral)
   vii. Postoperative placement of pedicular screw—not in spinal canal
7. Tumors (Chest metastasis, cortical destruction)—Osteoid osteoma.
8. Trochlear dysplasia—Patellar instability (TT-TG distance).

III. ADVANTAGES OVER MRI
1. Better imaging modality for bone tissue
2. Cheaper
3. Less time consuming
4. Can be done when MRI is contraindicated
   i. Cardiac pacemakers
   ii. Aneurysm chips
   iii. Cochlear implants.

IV. DISADVANTAGES
1. Poor soft tissue visibility.
2. High dose radiation hazard.

V. CONTRAINDICATIONS
1. Pregnancy
2. CT angiography
   i. Allergy to contrast
   ii. CKD

NUCLEAR MEDICINE SCANS

I. INTRODUCTION
Branch of medicine that deals with the use of radioactive substances in research, diagnosis, and treatment.

Diagnostic	Therapeutic
Radiation emitted from radiopharmaceuticals ↓ Detected by external detectors ↓ Gives its distribution in the body	Emitted radiation must be absorbed by targeted tissues

II. TYPES
1. Bone scan
2. Single-photon emission computed tomography (SPECT)
3. Positron emission tomography
4. Hybrid PET/CT.

A. Bone Scan "Bone Scintigraphy"

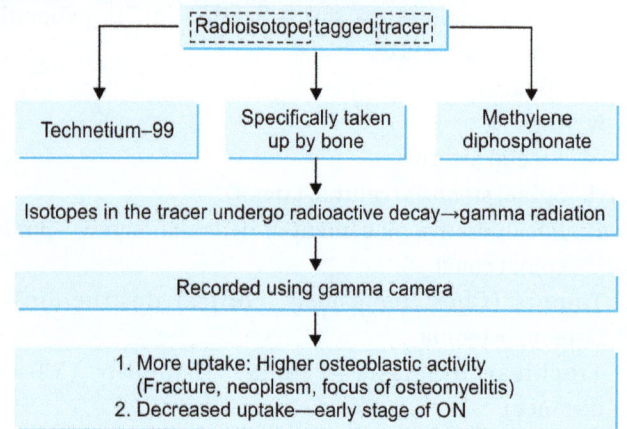

Other tracers used for bone scan:
1. Thallium-201
2. Gallium-67 Infection } Infection
3. Indium labeled leukocyte scan

A. Indications
1. *Bone tumors:* Malignant and nonmalignant
2. Metastatic bone disease (breast, lung, prostate)
3. ON of femur head
4. Infections
5. *Stress fractures:* IOC in B/L
6. *Metabolic bone disease:* Paget's, osteomalacia
7. Ruling out pathological fracture spine
8. Perthes disease
9. Sacroiliitis.

B. Triphasic Bone Scan
1. *Flow phase:* 2-5 seconds after injection. Reflects perfusion of the area (nuclear angiogram)
2. *Blood pool image:* 5 minutes-Vascularity of area
3. *Delayed phase:* 3 hours after injection-Metabolic bone turnover.
    a. *Osteoid osteoma*:
        i. Increased uptake—center due to nidus
        ii. Less increased uptake at periphery → Reactive sclerosis surrounding nidus
    b. Three phases differentiate between cellulitis and osteomyelitis.

B. PET
1. Functional imaging processes
2. Short $t_{1/2}$ life radionuclides like *nitrogen-13, oxygen-15, fluorine-18*
    ↓
3. Attached to naturally occurring compounds in the body like *glucose, water, etc.*
    ↓
4. *Most common: Fluorodeoxyglucose (FDG)*
5. Analogue of glucose → gets selectively taken up in areas of high metabolic activity.

6. *Principle:*

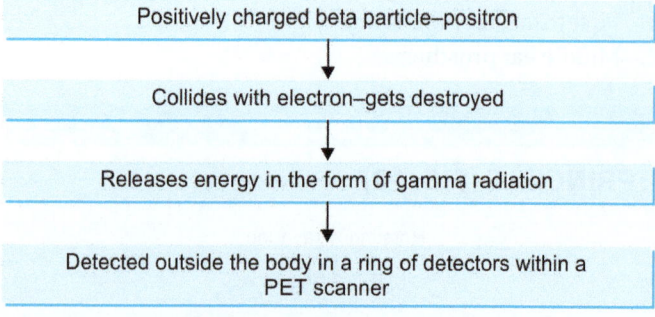

C. PET-CT/PET-MR

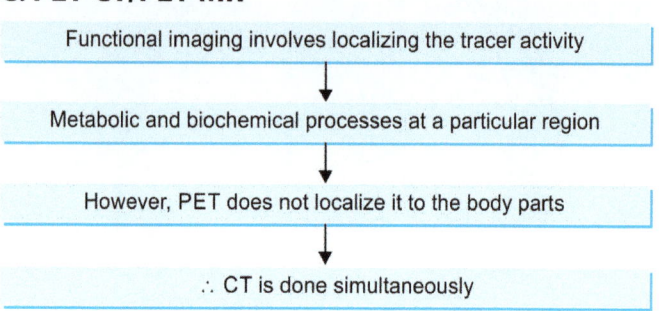

2. *Advantage:* CT scan of *low radiation dose* adequate for providing anatomical localization of PET positive functional abnormal.
3. *PET MRI:* Superior soft tissue discrimination.
4. *Indications:*
    i. *Spinal infections:* FDG-PET superior to MRI for detecting low-grade spondylitis.
       Limitation: Differentiation between infection and tumor
    ii. *Diabetic foot infections:* Differentiates OM, soft tissue infections from neuropathic disease.
    iii. *Prosthetic joint infections:* Aseptic loosening versus infection.
    iv. *Skeletal metastatic disease:*
        a. *Prognosis:* Successful treatment →↓ abnormal uptake
        b. *Detects extra-skeletal* disease and better bone marrow and lytic lesions.
        c. Better than bone scan for bone metastasis from breast Ca, lung Ca, lymphoma.

ULTRASOUND (US)

I. INTRODUCTION
1. US is a safe, cost-effective and noninvasive investigation.
2. It is user dependent → Subjective, experience dependant.

II. PRINCIPLE
1. US refers to mechanical vibrations which are essentially the same as sound waves but of higher frequency.

2. These waves are beyond the range of human hearing and are therefore called ultrasound. (> 20,000 Hz) (1 MHz = 10^6 Hz)
3. US frequency range
   i. 1-3 MHz → Therapeutic purposes
   ii. 2-10 MHz → Diagnostic purposes
4. Production of US waves is by Piezoelectric effect → Electric current applied to piezoelectric crystals placed in a transducer such as quartz, lead zirconate titanate (PZT).
5. The piezoelectric crystals deform → generating mechanical vibrations that produce US waves.
6. The frequency generated depends upon the probe used and the application that is desired.
7. **Echo sounding** or **Sonar** is the physics behind the working of an US machine.
8. US examination is based on how various tissues absorb and reflect sound frequencies.
9. US waves travel into tissue and are reflected back to the probe at a rate determined by the target tissue's consistency.
10. Reflections of sound that return to the probe are called echoes.
11. Images produced based on the echoes give structures and media their varying densities on the screen, referred to as echogenicity.
12. Structures with higher density reflect more sound and are considered more echogenic (white). Thus, bone and dense foreign bodies reflect sound fully and appear bright on the screen, whereas fluids such as water or urine reflect no sound to the probe and appear anechoic (black). Weak echoes appear grey.
13. When waves echo back to the probe from material such as bone and air, which cannot propagate sound, sound waves cannot pass to deeper tissue and a shadow behind the interface results.
14. A gel is used on the skin, which is free of acoustic impedance and helps in the transmission of sound waves from the probe onto the skin so that there is least echoing at the skin.

III.

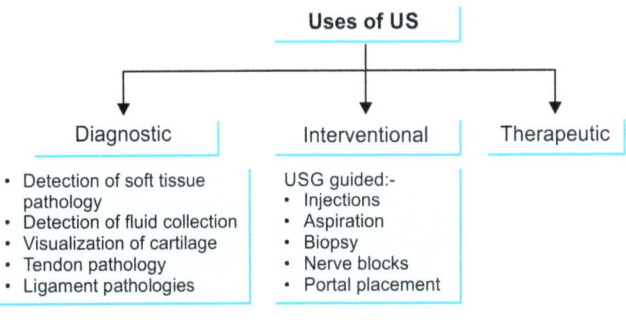

IV. DIAGNOSTIC USES

Various pathologies that can be diagnosed with the help of an US are:

A. Hip
1. Septic arthritis
2. DDH in infants

B. Knee
1. Septic arthritis
2. Effusion
3. Bursitis
4. Meniscal cysts
5. Assessment of extensor apparatus
6. Osgood-Schlatter disease
7. Baker cyst

C. Leg and Foot
1. TA tear
2. Ankle sprains
3. Plantar fasciitis
4. Retrocalcaneal bursitis
5. Haglund deformity
6. Tendinopathies

D. Shoulder
1. Calcific tendinitis
2. Rotator cuff tears, including dynamic studies
3. Adhesive capsulitis
4. Subacromial bursitis
5. Tendinitis
6. Septic shoulder

E. Elbow
1. Tendinopathies
2. Bursitis
3. Septic arthritis
4. Effusion
5. Loose body detection
6. Soft tissue tumors

F. Wrist and Hand
1. Tendon injuries
2. Ligament ruptures
3. TFCC injuries
4. Nerve compression syndromes: Carpal tunnel/Guyon's canal

V. THERAPEUTIC USES

A. Mechanism of Action
1. Acoustic streaming: Mechanical pressure wave causes fluid movement along the membranes of the cell.
2. Biological responses: Due to increased permeability of membranes, there is increased removal of pain producing peptides.
3. Mechanical responses:
   i. Sclerolytic effect: Improves extensibility of tendons (collagen)
   ii. Cavitation: Breaks adhesions
4. Thermal effects: Reduces muscle spasm and decreases joint stiffness
5. Types:
   i. Continuous → Thermal effects
   ii. Pulsed → Nonthermal effects

B. Method of Application
1. Direct contact: Transducer applied to skin surface with a thin layer of coupling gel.
2. Indirect contact: Hand or foot immersed in a plastic vessel with water above the levels of hand or foot. Probe is immersed in water just above the hand or foot without touching it. The probe should be at right angles to the skin
3. Duration of treatment:
   i. 1–8 minutes
   ii. 20 minutes for fracture healing
4. Dosage: 0.5–1 W/cm^2, maximum up to 3 W/cm^2

C. Indications
1. Paraspinal muscle spasm
2. Frozen shoulder
3. Bursitis
4. Tendinitis
5. Plantar fasciitis
6. Sprains
7. Metatarsalgia
8. Postinjury/Burn/Surgery scar tissue lysis
9. Fracture nonunions

D. Ultrasound in Fracture Healing and Nonunion (LIPUS: Low Intensity Pulsed US)
1. 1.5 MHz sine wave administered in a burst of 200 μs, with a pause of 800 μs (pulsed 1:4), repeated 1,000 times per second (rate of 1 KHz).
2. Administered through a nonmoving transducer for 20 minutes daily
3. Used for fresh fractures, delayed unions and nonunions.
4. Mechanism of action:
   i. Stimulates osteoblasts
   ii. Increased production of TGF-β
   iii. Increases calcium turnover at the fracture site, hence leading to active bone formation
   iv. COX-2 upregulation leading to increased production of PGE-2, which in turn stimulates bone formation
   v. Stimulates chondrocyte formation
   vi. Stimulates production of VEGF mRNA, NO, HIF-1α: They enhance union by increasing angiogenesis
5. It can be administered at any stage of fracture healing

E. Contraindications
1. Avoid in areas having implants like cardiac pacemakers, breast implants
2. Not applied directly over eyes
3. Open wounds
4. Avoided in tissues like ischemic tissues, neural tissues, reproductive tissues, suspected TB lesions

SECTION 13: Other Topics

BONE CEMENT

I. INTRODUCTION
1. Bone cements are polymers of methyl methacrylate.
2. "Cement" misnomer → Cement is used to describe a substance that bonds two things together.
   ↓
   Polymethylmethacrylate (PMMA) acts as a space filler that creates a tight space which holds the implant against the bone and thus acts as a "grout".

II. AIMS OF USING BONE CEMENT
1. Secure fixation of implant and bone
2. Mechanical interlock and space filling
3. Load transferring
4. Maintenance/restoration of bone stock.

III. CONSTITUENTS
1. *Powder:*
   i. Polymer: Polymethacrylate.
   ii. Initiator: Benzoyl peroxide (BPO)
   iii. Radio-opacifier: Barium sulfate ($BaSO_4$) or zirconia (ZrO_2).
   iv. Coloring agent → Chlorophyll
   v. Antibiotics: Gentamycin, tobramycin, colistin, etc.
2. *Liquid:*
   i. Monomer: Methyl methacrylate.
   ii. Accelerator: N,N-dimethyl-p-toluidine (DMPT)
   iii. Stabilizer: Hydroquinone (prevents premature polymerization)
   iv. Coloring agents: Chlorophyll (Easier visualization in revisions)

IV. PHASES
1. Mixing
2. Waiting
3. Working
4. Hardening

A. Mixing
1. Time taken to full integrate the powder and the liquid.
2. BPO + DMPT → Polymerization process
3. Mixing must be homogenous → Decreased pores.

B. Waiting
1. Achieves suitable viscosity for handling
2. "Dough time": Beginning of mixing till when the cement no longer sticks to the surgical gloves. Normal 3–4 minutes.

C. Working
1. Period during which cement is manipulated and prosthesis inserted.
2. Working time: Interval between the dough and the setting times. Normal = 5–8 minutes
3. The implantation of the prosthesis must end before the end of working phase.

D. Setting Phase
1. Cement hardens (cures) and sets completely
2. Temperature reaches peak due to chemical → Thermal energy
3. Hardening influenced by → Cement, body and OT temperature.
4. Setting time → Beginning of mixing till 50% of max temperature reached (**Fig. 1**).

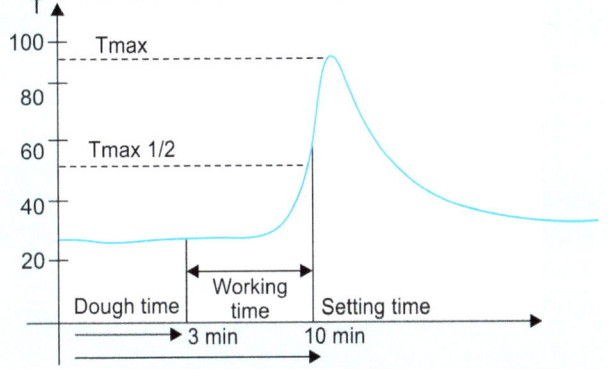

V. EVOLUTION OF CEMENTING TECHNIQUES

1. *1st generation (Charnley's original tech.):*
    i. Hand mixing of cement in bowls
    ii. Minimal femoral canal preparation
    iii. Cancellous bone left in situ
    iv. No cement restrictor → Finger pressurization
2. *2nd generation:*
    i. Meticulous removal of all cancellous bone using curette exposing solid endosteal surface.
    ii. Use of distal cement restrictor
    iii. Packing the canal with H_2O_2 soaked gauze.
    iv. Cement gun used to introduce cement in retrograde manner.
3. *3rd generation:*
    i. Vacuum centrifugation → Decreased pores
    ii. Femoral canal irrigated with pulsatile lavage and packed with adrenaline soaked swabs
    iii. Prosthesis inserted using both proximal and distal centralizers to ensure even cement mantle
    iv. Pressurized:
        a. Fills all endosteal space.
        b. No blood mixing with cement.

VI. TYPES OF CEMENT

A. Viscosity

Affects:
1. Bone cement handling characteristics.
2. Handling time
3. Penetration into cancellous bone.
   ↓
   Quality and longevity of fixation achieved.

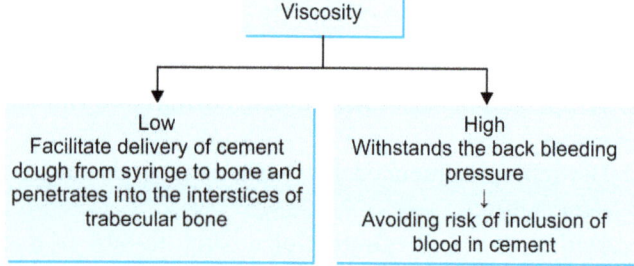

Types

1. *Low viscosity:* Long waiting phase → Short true working time
2. *Medium viscosity* → Dual phase cements can be both low and high depending on the time when it is delivered. They begin in low vicious phase, which allows easy mixing of powder and liquid.
3. *High viscosity* → Comprise of PMMA with practically no methyl methacrylate copolymer.
   Immediately after mixing → Cement doughy
   ↓
   Ready to apply by hand ← No runny state.

B. Antibiotics

1. Bone cements can act as modern drug delivery systems → delivering drugs directly to surgical site.
2. However not all antibiotics can be used.
3. *Properties:*
    i. Thermally stable
    ii. Water soluble
    iii. Bacterial
    iv. Gradual release into tissue → Eluting for long period of time
    v. Minimal local inflammation

    vi. No allergy
    vii. Does not affect mechanical integrity of cement
    viii. Broad antimicrobial coverage
4. *Commonly used antibiotics:*
    i. Gentamycin
    ii. Rifampicin
    iii. Tobramycin
    iv. Erythromycin
    v. Colistin
    vi. Vancomycin
    vii. Clindamycin
    viii. Meropenam
5. >2 g antibiotics → Alter mechanical properties.

VII. COMPLICATIONS

1. Hypotensive episode (Premature insertion of bone cement)
2. Thrombophlebitis
3. Trochanteric bursitis
4. Heterotopic ossification
5. *Bone cement implantation syndrome (BCIS):* Well-recognized complex of sudden physiologic changes that occur within minutes of implantation of bone cement.
    i. Hypoxemia
    ii. Increased pulmonary vascular resistance
    iii. Arrhythmia
    iv. Cardiac arrest
6. Bronchospasm
7. Hematuria, dysuria
8. Local neuropathy

VIII. DRAWBACKS

1. Stress shielding
2. Does not remodel
3. Neither osteoconductive nor inductive
4. Weak in tension **(Fig. 2)**.

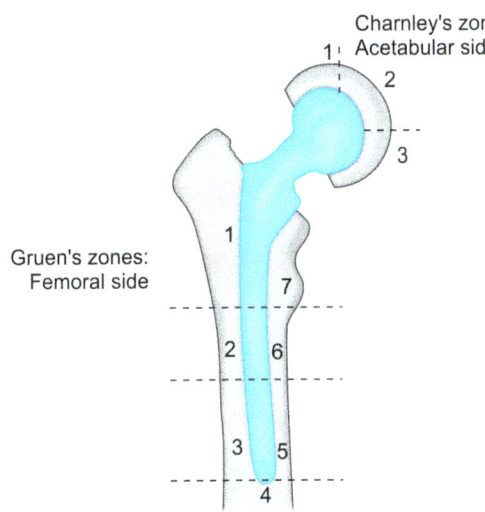

Fig. 2: Zones of cementing.

BONE BANK

Deals with procurement, storage and supply of bone.

I. GOALS

1. To preserve integrity of graft
2. To reduce immunogenicity
3. To ensure sterility

II. PROTOCOLS: FIVE COMPONENTS

1. Organization
2. Donor selection
3. Documentation
4. Storage and processing
5. Implementation

The HOD orthopaedics and their bone bank compose this protocol.

III. ORGANIZATION

1. HOD, orthopedics
2. Bone bank administrator
3. Trainer
4. Designated orthopaedics surgeon team
5. Hematological lab technician
6. Medical microbiologist
7. Anatomic pathologist
8. Clinical chemical analyst
9. Trained theatre nurse
10. Assistants: Maintenance and cleaning.

IV. DONOR SELECTION

A. General Exclusion Criteria

1. <18, >80 years
2. Active/recent systemic infection or sepsis
3. Recent (<4 weeks) vaccination with live virus
4. Malignancies (except BCC)
5. Collagen vascular disease
6. Metabolic bone disease
7. Consent not given by patients/relatives. (Transplantation of human organs, 1994)
8. Long-term steroids

B. Specific Exclusion Criteria

Positive serology for:
1. HIV: HIV Ag by PCR
   HIV 1, 2 → antibody
2. Hepatitis - A, C antibodies
   Hep B surface Ag and "B" core antibody
3. HTLV: 1, 2 - antibody
4. Syphilis: Rapid plasma reagin (RPR) antibody, fluorescent treponemal antibody
5. MSM: Men having sex with men
6. Hemophilic patients
7. History of IV drug abuse

V. HEMATOLOGICAL EXAMINATION

1. Blood group and typing
2. ESR → Males < 20, Females < 30

VI. STORAGE AND PROCESSING

1. Retrieval of femoral head is performed at the time of THR under aseptic conditions.
2. Removed femoral head → inspected → capsule and synovial tissue cultured.
3. Biopsy of 1 cm^3 cortico-cancellous bone, capsule taken for HPE to exclude malignancies and infections.
4. *Cadaveric donors:*
   i. Bone grafts as soon as possible
   ii. <12 hours → Unrefrigerated body
   iii. <24 hours → Refrigerated body
   iv. Pelvis is procured at the end to prevent contamination of bowel
5. Processing:
   A. **Fresh frozen allografts:**
      i. Blood and BM elements are washed away and graft cleaned → sterile water, isopropyl alcohol and H_2O_2
      ii. Storing at very low temperature (–70 to –80°C)

      Advantages:
      1. Simplicity of its preparation and storage
      2. High axial load bearing strength (retains structural integrity)
      3. Decreased immunogenicity

      Disadvantages:
      1. Need for graft to be frozen continuously at very low temperatures
      2. Freezers need to be continuously monitored to avoid thawing and spoilage.

3. Freezing alone doesn't destroy all the viruses and bacteria (especially spores)
↓
Needs secondary sterilization

B. **Freeze dried allograft:**
Involves removal of water from frozen tissue by **sublimation in vacuum**.
Advantages:
1. Storage at room temperature
2. Easy transportation
3. Longer shelf life

Disadvantages:
1. Process is time consuming, expensive and laborious.
2. Altered mechanical properties → Brittle.

C. **Demineralized bone:**
   i. Chemosterilized, antigen extracted, surface demineralized autolyzed, allogenic bone prepared from diaphyseal cortical bone
   ii. Lacks structural strength
   iii. High rate of resorption after grafting

6. **Secondary sterilization:**
   i. Gamma irradiation with 25 Gy from Co – 60
   ii. Irradiating graft at low temp (–80° C)
   ↓
   Less alterations in the mechanical properties by causing less collagen damage.
   iii. Ethylene oxide → Risk of subsequent elution of the agent from allograft → now unpopular

VII. DOCUMENTATION

1. Unique registration code is allocated to each allograft
2. Only bone bank administrator can trace the donor using this code
3. *For every registered allograft file:*
   i. Consent forms
   ii. Screening blood tests
   iii. Processing methods
   iv. Size
   v. Date of allocation, expiry
   vi. Replacement records

VIII. SOFT TISSUE ALLOGRAFTS

1. Patellar tendon bone allograft
2. Achilles tendon
3. Fascia lata
4. ACL
5. Peroneal tendon
6. Anterior and posterior tibialis tendons
7. Flexor tendons of hand
8. Meniscus → transplantation

AMPUTATION

I. INTRODUCTION

1. Transosseous removal of a limb or part of it.
2. Not failure of treatment, but
   ↓
3. 1st step towards return to a more comfortable and productive life.

II. INDICATIONS

1. Dead limb
2. Dangerous limb
3. Damned nuisance

A. Dead Limb
1. Severe trauma
2. Peripheral vascular disease
3. Burns
4. Frost bite

B. Dangerous Limb
1. Crush injury
2. Malignancy
3. Lethal sepsis
4. Forgotten tourniquet (>6 hours)

C. Damned Nuisance
1. Gross deformity
2. Recurrent sepsis
3. Loss of function

III. AIMS OF AMPUTATION

1. Preserving adequate length of stump
2. Ablation of diseased tissue (tumor/infection)
3. Reduce morbidity and mortality (tumor)
4. Securing rapid tissue healing.
5. Attaining maximum function of the residual portion of the extremity
6. Return patient to maximum level of independent function,

IV. PRINCIPLES OF AMPUTATION
A. Skin Flaps

1. Total length of flap (anterior + posterior)
   ↓
   Five times wide of stump
2. Flap → Semicircular for conical stump
3. Long posterior flap → BK amputation **(Fig. 3)**

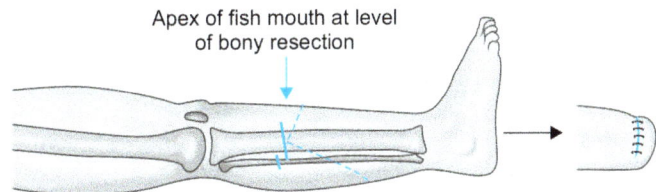

Apex of fish mouth at level of bony resection

4. Equal length anterior and posterior flaps → Upper limb and AK amputation.
5. Keep greatest skin length possible with muscle coverage, tension - free closure
   In open amputations → keeping in mind closure at a separate stage.
6. Scar should not be adherent to the underlying bone.
7. Large "dog ears" avoided → difficulty in prosthesis fitting.
8. Apex of fish-mouth → at the level of bony resection.

B. Muscles 4 Cs' (Contraction, Color, Consistency, Circulation)

1. Divide = 5 cm distal to bone resection.
2. Stabilization of muscle mass by adequate suturing

Myoplasty	Myodesis
Suturing of antagonists to each other over bony stump	• Suturing muscle to bone. • Contraindicated in ischemia • Useful in AK amputation • Stronger insertion maximizes strength and minimizes atrophy • Counterbalance antagonists → Prevent contractures and maximize residual limb function

3. Postoperative muscle exercises—prevents atrophy

C. Nerves

1. Isolate
2. Cut sharply under gentle tension
   ↓
   Allows retraction proximal to bone ends
3. Large nerves → ligate (due to contained vessels) (sciatic, median).

D. Blood Vessels

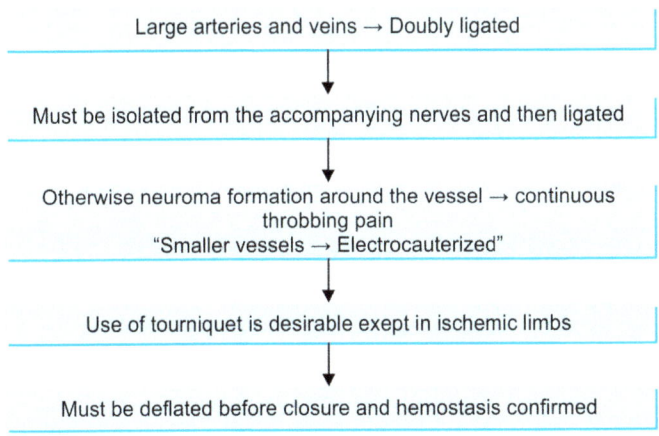

E. Bone

1. Avoid excess periosteal stripping, excess leads to ring sequestra and bone overgrowth (spur formation)
2. The bone ends must be smoothened using a file
3. Bony prominence that are not well padded by soft tissue → Resect
4. Protect soft tissue → Amputation shield.
5. Wash bone dust with saline.
6. Fibula 2 cm proximal to tibia.

F. Closure

1. Tension free
2. Interrupted sutures
3. Drains essential (Remove >48-72 hours)

G. Dressing

1. Soft dressing with crepe bandage.
2. Rigid dressing with POP
   ↓
   i. ↓ and prevents edema at surgical site
   ii. Enhance wound healing and early maturation of stump.
   iii. Decreases postoperative pain
   iv. Allows early mobilization and ambulation
   v. Prevents knee contractures in BK amputation.

H. Level of Amputation

1. *Factors deciding:*
   i. Zone of injury (trauma)
   ii. Adequate margins (tumor)
   iii. Adequate circulation (vascular disease)
   iv. Soft tissue envelope
   v. Bone and joint condition
   vi. Control of infection
   vii. Nutritional status
2. Metabolic cost of walking increases with more proximal amputations.
3. Conventional sites for amputation:
   i. Upper limb:
      a. AE: 20 cm from acromion → 4 cm below axillary fold
      b. BE: 18 cm from olecranon → 3 cm below biceps insertion
   ii. Lower limb   Minimum
      a. AK: 12 cm above knee   8 cm
      b. BK: 14 cm below knee   7.5 cm
4. The development of modern modular prosthesis has widened the possible sites of amputation

I. Ideal Stump

1. Optimum length
2. End of stump → Smooth and rounded

3. Vascularity of flaps well maintained
4. No projecting spurs of bone
5. Stump must be tension free
6. Position of scar free from pressure – not adherent to bone
7. Adjacent joint movements good
8. Adequate muscle padding
9. Healed completely

V. BELOW KNEE AMPUTATION (EXTRA POINTS)

1. Bone length: 2.5 cm for every 30 cm of body weight.
2. Stumps lacking quadriceps function – Not useful.
   (**Fig. 4:** Cross section of middle 1/3rd of the leg)

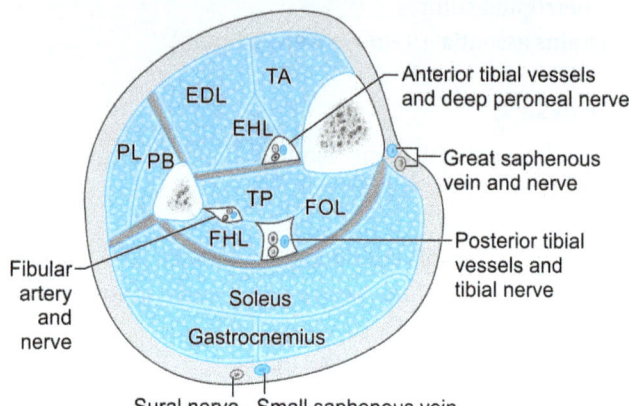

VI. BASIC FEATURES OF PROSTHESIS (FIG. 5)

1. Socket → Receptive area of stump, weight bearing
2. Suspension → Holds prosthesis to stump
3. Joints → Amputed joints replaced with artificial joints
4. Base → Contact with floor

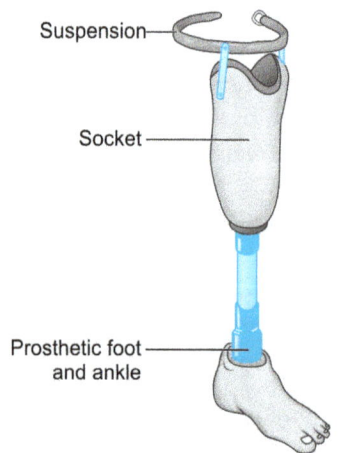

VII. SYME'S AMPUTATION (FIG. 6)

1. Amputation at the distal tibia and fibula 0.6 cm proximal to the ankle joint.
   ↓ (removal of foot with calcaneum)
2. Passing through the dome of the ankle centrally.
3. The tough durable skin of the heel flap → weight bearing.

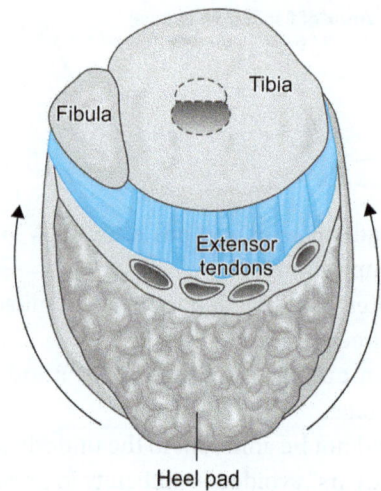

Fig. 6: Syme's amputation.

A. Disadvantages

1. Posterior migration of heel pad.
2. Skin slough resulting from trimming of dog ears.
3. Cosmesis: Stump is large and bulky (bulbous, elephant foot)
   ↓ due to
   Flair of distal tibia metaphysis

B. Technique

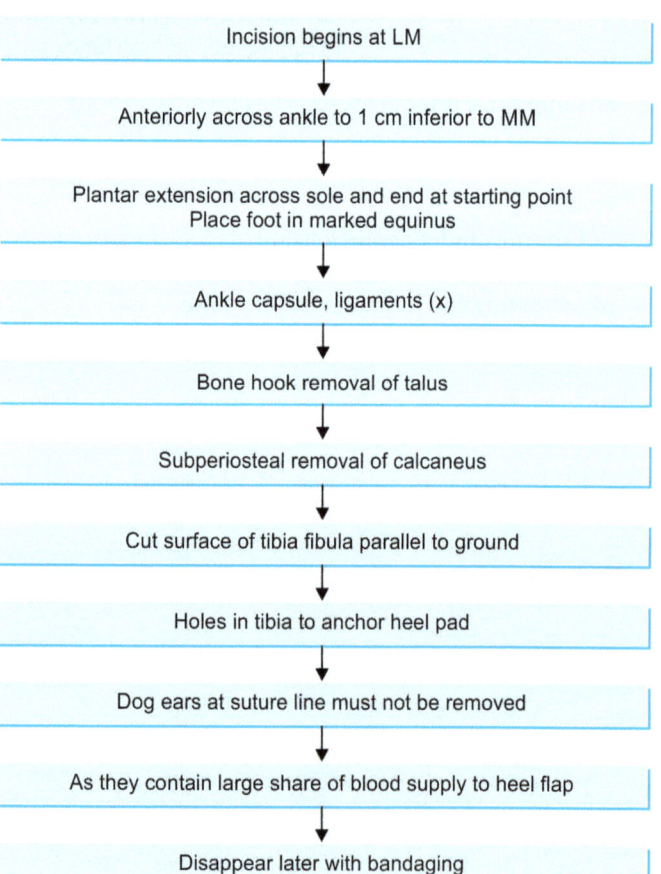

PERIPHERAL NERVE INJURIES AND NERVE CONDUCTION STUDIES

I. RELEVANT ANATOMY (FIG. 7)

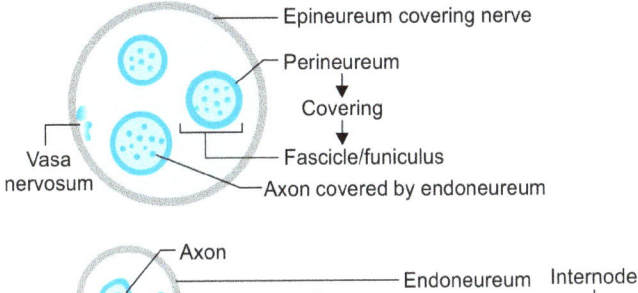

Peripheral nerves → Bundles of axons that use electrical and chemical signals to transmit sensory and motor impulses from one body part to another.

II. ETIOLOGY

1. *Trauma:*
    i. Crush/compression
    ii. Laceration
    iii. Sharp cut
    iv. Stretching
    v. Iatrogenic
    vi. Thermal → Burns
    vii. Electrical
2. Metabolic
3. Malignancy
4. Toxins
5. Ischemia → Freezing
6. Infection → Leprosy
7. Radiation

III. PATHOPHYSIOLOGY

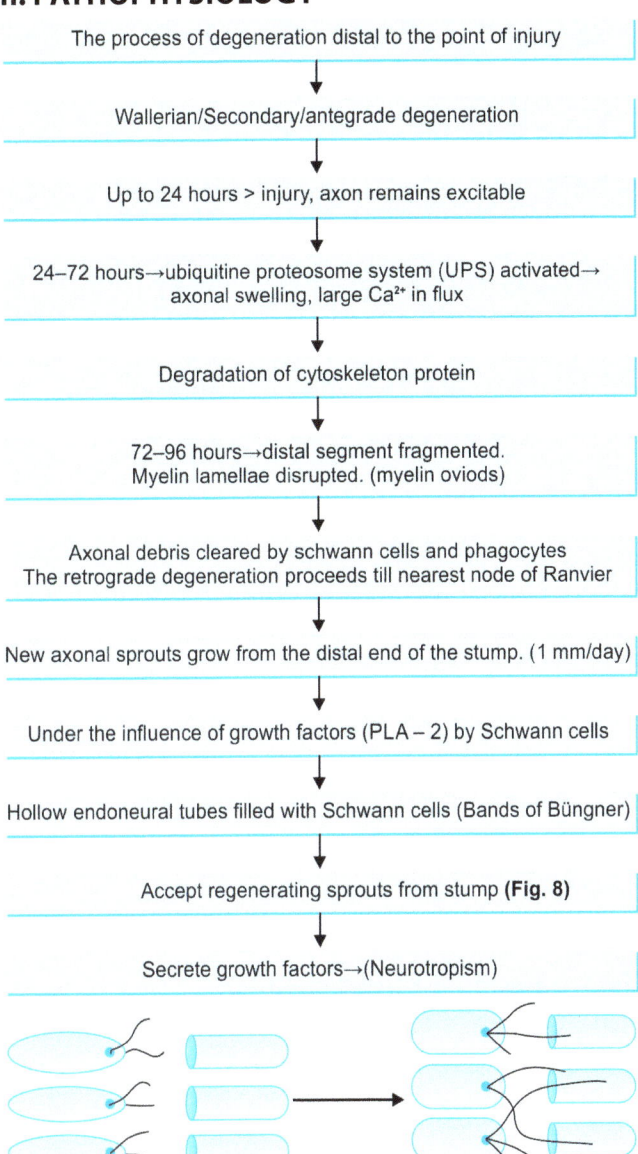

Fig. 8: Regenerating sprouts enter the hollow endoneural tubes.

Degeneration proximal to point of injury → Retrograde/Primary/Traumatic
↓
Loss of Nissl's granules, chromatolysis, nucleolar swelling.

IV. CLASSIFICATION
Sunderland and Seddon

	Histopathologic changes					Tinel sign	
Degree of injury	Myelin	Axon	Endoneurium	Perineurium	Epineurium	Present	Progresses distally
I Neurapraxia	±	−	−	−	−	−	
II Axonotmesis	+	+	−	−	−	+	+
III	+	+	+	−	−	+	+
IV	+	+	+	+	−	+	−
V Neurotmesis	+	+	+	+	+	+	
VI Various fibers and fascicle demonstrate various pathologic changes						+	±

V. CLINICAL PRESENTATION

1. *History:*
   i. Inability to move part of limb
   ii. Weakness
   iii. Numbness
2. *Examination:*
   i. **Attitude and deformity** — **Nerve injury**
      a. Wrist drop — Radial
      b. Foot drop — CPN
      c. Winging of scapula — Long thoracic nerve
      d. Claw hand — Ulnar and median
      e. Ape – thumb deformity — Median
      f. Pointing index — Median
      g. Policeman's tip deformity — Erb's palsy
   ii. Muscle wasting
   iii. Skin changes:
      a. Dry, glossy and smooth.
      b. Trophic disturbances → Brittle nails, atrophic skin.
   iv. Temperature: Cooler and drier
   v. Sensory: Dermatomal loss
   vi. Motor examination for muscles
   vii. Sweat test: To detect sympathetic function of the nerve.
      Presence of sweating in autonomous zone.
      ↓
      Complete interruption has not occurred

VI. DIAGNOSIS

Electrodiagnostic Studies (SAQ)

Diagnostic studies that measure the electrical activities of nerve and muscle (Neurophysiology)

Types:
1. Electromyography (EMG) ⎱ Nerve conduction studies (NCS)
2. NCV ⎰
3. Evoked potentials (SSEP)

A. Electromyography

Study of electrical activity of motor units and individual muscle fibers.

i. *Technique*

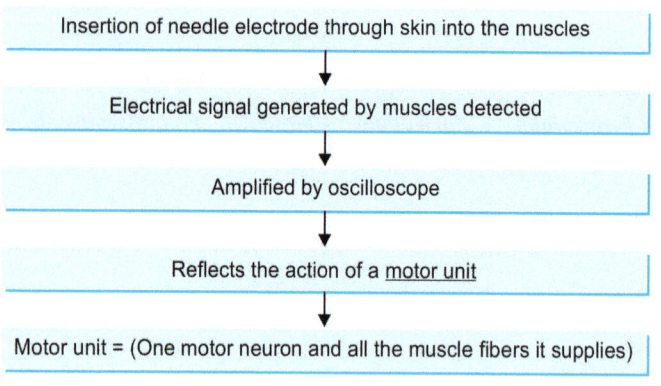

   ii. Application:
      1. Distinguishes a recent injury from a chronic condition that predates the injury (e.g., workers compensation)
      2. Differentiates between diseases of nerve roots, peripheral nerves or skeletal muscles.
      3. Used to evaluate NCV
      4. *Chronic muscle disorders:*
         i. Inflammatory myopathies
         ii. Muscular dystrophies
         iii. Congenital myopathies
         iv. Muscle trauma
      5. *Neurogenic disorders:*
         i. Radiculopathy
         ii. Axonal peripheral neuropathy
         iii. Entrapment neuropathies
         iv. Motor neuron diseases
   iii. *Types of activities* **(Fig. 9)**

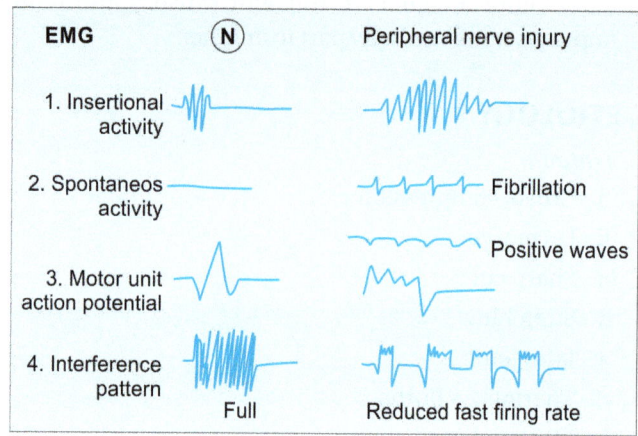

1. **Insertional**
   a. Brief burst of electrical activity upon electrode insertion.
   b. Fibrosis of muscle → No insertional activity
   c. Neuropraxia: Normal, spontaneous activity → silent.
   d. Axonotmesis, neurotmesis → ↑↑↑ spontaneous activity in the form of fibrillation
2. **Spontaneous:** Normal muscle is silent at rest.
   a. Fibrillations: Positive sharp waves due to lack of inhibitory (feedback) "stabilization" that nerves exert on muscle fibers. Seen in single muscle fibers.
   b. Fasciculation: Spontaneous discharge of group of muscle fibers.
3. Motor unit potential: Sum of the action potentials of all muscle fibers of a single motor unit.

B. Nerve Conduction Velocity

1. Test performed on peripheral nerves to determine their response to electrical stimuli.

2. Two sets of stimulating electrodes along the nerve trunk are tested.
3. A recording electrode is placed in the muscle belly innervated by the nerve to be tested.
4. Nerve is stimulated at two different points → time difference between evoked potential determined.
5. Since distance between the two electrodes is known → Velocity is calculated (**Fig. 10**).

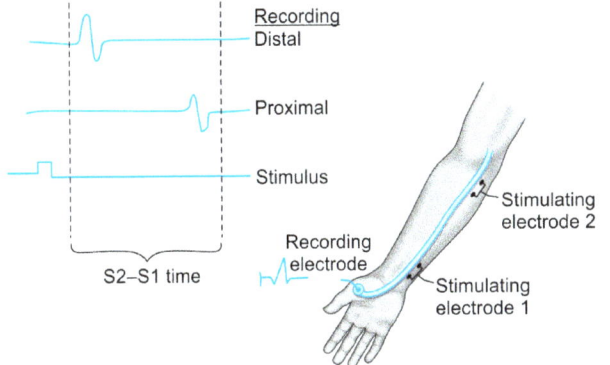

6. *NCV varies with*:
   i. Myelin thickness
   ii. Temperature
   iii. Age
7. NCV myelinated fibers → 50 m/sec
8. Unmyelinated fibers → 10 m/sec
9. *Age*: Newborn—50% of adult value
   1 year—75%
   5 years—100%
10. Amplitude – provides estimate of number of functioning axons and muscle fibers.
11. Neuropraxia → Delay at site of injury but otherwise EMG and NCV are normal.
12. Late responses evaluate proximal nerve lesions (near spinal cord: Guillain–Barré syndrome)
    → F-wave amplitude
    → H-reflex

VII. TREATMENT

A. Conservative
1. Observation with serial examination and EDS
2. Splinting the paralyzed in functional position
3. Preservation of mobility of joint
4. Physiotherapy
5. *Indications*:
   i. Closed fracture or dislocation
   ii. Neuropraxia
   iii. Axonotmesis.

B. Operative
i. Indications:
   1. Nerve injury (previously absent) secondary to manipulation of fracture.
   2. Open fracture: Taken up for surgery debridement.
   3. Fractures where satisfactory alignment is not possible by closed methods.
      ↓
      Exploration of nerve during fracture surgery
   4. Fractures with associated vascular injury.
   5. Sharp injury clearly transected the nerve → Primary repair.
   6. Abrading or blast wounds → Nerve condition unknown → Exploration → Marking nerve endings for later repair.
   7. Nerve deficit after closed injury with no clinical or electrical evidence of recovery after 3 months of injury.
ii. Techniques:
   1. Neurolysis
   2. Nerve repair (neurorrhaphy)
   3. Nerve grafting
   4. Nerve transfer
   5. Tendon transfer

1. *Neurolysis*
   i. External: Nerve is freed from enveloping scar.
   ii. Internal: Nerve sheath dissected longitudinally to relieve the pressure from the fibrous tissue within the nerve.
2. *Nerve repair*
   i. *Timing*: <8 hours: Primary
      First 7–18 days → Delayed primary
      3 weeks—secondary
   ii. Types based on extent (**Fig. 11**) → Partial
      → Complete

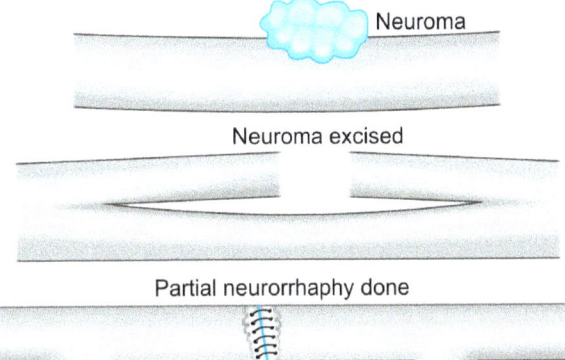

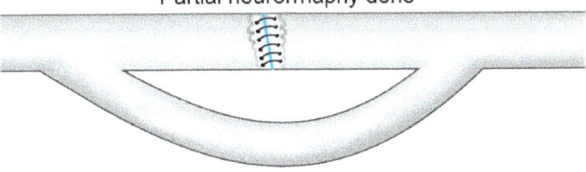

   iii. *Types*:
      a. Epineural
      b. Epiperineural
      c. Perineural
      d. Group fascicular (**Fig. 12**)

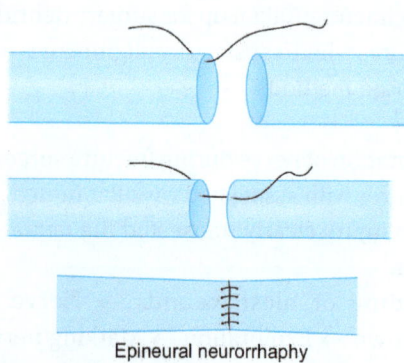

Epineural neurorrhaphy

- iv. *Reduction of nerve gap:*
  - a. Mobilization
  - b. Positioning of extremity
  - c. Transposition – changed anatomic course
  - d. Bone resection
- v. *Augmentation of repair:*
  - a. Using ensheathing materials
  - b. Fibrin clots
- vi. No tension at repair site must.
- vii. Normal excursion of nerve when extremity is moving should be considered.
  ↓
  ROM checked during repair
- viii. Epineural vessels must be preserved.
3. *Nerve grafting*
  - i. *Indication:*
    - a. Defect > 4 cm
    - b. Tension at repair site.
  - ii. *Graft options:*
    - a. Sural (MC) = 40 cm
    - b. Lateral antebrachial cutaneous nerve – brachial.
    - c. Medial antebrachial cutaneous nerve
    - d. Lateral cutaneous nerve of thigh
    - e. Terminal branch of posterior interosseus nerve (PIN)
    - f. Artificial conduits.
4. *Nerve transfer:*
  - i. *Proximal nerve injuries:* Delivers new axons and stimuli before motor end-plate degeneration.
  - ii. Shoulder Abduction and external rotation ⊗ → Spinal XI to suprascapular nerve
  - iii. Loss of elbow flexion → Oberlin transfer
    ↓
    FCU motor branch is transferred to musculocutaneous nerve
5. *Tendon transfers:*
  - i. *Indication:* Return of function through nerve regeneration not expected.
  - ii. Better outcome = <30 years age
    = Distal location
    Children → Neuroplasticity
  - iii. 1 grade of motor strength is lost after transfer.

BRACHIAL PLEXUS

I. INTRODUCTION

1. Somatic nerve plexus formed by the ventral primary rami of C5-T1
2. Network of nerve fibers from cervicoaxillary canal → supplying the upper limb.

II. PATHOANATOMY (FIG. 13)

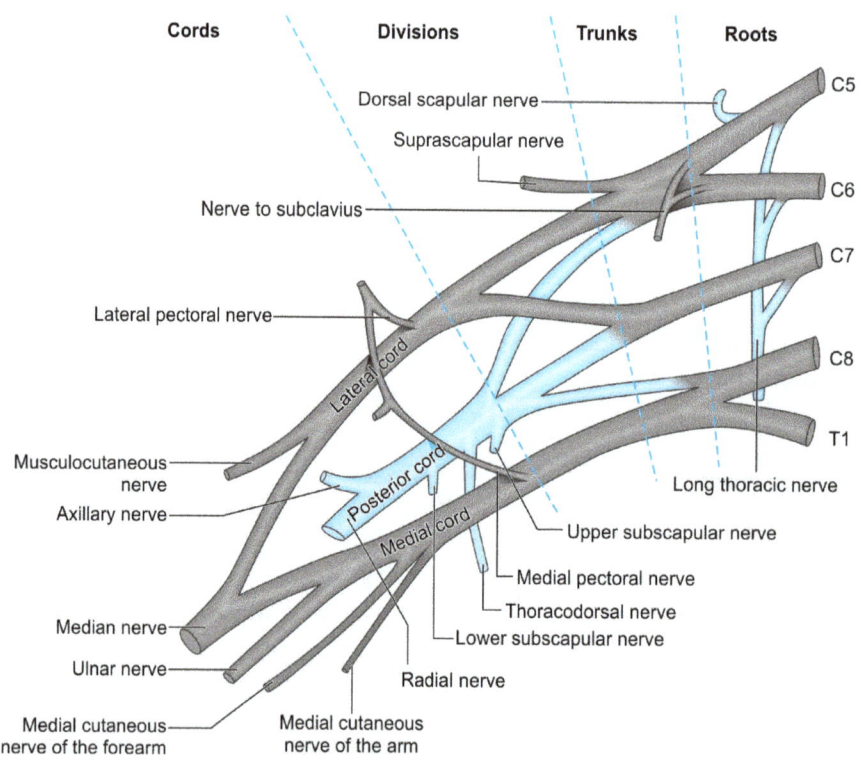

1. Brachial plexus consists of roots, trunks, divisions, cords and branches.
2. *Roots:*
   i. They are deep to the sternocleidomastoid muscle between scalenus anterior and medius muscle.
   ii. Origin of plexus may be prefixed: C4–C8, or post-fixed: C6–T2
3. *Trunks:*
   i. Derived from roots.
   ii. Situated in the anteroinferior part of the posterior triangle of the neck.
   iii. C5-6 → unite to form → Upper trunk
   iv. C7 → Middle trunk
   v. C8-T1 → Lower trunk
   vi. Each trunk ends by splitting into anterior and posterior divisions.
4. *Cords:*
   i. Posterior cord → formed from → Posterior divisions of all three trunks (C5-T1)
   ii. Lateral cord → Anterior divisions of upper and middle trunk (C5-C7)
   iii. Medial cord → Continuation of anterior division of the lower trunk (C8-T1)
5. Branches
   - Supraclavicular: From root or trunks
   - Infraclavicular: From cords
6. *From roots:*
   i. Dorsal scapular nerve (C5) → Rhomboids
   ii. Long Thoracic Nerve (C5-7) → Serratus anterior
7. *From trunk:*
   i. Nerve to subclavius (C5-6) → Subclavius
   ii. Suprascapular nerve (C5-6) → Supra and Infraspinatus
8. *Lateral cord (C5-7) (Mneumonic: LML):*
   i. **L**ateral pectoral nerve
   ii. **M**usculocutaneous nerve
   iii. **L**ateral root of median nerve
9. *Medial cord (C8-T1) (Mneumonic M 4 U):*
   i. Ulnar nerve
   ii. Medial pectoral nerve
   iii. Medial cutaneous nerve of arm
   iv. Medial cutaneous nerve of forearm
   v. Medial root of median nerve
10. *Posterior cord (Mneumonic: ULNAR):*
    i. Upper subscapular
    ii. Lower subscapular
    iii. Nerve to latissimus dorsi (Thoracodorsal nerve)
    iv. Axillary nerve
    v. Radial nerve

III. ETIOLOGY

Closed	Open

• Traction injury:
  – Avulsion
  – RTA
  – Sports
  – Obstetric palsy
• Radiation induced → Fibrosis
• Neoplastic:
  – Schwannoma
  – Neurofibroma
• Iatrogenic:
  – Intraoperative position
  – Tractions
• Infection: Viral plexopathy
• Nerve entrapment: Thoracic outlet syndrome
• Neuropathies
	• Gunshot wounds
	• Lacerations (RTAs)
	• Stab injuries
	• Surgeries:
	  – Surgical biopsy
	  – Sternotomy
	• Anesthesia related:
	  – Axillary
	  – Interscalene block
	• IV cannulas

A. Mechanisms
1. Traction
2. Penetration
3. Compression
4. Ischemia

IV. CLASSIFICATION
A. Leffert
B. Millesi
C. Anatomical

A. Leffert Classification
I → Open
II → Closed { IIa: Supraclavicular
              IIb: Infraclavicular
III → Radiation
IV → Obstetric { IVa: Erb's (Upper roots)
                 IVb: Klumpke's (Lower roots)

IIa: Supraclavicular
1. Preganglionic
   i. High speed injury → Avulsion of nerve roots
   ii. No proximal stump → ∴ No Neuroma formation: Negative Tinel's sign
   iii. Horner's syndrome
   iv. Pseudomeningocele
   v. Positive histamine test → Red reaction wheel and flare
   vi. Poor prognosis
2. Post-ganglionic:
   i. Traction injury → Roots remain intact.
   ii. Proximal stump + → Neuroma + : Positive Tinel's sign
   iii. No pseudomeningocele
   iv. Injury distal to ganglion

v. Negative histamine test
vi. Good prognosis after surgery

IIb: Infraclavicular → Trunk affected.

B. Millesi
1. Preganglionic
2. Post ganglionic
3. Trunk
4. Cord

C. Anatomical
1. Upper plexus palsy (Erb's) → C5-6, ±C7
2. Lower plexus palsy (Klumpke's) → C8-T1
3. Total plexus lesions (C5-T1)

V. CLINICAL FEATURES
1. Weakness of the affected muscles
2. Numbness → Burning, Paresthesia
3. Loss of sensation
4. Loss of movement (paralysis)
5. Neuropathic pain
6. Horner's syndrome: Ptosis, anhidrosis, miosis
7. Tinel's sign → Advancing - Recovering nerve injury
8. Erb's and Kumpke's findings (read in OBPP)

VI. INVESTIGATIONS
1. *X-ray:*
    i. Chest
    ii. C-spine
    iii. Clavicle and scapula
    iv. Shoulder
2. *CT* → Fracture, tumors
3. *CT myelography:*
    i. Absence of demonstrable rootlets in the subarachnoid space → Avulsion
    ii. Presence of meningocele → Arachnoid is torn at given root level.
4. *MRI:*
    i. Pseudomeningocoele
    ii. Empty nerve root sleeves
    iii. Cord shift away from midline
5. *EMG/NCV:*
    i. Fibrillation potentials and positive sharp potentials → Denervated muscles → regenerating axons have reached the motor end plates **(Fig. 14)**.

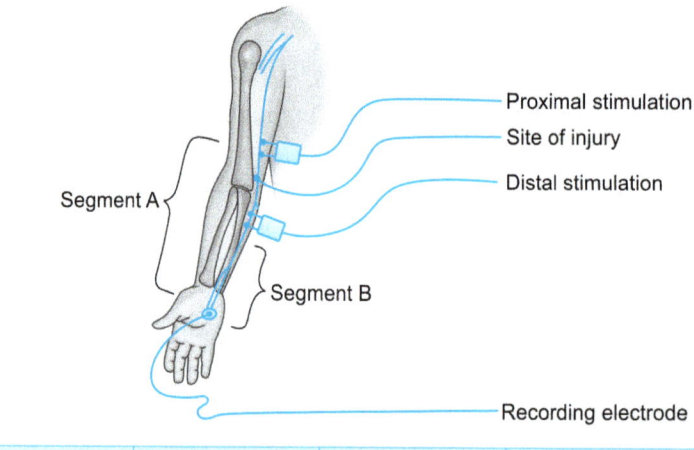

i.

VII. MANAGEMENT
1. Physiotherapy and rehabilitation → Prevent contractures
2. Splints
3. Preganglionic injury → Neurotization

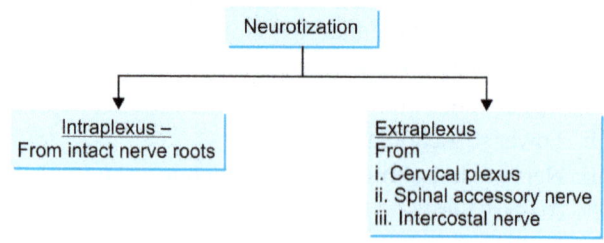

ii. Oberlin: Part of ulnar nerve transferred to innervate biceps (C5–C6 avulsion)
4. Postganglionic injury →
   i. Follow-up and observation → for spontaneous recovery
   ii. EMG/NCV at 3–4 weeks
   iii. Exploration of nerve is considered if clinical or electrical recovery is not evident by 4–5 months.
5. *Basic aim of surgery:*
   Surgeon's priority should be in following order:
   i. Elbow flexion
   ii. Shoulder instability:
       a. Abduction
       b. ER
       c. Adduction
   iii. Sensation: Median nerve territory
   iv. Wrist extension/finger flexion
   v. Wrist flexion/finger extension
   vi. Intrinsic function
6.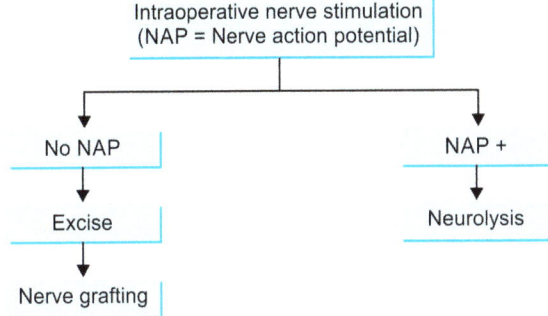
7. Tendon transfers in brachial plexus injury
   i. Trapezius → Deltoid → El Hassan
   ii. Lateral dorsi → ER → L'Episcopo
8. Erb's and Klumpke's management: (Read from OBPP)

OBSTETRIC PARALYSIS

I. INTRODUCTION
1. Injury to the brachial plexus during birth.
2. *Erb's palsy:* Upper brachial plexus (C5, C6, C7) with injury at the

   Erb's point
   ↓
   Point where C5 and C6 meet.

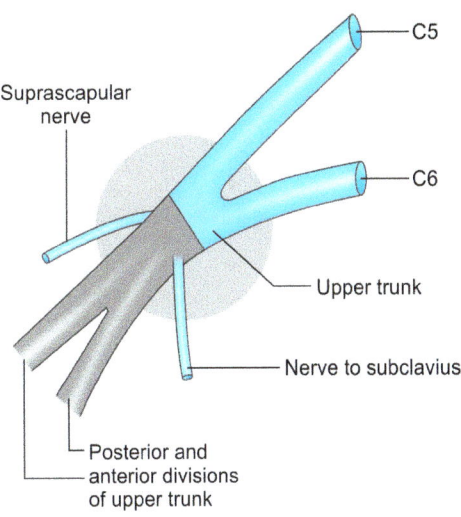

3. *Klumpke paralysis:* Lower brachial plexus paralysis involving (C8 and T1) **(Fig. 15)**.

II. RISK FACTORS
1. Macrosomia (large for gestational age)
2. Multiparous pregnancies
3. Previous delivery with OBPP
4. Prolonged labor
5. Breach delivery
6. Assisted delivery (vacuum/forceps)
7. Difficult deliveries
8. History of shoulder dystocia

III. PATHOPHYSIOLOGY
1. Traction across the brachial plexus is the most common mechanism of injury.
2. Forceful widening of the interval between the head and the shoulder.
   i. Laterally, flexing the head when shoulder is caught behind symphysis pubis.
   ii. In breech delivery, the after coming head is fixed behind the bony rim.
3. Upper portion of the brachial plexus affected. Most commonly → Erb's point.

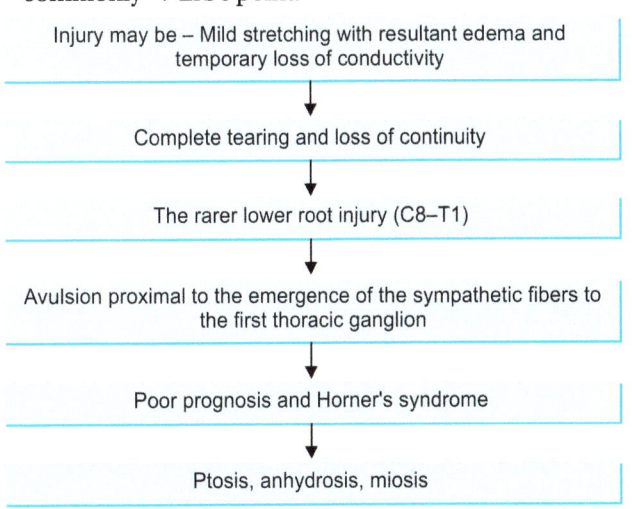

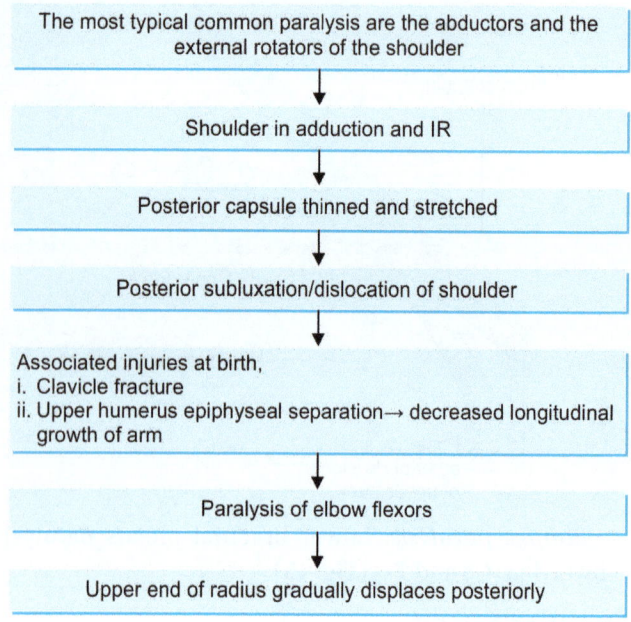

IV. CLINICAL FEATURES

1. Newborn lies with extremity lying limp at the side.
2. Infant cries at attempts to move extremity passively.
3. Some amount of muscle activity returns over few hours/days and swelling and sensitivity to passive movement disappear.
4. *Erb's palsy:* Policeman's/Waiter's tip position→
    i. Shoulder abducted and IR
    ii. Elbow extended
    iii. Forearm pronated.
5. *Klumpke palsy:*
    i. Intrinsic muscles of hand ⊗ → Claw Hand
    ii. Medial aspect of arm/forearm anesthetized
    iii. Horner's syndrome
6. Residual paralysis unfolds gradually over 3–4 months → further improvement unlikely
7. Deltoid is thinned
8. With time, the acromion process becomes prominent and curves anterolaterally
9. Fracture Clavicle → Crepitus, palpable

V. DIFFERENTIAL DIAGNOSIS

1. Sepsis → Pseudoparalysis
2. Tumor of spinal cord or plexus
3. Brachial plexus neuritis
4. Cerebral palsy.

VI. TREATMENT

1. Multidisciplinary approach → Optimal rehabilitation.
2. Initial treatment → Nonoperative
    ↓
    i. Maintaining full passive range of motion in all affected joints
    ii. Maintaining glenohumeral motion by passive stretching → prevent contractures
    iii. Orthosis as required (wrist drop splint)
3. If antigravity muscle power (shoulder abductors and biceps) returns within 3 months of life → Prognosis good and therefore continue nonoperative management.
4. *Microsurgery:* Timing controversial.
    i. Early surgical intervention → Best results.
    ii. Absence of biceps function at 3 months → Indication for surgery.
5. *Surgeries:*
    i. Neurolysis
    ii. Neuroma resection
    iii. Nerve grafting → sural nerve
    iv. Nerve transfers
6. Nerve repair → Not performed
7. Lesions affecting entire BP → Nerve transfers
    ↓
    Thoracic intercostals, spinal accessory, contralateral C7
8. No possible repair for preganglionic injuries.

VII. RECONSTRUCTIVE PROCEDURES FOR SEQUELAE OF OBPP

1. *Objectives:*
    i. Restore muscle balance
    ii. Release contractures
    iii. Overcoming deformity
2. **Fairbank:** Pectoralis major and subscapularis

    Tendon of insertion sectioned.
    Anterior capsule divided → Predisposes anterior shoulder dislocation.
3. **Severs:**
    i. Modification of fairbanks
    ii. Avoids opening capsule → No instability
    iii. Coracobrachialis and short head of biceps tendon released if contracted
    iv. Most commonly performed operation
4. **L'Episcopo:** "Sever's" operation + Teres major transferred posteriorly and attached to lateral aspect of humerus.
    IR → ER
5. **Green:** Incomplete division of pectoralis major and subscapularis → Lengthened (IR maintained). Both Latissimus dorsi and Teres major rerouted posterolaterally to act as ER.
6. steotomy of humerus → to correct IR
7. Derotation osteotomy for posterior torsion/subluxation

MEDIAN NERVE

Labrourer's nerve: C5 C6 C7 C8 T1
Lateral cord: C5 C6 C7

Medial cord: C8 T1 (**Fig. 16**)

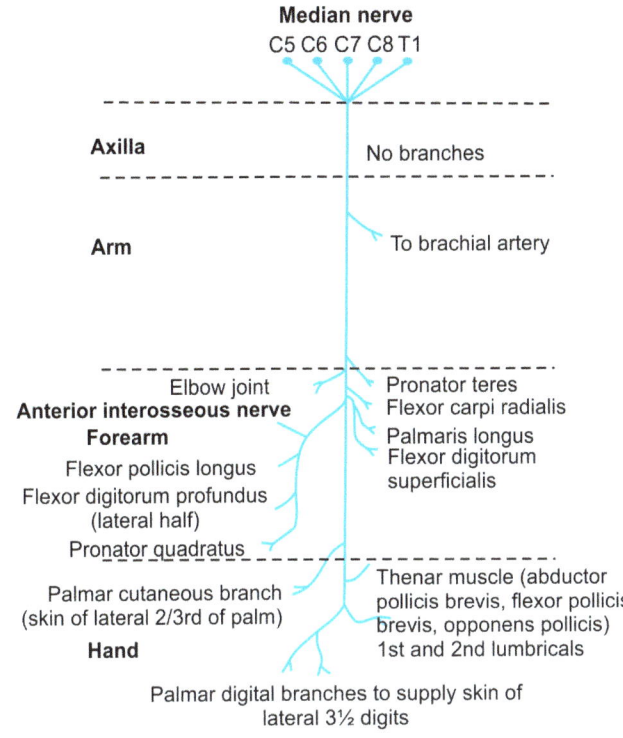

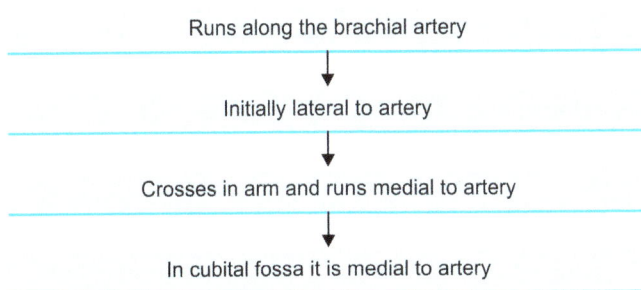

Median nerve innervates:
1. Pronator teres
2. FCR
3. FDS
4. PL

Anterior interosseous nerve (AIN):
1. FDP (lateral half)
2. FPL
3. Pronator Quadratus.

Terminal branches:
1. Abductor pollicis brevis
2. Flexor pollicis brevis
3. Opponens pollicis
4. 1st and 2nd lumbricals

Sensory:
1. Palmar cutaneous branch
2. Palmar digital branch

Compression sites for median nerve:
1. Ligament of struthers
2. Lacertus fibrosis thickening → Thick fibrous band extending from biceps tendon to forearm fascia
3. Hypertrophied pronator teres
4. Tight fibrous arch of FDS
5. Kiloh–Nevin syndrome (anterior interosseous syndrome) → Compression of AIN
6. Carpel tunnel syndrome

Clinical features:
1. Thenar muscle atrophy
2. Ape thumb deformity: Loss of opponens pollicis
3. Pointing index ⎫
4. Benediction hand ⎬ FDS
5. Ochsner's clasp test ⎭
6. Pen test: Abductor pollicis brevis
7. Sensory loss → Lateral 3½ digits volar aspect

MEDIAN NERVE PALSY

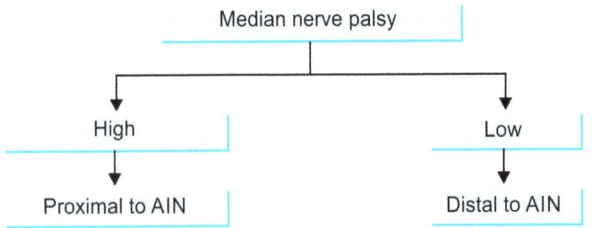

A. Low Median Nerve Palsy

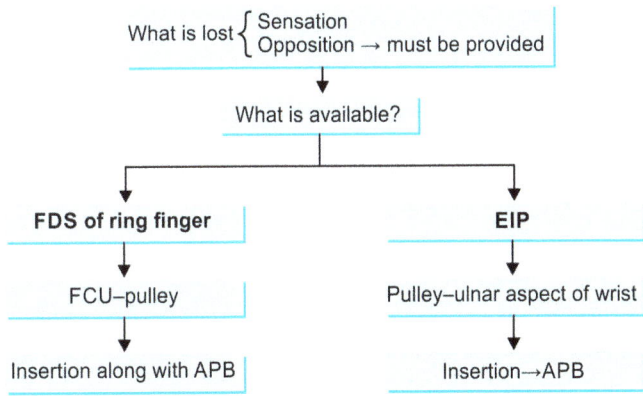

B. High Medial Nerve Palsy

What is lost →
1. Sensation
2. Thumb opposition: OP
3. Thumb IP joint flexion: FPL
4. Index finger MCP and IP joint flexion

What is available?
1. **EIP** → Opposition.
2. **Brachioradialis** → FPL
3. FDP of 4th and 5th to 2nd and 3rd

ULNAR NERVE

I. COURSE (FIG. 17)

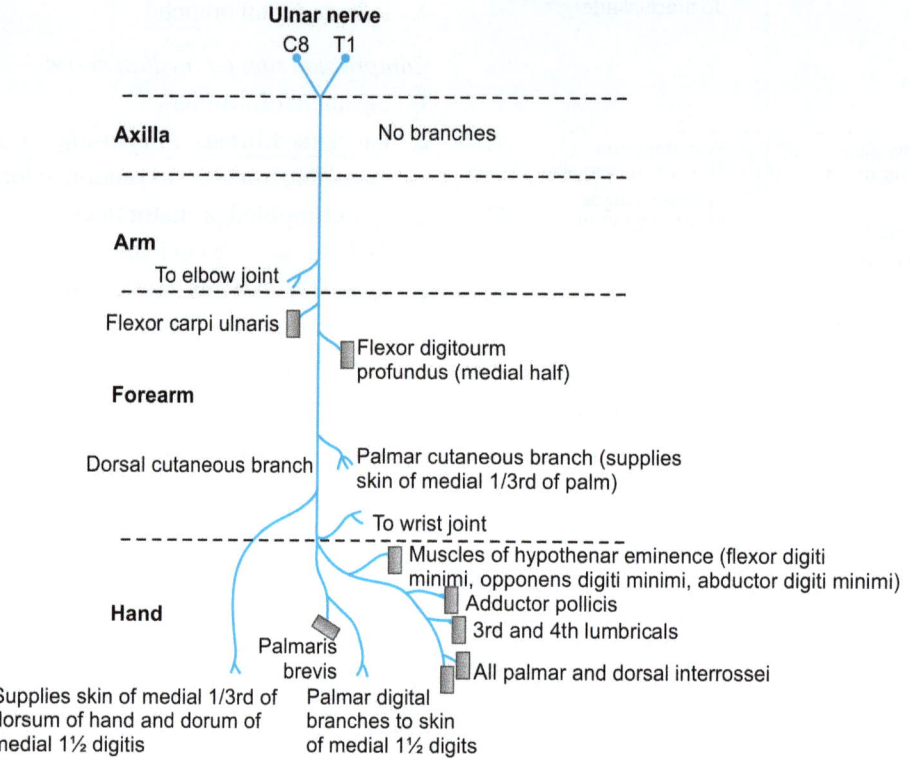

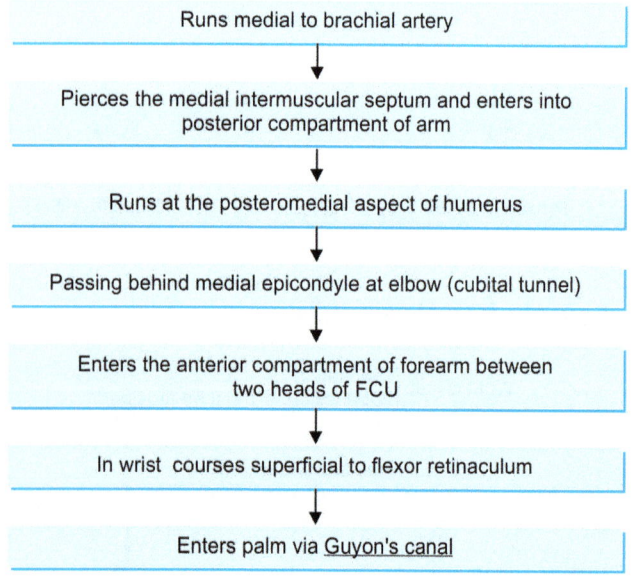

1. *Motor supply:*
   i. FCU
   ii. FDP (medial half)
   iii. Lumbricals of 4th and 5th digits
   iv. Hypothenar muscles:
      a. Flexor digiti minimi
      b. Opponens digiti minimi muscle
      c. Accessory abductor digiti minimi muscle
   v. Interossei → Palmar
                  → Dorsal
   vi. Adductor pollicis
   vii. Palmaris brevis.
2. *Sensory supply:*
   i. Palmar cutaneous branch
   ii. Dorsal cutaneous branch
3. *Special tests:*
   i. Card test: Palmar interossei
   ii. Egawa test: Dorsal interossei
   iii. Froment's sign (Book test): Adductor pollicis
   iv. Ulnar paradox → Claw hand is more severe in low ulnar nerve palsy as compared to high ulnar nerve palsy due to retention of medial half of FDP function.

II. LOW ULNAR NERVE PALSY

What is lost →
1. MCP joint flexion: Lumbricals

2. Finger adduction–abduction: Interossei
3. Thumb adduction: Adductor pollicis
   ↓
What must be replaced →
1. MCP joint flexion
2. Thumb adduction

A. MCP Joint Flexion

1. *Static*:
   i. Zancolli's capsulodesis
   ii. Fowler's tenodesis
2. *Dynamic*:
   i. ECRL
   ii. ECRB
   iii. FCR

B. Thumb Adduction

1. Smith technique → ECRB
2. Boyd's technique → ECRB/BR
3. Modified Royle – Thompson transfer → FDS
   ↓
   For restoration of adduction and opposition.

RADIAL NERVE

I. COURSE (FIG. 18)

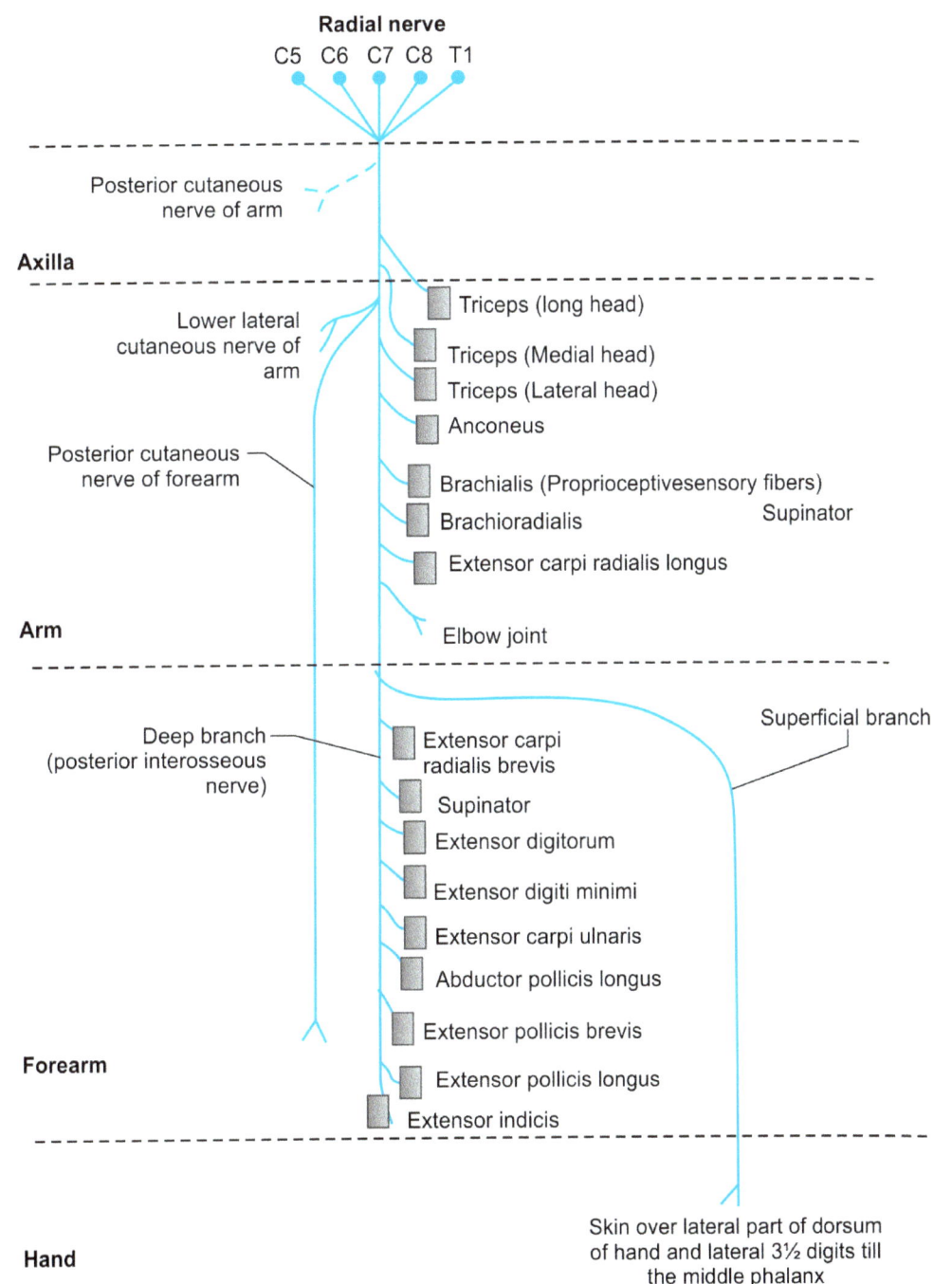

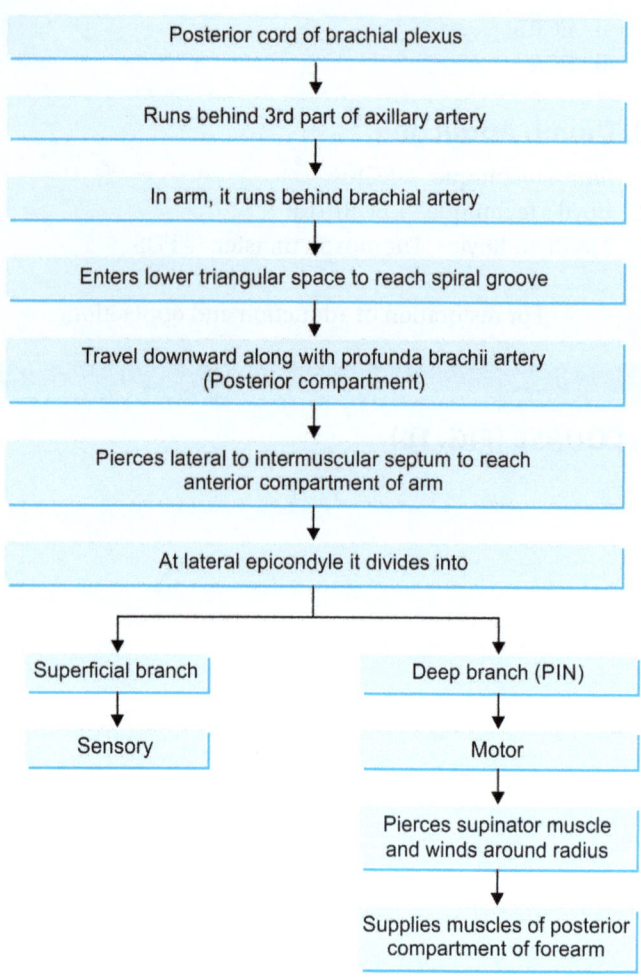

A. Radial Nerve Supplies

1. Long head of triceps
2. *Triceps*:
   i. Medial
   ii. Lateral
3. Anconeus
4. BR
5. ECRL

B. Posterior Interosseous Nerve

1. ECRB
2. Supinator
3. EDC
4. ECU
5. EDM
6. EPL
7. EIP
8. Abductor pollicis longus
9. EPB

C. Sensory

1. Posterior cutaneous nerve of arm
2. Posterior cutaneous nerve of forearm
3. Lateral cutaneous nerve of arm.

4. Superficial radial nerve
   ↓
   Sensory supply to dorsum of hand.

D. What is Lost?

1. Wrist extension
2. MCP joint extension   } All three must be provided
3. Thumb extension and abduction

E. What is Available?

Jones Transfer

1. PT → ECRL, ECRB
2. FCU → EDC
3. FCR → EIP, EDC, EPL

Modified Jones

1. PT → ECRL, ECRB
2. FCR → EDC
3. PL → EPL

If PL is not available,
FDS → EPL

NONUNION (NU)

I. INTRODUCTION

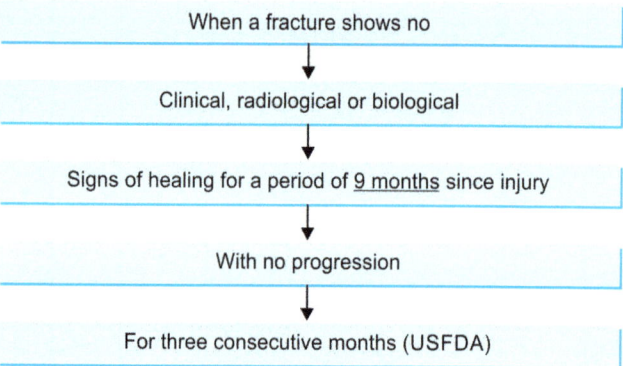

Permanent failure of fracture to unite, unless a radical change in intervention is initiated.

II. ETIOLOGY

A. Patient Related

1. Age: Elderly
2. Malnutrition (Albumin <3 g/dL, WBC → <1,500/mm^3)
3. Long term steroid therapy
4. Immunosuppressive treatment (Inflammatory and cancer)
5. Renal and hepatic systemic diseases
6. DM
7. Metabolic bone diseases
8. Anticoagulants
9. Long-term NSAID intake

10. Smoking
11. Alcohol
12. Radiation

B. Fracture Related
1. Open fractures → loss of soft tissue → ↓ Blood supply
2. Infected
3. Site → Neck of femur, scaphoid, lateral condyle humerus, talus neck
4. Comminuted
5. Segmental
6. Soft tissue interposition

C. Treatment Related
1. Inadequate immobilization
2. Inadequate reduction or distraction
3. Excessive periosteal stripping
4. Disrespect to surrounding soft tissue
5. Inadequate fixation

III. CLASSIFICATION

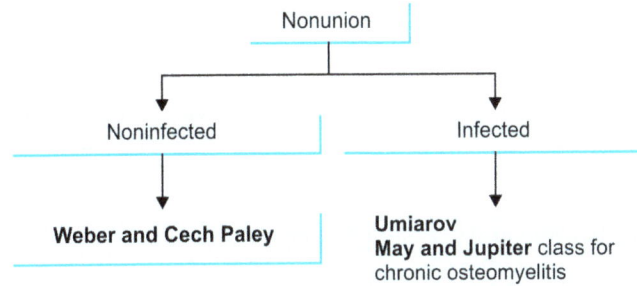

A. Noninfected

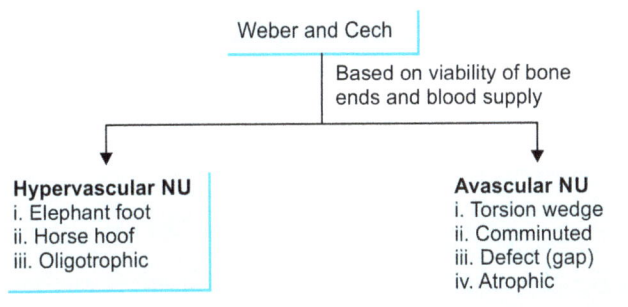

Elephant foot **(Fig. 19)**

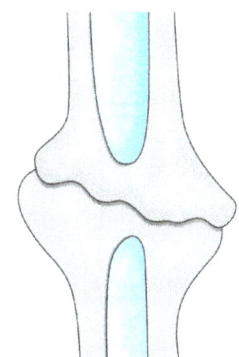

Hypertrophic callus due to inadequate fixation, immobilization or early weight bearing.

Horse-hoof (Fig. 20)

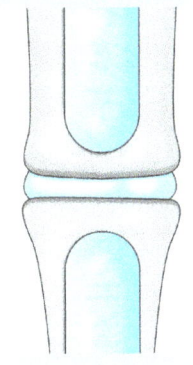

Mildly bulbous, exceeding thickness of bone.

Oligotrophic (Fig. 21)

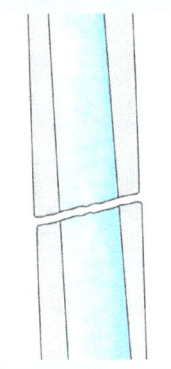

Not hypertrophic, but callus is absent, due to displaced fragments with adequate vascularity

Torsion-wedge (Fig. 22)

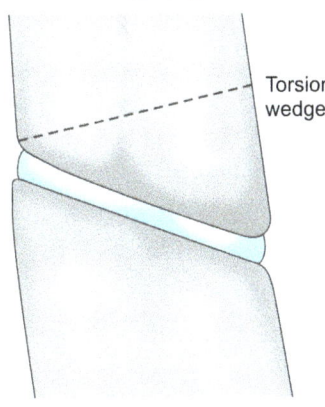

Butterfly fragment heals to one main part of bone, but not the other due to compromised blood supply

Comminuted (Fig. 23)

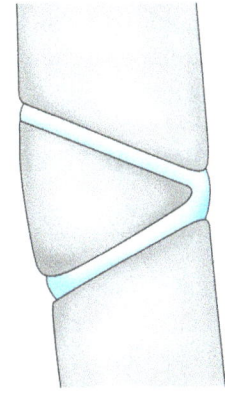

One or more necrotic fragment in between fails to unite

Defect (gap) (Fig. 24)

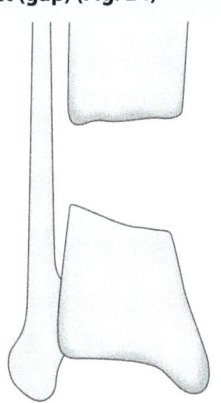

Intermediate fragment of bone →lost in full circumference
↓
Open fracture
Chronic osteomyelitis
(Sequestrum)

Atrophic (Fig. 25)

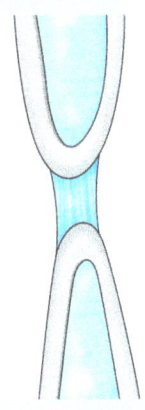

Ends of bone osteoporotic and atrophic due to lack of trophic factors and ↓ blood supply

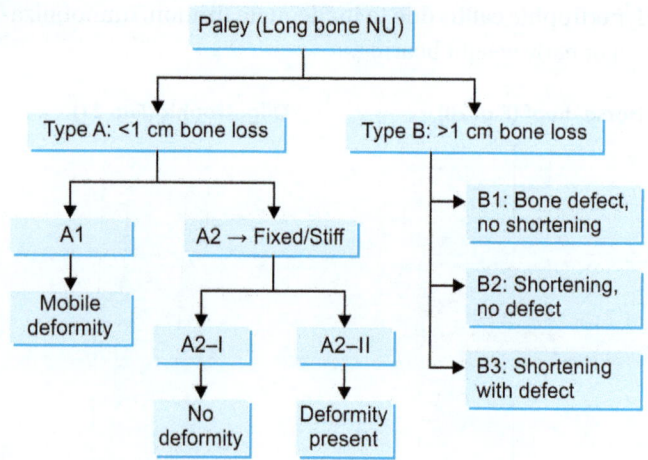

B. Infected NU

Umiarov (Viability of Bone Ends)

1. Normotrophic without shortening
2. Hypertrophic with shortening
3. Atrophic with shortening
4. Atrophic with bone and soft tissue defect usually with shortening

IV. CLINICAL FEATURES

A. Symptoms

1. Persistence of pain/maybe painless too
2. Inability to bear weight
3. Unable to perform functions of daily living from the affected limb
4. Discharging sinus

B. Signs

Inspection

1. Scar   i. Primary or secondary intention healing
         ii. Tethered to underlying skin
2. Sinus i. Discharging
         ii. Bone fragment
        iii. Color of discharge
         iv. Continuous or intermittent
3. Discoloration: Hyper/hypopigmentation
4. Muscle atrophy
5. Limb lengthening discrepancy
6. Deformity

Palpation

1. Warmth, tenderness: Irritation to periosteum due to screws - infected nonunion.
2. Loss of transmitted movements.
3. Abnormal mobility at fracture site. (In two perpendicular planes)
4. Swelling → Callus, irregular bone surface
5. Crepitus
6. ROM → Restricted of surrounding joints.
7. ↓ Girth compared to normal side.
8. Implant palpation.

V. INVESTIGATIONS

i. Radiograph:
   1. Marked sclerosis of bone ends – with rounding off
   2. Closed medullary canal
   3. Diffuse osteoporosis of bone fragments
   4. Fracture gap ±
   5. Proximal end convex and distal end concave
ii. *CT scan:* Doubt for cortical continuity.
iii. *MRI:*
   1. Vascularity of fragments and small bones
   2. ON: Head of femur, scaphoid, talus
iv. *Bone scan:*
   1. Synovial pseudoarthrosis: Cold cleft between two areas of high uptake.
   2. Hypervascular active nonunion versus nonresponsive avascular nonunion
v. *PET:* Infection ±, Vascularity ± Costly

vi. *Laboratory investigations:*
1. CRP, ESR ↑
2. Pus culture and sensitivity: Identify the causative organism and antibiotic susceptibility.

VI. TREATMENT

A. Principles

1. Eradication of infection and healing of soft tissue → Infected NU
2. Removal of implants, if any
3. Correct the alignment
4. Correct any associated LLD
5. Provide stability
6. Adding biological stimulus → BG, BS
7. Rehabilitation → Improve muscle strength and joint ROM
8. Regain functional limb to carry out activities of daily living

B. Operative Management

Hypervascular NU of long bones (Diaphysis):
1. Exchange nailing using a larger diameter nail
2. Autograft → Reaming at endosteal site
   ↓
3. Stimulation of osteogenesis
   ↓
4. Blood flow centripetal, from centrifugal

5. Debrides the fibrous tissue → New callus formation
6. Back slapping of new nail → Compression
7. Torsional instability → unicortical auxillary plate ± BG

Metaphysis:
1. Distal Femur → Locking plate fixation with BG → fibula ±
2. Proximal Femur → PFN + BG
3. Neck of femur → Valgus intertrochanteric osteotomy, THR
4. Shortening up to 4 cm → Shoe raise
   >4 cm → Ilizarov, monolateral distracters
5. NU too close to joint → arthroplasty

C. Surgical Methods

1. Osteosynthesis → External
                 → Internal
2. Compression distraction osteogenesis bone transplant.
3. Bone grafts.
4. Bone substitutes
5. Masquelet technique
6. Adjunctive measures → BM injection
                      → PRP
                      → BMP

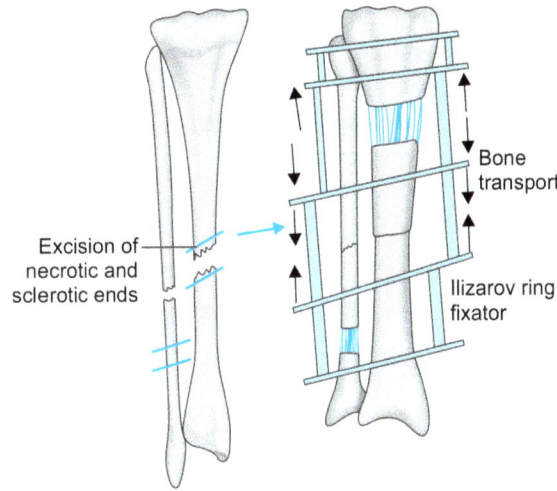

i. Scaphoid NU → Headless compression screw + BG
ii. Comminuted NU → Cancellous BG
iii. Shingling

D. Nonoperative Adjunctive Methods

1. Extracorporeal shockwave therapy
2. Ultrasound
3. **Electrical stimulation (SAQ)**

I. INTRODUCTION

1. Electrical stimulation is a medical procedure to promote bone growth and thus enhances fracture healing.
   ↓
   By application of low electrical currents to the fracture site.
2. Mechanical stressed bone generates an electric potential.
   Area of compression → Electronegative
   Tension → Electropositive
3. This stress generated potential is due to
   i. Piezoelectric property.
   ii. Streaming potentials.

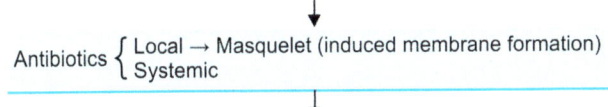

II. DEVICES (FIG. 27)

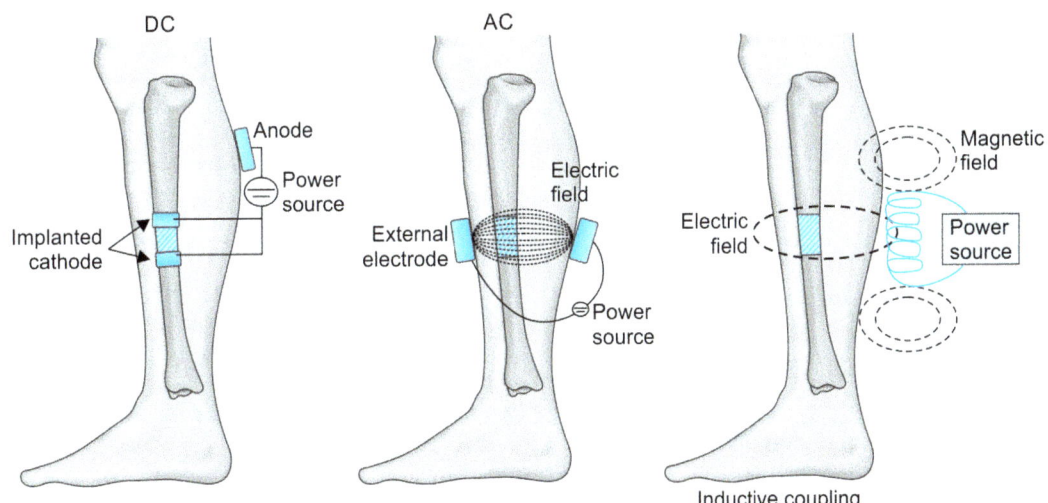

Inductive coupling

1. Direct current
2. Capacitive coupling (Alternating current)
3. Inductive coupling →
    i. Pulsed electromagnetic
    ii. Controlled magnetic

III. MECHANISMS
A. Direct Current
1. Invasive
2. ≥1 insulated cathodes at fractured site implanted, anode at skin surface

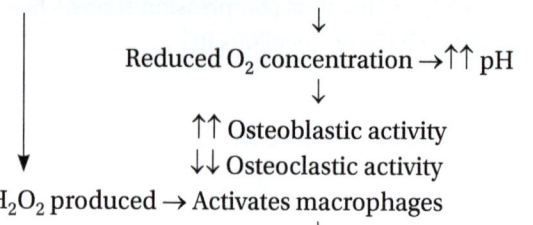

3. Bone growth occurs under electronegative potentials
4. Electrochemical reaction

↓
Reduced O_2 concentration → ↑↑ pH
↓
↑↑ Osteoblastic activity
↓↓ Osteoclastic activity
H_2O_2 produced → Activates macrophages
↓
↑ Bone healing ← ↑↑ VEGF, angiogenic factor

B. Capacitive Coupling
1. Noninvasive
2. Two capacitor electrodes on opposite side of fracture bone **(Fig. 28)**.

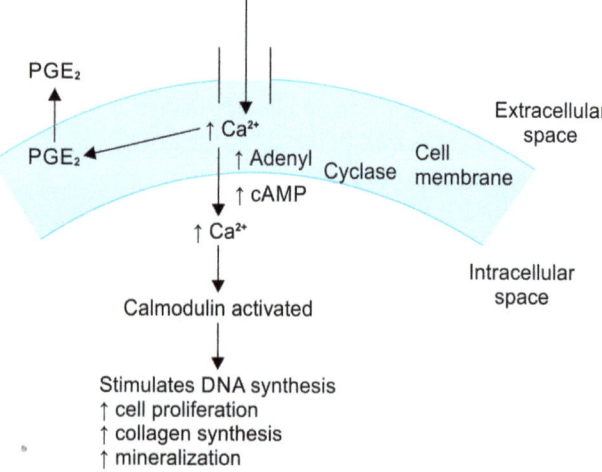

C. Inductive Coupling
1. Noninvasive
2. Electric current through electromagnetic coil
↓
Pulsed magnetic field
↓
Electric field induced in region of fracture
3. Accelerated calcification of fibrocartilage

IV. USES
1. Nonunion (hypertrophic)
2. Pseudoarthrosis
3. Failed fusion (spinal)
4. Enhancement of fresh fracture healing
5. ON (Controversial)

V. CONTRAINDICATIONS
1. Coexisting deformity
2. Avascular nonunion
3. Fractures with large gaps
4. Synovial pseudoarthrosis
5. Infected nonunion

VI. COMPLICATIONS
1. Skin irritation
2. Anode causes local tissue necrosis
3. Infection with implanted electrodes
4. Incorporation of electrode in new bone → Removal

LLD/LIMB LENGTHENING/ILIZAROV

1. Limb length discrepancy or anisomelia
↓
Condition in which paired lower extremity limbs have unequal length.
2. Cosmetic + Functional concern.
↓
3. Short leg gait → Not acceptable.
4. ↑ Energy expenditure due to excessive vertical rise and fall of pelvis.

I. ETIOLOGY
A. Undergrowth
1. *Congenital:*
    i. PFFD
    ii. Tibial hemimelia
    iii. Fibular hemimelia
    iv. Pseudoarthrosis of tibia
    v. Unilateral CTEV
2. *Trauma:*
    i. Physeal injuries: Growth arrest
    ii. Malunion
3. *Developmental:*
    i. DDH
    ii. Perthes disease
    iii. Infantile ⎫
    iv. Adolescent ⎬ Tibia vara
4. *Neurological:*
    i. Poliomyelitis
    ii. Cerebral palsy

5. *General:*
   i. Infection–pathological hip dislocation, septic hip sequelae (Tom–Smith arthritis)
   ii. Neoplasia
   iii. Radiation
   iv. Iatrogenic–treatment of injuries near physis
   v. Russel silver syndrome.
   vi. Idiopathic nonsyndromic hemiatrophy

B. Overgrowth

1. *Reactive overgrowth:*
   i. Post-traumatic overgrowth
   ii. Osteomyelitis
   iii. Inflammatory arthritis
2. *Overgrowth syndromes:*
   i. Gigantism with NF
   ii. Klippel-Trenaunay syndrome
   iii. Proteus syndrome
   iv. Beckwith-Wiedman syndrome

C. Others

1. Neglected hip dislocation
2. OA hip (severe)

II. CLASSIFICATION
A. McCaw and Bates

1. Mild = <3 cm
2. Moderate = 3–6 cm
3. Severe = >6 cm

B. LLD

Structural/Anatomical	Functional/Apparent
Inequality in bone structure ↓ Actual shortening/lengthening between head of femur and ankle	Factors other than actual bone shortening/lengthening No osseous component in the discrepancy

III. CLINICAL FEATURES

1. Short limb gait.
2. *Leg-length measurement:*
   i. Apparent length: Xiphisternum to medial malleolus (MM) with both lower limbs parallel.
   ii. True length: ASIS to MM. ASIS at same level.
3. Coronal plane deformity: Abduction, adduction contracture of hip
4. Sagittal → Hip flexion contracture, equinus contracture at ankle.
5. Structural Scoliosis → Suprapelvic LLD
6. Wood block test: Block added below short limb till pelvis at same level.
7. Galeazzi test
8. Backache
9. Early hip and knee arthritis
10. Callosities

IV. RADIOGRAPHIC EVALUATION (FIG. 29)

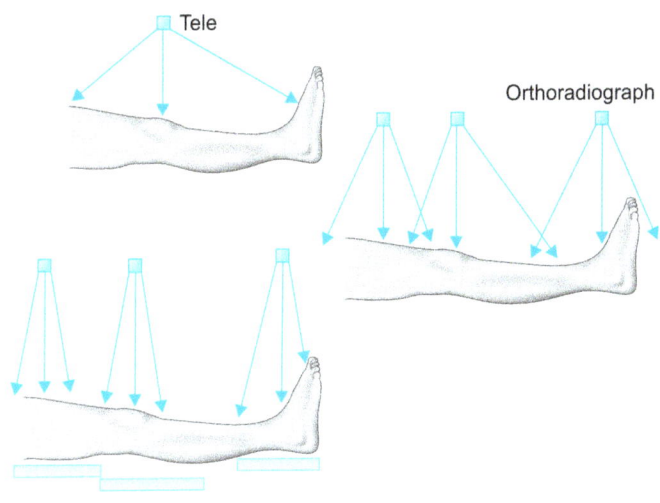

1. *Teleradiograph:* Single exposure of both limbs from 6 ft.
2. *Orthoradiograph:* Separate exposure of hip, knee and ankle → Central beam passes through joints.
3. *Scannogram (radiograph):* Separate exposure but reduces the size of the resulting film by moving the film cassette between exposures.
   CT scan scannogram: Single exposure, fast and accurate

V. LLD CALCULATION

In skeletally immature (one must know)

Normal growth rate	Predict LLD at skeletal maturity	Appropriate time for intervention

↓

1. Menelaus method
2. Green and Anderson method
3. Moseley's chart
4. Paley's multiplier method

A. Menelaus Method

1. Chronological age rather than skeletal
2. Proximal femur = 3 mm/y
3. Distal femur = 9 mm/y
4. Proximal tibia = 6 mm/y
5. Distal tibia = 3 mm/y
6. Growth cessation: G = 14–15 y
   B = 16–17 y

B. Green and Anderson
1. Uses skeletal age
2. Growth potential in DF and PT at different skeletal ages.

C. Moseley Chart
Straight line graph method.
Three measurements done 3 times over 3 months
1. Long leg length
2. Short leg length
3. Skeletal age

D. Paley
1. LLD at skeletal maturity = current LLD × multiplier
2. Multiplier for boys and girls for chronological and skeletal age

VI. MANAGEMENT

Goals
1. Equalize limb lengths
2. Correct mechanical weight bearing axis
3. Balanced spine and pelvis

Guidelines as per Degree of Shortening: LLD
1. <2 cm: No treatment or shoe lift.
2. 2–5 cm
   - Skeletally immature → Growth modulation by epiphysiodesis
   - Skeletal mature → Shoe lift or shortening of longer limb
3. 6–15 cm: Lengthening of shorter limb
4. ≥15 cm: Prosthesis or amputation

Shoe Lift
1. Patients who do not wish or not appropriate for surgery
2. >5 cm → Poorly tolerated

Epiphysiodesis
1. Growth arrest of physis of longer limb.
2. Allowing time for short leg to catch up.

Indications:
1. Sufficient growth remaining
2. Discrepancy between 2–5 cm
3. Patient agreeing for consistent follow-up.

Techniques:
1. Phemister epiphysiodesis
2. Blount's staple epiphysiodesis
3. PETS: Percutaneous epiphysiodesis using transphyseal screw
4. Tension plate epiphysiodesis **(Fig. 30)**

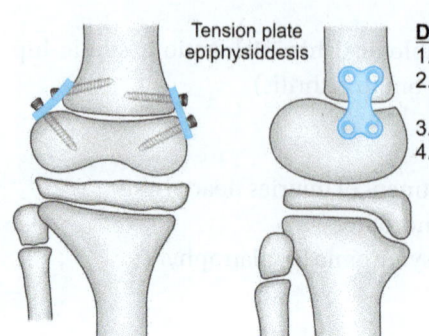

Tension plate epiphysiddesis

Disadvantage
1. Normal limb operated
2. Deformity of pathological limb cannot be treated
3. Under/over-correction
4. Asymmetric

Limb-shortening
Indications:
1. Skeletally mature
2. Max shortening = Femur: 5 cm } without affecting muscle
   Tibia: 3 cm } function.
3. Patient height > 50th percentile
4. 2–5 cm
   ↓

Shortening of normal limb better than lengthening → less complications such as joint stiffness.

2 types → Wagner's limb shortening of femur and tibia
        → Winquists → closed technique for diaphyseal shortening.

Femoral shortening	Tibial shortening
Only one bone involved	Two bones
↓ NU	↑ NU, ↑ Neurovascular injuries
Muscle recovery faster	Slower

Femoral shortening preferred over tibial

VII. LIMB-LENGTHENING (LAQ)

A. Indications
1. Shortening >6 cm
2. Nearing skeletal maturity (Epiphyseal arrest would not produce satisfying results)
3. Discrepancy is more in a single bone due to trauma or infection.
4. Associated with deformity.
5. Not for <6 cm → ↑ morbidity (joint stiffness)
6. Femur up to 10 cm, tibia up to 7 cm
   Not >15 cm (Femur + Tibia)
   ↓

Risks > benefits combine with shortening of other limb. Child and adult can be done in both

B. Prerequisites and Features
1. Neighboring joints → Near normal ROM
2. Absence of scarring of skin/soft tissue
3. Bone must be normal. Fracture if any should be united

4. Distraction stopped when goal achieved or unresolved complications
5. Maintaining extension is essential. Stop lengthening if knee FFD > 10 or ROM <30. Start again after this achieved.
6. Corticalization (3 cortices on 2 radiographs) → adequate strength → remove

C. Types

	Limb lengthening
Acute (Rare)	Gradual (Common)

→ Transiliac	• External fixators
	  – Ilizarov
	  – Hybrid
	  – Taylors spatial frame
	  – LRS
	• Combined internal+ internal devices
	• Implantable internal lengthening devices

i. <u>Acute</u>: Trans-iliac (Millis and Hall) **(Fig. 32)**

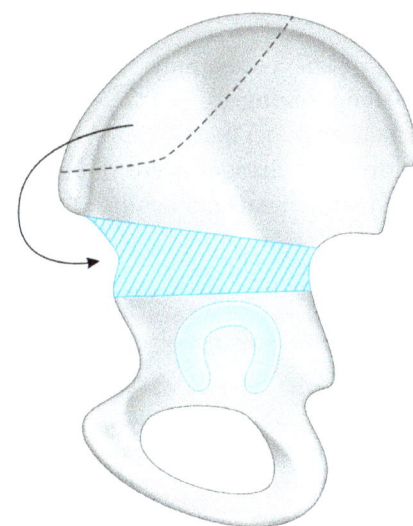

1. For shortening of 2–3 cm
2. Salters osteotomy modification
3. Suitable for patients with acetabular dysplasia

ii. <u>Gradual</u>

ILIZAROV (LAQ)

I. INTRODUCTION

1. Prof. Gavril Abramovich Ilizarov was born in Soviet Union (1921–1992)
2. 1950: Sent to kurgan as a surgeon → to treat wounded soldiers.
3. Inspired by the shaft of bow harness on horse carriage.
   ↓
   Used spokes of bicycle from local shop
   → devised the ring external fixator.
4. Accidentally found new bone formation radiologically → Patient turned rods between rings in distraction rather than compression.
5. Thus, his three main contributions were the discovery and invention of:
   i. Distraction histogenesis
   ii. Corticotomy
   iii. Versatile ring fixator

II. PRINCIPLES

1. **Wolff's law**

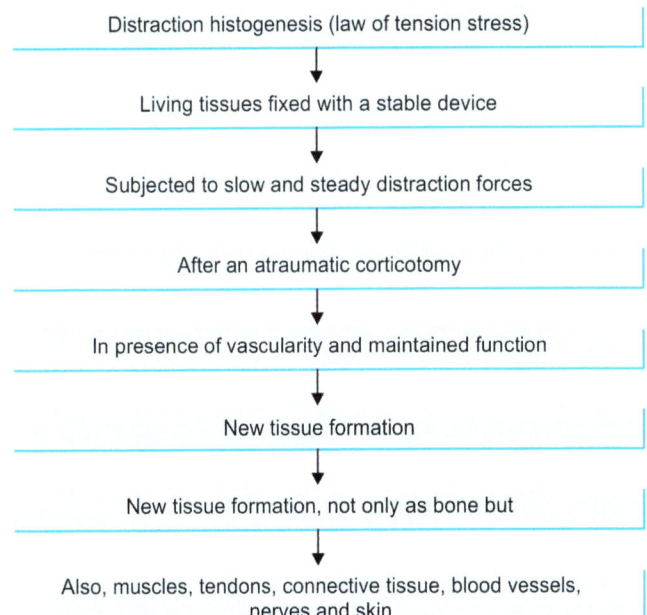

2. **Law of tension stress**

3. **Stability of fixation**
   i. Permits pain free mobilization and weight-bearing
      ↓
   ii. Essential for formation of new regenerate.
   iii. Enhanced by → More fixation pins
                    → More circular rings
                    → Smaller diameter rings
4. **Atraumatic corticotomy** (SAQ) **(Fig. 33)**

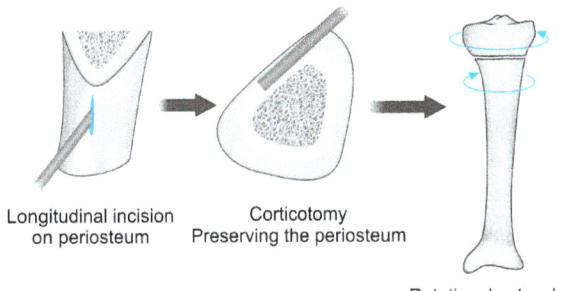

Longitudinal incision on periosteum   Corticotomy Preserving the periosteum

Rotational osteoclasis

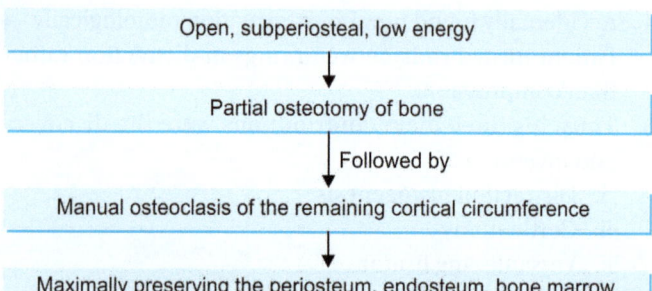

Types: Monfocal/Bifocal

Principles:
1. Low energy injury force
2. Minimal incision: Only slightly longer than width of osteotomy.
3. Periosteum incised longitudinally and preserved all around corticotomy site.
4. Saline used for continuous cooling during drilling of holes →↓↓ Thermal necrosis
5. Twisting the osteotome to join hole, thus breaking the posterior cortex.
6. No communition
7. Metaphyseal in location
8. Fixed in anatomical position with gap <2 mm

Techniques:
1. Percutaneous osteotomy: Posterior cortex by rotational osteoclasis. (Max. preservation of endosteum and intramedullary blood supply)
2. Drilling of posterior cortex: Joining the holes using osteotome
3. Gigli saw method
4. Oblique osteotomy: ↓ tendency for axial deviation

Types:

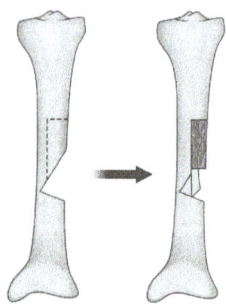

1. *Transverse:*
   i. Lengthening
   ii. Deformity correction
   iii. Bone transport
2. *Longitudinal:*
   i. To widen the bone
   ii. Improve shape of thin atrophic limb
3. *Splinter:* Splints off a piece of bone with attached periosteum, soft tissue and skin.
   i. Bridging NU
   ii. Eliminate partial bone defects **(Fig. 34)**
4. *S-shaped:* Chronic OM
5. *Partial:* To correct bow or curved defect in bones, e.g., OI

Complications:
1. Neurovascular injury
2. Displacement corticotomy
3. Incomplete corticotomy
4. Premature consolidation
5. **Latency period:** 5–7 days – needed for tissue to recover following corticotomy

   Poor vascularity
   Thin soft tissue cover } Delay distraction further

6. **Rate of distraction:** 1 mm/day
7. **Rhythm of distraction:** 4 distraction turns of 0.25 mm spread out over one day.
8. **Intact vascularity:** New vessel formation in the regenerate gap as well as rest of the limb.
9. **Preserved function:** New bone formation is best
   ↓
   When patient walks and retains function
10. **Amount of lengthening:**
    i. Principally no upper limit.
    ii. But permanent changes occur in nearby joints and muscle tissue if tibial lengthening >11%
11. **Dynamization:**

    i. Trampoline effect: Tensioned wires elastically compress and distract regenerate with movements and axial loading of the limb Cyclic loading of the regenerate promotes osteogenesis
    ↓
    ii. Accordion maneuver: Alternating cycles of compression and distraction (daily/weekly) during the consolidation phase

12. **Consolidation:** A period equal to that of lengthening → to allow regenerate bone to develop adequate strength.
    ↓
    Removal of fixator
13. **Lengthening index:** No. of months of fixator for 1 cm of lengthening 1 cm → 1–1.5 months

III. BIOMECHANICS AND INSTRUMENTATION

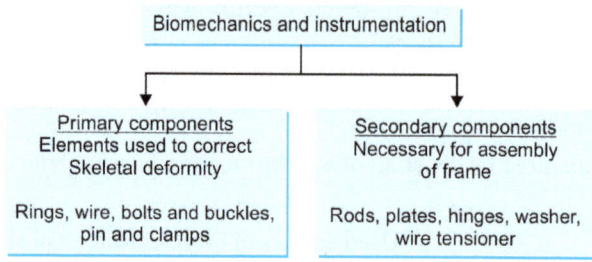

A. Rings (Fig. 35)

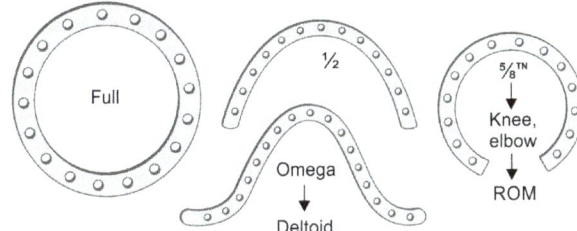

Principle component:
1. All rings placed perpendicular to long axis of bone
2. Material → stainless steel
   → carbon fiber
3. Internal diameter → 80–240 mm
4. Increased stability of assembly →
   Numbers (increases), size (decreases) and position of ring
5. Rings on either side of the fracture must be close → ↑ stability
6. 2 cm = Between ring and skin → for swelling, hygiene
7. "Dummy rings": To minimize unsupported length between rings.
8. Arches → Larger diameter than half ring
   → Proximal femur and humerus (Fig. 36)

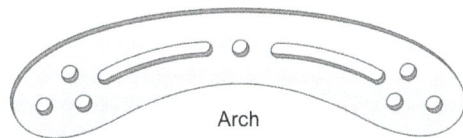

B. Wires

1. Smooth, thin (1.5-Pediatrics, 1.8-Adults) → Cross Kirschner wires
2. Circumferential, multilevel, multiplane, multidirectional, transosseous osteosynthesis.
3. Tensioned → Greater the tensioning → ↑ Stability
4. Olive wires → Metallic lead in wire. Use: Interfragmentary compression, translation of fragment (Fig. 37)

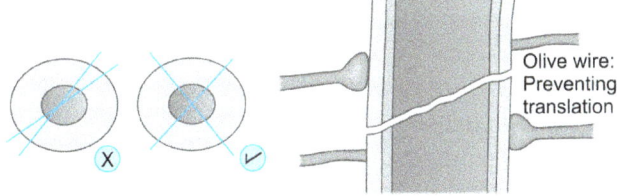

5. ↑ Wires → ↑ Stability
6. Minimum 2, preferably 3 to each ring

C. Bolts (Fig. 38)

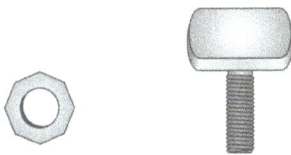

1. Hexagonal head = 10 mm, threaded shaft diameter = 6 mm, pitch = 1 mm, length = 10, 16, 30
2. Longitudinal slots under head → to fix wires to rings
3. *Nuts (Diameter = 6 mm)* → ¼ turn for distraction compression
   ↓
   Driving force in Ilizarov system

D. Rods

6 mm thickness, 4 rods at equidistance connect 2 rings

E. Plates

i. *Short plates*: Extension of ring
ii. *Twisted plates*: Connect two components at right angles

F. Support Post (Fig. 39)

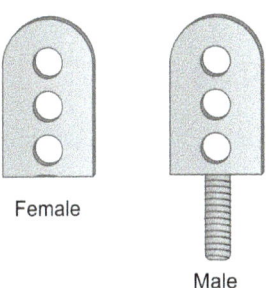

i. Male: Threaded projection fixed with nut
   Female: Threaded hole fixed with bolt
ii. Third wire can be connected to post
iii. Can work as hinge

G. Tensioner → Standard wire tensioner
→ Dynamometer → Has scale (Fig. 40)

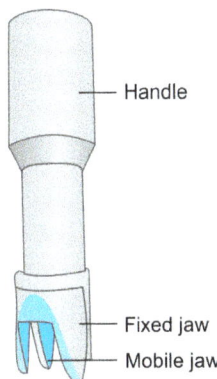

H. Ring positioning (Fig. 41)

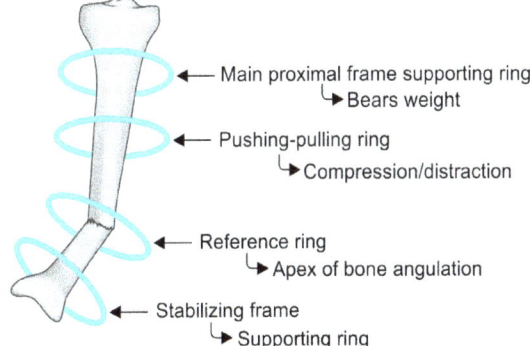

IV. USES

1. Fracture NU → Infected
               → Noninfected
2. Limb lengthening
3. Long bone deformity correction
4. Open fractures
5. Malunion (cubitus varus)
6. Correction of joint contractures
7. Congenital deformity → CTEV
                        → CPT
                        → Hemimelia
                        → Club hand
8. Reconstruction of bone defect
9. Vascular insufficiency (TAO, Buerger's disease)

V. COMPLICATIONS

Early	Late
1. Vascular, neurological ⊗	1. Pin site infection
2. Fracture of corticomized bone	2. Pain at corticotomy site
3. Local skin tightness	3. Soft tissue contractures
4. Psychological incompatibility	4. Joint stiffness
	5. RSD
	6. Osteoporosis
	7. Compartment syndrome
	8. Joint stimulation
	9. Premature consolidation
	10. Progression of angular def.

VI.

Advantages	Disadvantages
1. Minimally invasive	1. Bulky
2. 3-dimensional def. correction	2. Not accepted by patient.
3. Early mobilization and weight bearing	3. Long duration of Rx
4. Bone graft not necessary	4. Long surgery
5. Simple hardware removal	5. Long learning curve
	6. Laborious

VII. RECENT ADVANCES

1. *Taylor's spatial frame:* 2 carbon rings connected by 6 telescopic rods called Strut → hinge joint at both ends **(Fig. 42)**

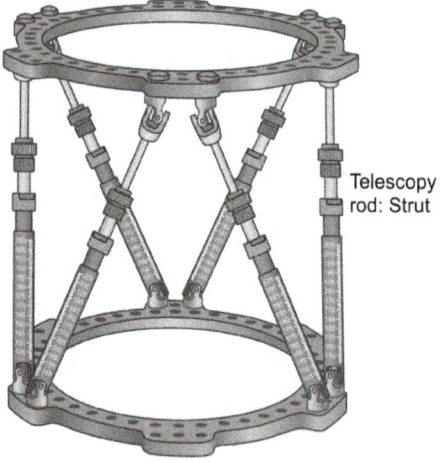

Telescopy rod: Strut

   i. Can be applied with Ilizarov
   ii. Allows 3-dimensional bone movements
2. *Hybrid fixator:* Proximal ring connected to 2–3 pins with connecting rods.
   Use: Proximal tibia fracture
3. *Internal bone transport:* Using IM nail with external remote control (ERC)
4. *GLONE:* Gradual lengthening over nail using external fixator **(Fig. 43)**

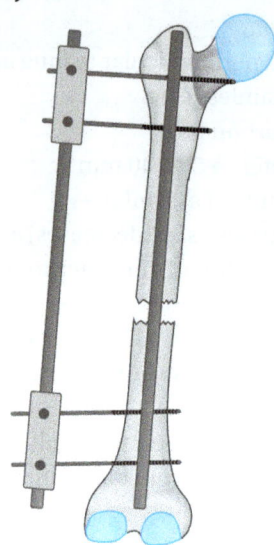

MASQUELET TECHNIQUE

I. INTRODUCTION

1. First described by Masquelet in 1986, it is also known as "Induced Membrane Technique".
2. It is a two-stage technique for managing critical bone defects (up to 25 cm) and nonunions by induced membrane osteogenesis.

II. INDICATIONS

Bone Defect Reconstruction due to:
1. Infected bone (Chronic Osteomyelitis)
2. Severe Trauma
3. Debridement of devitalized bone
4. Septic Nonunion
5. Aseptic Nonunion
6. Pseudoarthrosis (Congenital, Acquired)
7. Tumor Resection

III. STAGES

A. First Stage (Membrane Induction)
   1. Radical debridement of the infected soft tissue and bone.
   2. Multiple culture samples are sent.
   3. Bone edges must be healthy with viable bleeding.
   4. PMMA cement spacer (with or without antibiotics) is inserted into the bone defect.

5. The long bone is stabilized with either an internal (Intramedullary K-wire) or external fixation.
6. Soft tissue reconstruction in the form of skin graft or flap if required.
7. The cement spacer induces the formation of an encapsulation membrane around it in about 3-4 weeks.

B. Second Stage (Bony Reconstruction)
8. Performed 6-8 weeks later.
9. Membrane must be incised with care and minimally disturbed.
10. Cement spacer is removed with caution.
11. The cavity (now lined by an encapsulation membrane) is filled with autogenous cancellous bone graft harvested usually from the iliac crest.
12. If the quantity of autogenous cancellous bone graft is insufficient, then allograft can be added in the ratio of 1 part of allograft to 3 parts of autograft.
13. Internal fixation is in the form of bridge plating or intramedullary nailing.
14. External Circular fixator → If skin condition is poor.
15. Bone Formation and union → 8-9 months

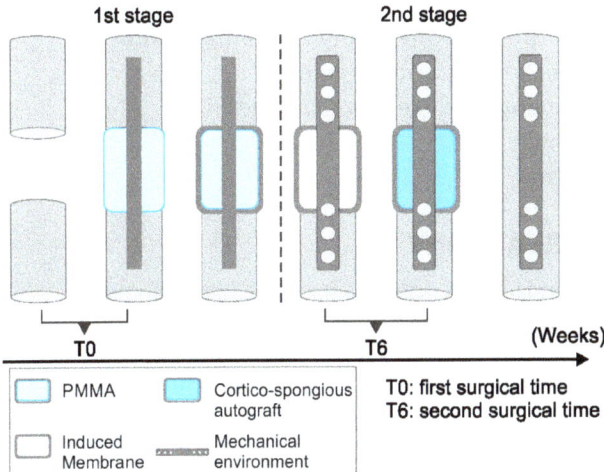

IV. EFFECT OF THE INDUCED MEMBRANE

A. Mechanical
1. Preservation of limb length
2. Appropriate soft tissue tension
3. Prevention of encroachment by adjacent soft tissues into the bone defect.
4. Creates a confined space for bone graft placement.
5. Prevention of resorption of bone graft material

B. Biological
1. It is a pseudosynovial membrane that has the properties of being both hypervascular and impermeable.
2. Rich in Type 1 collagen, fibroblasts and myofibroblasts.
3. VEGF → promotes angiogenesis (hypervascular)
4. TGF-β, BMP-2, IL-6, IL-8, IGF-1, PDGF → Osteogenesis
5. This produces a combination of Intramembranous and Enchondral Ossification leading to a progressive healing response.

V. CONTRAINDICATIONS

1. Significant Limb Length discrepancy
2. Soft Tissue coverage not possible
3. Graft unavailable

VOLKMANN ISCHEMIC CONTRACTURE

I. INTRODUCTION

1. A condition which is characterized by ischemic necrosis of the structures in the forearm (extending to lower arm and hand) and subsequent crippling contractures associated with varying degree of neurological deficit.
2. 1st described by Richard van Volkmann in 1881

II. CAUSES

1. Compartment syndrome due to:
   i. Prolonged external compression
   ii. Internal bleeding
   iii. Burns
   iv. Snake bites
   v. Regional anesthesia, i.e., Bier's block
2. 2nd most common cause especially in children is ischemic contracture following **Supracondylar Humerus fracture**
3. Crush injuries
4. Severe contusion of forearm
5. Chronic infections
6. Congenital
7. Idiopathic

III. PATHOGENESIS

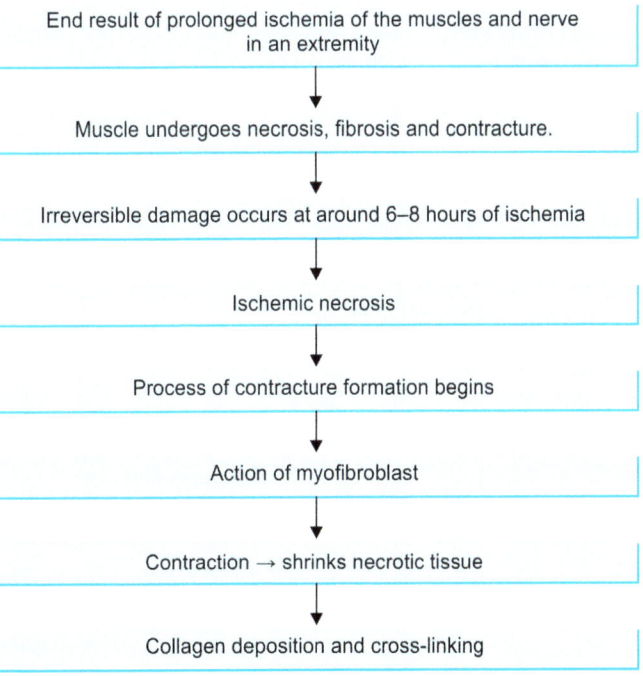

1. **FDP and FPL** are most common muscles involved **(Seddon's Ellipsoid)**
   ↓
   With increasing severity, FDS, PT also involved.
2. **Median nerve** is most common nerve involved.

IV. CLASSIFICATION
A. Tsuge Modification of Seddon Classification
1. *Mild:*
   i. Deep flexor muscles are partly degenerated.
   ii. Ring and long finger most commonly involved.
   iii. Joints are spared.
   iv. Cord like induration on volar forearm
   v. No sensory disturbance
   vi. Volkmann's sign +ve
2. *Moderate:*
   i. All deep flexors are degenerated with partial involvement of FDS and wrist flexors.
   ii. Flexion contractures of all fingers and thumb.
   iii. Neurological signs (+), most common median nerve.
3. *Severe*:
   i. Necrosis, fibrosis, paralysis with deformity.
   ii. Wrist extensor muscles involvement.

B. Zancolli Classification
Based on the condition of the intrinsic muscles of the hand.

Normal intrinsic muscle type	Paralytic intrinsic muscle type	Retracted intrinsic
Type I • Simple digital claw • Contracture is limited to forearm muscles • Joint spared • No stiffness	Type II • Intrinsic claw hand • Simple →Flexed position of wrist, contracture of long flexors of wrist • Complex → severe intrinsic paralysis associated with digital joint stiffness • Totally rigid → Flexed IP joint + MCP joint extension	Type III • MCP joints flexed + IP joints are extended • Distal IP joint is in flexion due to FDP contracture • Wrist flexion

C. Holden's Classification

Level I	Level II
• Injury is proximal to ischemia and later contracture. ↓ • Brachial artery injury by SCH # • Tsuge type 1	• Ischemia is directly under the injury usually by tight bandages and casts ↓ • Moderate to severe type of Tsuge

V. FUNCTIONAL EVALUATION
1. *Volkmann's sign:*
   i. Inability to actively extend fingers (at IP and MCP joints) without flexing wrist.
   ii. Passive extension of fingers possible only with wrist flexion.
2. *Bouvier's maneuver:* Fingers actively tend to extend, when the wrist is flexed and hyperextension of the proximal phalanx is prevented
3. Wrist flexion
4. Pronated forearm
5. Wasting
6. Flexed elbow
7. Cord like induration on flexor side
8. Paraesthesia/anesthesia in the hand and fingers
9. Fixed and adducted thumb
10. Claw hand
11. Deformity and tropic changes due to ulnar and median nerve involvement

VI. DIFFERENTIAL DIAGNOSIS
1. Post-traumatic hematoma, resulting contracture
2. OM and muscle involvement
3. Hemangioma of forearm muscles
4. Pseudo – VIC
5. Burns

VII. TREATMENT
1. Exercises and orthoses for wrist, hand, fingers
2. Turnbuckle splint
3. *Excision of fibrous tissue*:
   i. Capsulotomy
   ii. Neurolysis
   iii. Tenolysis
4. *Proximal "muscle slide" of max page:*
   i. If there is clinically good finger flexion available
   ii. No need to excise the muscle sequestrum while doing slide.
5. *For involvement of multiple tendon units:*
   i. Tendon lengthening
   ii. Tendon transfer
   iii. Nerve grafting
   iv. Free, vascularized, innervated musculocutaneous flaps

Gracilis ↓ • Minimal donor site morbidity and consistent pedicle • 1st choice	Latissimus dorsi (LD) • 2nd choice • Longer pedicle	Rectus femoris (RF) • Donor site morbidity is high • 3rd choice

6. *Mild*:
   i. Correct wrist contracture by releasing FCR, FCU
   ii. Tendon transfer/lengthening when there is loss of muscle mass
      ↓
      → Z-plasty
      → Motorization of FDP
   iii. Max page operation
7. *Moderate:*
   i. For preserved muscle mass
      ↓
   ii. Maxpage sliding operation + neurolysis of median and ulnar nerve
   iii. No useful finger flexion left
      ↓
   iv. BR and ECRL tendon transfers to flexors and complete release of contracture and neurolysis
   v. **Garre's operation** → Proximal row carpectomy or forearm shortening by 2-3 cm
8. *Severe:* Two stage procedure:
   i. Early excision of all necrotic tissue with complete neurolysis of ulnar and median nerves
      ↓
      Followed by aggressive mobilization of joints of wrist and hand to prevent deformity and retain mobility.
   ii. Reconstruction is done in 2nd stage by tendon transfer.

CHRONIC REGIONAL PAIN SYNDROME (CRPS)

I. INTRODUCTION

Idiopathic disorder caused by an aberrant inflammatory response that leads to sustained sympathetic activity in a perpetuated reflex arc.
1. *Complex:* Variable clinical presentation
2. *Regional:* Symptoms affect particular region
3. *Pain:* Disproportionate to the severity of injury
4. *Syndrome:* A cluster of symptoms and signs

II. EPIDEMIOLOGY
1. F > M: 4:1
2. Increases with age until 70 years
3. UL: 60%, LL: 40%

III. RISK FACTORS
1. Trauma
2. Surgery
3. Prolonged immobilization
4. Anxiety or depression
5. Use of ACE inhibitors at the time of trauma
6. History of migraines or asthma
7. Smoking
8. Fibromyalgia
9. Genetic predisposition

International Association for the Study of Pain Classification	
Type I (RSD)	• CRPS without demonstrable nerve damage • Most common
Type II (Causalgia)	• CRPS with evidence of identifiable nerve damage • Minimal positive response with sympathetic blocks

IV. PATHOPHYSIOLOGY
1. Aberrant inflammatory response
2. Vasomotor dysfunction
3. Maladaptive neuroplasticity

V. CARDINAL SIGNS
1. Exaggerated pain
2. Swelling
3. Stiffness
4. Skin discoloration

VI. PHYSICAL EXAMINATION
1. Vasomotor disturbance
2. Trophic skin changes→ Loss of hair, thin, shiny, ulceration
3. Hyperhidrosis
4. "Flamingo gait" if the knee is involved
5. Equinovarus deformity if the ankle is involved
6. Muscle atrophy
7. Involuntary movements → Tremors, muscle spasms, dystonia
8. Sweat test

Lankford and Evans stages of RSD			
Stage	Onset	Exam	Imaging
Acute	0–3 months	Burning pain; redness, swelling, warmth, hyperhidrosis, hyperesthesia, cold intolerance, joint stiffness	Normal X-rays, positive three-phase bone scan
Subacute (dystrophic)	3–12 months	Worsening pain, cyanosis, dry skin, stiffness, skin atrophy	Subchondral osteopenia on X-ray
Chronic (atrophic)	>12 months	Diminished pain, glossy skin, fibrosis, joint contractures, loss of hair and nails	Extreme osteopenia on X-ray

Acute → Warm → Good prognosis

VII. RADIOLOGY
1. *X-ray:*
   i. Osteopenia-affects the patella if the knee is involved
   ii. Soft tissue swelling

iii. Subperiosteal bone resorption
iv. Preservation of joint spaces
2. Three-phase bone scan-can help to rule out CRPS type I (has high negative predictive value):
   i. Phase I (2 minutes): Extremity arteriogram
   ii. Phase II (5-10 minutes): Cellulitis and synovial inflammation
   iii. Phase III (2-3 hours): Bone images
   iv. Phase IV (24 hours): Differentiate osteomyelitis from adjacent cellulitis
      → Findings: Increased uptake in all phases → phase III is most sensitive
3. Thermography: Used to quantify temperature differences between the limbs
4. EMG/NCV: Slowing in known nerve distribution (e.g., slowing of median nerve conduction for CRPS type II in the forearm)

VIII. BUDAPEST DIAGNOSTIC CRITERIA

1. Continuing pain → disproportionate to any inciting event
2. At least 1 symptom in 3 (clinical Dx criteria) or 4 (research Dx criteria):
   i. Sensory: hyperesthesia or allodynia
   ii. Vasomotor: temperature asymmetry, skin color changes, or skin color asymmetry
   iii. Sudomotor/edema: edema, sweating changes, or sweating asymmetry
   iv. Motor/trophic: decreased range of motion, motor dysfunction (weakness, tremor, or dystonia), or trophic changes (hair, nails, or skin)
3. Must display at least one sign at time of diagnosis in 2 or more: (Same as above)
4. No other diagnosis better explains the signs and symptoms

IX. DIFFERENTIAL DIAGNOSIS

1. Soft tissue infection
2. Malingering
3. Psychiatric disease (e.g., Clenched Fist syndrome)
4. Neuropathic pain
5. Chronic pain
6. Raynaud disease
7. Thoracic outlet syndrome
8. Arterial insufficiency
9. Erythromelalgia

X. MANAGEMENT
A. Physiotherapy

1. Gentle physiotherapy exercises
2. Tactile discrimination training
3. Graded motor imagery and mirror therapy

B. Medications
1. NSAIDs
2. Corticosteroids
3. Vitamin C → 500 mg × 50 days
4. Alpha blockers → phenoxybenzamine, prazosin
5. Beta blockers → propranolol
6. Antidepressants → Nortriptyline
7. Anticonvulsants
8. Calcium channel blockers
9. GABA agonists → gabapentin
10. Bisphosphonates
11. Calcitonin

C. Nerve Stimulation: Programmable Stimulators Placed on Affected Nerves
1. Transcutaneous electrical stimulation (TENS)
2. Peripheral nerve stimulation
3. Spinal cord stimulation

D. Nerve Blockade and Chemical Sympathectomy
1. *Types:*
   i. Sympathetic:
      a. Stellate ganglion (for upper extremity)
      b. Lumbar spinal (for lower extremity)
   ii. Peripheral nerve
   iii. Neuraxial/epidural
2. *Blocking agents:*
   i. Anaesthetics → lidocaine or bupivacaine +/- epinephrine
   ii. Sympatholytic → Bretylium, guanethidine
3. Chemical → Phenol, alcohol

E. Surgical Sympathectomy
Indicated in patients showing response to sympathetic nerve blockade.
1. Excision
2. Electrocautery

HETEROTOPIC OSSIFICATION
I. INTRODUCTION
1. Abnormal formation of mature lamellar bone in soft tissues.
2. Reactive lesion occurring in Extra-skeletal tissues characterized by fibrous, osseous and cartilaginous proliferation by metaplasia.
3. Most common location → Between muscle and joint capsule.

II. ETIOLOGICAL CLASSIFICATION

Traumatic HO (Myositis ossificans)	Neurogenic HO	Genetic HO (Munchmeyer's diseases)
• Fracture • Dislocations • Surgery • Burns Common sites: • Hip–fracture, ORIF, THR • Elbow • Shoulder • Knee • Ankle • TM joint	• After CNS insult ↓ – Head injury – Spinal trauma • Infections: – Encephalitis – Meningitis – Myelitis – Tetanus	• Fibrodysplasia ossificans progressiva • Progressive osseous hyperplasia • Albright hereditary osteodystrophy • Autosomal dominant Begins in childhood ↓ ∴ Progressively increases *GNAS*, gene mutation ↓ Decreased expression/dysfunction of α-subunit of stimulatory G-protein of adenylyl cyclase

Type IV: Bony ankylosis **(Fig. 44)**

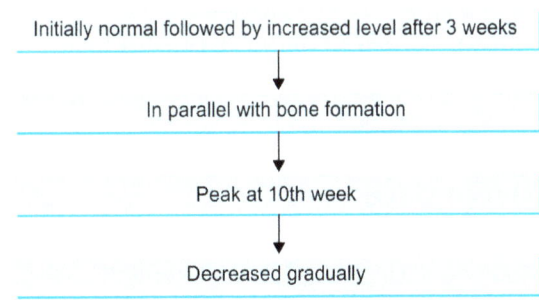

III. PATHOPHYSIOLOGY

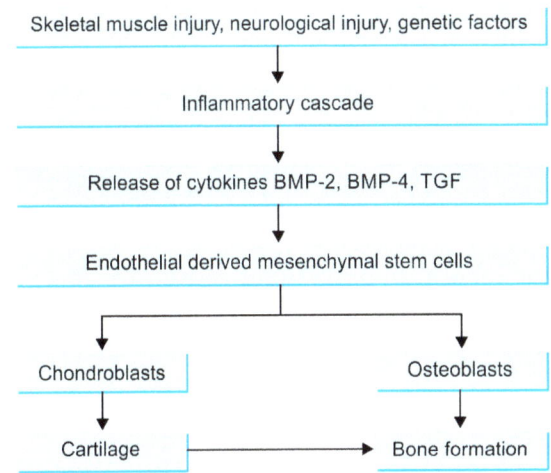

IV. CLINICAL FEATURES

1. M:F – 2:1
2. Typically asymptomatic → Detected as incidental finding on X-ray
3. When symptomatic → Decreased ROM
   ↓
   Complete ankylosis (in severe cases)
4. Local pain
5. Warmth
6. Swelling
7. Erythema
8. Peripheral neuropathy

V. BROOKER'S CLASSIFICATION [HO AROUND HIP JOINT (AFTER HIP SURGERY)]

Type I: Island of bone within soft tissue
Type II: Bone spur from pelvis or proximal femur leaving at least 1 cm gap between opposing surface.
Type III: Gap < 1 cm

VI. INVESTIGATIONS

A. Laboratory Findings

1. Serum alkaline phosphatase (ALP) (>250 IU/L)

   Initially normal followed by increased level after 3 weeks
   ↓
   In parallel with bone formation
   ↓
   Peak at 10th week
   ↓
   Decreased gradually

2. *Acute phase reactants:*
   i. CRP
   ii. ESR

B. Imaging

1. *X-ray:*

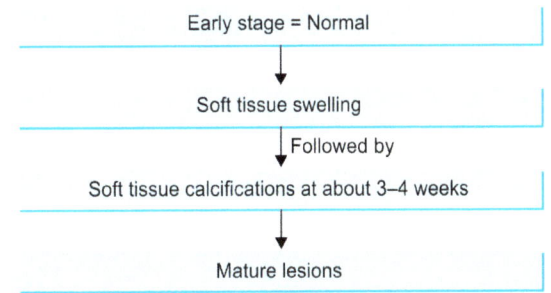

   i. Densely calcified peripheral rim with lucent center → Zonal pattern of calcification
   ii. Maturity of HO:
      a. Appearance of a bony cortex

b. Sharp demarcation from surrounding tissue
c. Trabecular pattern
2. *Ultrasonography:*
   i. Cheap
   ii. Easily available
   iii. No radiation
   iv. Differentiates between cystic and solid lesions
3. Bone scintigraphy:
   i. Triphasic bone scan helps in diagnosis
   ii. Monitors activity
4. *CT scan:*
   i. Best modality to assess zonal pattern of calcification
   ii. Can detect HO before X-ray
   iii. Egg-shell appearance
5. *MRI:*
   i. Best modality for imaging soft tissue masses
   ii. Peripheral enhancement with gadolinium
6. *Biopsy:*
   i. Core
   ii. Incisional
   iii. Excisional
7. Gross → Soft center with hard bony periphery
8. *Microscopy:*
   i. Immature central zone → Highly cellular
   ii. Intermediate zone → Fibrotic
   iii. Mature peripheral zone with lamellar bone.
       (Reverse Zonal phenomenon → Osteosarcoma)

VII. MANAGEMENT

A. HO Prophylaxis

1. *NSAIDs:*
   i. Indomethacin 25 mg TDS × 5–6 weeks

   ii. Oral
   iii. Low cost
   iv. Adverse effect:
       a. Gastritis
       b. Peptic ulcer
       c. Nonunion of fracture
2. *Radiation therapy:*
   i. 20 Gy in 10 fractions
   ii. Within 4 days of surgery

B. Surgical Excision

1. *Indications:*
   i. Severe loss of motion
   ii. Restricted activities of daily living.
2. *Timing:*
   i. Normalization of ALP
   ii. ↓↓ in Bone scan activity
   iii. 1–2 years after initial traumatic event

VIII. COMPLICATIONS

1. Hematoma
2. ↑ Intraoperative bleeding
3. Fractures of osteoporotic bone
4. Recurrence
5. Osteonecrosis

NEUROGENIC BLADDER

I. DEFINITION

Dysfunctional urinary bladder caused by an injury to the central or peripheral nervous system controlling urination.

II. PATHOANATOMY (FIG. 45)

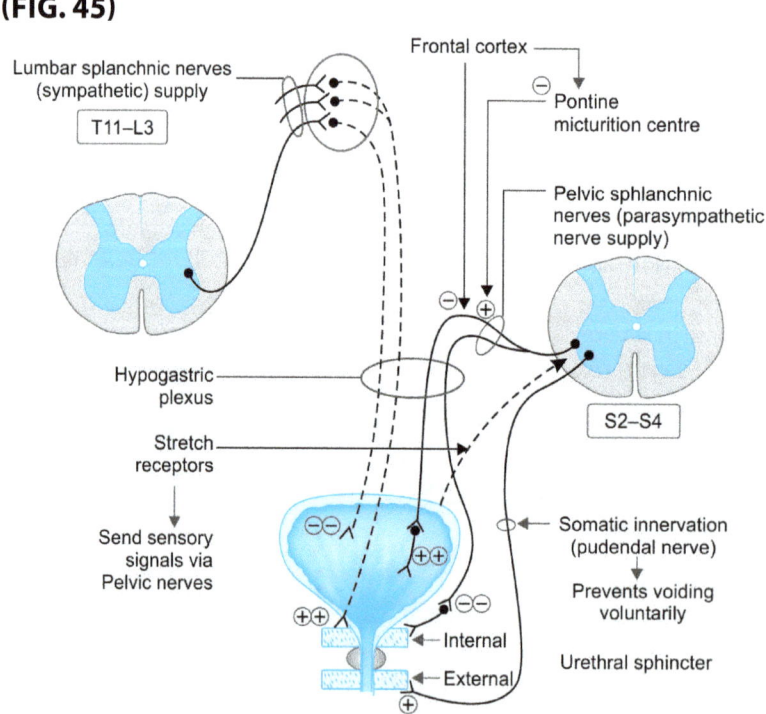

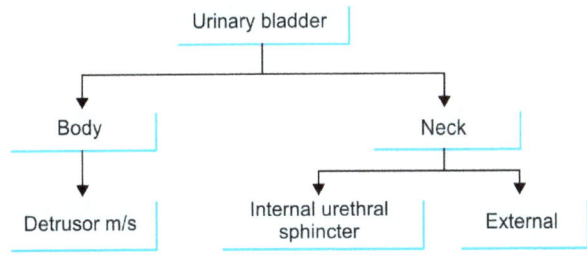

III. PATHOPHYSIOLOGY

1. PNS (S2–S4) → Pro-micturition
   i. Motor to detrusor
   ii. Inhibitory to Internal urethral sphincter
2. Sympathetic (T11–L3) → Antimicturition
   i. Relaxation of detrusor
   ii. Contraction of internal urethral sphincter
3. Micturition reflex → Spinal cord reflex
   ↓
   Inhibited and Facilitated by frontal cortex.

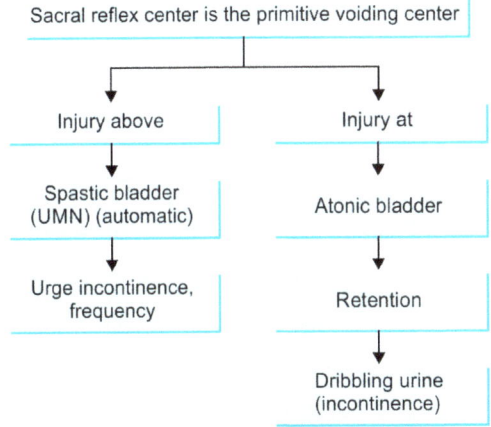

IV. LAPIDES CLASSIFICATION

1. Sensory neurogenic:
   Lesion → Posterior column of SC
   → Afferents from bladder to SC
   Overdistension and Hypotonicity
2. Motor paralytic – Motor neurons of bladder
3. Uninhibited: Incomplete lesion above S2
4. Reflex (automatic) – Complete lesion above S2
5. Autonomous – LMN lesion overtime develops intramural reflexes → bladder contracts due to direct stimulation.

V. LABORATORY INVESTIGATIONS

1. Urine analysis and culture: UTI
2. Voiding diary
3. Pad test
4. Urodynamic tests:
   i. Post-void residual urine (USG)
      If high → Bladder not contracting properly.
   ii. Uroflowmetry
   iii. Filling cystometrogram: Bladder capacity
      ↓
      Voiding → Pressure flow study.
   iv. EMG → DSH-DH (Detrusor sphincter dyssynergia with detrusor hyper-reflexia)

VI. MANAGEMENT

1. *Goals:*
   i. Prevention of infection
   ii. Prevent overdistension
   iii. Prevent renal damage
   iv. Promotion of independence.
2. *Acute phase:*
   i. Indwelling catheter
   ii. Suprapubic catheter
   iii. CSIC
3. *Pharmacotherapy:*
   i. Detrusor activity

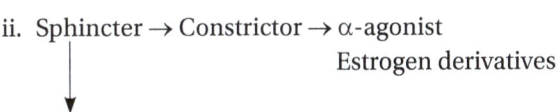

Inhibitors – anti-cholinergics	Enhancers
1. Oxybutynin	Cholinergics
2. Dicyclomine	

   ii. Sphincter → Constrictor → α-agonist
                                  Estrogen derivatives

   Relaxers → α-blockers
4. *Surgical:*
   i. Sphincterotomy
   ii. Sphincteric stent
   iii. Sling procedures
   iv. Botulinum toxin injection.

OBTURATOR NEURECTOMY

1. Surgical procedure involving removal of a part of the obturator nerve for the adductor spasm in spastic paralysis.
2. *Course (Fig. 46):*

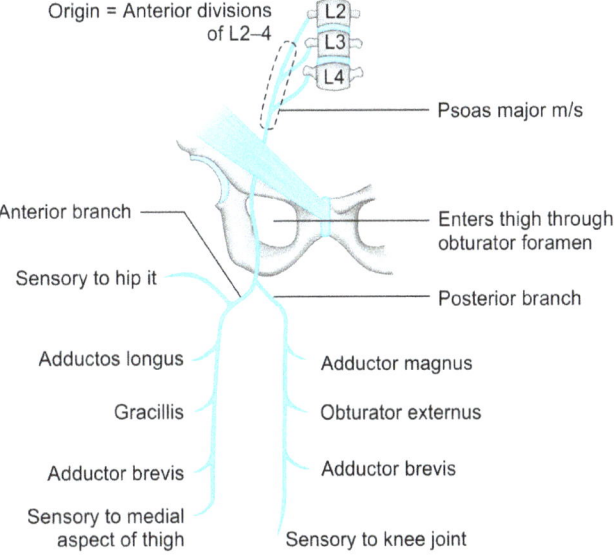

Origin = Anterior divisions of L2–4

3. *Rationale:*

   Adduction contractures → Scissoring of legs
   ↓
   i. Abnormal gait
   ii. Imbalance
   iii. Hygiene care difficulty (Perineal)
   iv. Pathological dislocation of hip
   v. Unable to sit on a wheelchair
   vi. Sexual intercourse

   → Pain arthritis of hip (archaic indication)

4. *Indications* (All causes of spastic paraplegia):
   i. Spinal cord injury
   ii. Cerebral palsy
   iii. Stroke
   iv. MS
   v. Motor neuron disease
   vi. Cervical myelopathy

5. *Principles:*
   i. Decrease pain
   ii. ↑ Function and autonomy
   iii. ↑ Comfort and better rehabilitation
   iv. Prevent complications
   v. Re-equilibrate the tonic balance between agonist and antagonist muscle at hip.

6. *Neurectomy:*
   i. Complete: done in the past
   ↓
   Leads to uncontrolled hip abduction contracture.
   ii. Selective: Only anterior branch
   iii. Combined with adductor tenotomy → in severe cases.

7. There are two approaches:
   i. Intrapelvic → Pfannenstiel incision just above symphysis
   ii. Extrapelvic: Along adductor longus tendon medial aspect of thigh. Nerve identified by stimulation → Adductor longus contraction

8. 2–3 cm of nerve excised.
9. Hemostasis is achieved
10. Obturator vessels are protected.
11. *Indications:* Failure of conservative and medical management
12. *Advantages:*
    i. Simple
    ii. Cost-effective in long run
    iii. Fast procedure.

PROSTHESIS

Devices designed to replace a missing limb and to restore the function.

I. FUNCTIONS

1. Replace missing part of the body
2. Provide variable range of physical activity
3. Provide variable range of professional activities
4. Mental satisfaction to the individual
5. Increased social acceptance of patient

II. CHARACTERISTICS

1. Comfortable
2. Convenient to wear and remove
3. Mechanically efficient
4. Needing minimal maintenance
5. Cosmetically acceptable
6. Light weight, durable

III. CLASSIFICATION

1. Exoskeletal
2. Endoskeletal

A. Exoskeletal

1. Gains structural strength from the outer laminated shell, through which the weight of the body is transmitted.
2. Shell made of → Resin socket. Filler material → Wood, foam.
3. Whole prosthesis is shaped and colored with reference to the opposite limb **(Fig. 47)**.

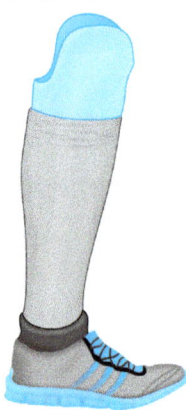

B. Endoskeletal

1. Gains structural integrity from the inner endoskeleton: A pylon made of metal or carbon fiber and provides weight bearing.
2. Cosmetic appearance by shaped foam covering the modular components **(Fig. 48)**.

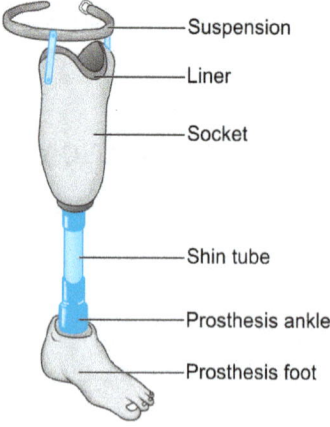

IV. PARTS

1. Socket
2. Body
3. Suspension
4. Terminal device: Hand - UL, Foot - LL

MYOELECTRIC PROSTHESIS

I. INTRODUCTION

1. Prosthesis is an artificial device that replaces a missing body part, which may be lost through trauma, disease, or congenital conditions.
2. "Myoelectric" is the term for electric properties of muscles.
3. A myoelectric-controlled prosthesis is an externally powered artificial limb that can be controlled with the electrical signals generated naturally by the patient's muscles.

II. PRINCIPLE

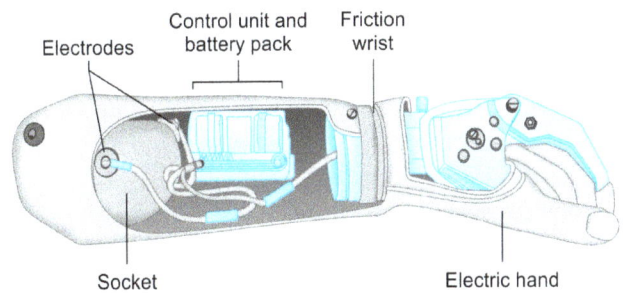

1. The prosthesis consists of
   i. A set of Electrodes
   ii. Circuit which consists of → Operational amplifiers, filters, comparators, transmitters, battery and feedback systems.
   iii. A relay system between the circuit and the robotic arm.
2. It uses electromyography signals/electric potentials from voluntarily contracted muscles within a person's residual limb to control movements of the prosthesis.
3. Sensors fabricated into the prosthetic socket receive electrical signals when the patient intentionally engage specific muscles in the residual limb.
4. Sensors relay information to a controller, which translates the data into commands for the electric motors and moves the mechanical joints.
5. A battery in the prosthesis provides the power.

II. INDICATIONS

1. Amputation due to:
   i. Trauma
   ii. Severe Infections
   iii. Tumors
2. Congenital Limb Deficiencies

III. PHASES OF TRAINING (3 STAGES)

1. Signal Training:
   i. In this initial phase, amputees learn to control specific muscles to operate the myoelectric arm by producing and inhibiting signals.
   ii. Electrodes and trainers provide feedback as they contract muscles, facilitating skill development in signal production and inhibition.
2. Control Training:
   i. Amputees progress to learning how to control muscles appropriately for various functions, aided by feedback from computer games or actual artificial limbs.
   ii. For children, modified toys like toy trains can engage them in muscle control exercises, fostering motor skill development.
3. Functional Training:
   i. The most intensive phase involves ensuring proper fit of the artificial limb before training commences.
   ii. Through repetitive tasks and problem-solving approaches, amputees become proficient users, integrating the artificial limb into their body image and daily activities with guidance from occupational therapists and prosthetists.
   iii. Children benefit from consistent wear, gradual increases in wearing time, and engaging activities to reinforce positive associations with the myoelectric arm.
   iv. Frequent review and booster sessions may be necessary for optimal function.

IV. ADVANTAGES

1. Movements include:
   i. Elbow flexion/extension
   ii. Wrist supination/pronation
   iii. Opening/closing of fingers
2. Less bulky compared to a body powered prosthesis
3. Quick reflexes
4. Secure hold
5. Grasping objects
6. Available in different sizes
7. Flexible in functioning
8. Can be given to a child at the age of 18–24 months.
9. 1–2 year guarantee available.

V. DISADVANTAGES

1. Motor and drive last about 2–3 years.
2. With high level of activity, the entire prosthesis may need to be replaced after only 4 or 5 years.
3. When used on a child, the sockets need to be replaced every year due to growth.
4. The material used in making it may result in skin irritations, inflammations, infections in the initial days.
5. Relatively expensive.

JAIPUR FOOT

Prosthesis → Replacement of a missing part of the body.
Classification (Lower limb)

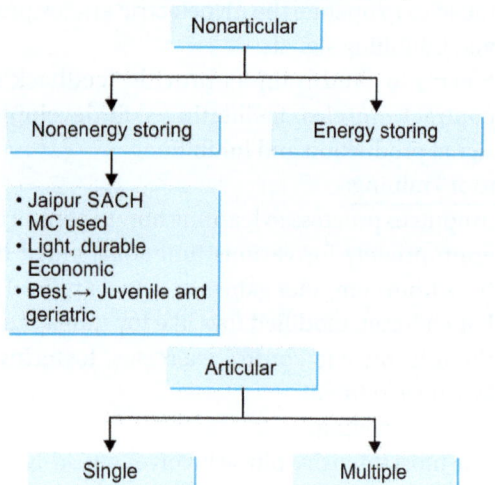

Jaipur foot – by Dr Pramod Sethi (**Fig. 49**):

1. Raw material easily available
2. Looks like normal foot
3. Water resistant
4. DF, PF inversion, external rotation → Possible
   ↓
5. ∴ Walking on uneven surfaces and bare foot possible
6. Squatting possible. Also, cross-leg.

SPINAL ORTHOSES

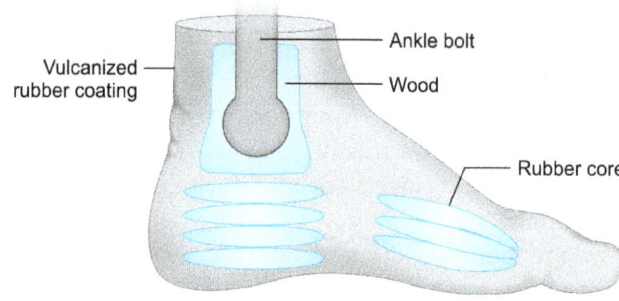

Fabric spinal orthroses	Rigid spinal orthoses	
Restricts only the extremes of forward flexion and extension	Constructed on the basis of metal frame which takes firm support from the pelvis	
1. Spinal belts, corsets	1. Taylor spinal brace	1. Milwaukee brace
2. Sacroiliac orthosis	2. Fisher spinal brace	2. Boston brace
3. Lumbo-sacral orthosis	3. Thomas spinal brace	
4. Thoraco – lumbar orthosis	4. Anterior hyperextension spinal brace (ASH)	

I. FUNCTIONS

1. To relieve pain
2. To support weakened or paralyzed muscles and unstable joints
3. To immobilize the vertebral column in the best functional position while healing occurs
4. To prevent the occurrence of deformity
5. To correct an existing deformity

PTB CAST

I. INTRODUCTION

1. Closed method of fracture treatment using plaster cast
2. Also known as "functional cast bracing"
3. "Sarmiento brace"

II. PRINCIPLE

Based on the belief that continuing function while a fracture unites does three things:
1. Enhances osteo-synthesis
2. Promotes healing of fracture
3. Prevent complications like joint stiffness

III. MECHANISM OF ACTION

"Based on Pascal's law":
1. When limb is loaded there is generation of intra-compartmental pressure around fracture site
   ↓
   That exerts pressure on wall of fascial compartment
2. As there is rigid cast around limb, the similar amount of pressure starts working in opposite direction
   ↓
   That maintains reduction of fracture (**Fig. 50**)

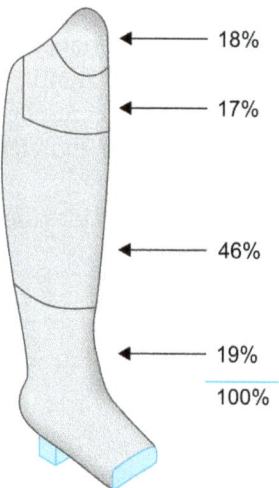

IV. PREREQUISITES

1. Fracture should be treated first by conventional methods
2. Angular and rotational deformity must be corrected
3. No pain at fracture site on minimal movements
4. No deformity at fracture site
5. There should be reasonable resistance to telescopy
6. Shortening should not exceed 0.25″ for tibia and 0.5″ for femur

V. USES

1. Distal femur fractures
2. Proximal tibia fractures
3. Tibia shaft fractures
4. Distal tibia fractures
5. Fracture shaft of humerus

VI. CONTRAINDICATIONS

1. Noncompliant patient
2. Neuromuscular disorder (NMD)
3. Altered sensitivity of limb
4. Isolated tibia fracture (fibula intact)
5. Proximal femur fracture
6. Both bone forearm fracture

TRACTION IN ORTHOPEDICS

A mechanical force applied against a resistance to overcome deforming forces on a pathological joint or a fractural fragment.

I. APPLICATIONS

1. Reduce a fracture → Promotes healing
2. Reduce dislocation of a joint (cervical spine facet, elbow)
3. Relieve pain
4. Rest limb in functional position
5. Aid in bone healing
6. Overcome muscle spasm
7. Correction of soft tissue contractures
   ↓
   Prevents and corrects deformities

II. METHODS

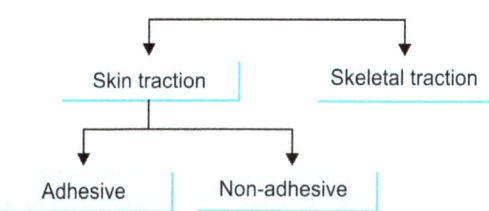

A. Skin Traction

1. Traction force applied over a large area of skin.
   ↓
2. Load is spread → ↑ Comfort and efficiency.
3. Weight → 1/10th body weight, around 6.7 kg
4. Adhesive → Zinc oxide, acrylic
5. *Contraindications:*
   i. Abrasions and lacerations
   ii. Dermatitis
   iii. Skin fragile
   iv. Impeding gangrene
   v. Allergy to adhesive

B. Skeletal Traction

1. Applied directly to the bone by means of:
   i. Steinmann pins
   ii. Denham pin **(Fig. 51)**

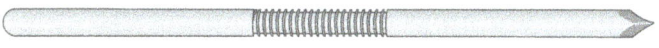

   iii. K-wire
2. Direction of pin → The entry point must always be where the neurovascular bundles are
   Because there is control over pin at entry point, but not at exit point.
3. *Complications*:
   i. Pin track infection
   ii. Physeal injury
   iii. Ligamentous damage
   iv. Distraction at fracture site
   v. Neurovascular injury
4. *Pin entry sites:*
   i. Lateral upper femoral: 2.5 cm below the most prominent point of GT, midway between anterior and posterior border of shaft of femur.
   ii. Distal femoral traction: Meeting of two lines,
      a. Along anterior border of head of fibula.
      b. Along upper border of patella. (Anterior to Posterior)
   iii. Proximal tibia: (Lateral to medial)
      2 cm below and behind the tibial tubercle **(Fig. 52)**.
   iv. Distal tibia: 5 cm above ankle joint.
   v. Calcaneal: 3 cm below and behind medial malleolus
   vi. Olecranon: 3 cm distal to tip of olecranon.

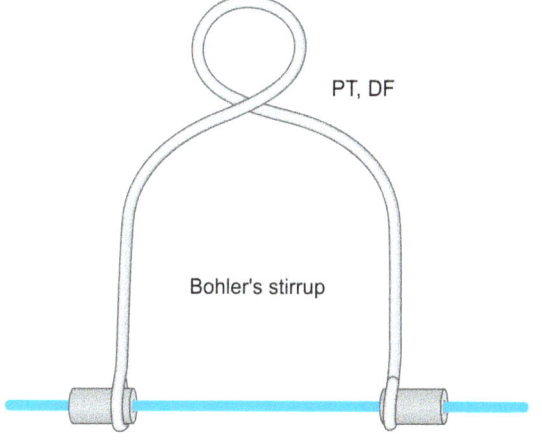

Bohler's stirrup: Used for skeletal traction in distal femur and proximal tibia fractures.

III. EXAMPLES

1. Bucks traction → NOF, acetabulum (skin)
2. Perkin's: Femur shaft fracture skeletal traction
3. Bryant's/Gallows → <2 years, femur shaft fracture
4. Dunlop's: Supracondylar humerus fracture
5. Pelvic traction: Lumbar PID
6. Cervical traction → Cervical PID, cervical dislocation
7. Ninety-ninety: Proximal femur fracture
8. Russel traction: Triple deformity, femur shaft (pediatrics)
9. Agnes-hunt: Hip FFD **(Fig. 53)**

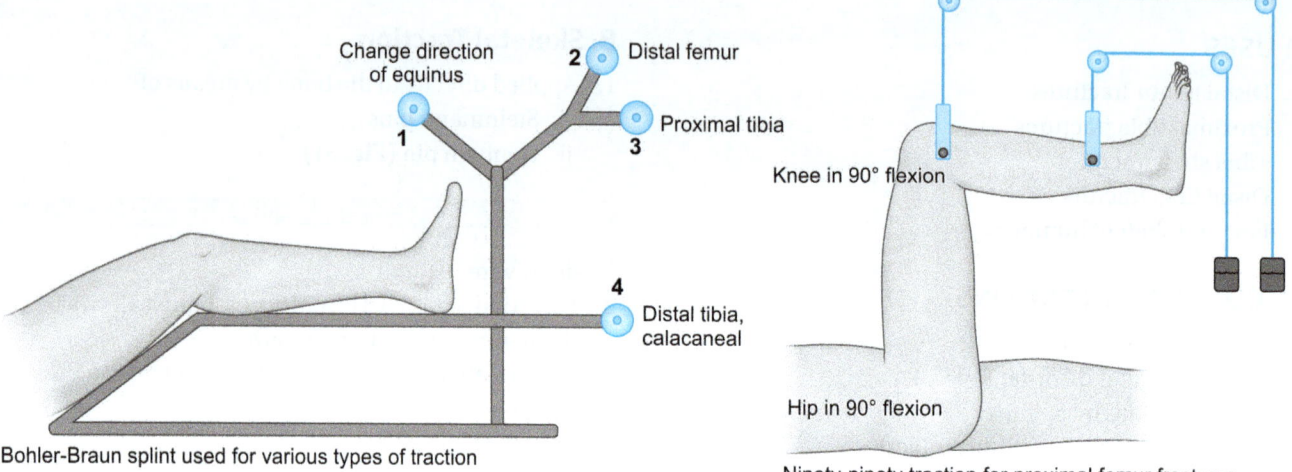

Bohler-Braun splint used for various types of traction

Ninety-ninety traction for proximal femur fractures

IV. TYPES

1. *Fixed:* Counter traction achieved by an appliance by taking purchase on a part of the body. For example, Thomas splint.
2. *Sliding:* Counter traction achieved by weight of the body under the influence of gravity by elevating the bed so that patient slides in opposite direction. For example, Bucks traction.

GALLOW'S/BRYANT'S TRACTION

I. APPLICATION (FIG. 54)

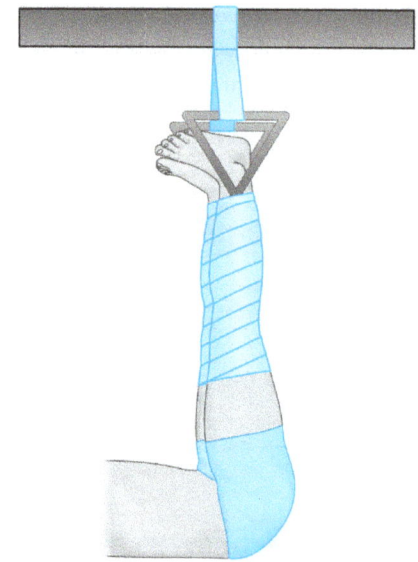

1. Apply adhesive skin traction on both lower limbs.
2. Traction cord ties to overlying frame.
3. Traction cords tightened sufficiently to raise the child's buttocks first to clear the mattress.
4. Counter traction obtained by the weight of pelvis and buttocks.

II. INDICATIONS

1. Femur shaft fracture <2 years
2. Weight <18 kg

III. CIRCULATION STATUS

1. Most important in first 24 hours.
2. Color, temperature, passive stretch pain, pulse, capillary refill, edema, sensation of foot.
   Position tolerated by children
   ↓
   Bone unites rapidly → Traction not > 4 weeks

IV. BLOOD SUPPLY EFFECT

<2 years → Insignificant
2–4 years → Precarious
>4 years → Compromised, definite contraindication

V. MODIFIED BRYANT'S

1. DDH
2. Initial 5 days → Vertical position of limb

3. Alternate days →10° abduction of each limb
4. In 3 weeks → Full abduction

THOMAS TRACTION SPLINT

I. INTRODUCTION

Designed by Hugh Owen Thomas.
↓
Immobilization of tuberculosis of knee.
↓
Later used in the world war I to transport injured soldiers by Robert jones.

II. COMPONENTS (FIG. 55)

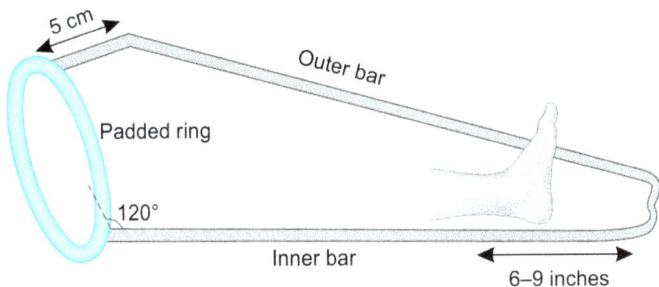

1. Well-padded circular ring
2. Outer bar with proximal angulation
3. Inner bar
4. W-shaped joint of 2 bars

III. MEASUREMENT

1. Length → Crotch to heel, add 6–9″ to it.
2. Circumference (oblique) → taken just below gluteal fold and ischial tuberosity.
   Normal thigh → Oblique circumference of thigh and addition of 2 inches to it.
   Affected thigh → Oblique circumference equal to internal circumference of the padded ring.

IV. WRAPPING AND PREPARATION (FIG. 56)

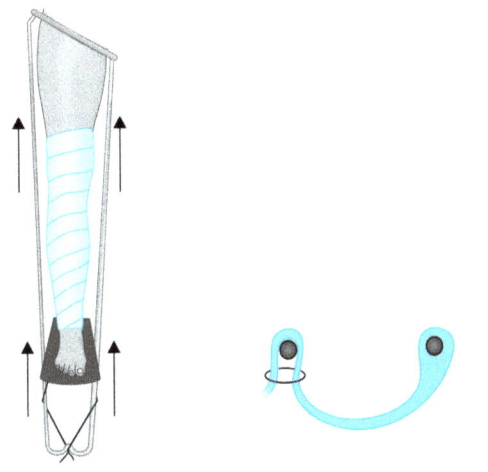

1. Sling wrapped between side bars in a "U-manner" with a 6″ roller bandage on which the limb can rest.
2. Master pad of Henry → A gamgee roll is placed under the lower part of thigh to maintain the anterolateral angulation of femur.
3. Windlass → to tighten the traction cards.

V. USES

1. For transportation of fracture lower limb:
   i. Subtrochanteric femur fracture
   ii. Femur shaft
   iii. Distal femur
2. Awaiting surgery
3. Fixed or sliding traction → Pediatric shaft femur

VI. COMPLICATIONS

1. Skin abrasions
2. NV complications: Tight bandage

Other Emergency Splints in Trauma

1. Cervical hard collar
2. Philadelphia collar
3. USI
4. Elbow pouch
5. Pelvic binder

SKULL TRACTION

I. METHODS

1. Garden well tongs
2. Crutchfield tongs
3. Barton tongs
4. Cervical Halo

II. CRUTCHFIELD (FIG. 57)

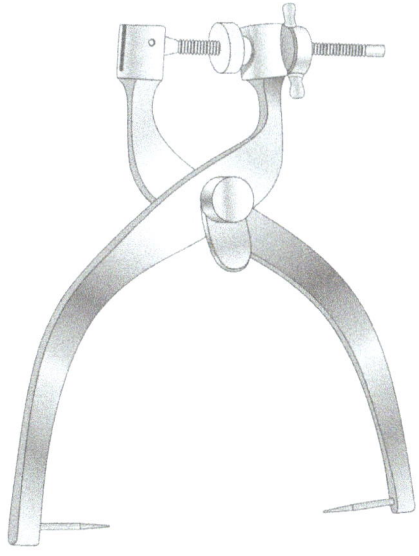

→ Fit into partial bone (Outer-table)
→ A special drill bit with shoulder
⬇
To enable accurate depth of hole to be drilled.

A. Application

1. Patient is sedated.
2. Scalp shaved locally.
3. *Entry:* Three finger-breadths above pinna in the line of mastoid
4. *Penetration:* 3 mm – Children
   4 mm – Adults.
   Tighten the adjustment screw for the first 3–4 days.
5. Infiltrate the area
   ⬇
   Including the periosteum with LA.
6. Elevate head end for counter-traction.

B. Weight

2.5 kg for head, 1/2 kg for each vertebra (**Fig. 58**).

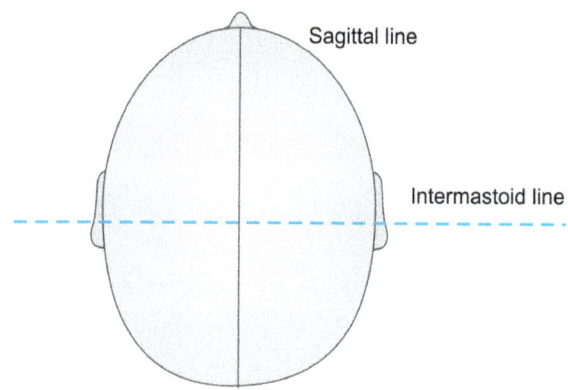

C. Complications

1. Hematoma
2. Infection
3. Meningitis
4. Failure of traction
5. Occipital ulcer
6. Ligamentous injury

D. Use

1. Reduction of fracture: Dislocation of C. spine
2. Maintenance of reduction
3. Before and after operative fusion
4. Cervical spondylosis with severe nerve compression

E. Contraindication

1. Hangman's fracture
2. Flexion distraction injury with disk herniation and ND

BONE PLATES

Bone plates are like internal splints holding together the fractured ends of a bone.

I. TWO MECHANICAL FUNCTIONS

1. Transmit forces from one end of a bone to the other, bypassing and thus protecting the area of fractures.
2. Hold the fracture ends together while maintaining the proper alignment of the fragments throughout the healing process.

II. CLASSIFICATION (BASED ON FUNCTION)

1. Neutralization/Protection plates
2. Compression plates
3. Buttress plates
4. Tension band plates
5. Bridge plates
6. Condylar plates

A. Neutralization

1. Plate used in combination with a lag screw → Merely protects the lag screw.
2. *Use:* Oblique, spiral, butterfly fragment #.

B. Buttress Plate

1. Mechanical function → strengthen (buttress) a weakened area of cortex.
2. Prevents the bone from collapsing during the healing process.
3. Usually designed with a large surface area → wider distribution of the load.
4. Insufficient to resist the axial loading forces that are applied to joint surfaces during weight bearing and other muscular activities.
5. To prevent shearing at the fracture site, or displacement of the fracture fragments bringing about widening of the articular surface, it is necessary to apply a plate that extends from the diaphysis across the outer surface of the metaphyseal-epiphyseal fragment.
6. Must be firmly anchored to the main fragment.
7. Must be contoured accurately to the segment of bone.
8. The fixation begins in the middle of the plate closest to the fracture site on the shaft.
9. Screws then be applied one after the other, toward both ends of the plate.
10. Maintain the bone length and supports the depressed fracture fragments.
11. *Use*: Epiphyseal and metaphyseal fractures. Distal Radius, Proximal Tibia, Distal Femur, tibial pilon, Distal Humerus

12. *Example*: T, L or hockey plate.
13. Special application "anti-glide plating" → one-third tubular plate prevents the displacement of the tip of an oblique fracture.

C. Bridge Plate → Acts as a "Bridge"

1. Transmits forces from one end of the bone to the other, bypassing the area of the fracture.
2. Main function → mechanical link between the healthy segments of bone above and below the fracture.
3. Does not produce any compression at the fracture site.
4. Plate span ratio – Plate length/Fracture width
   N = simple fractures = 10:1, multi-fragmentary = 3:1
5. Plate screw density = Number of screws/Number of plate holes
   Simple – 0.7, multi-fragmentary – 0.4–0.5
6. *Indications*:
   i. Comminuted #
   ii. Osteoporotic #

D. Compression Plate

1. A compression plate produces a locking force across a fracture site to which it is applied.
2. Basis → Newton's Third Law (action and reaction are equal and opposite).
3. Plate attached to a bone fragment → then pulled across the fracture site by a device → producing tension in the plate. As a reaction to this tension, compression is produced at the fracture site across which the plate is fixed with the screws. The direction of the compression force is parallel to the plate.

I. Role of compression

1. Compaction of the fracture to force together the interdigitating spicules of bone → increase the stability of the construct.
2. Reduction of the space between the bone fragments → decreases the gap to be bridged by the new bone.
3. Protection of the blood supply through enhanced fracture stability.
4. Friction resists the tendency of the fragments to slide under torsion or shear. Advantageous as plates are not particularly effective in resisting torsion.

II. Static and dynamic compression

1. A plate applied under tension produces static compression at a fracture site → exists when the limb is at rest or is functioning.
2. Dynamic compression is a phenomenon by which a plate can transfer or modify functional physiological forces into compressive forces at the fracture site.
3. A compression plate on the lateral side of the shaft of the femur exerting static compression both when the limb is at rest and when it is functioning. When functional activity begins, the physiological forces, which are normally destabilizing for a fracture, are converted to a stabilizing and active force by the same plate, which now acts as a tension band. A dynamic compression is thus exerted at the fracture site.
4. With cessation of physiological activity, this dynamic compression force will cease but the static compression force will continue to act.

III. Methods of achieving compression

1. *Self-compressing plate: (DCP, LCDCP)*:
   i. Dynamic Compression Plate → Misnomer
   ii. Developed to improve the former plating techniques with round hole plates.
   iii. Converts the torque (turning force) applied to the screw head to a longitudinal force which compresses the fractured bone ends.
   iv. The special geometry of the plate hole allows for self-compression and a congruent fit between screw head and plate hole at different angles of inclination. The plate can thus fulfil different plate functions, e.g., compression plating, tension band plating, neutralization (protection) plating, and buttress plating.
   v. Plate hole and sliding gliding principle
   vi. The plate hole can best be described as a part of an inclined and horizontal cylinder in which a sphere can be moved downwardly and horizontally to the intersection of the two cylinders.
   vii. The cylinders represent the plate hole and the sphere represents the screw head.
   viii. Axial compression between fragments can be achieved by using this feature of the plate holes.
   ix. A screw placed at the inclined plane, i.e., eccentrically (load position), will move the underlying bone horizontally in relation to the plate until the screw head reaches the intersection of the two cylinders.
   x. At this point the screw has optimal contact with the hole, ensuring maximal stability. The horizontal "cylinder" prevents jamming as well as undesired distraction.
2. *Tensioning device:*
   i. A special tensioning device can be attached between the bone plate and the adjacent bone cortex.
   ii. A bolt is then tightened to pull the plate across the fracture site. This produces tension in the plate and large compressive forces across the fracture. The attachment of the device to the bone necessitates a larger surgical exposure.
3. Lag screw

IV. Advantages of DCP

1. Inclined insertion of the screw with hemispherical screw head is possible up to an angle of 25° longitudinally 7° sideways.
2. Placement of a screw in neutral position without the danger of distraction of fragments.

3. Insertion of a load screw into the hole positioned most favorably for a given fracture. All holes permit compression.
4. Usage of two load screws in the main fragments for axial compression. After one screw has been inserted in load position → 1 mm displacement, the horizontal track in the hole still permits a further 1.8 mm of "gliding".
A second load screw can therefore be inserted in the next hole without being blocked by the first screw. The first screw slightly loosened before the further 1 mm compression can be produced by the second screw.

V. LCDCP → Improved design over DCP

1. The evenly distributed undercuts reduce the contact area between bone and plate to a minimum → reduces impairment of the blood supply of the underlying cortical bone → prevents consequent demineralization beneath the plate.
2. The undercuts also allow for the formation of a small callus bridge →increases the strength of the bone at a very critical location.
3. The enlarged cross section at the plate holes and the reduced cross section between holes → constant degree of stiffness along the long axis of the plate → No stress concentration at the holes when exposed to a bending load or during the contouring.
4. Trapezoid cross section → smaller contact area between plate and bone. A broad and low lamella along each side of the plate is formed → less likely to be damaged at plate removal.
5. The plate holes are uniformly spaced, which permits easy positioning of the plate.
6. *Undercut plate holes:* Undercut at each end of the plate hole allows 40° tilting of screws both ways along the long axis of the plate. Lag screw fixation of short oblique fractures. Screws can be tilted ±7° in the transverse plane. Furthermore, the undercuts reduce the contact area between plate and bone even more.
7. Disadvantage - Larger plate for same screws.

TENSION BAND PRINCIPLES

I. INTRODUCTION

1. Tension band technique converts a tensile force into a compressive force.
2. "Tension band" is a device which exerts a force equal in magnitude, but opposite in direction to the distracting tensile force.

II. RATIONALE (FIG. 59)

Bending force applied eccentrically to a column (Bone)
↱ Tensile
↳ Compressive
Tension band resists then tension of the eccentric load.

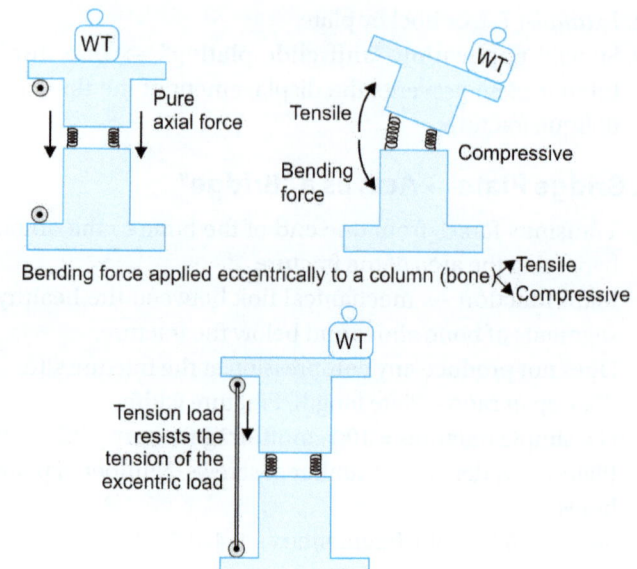

III. TENSION BANDS

1. Stainless steel wires with K-wires
2. Plates
3. External fixators
4. Metal cables
5. Nonabsorbable polyester sutures (Ethibond)

IV. PREREQUISITES

1. Bone must be able to withstand compression.
2. Intact cortex on the opposite surface.
3. Strong plate to withstand tensile forces.
4. Device placed on the tensile surface of bone.

V. GOALS

1. To achieve anatomic reduction
2. To create absolute stability
3. To achieve primary fracture healing

VI. <u>TYPES</u>

Static	Dynamic
Compression forces mainly at time of application → Forces at fracture site remain fairly constant during movement. For example, MM	Compression forces increases with movement.

VII. INDICATIONS – MUSCLE PULL DISTRACTS THE FRACTURE

1. Patella
2. Olecranon
3. Medial malleolus
4. Lateral malleolus
5. GT - Humerus
6. GT - Femur
7. Lateral end of clavicle

8. Plating in eccentrically loaded bones—femur, humerus
9. Angular deformity creating a tensile side.
10. Arthrodesis → Thumb
                   Wrist

VIII. CONTRAINDICATIONS

1. Communition at compression site **(Fig. 60)**
2. Sepsis
3. Osteoporosis
4. TBW:
   i. Hardware irritation
   ii. K-wire back out
   iii. Joint stiffness
5. Infection
6. Nonunion.

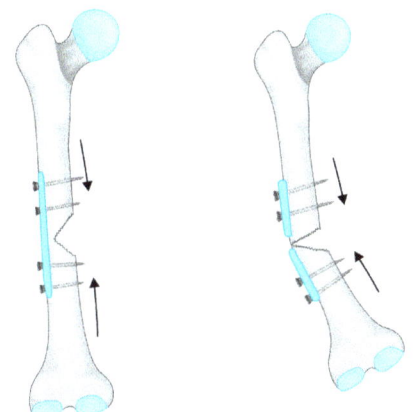

5. Core diameter of locking screw is larger than conventional screws : Therefore, ↑ Bending strength
6. Locking Head Screw (LHS):
   i. Always used in combination with plate
   ii. Never used as lag screw
   iii. Never to cross an unreduced fracture with a LHS
7. Types → Fixed angle: Perpendicular to plate
         → Variable angle: Angulation up to 30°
         ↓
   Adapts to different fracture patterns, but
   i. ↓ bending strength than fixed angle.
   ii. Thicker implant → undesirable near joint.
8. Generations
   i. 1st => Only locking holes
      ↓
      Highly rigid implant → Nonunion
   ii. 2nd => Alternate holes => Cortical and locking

LOCKING PLATE

I. INTRODUCTION

Fracture fixation devices with threaded screw holes, which allow the screws to get locked to the plate and function as one stable fixed angle device.

II. PRINCIPLES

1. Follows the principles of external fixators.
   ↓
   Without its disadvantages
2. Locking the screw into the plate →
   i. Angular and axial stability
   ii. Abolishes the possibility of screw to toggle, slide or dislodged, loosening.
   iii. Eliminates risk of post-op loss of reduction
   iv. Cannot be overtightened.
3. Plate need not be pressed against the bone.
   ↓
   i. Blood supply preserved.
   ii. Reduced compression pf periosteum.
   iii. Callus formation and bone healing under the plate.

4. Functions as a single beam construct **(Fig. 62)**

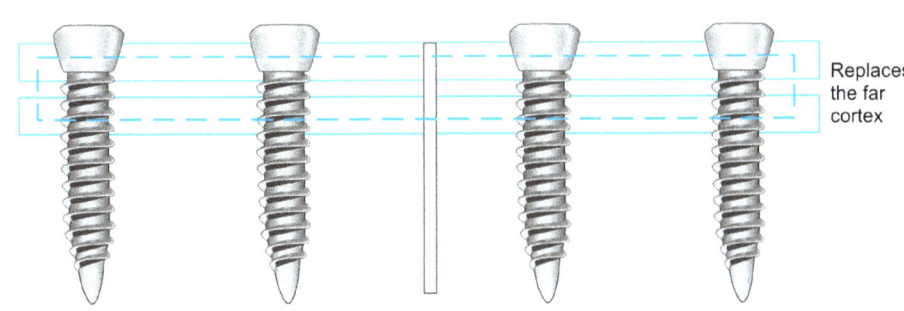

   iii. 3rd => Combi-hole
        ↓
        Advantages of both.
9. Unicortical insertion is possible as it eliminates far cortex. But only if bone quality is good.
   Torsional strength of unicortical is less. **(Fig. 63)**

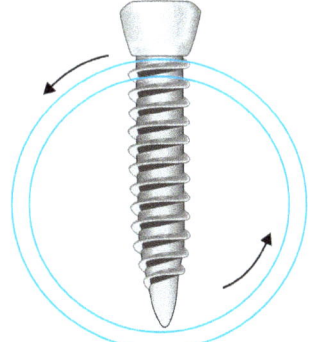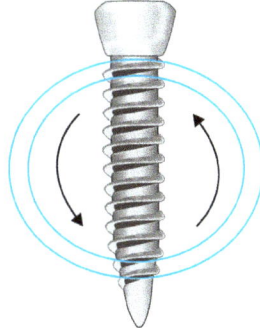

10. Can be used as MIPO → ↓ Invasive.
    ↙ ↓ Soft tissue injury
Therefore, Faster healing, smaller size.
11. Can be applied to all three modes
    i. Compression
    ii. Bridging
    iii. Neutralization
12. Construct stability increases with
    i. ↑ No. of screws
    ii. Longer plate
    iii. <50° screw divergence
13. Transfer of load
    BONE → SCREW → PLATE → SCREW → BONE

III. INDICATIONS

1. Intra-articular fractures of
    i. Distal femur
    ii. Proximal tibia
    iii. Distal radius
    iv. Distal humerus
2. Short, extra-articular metaphyseal fractures
   IM → fail to control.
3. Periprosthetic fractures ┌→ Below THR
                            └→ Above THR
4. Proximal humerus fractures
5. Osteoporotic bones
6. Fixation of corrective osteotomies => Angular stability
7. Malunion, Nonunion, Failed fixation
8. Orthopedic oncology => Stability of locking plate independently of bone quality.

IV. LIMITATIONS

1. Rigid construct => Nonunion if fracture not reduced and compressed => Diaphyseal
2. No angular stability if screw improperly inserted.
3. Implant removal difficult ┌→ Cold welded
                              └→ Bone graft over
4. Feel of bone quality during insertion absent
   ↓
   No screw length judgement
5. 2° loss of fixation with varus collapse → Inadequate screw length and improperly inserted.
6. Costly
7. Short working length → Failure

V. CONTRAINDICATIONS

1. Simple diaphyseal fractures => Do Conventional plating
2. Lower limb → IMN
3. Without reducing intra-articular fracture.

EXTERNAL FIXATOR

I. INTRODUCTION

1. External fixator is a device placed outside the skin that stabilizes bone fragments by means of pins or wires passing through the bone and connected to bars or rings.
2. *Two types mainly:*
    i. Pin
    ii. Ring
3. Other fixators → JESS, Taylors spatial frame, LRS, UMEX (universal mini ex fixator)

II. CLASSIFICATION (FIG. 64)

Type	Frame
1	Unilateral
1A	Unilateral uniplanar
1B	Unilateral biplanar
2	Bilateral
2A	Bilateral uniplanar
2B	Bilateral biplanar (3D)
3	Modular

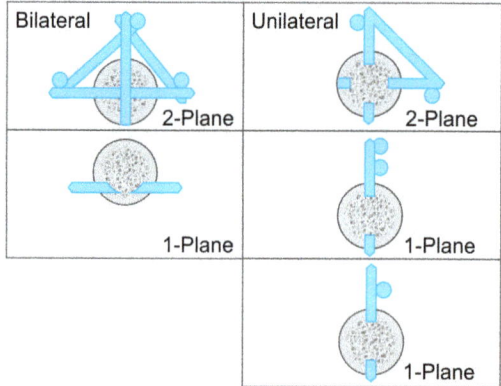

III. INDICATIONS → EMERGENCY OR ELECTIVE

1. Open fractures → Gustilo Anderson IIIB, IIIC
2. Polytrauma → Damage control
3. Poor soft tissue condition
4. Impending compartment syndrome after fasciotomy
5. Pelvic Fractures → Controls hemorrhage
6. Distracting fixator for ligamentotaxis
7. Infection - OM - Skeletal stabilization
8. Deformity correction
9. Limb length discrepancy
10. Fixation after radical tumor excision
11. Arthrodesis

12. Bone transport
13. Infected nonunions
14. Congenital pseudoarthrosis
15. Joint contractures
16. Fixation of complex comminuted fractures.

IV. COMPONENTS OF A PIN FIXATOR

1. Bone pins
2. Clamps
3. Connecting rods or tubes
    i. Pins → Tip, thread, core, shaft
    ii. Short Thread → Diaphysis, long → Metaphysis
    iii. In diaphysis only distal cortex engaged by threads → shaft of pin has greater core diameter for near cortex
    iv. Clamps → provides multiplanar adjustment of the pin Pin to rod, rod to rod, pin to rod

V. ADVANTAGES

1. Minimal damage to blood supply
2. Minimal damage to soft tissues
3. Fixation is away from site of injury
4. Good option when significant infection risk

VI. DISADVANTAGES

1. Restricted joint motion
2. Pin tract infection
3. Cumbersome
4. Inadequate stability for certain fractures

VII. STIFFNESS OF A FIXATOR—FACTORS (FIG. 65)

1. Distance between the bone and the connecting rod
    i. Closer the pin clamps can be to the pin-bone interface —more rigid fixation
    ii. Optimal distance—4 cm
    iii. 2 rods increases the stiffness (Instead of 1)
    iv. Stiffness of the connecting rod
2. Pin clamp interface
3. Slippage of clamp decreases stiffness
4. Periodic tightening
5. ↑ thickness of Schanz screw
6. Thread design → HA coating ↑ stiffness
7. Number of pins used
    i. More number of pins: More stability
    ii. 2 pin/segment for tibia and 3 for femur
    iii. Pins closer to fracture: More rigid
    iv. More pin to pin distance in a segment: More is the bending stiffness
    v. Pin angled at 90°—increases torsional stiffness
8. Pin diameter
    i. 4.5 mm to 5.5 mm for tibia and femur,
    ii. 3.5 mm for radius ulna
    iii. 2.5 mm for metacarpals or metatarsals
    iv. More the diameter: More is the stiffness

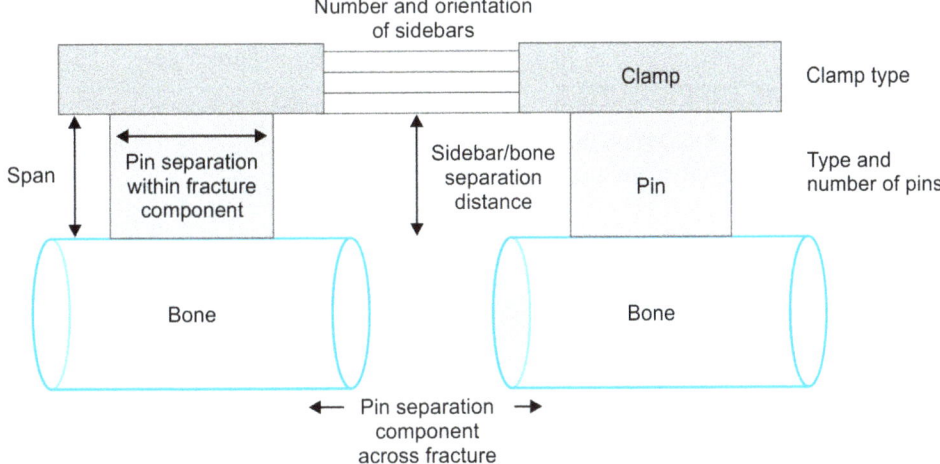

VIII. COMPLICATIONS

1. Neurovascular injury
2. Pin loosening
3. Pin tract infection
4. Joint stiffness
5. Malalignment
6. Malunion
7. Nonunion
8. Cosmetically unacceptale

IMPLANT REMOVAL

I. INDICATIONS

1. Pediatric patients: To avoid interference with growth
2. Pain around the region bearing the implants
3. Protruding implant through skin or into joint → prevent future chondrolysis
4. Post-operative infection
5. Broken implants

6. Screw cut out into the joint
7. Screw loosening and backout
8. Threatening integrity of adjacent vital structures
9. Joint arthroplasties: Implant loosening and wear for revision
10. Temporary implant in a staged surgery when purpose is served → Spacers, square nails in masquelet
11. Patient's request

II. TIMING – FRACTURES

1. As a general rule, implants must be removed once the fracture has solidly united on orthogonal films of radiograph.
2. *Pediatrics:*
   i. Supracondylar and Lateral condyle: 3-4 weeks
   ii. TENS nail: Depending on the age: 5-6 months
3. *Adults:*
   i. 3 months: Wires and screws
   ii. 18 months: Plates of long bones, periarticular plates, intramedullary implants

III. DIFFICULTIES

1. Incision: Generally along the same previous incision line
2. Distorted anatomy
3. Fibrous tissue
4. Neurovascular structures tethered and at risk
5. Wound closure
6. Cortical growth over the implant
7. Cement in Joint arthroplasties

IV. METHODS TO OVERCOME DIFFICULTIES

1. If surgery at a different center or primary surgeon unavailable → details of surgery evaluated from hospital papers.
2. Multiple set of implant removal instruments from different companies if status not known.
3. Experienced surgeon – preferably same.
4. Use of fluoroscopy guidance intraoperatively
5. IMN: Backslapping hammer
6. May need Burr for spinal implants and when cortical growth over plates
7. Metal debris is produced while removing screws → Copious Wash
8. For Removal of cement after implant removal (TKA, THA) → extended trochanteric osteotomy, tibial tuberosity osteotomy.
9. Confirm the number of screws removed with the preoperative X-rays.
10. Screw heads with destroyed recesses may need pliers and osteotomes.
11. Send implants for culture when indicated

12. Postoperative immobilization → integrity of bone questionable
13. Orthotic devices

V. COMPLICATIONS

1. Neurovascular Injury
2. Refracture
3. Wound sepsis
4. Further soft tissue trauma

PREOPERATIVE PREPARATION OF PATIENT

I. INTRODUCTION

1. *Aim:* Identify and quantify comorbidities that may impact surgical outcome.
2. *Goal:* Preoperative optimization for the best surgical outcome
3. Multidisciplinary approach → Surgeon, anesthetist, nurse
4. Thorough history and physical examination
5. Specialist reference in case of comorbidities impacting surgical outcome

II. INVESTIGATIONS (ROUTINE)

1. CBC
2. RFT
3. LFT
4. Sr. electrolytes
5. PT-INR
6. Blood Grouping and cross matching
7. Blood sugar → Diabetics
8. HHH
9. RT PCR → COVID
10. Chest X-ray
11. ECG → 2D ECHO
12. ABG

III. RADIOLOGY

1. Radiograph: Planning
2. Scannogram: HTO, TKR
3. CT scan: Complex fractures
4. CT Angio: Cervical spine → Course of vertebral artery
5. MRI → Spine: Level of PID
   Knee: ACL, Meniscus injuries, etc.
   Shoulder: Rotator cuff tears

IV. SPECIAL CASES

1. Pulmonary function Tests → Scoliosis
2. Cervical spine movement and Mallampati score: Ankylosing spondylitis
3. Antibiotics stopped 2 weeks prior → Infection
4. Achieving ROM before surgery → ACL reconstruction

V. PREOPERATIVE INSTRUCTIONS AND PROTOCOLS

1. Implant ordering and instruments autoclaved
2. Nil by mouth: 8 hours solid, 6 hours liquid
3. Bowel preparation → Pelvis and Acetabulum surgeries
4. HTN → anti-HTN on the day of surgery
5. Blood sugar control
6. Shaving just prior to surgery → Least bacterial colonization
7. Patient must mark a big cross on the normal limb himself
8. Medications continued or stopped as per requirement. Conventional DMARDs can be continued perioperatively. Only biologicals must be discontinued 3 weeks prior.
9. Clopidogrel stopped 5 days before surgery
10. Aspirin low dose continued
11. Consent from patient, guardian in their language
12. Antibiotic prophylaxis → 30 minutes before incision and before tourniquet is applied
13. X-rays in the OT room
14. Confirmation of side by announcing loudly in the OT before incision.

REHABILITATION OF A PARAPLEGIC PATIENT

I. INTRODUCTION

1. Paraplegia is the impairment in motor and/or sensory function of the lower extremities.
2. Rehabilitation → Restoring the patient to the optimal physical, mental, social, vocational and economic capacity of which he/she is capable.
3. *Multidisciplinary team:*
   i. Orthopaedician
   ii. Physical therapist
   iii. Occupational therapist
   iv. Psychiatrist
   v. Social worker
   vi. Dietician

II. PREVENTION OF BED SORES

1. Occur on sacrum, ischial tuberosity, trochanter and heel
2. Patient position change every 2–3 hours
3. Air beds
4. Early mobilization → Wheel chair
5. Keep skin clean and dry → Prevent soiling with urine and stool

III. PHYSICAL THERAPY EXERCISES

1. Most important part of Rx program at rehab center.
2. *Goals:*
   i. Reducing muscle tone
   ii. Maintaining and improving range of motion and mobility
   iii. Increasing strength and coordination
   iv. Improving comfort
3. Maintains bone density → Paraplegic patients are prone to osteoporosis.
4. Prevent complications → Contractures, Frozen joints, Bed sores
5. Balance and coordination → transfer training → Bed to wheel chair, wheel chair to car
6. *Three types:*
   i. **Stretching:**
      a. Slow, sustained lengthening of muscle
      b. Improves flexibility → Full range of motion.
      c. ↓ Muscle spasticity and cramps, tendonitis and bursitis.
      d. Regularly and twice a day.
      e. Stretch as far as muscle can
         ↓
         Hold for 10 seconds → Ease
      f. Must also be done before and after other exercises.
         ↓
         Prevents soreness and injuries.
   ii. **Aerobics:**
      a. Utilizes large muscle groups
      b. Strengthens heart and lung
         ↓
         Improves body's ability to use O_2
      c. Reduces fatigue, increases energy levels → Better sleep, weight control.
      d. 3–4 sessions/week → 15–60 minutes
      e. Aquatic exercises and swimming (hydrotherapy)
         ↓
         Eliminating effect of gravity
         ↓
         ↑ Strength and endurance
      f. Warm water → Stiff joints
      g. Stationary bicycling
   iii. **Strengthening:**
      a. Repeated muscle contractions → until muscles tires.
      b. Increase muscle tone
      c. Strong glutei, Quadriceps → to stand
      d. Core and back muscles → Erect posture

IV. GAIT TRAINING AND ASSISTIVE DEVICES

1. Knee ankle foot orthosis (KAFO) with pelvic belt
   +
   Elbow crutches
2. Treadmill training
3. Cane: Supports 25% BW
4. Wheelchair
5. Thoracolumbar brace
6. Walker: 50% BW

V. THROMBOEMBOLIC DISEASE

1. Due to venous stasis and hypercoagulability
2. Pneumatic compression devices
3. DVT stockings
4. LMW heparin

VI. BLADDER MANAGEMENT

1. Acute → Indwelling catheter
2. Clean, intermittent catheterization
   ↓
   Good hand function, good assistants
   ↓
   Catheterized every 6–8 hours
3. Suprapubic catheter

VII. BOWEL MANAGEMENT

1. Prolonged colonic transport time
   ↓
2. Hard, drying of stool
3. Adequate fluid and fiber intake
4. Docusate sodium (100 mg BD)

VIII. NEUROPATHIC PAIN

1. At or below level of SCI
2. Gabapentin 100 mg TDS
3. TCA → Nortriptyline

IX. ORTHOSTATIC HYPOTENSION

1. Gradual tilting and getting up
2. Abdominal binders
3. Elastrocrepe bandages for LL
4. T. Ephedrine 30 mg

X. SEXUAL HEALTH – ERECTILE DYSFUNCTION

1. Vacuum devices
2. PDE: 5 inhibitors
3. Implantable penile prosthesis

XI. SPASTICITY

1. Baclofen, tizanidine, dantrolene, diazepam
2. POP casts, phenol, botulinum

XII. PHYSICAL AGENTS

1. Thermotherapy
2. Electrical therapy

XIII. VOCATIONAL REHABILITATION

1. Change of occupation
2. Desk job

SECTION 14

Recent Advances

BONE SUBSTITUTES

I. RATIONALE
1. Current gold standard → Autograft ↓
2. As it has all characteristics of new bone growth →
    i. Osteogenesis
    ii. Osteoconductivity
    iii. Osteoinductivity
3. However, limitations
    i. Donor site morbidity
    ii. Limited supply
    iii. Increased OT time, anesthesia, blood loss
    ↓
    Therefore, bone graft substitutes (BGS).
    ↓
    An ideal BGS must be:
    a. Osteoinductive (OI)
    b. Osteoconductive (OC)
    c. Biocompatible
    d. Bioresorbable
    e. Structurally similar to bone
    f. Easy to use
    g. Cost effective

II. CLASSIFICATION (LAURENCIN ET AL.)

	Class	Description
1	Allograft-based	Allograft bone used alone or in combination with other materials
2	Cell based	Utilize cells to generate new tissue either alone or seeded onto a support matrix
3	Factor based	Natural and recombinant growth factors
4	Ceramic based	Calcium phosphate, $CaSO_4$, bioactive glass
5	Polymer based	Degradable or non-degradable polymers

A. Allograft Based
1. Most commonly bone substitute
2. Osteoconductive more than osteoinductive
3. Degree of osteoconduction depends on:

    Processing method   Type of graft
    i. Fresh frozen → OI + OC   Cancellous > Cortical
       a. Due to preservation of BMP
       b. But needs secondary sterilization
    ii. Freeze dried → OC only
       a. As BMP is depleted
       b. ↓ Structural integrity
       c. ↓ Disease transmission
4. Demineralized bone matrix (DBM)
    i. Acidic extraction of bone matrix from allograft, Chemosterilized and Ag extracted
    ↓
    ii. Removes minerals but leaves the collagenous and non-collagenous structural proteins.
    iii. Osteoconductive without structural integrity.
    iv. Minimally osteoinductive due to BMP, TGF-B
    v. Available as chips, gels, pastes.

B. Cell Based
1. Most commonly used cell based → Autologous bone marrow aspirate.
2. Mesenchymal stem cells → Depending on the environment develop into osteoblasts, chondroblasts, myoblasts.
3. MC site → Iliac crest
4. Centrifugation of aspirate done on cell separator.
    ↓
    Produces buffy coat → contains progenitor cells → Angiogenic and osteogenic cytokines.
5. Buffy coat taken into a syringe for intraosseous injection

C. Factor Based
1. Growth factors regulate cellular activity.
2. Includes TGF-B, IGF-I and II, PDGF, FGF and BMP
3. BMP → Discovered by Marshall Urist (1965) → BMP-7 (Osteogenic protein-7)

4. Osteoinductive only → Stimulates undifferentiated perivascular mesenchymal cells to differentiate into osteoblasts.
5. FDA approved → rhBMP-2 (acts on MSCs) and rhBMP-7 (acts only on pre-osteoblast)
6. BMPs are water soluble → Need carrier → Interconnected porous Ca hydroxyapatite ceramics used as carriers

D. Ceramic Based (Separately Asked as SAQ)

Ceramics are inorganic non-metallic solids that have been created by heating non-metallic mineral salts at temperatures >1,000° (sintering).

Ceramics are:
- Hard and brittle
- Have high compressive strength

Bioceramics are especially designed ceramics for the repair and reconstruction of the diseased or damaged parts of bones and joints.

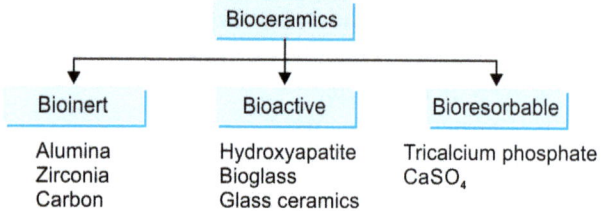

1. Applications
i. Orthopedic load-bearing coatings
ii. Bone graft substitutes
iii. Bones cements

2. Advantages
i. Biocompatible
ii. Wear resistant
iii. Lightweight
iv. No disease transmission
v. Less stress shielding

3. Disadvantages
i. Low tensile strength
ii. Low toughness
iii. Not resilient

A. Bioinert
1. Maintain physical and mechanical properties while in host.
2. Resist corrosion and wear.
3. Two types → Nonporous and porous
   i. Nonporous → Attach by bone growth into surface irregularities, by press fitting into defect. → Morphological fixation
   ii. Porous → Bone ingrowth occurs mechanically attaching the bone to the material. Biological fixation (Fig. 1)

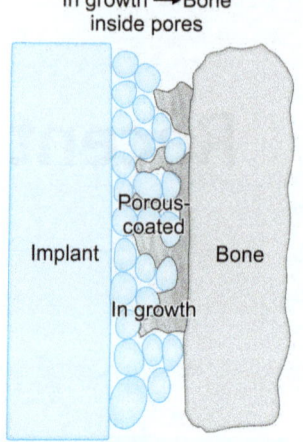
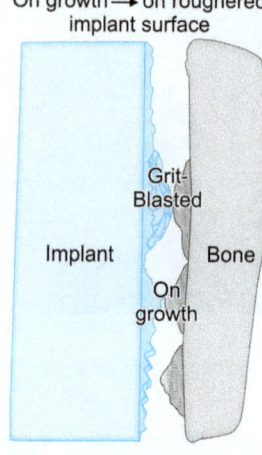

Use:
1. Hip arthroplasty → Femoral head
2. Knee prosthesis
3. Bone screws
4. Implant coating
5. Load-bearing implant

B. Bioactive
1. Surface reactive ceramics
2. Direct and strong chemical bond with tissue (biologically active)
3. Formation of hydroxycarbonate apatite
4. Bonding at the interfacial zone between material and tissue.
5. The interfacial strength of adhesion > cohesive strength of the implant or tissue. Failure occurs in implant or bone but not interface.
6. The collagenous portion of the soft tissue strongly adheres to bioactive silica glass.

C. Bioresorbable
1. Chemically broken down by the body and degrade.
2. Slowly replaced by bone.
3. Chemical produced as the ceramic is resorbed, must be able to be processed through body's metabolism.
4. Synthesized from chemicals (synthetic ceramics) or Natural sources (natural ceramics) → Coralline HA
5. Available as pastes, putties, granules, etc.
6. Most widely used → Calcium phosphate → As it occurs naturally in bones in the form of HA.
7. $CaPO_4$ stable phase depends on water, pH and temperature
8. Used in the form of:
   i. Cement
   ii. Coating on implants
   iii. Powders
9. Calcium sulfate
   i. Osteoconductive bone void filler
   ii. Filing of cysts, bone cavities, benign bone lesions, segmental defects.
   iii. Spinal fusion
   iv. Filling of bone graft harvest sites

D. Polymer Based
1. Natural or synthetic
2. Biodegradable or non-biodegradable → Composites of polymer + Ceramic
3. Polyglycolic acid or polylactic acid

ORTHOBIOLOGICS AND BMP

INTRODUCTION

Orthobiologics are biologically derived substances that naturally occur in body and are used in:
1. Optimization of the healing environment
2. Regeneration and repair of muscle tissue

I. RATIONALE

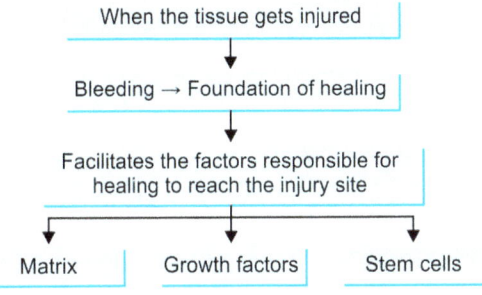

1. *Matrix:*
   i. Serves as building blocks → help to fill tissue gaps
   ii. It forms the framework of the bones, tendons or ligament where the cells are present and multiply.
2. *Growth factors:*
   i. Regulate cellular activity
   ii. TGF-β, IGF-1, PDGF, FGF, BMP
3. *Stem cells:* Depending on the environment stem cells develop into osteoblasts, chondroblasts, myoblasts.
4. If any of the above mentioned three are deficient → healing is affected.

II. TYPES

i. Bone Grafts (BG)
1. Autologous bone graft
2. Allogenic
3. BG substitutes
4. Demineralized bone matrix
5. Bone marrow aspirate

ii. Growth Factors
1. BMP
2. VEGF
3. PDGF

iii. Stem Cell Therapy
1. Bone marrow aspirate concentrations
2. Amniotic tissue products
3. Embryonic tissue products

iv. Blood-based Preparations
1. Pure platelet rich plasma (PRP)
2. Leukocyte and platelet rich plasma

v. Viscosupplementation and Scaffold Based
1. Hyaluronic acid injections
2. Autologous Chondrocyte implantation
3. Matrix induced stem cell transplantation (MAST)

BMP (BONE MORPHOGENIC PROTEIN)

I. INTRODUCTION

1. Morphogens are extracellularly secreted signals governing morphogenesis during epithelial mesenchymal interactions.
2. BMPs are growth factors that work by inducing the mesenchymal stem cells to differentiate into bone forming cell lines.
3. Also known as osteogenic proteins, BMP play a critical role in **cell growth, differentiation, and apoptosis** in a variety of cells including osteoblasts and chondrocytes.
4. Maintain adult tissue homeostasis:
   i. Maintenance of joint integrity
   ii. Initiation of fracture repair
   iii. Vascular remodeling
   iv. Inflammatory response
   v. Immune response
   vi. Oncogenesis
5. Marshall Urist in 1965, coined the term when he saw the crude bone extracts had the ability to induce bone formation at an ectopic site.
6. Structural properties and MOA
   i. Members of TGF-β superfamily.
   ii. In the bone, secreted by osteoprogenitor cells, osteoblasts, platelets
7. Carriers

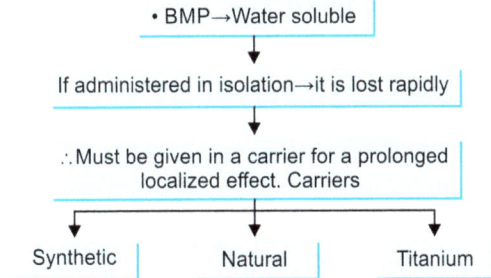

   i. Synthetic → Ceramics: HA and $CaPO_4$
      → Nonceramic: Polymers
   ii. Natural: Collagen → MC carrier: Agarose, chitin
   iii. Titanium → Implants treated with BMP
8. USES
   i. Two recombinant forms currently in use rhBMP-2 and rhBMP-7
   ii. Osteoinductive → *Nonunions*

iii. Also used in fresh open fracture of tibia, → infection rates probably due to increased stability.
iv. Approved by FDA for lumbar interbody spinal fusion cages
↓
To eliminate the need for autograft **(Fig. 2)**

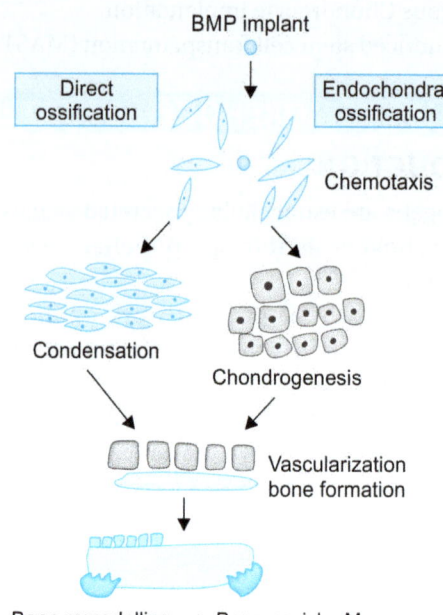

II. DRAWBACKS AND COMPLICATIONS

1. Ectopic bone formation → Spinal canal heterotopic ossification
2. Extremely costly
3. Increased postoperative pain and radiculitis
4. ↑ Postoperative swelling
5. ↑ Risk of malignancy

III. CONTRAINDICATIONS

1. Hypersensitivity to rhBMP
2. Pregnancy
3. Active infection
4. Skeletally immature (<18 years)
5. Malignancy

IV. PLATELET RICH PLASMA

1. Platelet-rich concentrate, autogenous platelet gel
2. Autologous suspension of platelets
↓
from whole blood via double centrifugation technique
3. Normal platelet count → 150,000–450,000/µL
↓
4. Must be 4–5 times [N] of baseline = PRP
>5 → inhibits healing

5. *Key growth factors:*
   i. PDGF
   ii. TGF
   iii. IL-1
   iv. Platelet-derived angiogenesis factor
   v. Epidermal growth factor
   vi. Platelet-derived endothelial GF
   vii. VEGF
   viii. IGF-1, 2
   Functions:
   i. ↑ ECM deposition
   ii. ↓ Pro apoptotic signals
   iii. Minimize joint inflammation
7. After extraction and before application, the platelets are activated with $CaCl_2$ and resultant clot applied to site of injury.
8. Platelets begin secreting these proteins within 10 minutes of clotting.
9. *Use:*
   i. Lateral epicondylitis.
   ii. Rotator cuff tears
   iii. Subacromial impingement.
   iv. Shoulder OA
   v. Patellar tendinosis
   vi. OA knee
   vii. Tendoachilles tear
   viii. Plantar fasciitis
   ix. Nonunion
   x. Topically to control bleeding > TKR

Animal studies have shown enhanced fracture healing, however not in humans as of now.

LAMINAR AIR FLOW

1. An airflow in which the entire body of air within a confined area moves with uniform velocity along parallel flow lines (i.e., laminar) with a minimum of eddies.
2. LAF systems were originally designed by national aeronautics and space administration (NASA) to create an ultraclean environment for assembly by missle parts.
3. Later applied in:
   i. Laboratories
   ii. Pharmaceutical research facilities
   iii. Operation theaters
   iv. As cabinets: tissue cultures
   v. Electronic and industrial sector
4. The OR therefore has → Conventional air flow
                         → Laminar airflow systems
5. LAF provides **unidirectional** airflow that moves at a **uniform velocity** (0.5 m/s) and pressure (>15 Pa)
6. In the OT, thus occurs within a central enclosed space formed by vertical panels extending from the ceiling.
7. Air is drawn through a series of filters, most importantly **HEPA filters** (high efficiency particulate air)

8. LAF may be:
   i. Horizontal
   ii. Vertical **(Fig. 3)**

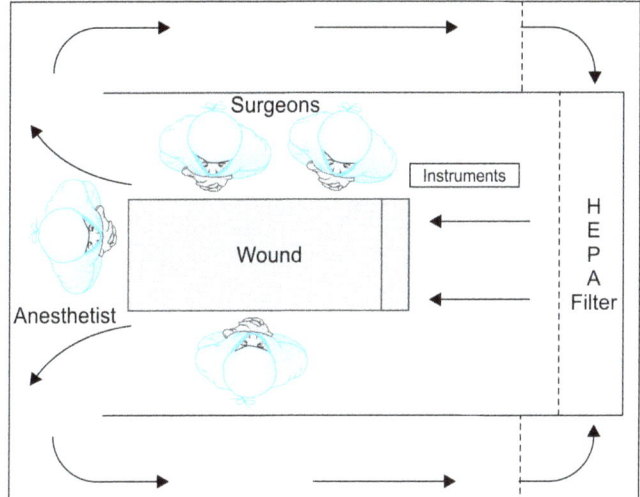

Horizontal LAF (Top view)

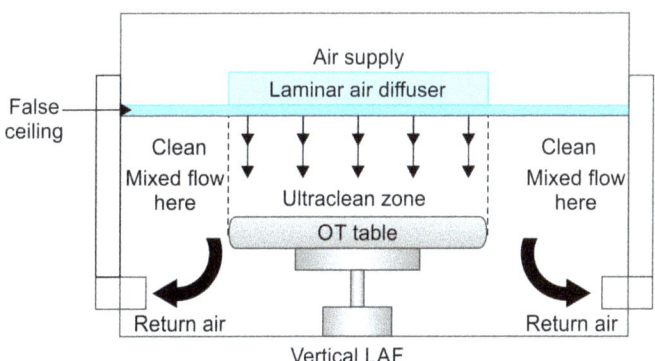

Vertical LAF

9. HEPA filters → Remove 99.97% airborne particles up to size of 0.3 µm
10. Each HEPA filter has a regulatory manometer that measures the resistance to filtration as a result of becoming blocked.
11. Filters must be positioned as close to air supply as possible
    ↓
12. To ensure that particles are filtered out well before entering the OT
13. "Ultraclean" air produced by LAF systems (<10 CFU/m^3)
14. Compared to conventional systems, LAF more efficiently reduces contaminated air from peripheral areas entering the ultraclean area as
    ↓
    Positive pressure air currents are targeted directly on the surgery site.
15. LAF air changes → 300 times/h
    Conventional → 20 times/h
16. Main drawback → Turbulence
17. Physical barriers (staff, OT lights, C-arm, etc.) obstruct and divert the contaminated air flow currents toward the incision.
18. Exponential airflow modification → Air flow is in form of upside-down trumpet.
19. Recommendation for effective LAF use:
    i. Minimize no. of personnel in the OR.
    ii. Door openings strictly minimized on surgery starts.
    iii. Instrument and implant trays only to be opened prior to use.
    iv. Ceiling lamps not directly above surgical site
    v. Decreased time that image intensifiers are within "ultraclear" zone.
    vi. Gloves not to be changed over surgical site
    vii. Physical movements of theatre personnel ↓ **(Fig. 4)**

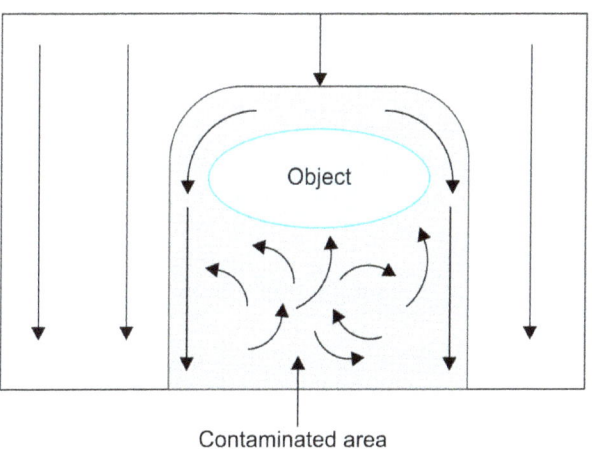

REAMER IRRIGATOR ASPIRATOR

I. INTRODUCTION
RIA is an innovative reaming system developed for aspiration of the reaming debris along with continuous irrigation.

II. INDICATIONS
1. To clear the medullary canal of BM and debris
2. To effectively size the medullary canal for the acceptance of an intramedullary implant or prosthesis.
3. To harvest finely morselized autogenous bone and bone graft marrow for any surgical procedures requiring bone graft.

   To facilitate fusion   Fill bone defects
4. To remove infected and necrotic bone and tissue from the medullary canal in the treatment of OM.
5. Stabilization of B/L femoral fractures in one surgical setting.
6. IM reamed nailing in polytrauma patients with chest injury.

III. PARTS (FIG. 5)

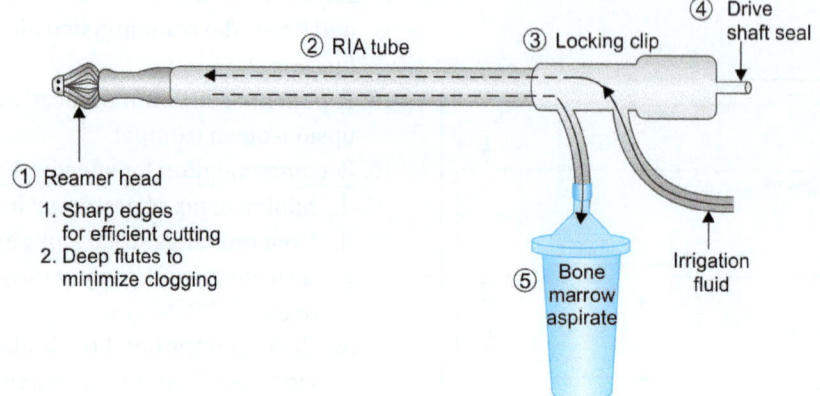

1. Reamer head:
   i. Sharp edges for efficient cutting
   ii. Deep flutes to minimize clogging.
2. RIA tube
3. Locking clip
4. Drive shaft seal
5. Bone marrow aspirate
6. Irrigation fluid

IV. STEPS

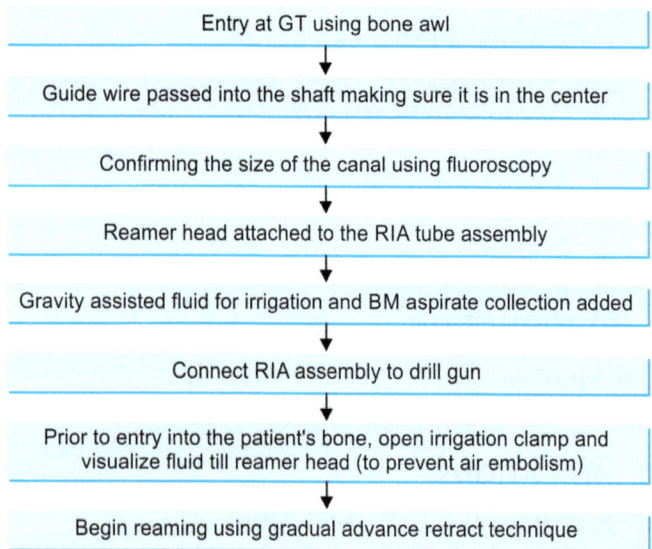

V. ADVANTAGES

1. Reduces heat generation
2. Removal of infected tissue
3. Reduces potential for air embolism
4. Reduces intramedullary pressure

VI. CAUTION

1. Eccentric reaming can lead → Iatrogenic femur fracture.
2. Reamer stuck in the shaft.
3. Sharp reamer head → injury to operating surgeon → use tip protector.

4. Never ream when there is no irrigation or aspiration
   ↓
   The irrigation fluid decreases reamer head temperature
5. Hematoma formation
6. Considerable blood loss

VII. CONTRAINDICATIONS

A. Specific
1. Metabolic bone disease
2. Active metastatic bone disease

B. Relative
1. Osteoporosis
2. Advanced age
3. Bleeding disorder

FIBRIN GEL

I. INTRODUCTION

Fibrin gel is a network of proteins produced naturally by the body after the injury.
↓
And it has been bioengineered as a sealant for homeostasis and a tissue substitute to speed healing.

II. COMPOSITION

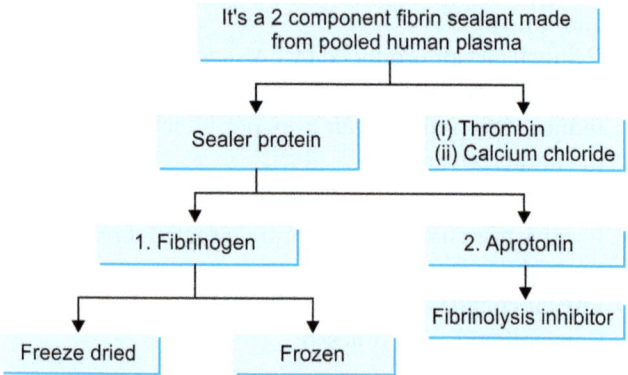

III. MECHANISM OF ACTION

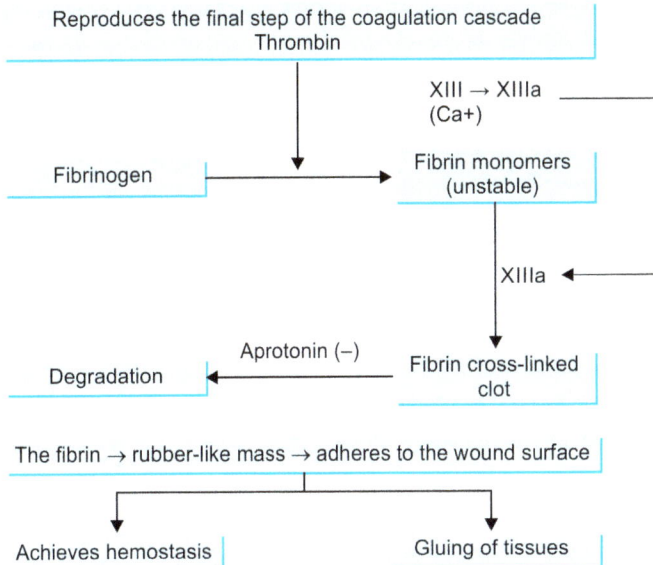

IV. USES

1. To reduce blood loss in arthroplasties and spine surgeries.
2. *Blood conservation*: The decrease perioperative BL translates into less blood transfusion.
3. To seal suture holes in dural tear in spine surgeries
4. Enhances the repair of osteochondral defect and other articular cartilage and tendon injuries (Achilles)
5. As an antibiotic delivery system
6. Composite bone substitute (Polymer + Fibrin scaffold)
7. RhBMP + Osteoinductive
   ↓
   It prevents rhBMP spread which decreases ectopic bone formation
8. Autologous chondrocyte implantation (ACI)
9. Aseptic Nonunions → ↑ bone healing and induction of bone fusion
10. Benign cystic tumors
    Synovial cysts and hemophilic pseudotumors
    ↓
    Closes off tumor/cyst at its neck preventing reformation
11. TKR
    Increased ROM postoperative
    Decreased length of stay
    Decreased postoperative infection
    Stunted rate of arthrofibrosis
    Significantly elevated postoperative Hb

V. ADVANTAGES

1. Can be used in heparinized patients
2. In TKR, when IV tranexamic acid is contraindicated
3. Can be used in pediatric patients (>1 month)
4. Naturally produced in the body therefore,
   ↓
   Decreased inflammation
   Decreased immune reaction
   Nontoxic degradation products
   Good cell adhesion

VI. ADR

1. Hypersensitivity
2. Hypotension
3. Inadvertent IV application → Life-threatening thromboembolism
4. Angioedema, erythema
5. Bronchospasm
6. Paresthesia

VII. PRECAUTIONS

1. Not to be used for treatment of severe or brisk arterial or venous bleeding
2. Only topical, never IV
3. Only to be applied as a thin layer
   ↓
4. Excess clot thickness negatively affects wound healing
5. Must be used within 4 hours of reconstitution.

LASERS

I. INTRODUCTION

Light amplification by stimulated emission of radiation

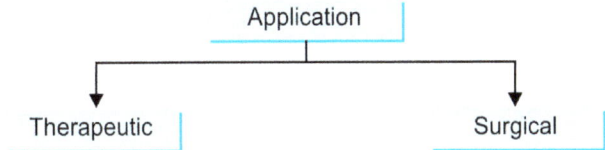

II. THERAPEUTIC

1. Low energy (30–100 Mw)
2. Produced from laser diodes
3. Relieve pain and resolve inflammation
4. ↑ Speed, quality and tensile strength of tissue repair
5. Phase → Pulsed
          → Continuous
6. *Indications:*
   i. Fibromyalgia
   ii. Myofascial plane
   iii. Cervical neck pain
   iv. Lower back pain
   v. Joint pain
   vi. Trigeminal neuralgia
   vii. Rheumatoid arthritis

    viii. Carpal tunnel syndrome
    ix. Tendonitis, tendon rupture
    x. Bursitis
    xi. Plantar fasciitis
    xii. Sprains
7. *Contraindications*:
    i. ≤6 months of radiotherapy
    ii. Epilepsy
    iii. Fever
    iv. Pregnancy
    v. Malignant tumors

III. SURGICAL LASERS

1. High energy → 10–60 W
2. *4 basic components*:
    i. *Laser medium:* Solid, liquid or gas that determines the wavelength of LASER.
       → CO_2, Argon gases
       → YAG (Yttrium aluminum garnet) crystals
    ii. *Resonator cavity:* Sandwiches the medium between 2 mirrors.
    iii. *Excitation source:* Pumps high energy electrical or optical energy into medium.
    iv. *Cooling system:* Removes excess thermal energy.
3. Continuous waves → conduct heat to surrounding tissues.
    ↓
4. Large peripheral zones of thermal damage.
5. Pulsed → High intensity light over short time intervals.
    ↓
   Time between pulses allows for dissipation of thermal energy.
    ↓
   Prevents excessive damage due to thermal conduction.
6. *Surgical laser mechanisms*:
    i. Photothermal: Tissue ablation by heating > 100°C → Explosive release of vaporized tissue contents.
    ii. Photochemical: Cold excimer laser
        Dissociates molecular bonds → nonthermal cutting.
    iii. Photomechanical: Thermal energy and rapid expansion of vaporization contents.
        ↓
        High pressure within the tissue
        ↓
        Shock waves that create damage at large distances from the site
7. Commonly use lasers:
   Nd-YAG (Neodymium)
   Ho-YAG (holmium)
   Xenon chloride excimer
8. *Uses*:
    i. Meniscectomy
    ii. Lateral retinacular release
    iii. Laser-induced capsular shift (tightening)
    iv. Laser discectomy.
    v. Synovectomy
    vi. Shoulder arthroscopic debridement
    vii. Subacromial decompression
    viii. Shoulder capsulorrhaphy
9. *Experimental uses*:
    i. Removal pf PMMA cement.
    ii. Laser osteotomy
    iii. Tissue welding.
    iv. Biostimulation → ↑ Cellular metabolism
    v. Photodynamic therapy (PDT) → RA
10. *Disadvantages*:
    i. ON due to Nd:YAG
    ii. Extensive subchondral damage
    iii. *Photoacoustic effect:* Damage remote from laser site
    iv. Better outcomes not demonstrated

GENE THERAPY

1. Gene therapy involves *genetic modification* of cells to produce a therapeutic effect.
2. *Mechanisms*:
    i. Replacing a disease-causing gene with a healthy copy.
    ii. Inactivating a disease-causing gene.
    iii. Introducing a recombinant or modified gene to treat the disease.
3. Gene for specific growth factor can be transferred.

Directly	Indirectly
Vector with gene is injected into the injured tissue	Cells taken by biopsy from injured tissue → cultured in vitro → Vector injected into stabilized cells

4. *Gene therapy*:

Germline	Somatic
i. Possibility of transmission to future generations ii. Ethical issues	Exclusively benefit the patient Not passed to next generation

5. *Vectors*: Carriers that target specific tissues, serve as delivery systems.

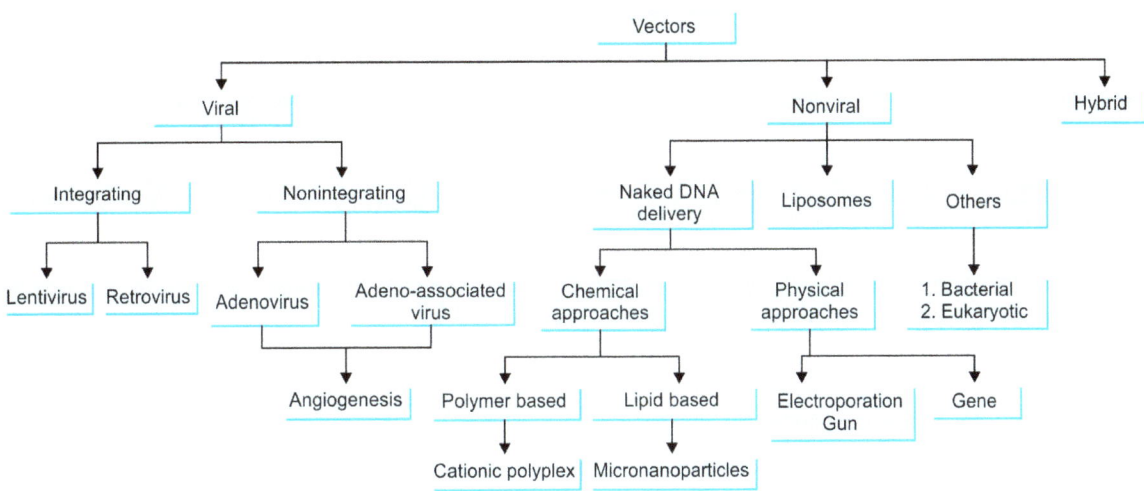

6. **Applications:**
   i. *Fracture healing and nonunion*
      Transfers of genetic sequence with one of the growth factors → BMP, LMP-1, TGF-β
   ii. Osteoporosis: Growth factors
   iii. *Cartilage defects:*
      a. Enhancement of chondrogenesis → TGF-β, BMP-2
      b. Autologous chondrocytes → harvested and cultured → with vectors containing growth factor genes →Reimplanted into articular defect.
   iv. *Osteoarthritis:*
      a. Target cells in OA →Chondrocytes, osteocytes, cells of synovial lining, progenitor cells, surrounding muscles.
      b. Interleukin receptor antagonist protein (IL – Ira) → Chondroprotective.
   v. *Rheumatoid arthritis:*
      a. Intra-articular gene therapy → allows local production of therapeutic molecule.
      b. *Ex vivo gene therapy:* Cells presenting antigens → Dendritic, macrophages, B cells
         ↓
         Regulated to alter immune response in RA
   vi. *Degenerative disc disease:*
      Direct delivery of TGF-β1 to nucleus pulposus → ↑ Proteoglycan synthesis.
   vii. *Spinal fusion:*
      Adenovirus mediated BMP-2 gene transfer
   viii. *Skeletal muscle healing:*
      a. Indirect gene therapy → Basal lamina of muscles cannot be penetrated by virus
      b. IGF-1, NGF improve muscle healing
   ix. Osteogenesis imperfecta: Experimental
7. *Limitations*:
   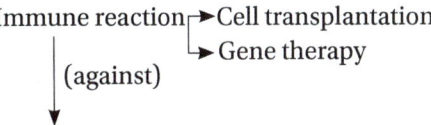

   i. Viral coat
   ii. Viral vector proteins
   iii. MHC
   iv. Culture medium
   v. Gene product
8. *Solutions to immune reactions*:
   i. Immunosuppression
   ii. Developing immune tolerance:
      → Antigens/vector in thymus
      → Antibodies
      → Autologous cell transplantation

SHORT WAVE DIATHERMY

I. INTRODUCTION
Therapeutic modality that produces deep heating within the body via conversion of electromagnetic energy to thermal energy. ("Dia" – through, "thermy" – heat)

II. PRINCIPLE
Normal dipole molecules of the body tissue are arranged based on polarity.
↓
Tissue damage → dipole distribution becomes irregular
↓
Under electric field of influence
↓
Rotate according to polarity.
↓
Rearranged and previous state of polarity restored.
Diathermy uses electric current to produce heat deep inside the target tissue.
↓
Does not apply heat directly to the body.
↓
Current from the machine allows the body to generate heat from within the targeted tissue.

III. EFFECTS
1. Pain relief
2. Better flexibility
3. Improves circulation (vasodilatation)
4. Accelerates healing

IV. MODALITIES

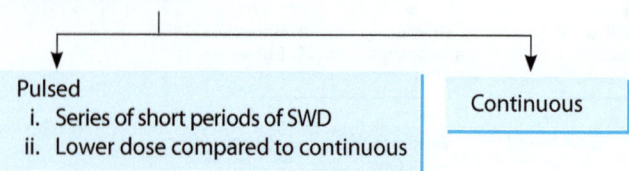

- **Pulsed**
  - i. Series of short periods of SWD
  - ii. Lower dose compared to continuous
- **Continuous**

iii. SWD frequency = 10–100 MHz (27.12 MHz)
iv. 20 minutes at maximum tolerable dose

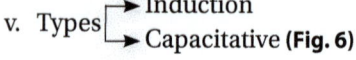

v. Types → Induction, Capacitative **(Fig. 6)**

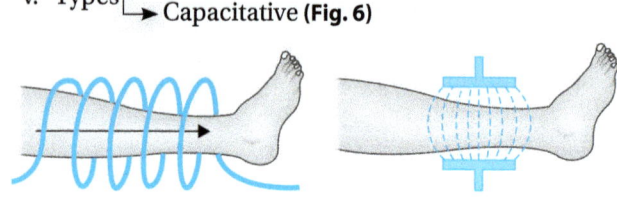

Induction	Capacitative
Body part placed in a coil producing electromagnetic field	Patients tissue as a part of the circuit. Tissue electric resistance produces heat

V. PHYSIOLOGICAL EFFECTS
1. Increased metabolism
   Heating → ↑ O_2 consumption → ↑ metabolism
2. Increased blood supply → heat → stimulates nerve endings → vasodilatation
   ↑ Metabolism → ↑ Acidosis → Vasodilatation
3. Rise in temperature → Muscle relaxation
4. Fall in blood pressure = ↓ reduced PVR from heat
5. Better local immune response
   Vasodilatation → ↑ WBCs and Ig → ↓ Infection
6. Faster healing
7. *Pain relief*:
   i. Counter irritation
   ii. Resolution of inflammation
   iii. Clearance of toxic metabolites

VI. APPLICATIONS/USES
1. Degenerative joint disorders: OA
2. Inflammatory arthritis: RA
3. Muscle sprain
4. Ligament strain
5. Hematoma
6. Muscle and tendon tears
7. Capsule lesions
8. Infected surgical incisions
9. Low back ache → PID, annular tears

VII. **CONTRAINDICATIONS**
1. Mental implants and jewelery
2. Cardiac pacemakers
3. Ischemic areas
4. Peripheral vascular disease
5. Pregnancy
6. Fever
7. Sensory loss
8. Tumors
9. Epiphyseal plates in children

VIII. SIDE EFFECTS
1. Burns → Hypersensitivity to skin, Lead touching skin, Excess current
2. Precipitation of gangrene
3. Electric shock
4. Giddiness

INTERFERENTIAL THERAPY

INTRODUCTION
1. Transcutaneous application of alternative electric currents for therapeutic purpose.
2. *Principle*: To cause 2 medium frequency currents of slightly different frequencies to interfere with one another.
3. Involves utilization of effects of low frequencies without painful or unpleasant side effects.
4. *Advantage*: Produces effects in tissues exactly where required without unnecessary and uncomfortable skin stimulation.
5. *Mechanism*:
   i. Increased circulation, relieves pain, decreases edema.
   ii. Stimulate large diameter A - beta fibers, and inhibit transmission of small - diameter nociceptive traffic (C and A - delta)
6. *Frequency*: 100–150 Hz
7. *Uses*: Pain relief in:
   i. Causalgia, HZV, neuralgia
   ii. Cervical spondylosis
   iii. OA knee
   iv. Ankylosing spondylosis
   v. RA
   vi. Frozen shoulder
   vii. Disc herniation
   viii. Spinal stenosis
   ix. Muscle injuries
   x. Ligamentous injuries
   xi. Reduction of edema

8. *Contraindications*:
    i. Infective etiology
    ii. Malignancy
    iii. Pacemakers
    iv. Loss of sensation
    v. Danger of hemorrhage
    vi. Large open wounds
    vii. Pregnant uterus

NEGATIVE PRESSURE WOUND THERAPY (NPWT)

1. Therapeutic technique which uses a device to remove excess exudates and promote healing of wounds.
2. Controlled application of subatmospheric pressure to the local wound.
3. **Parts (Fig. 7)**

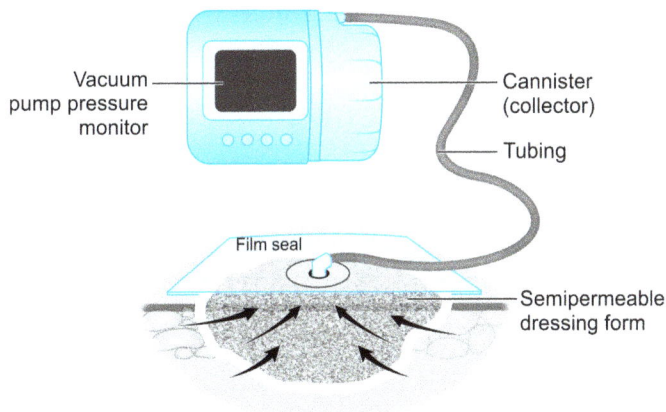

Macrodeformation

4. **Mechanism of action**
    i. *Macrodeformation*: Wound contraction.
    ii. *Microdeformation*:
        a. ↑ Thermoregulation.
        b. ↑ Differentiation → ↑ Bloody supply
        c. Neurocutaneous activation
        d. Inflammatory modulation
    iii. *Fluid removal*:
        a. ↓ Bacterial load, ↓ edema
        b. Shear forces
    iv. *Optimized wound environment*:
        a. Closed and moist
        b. ↓ Interstitial fluid
        c. Promotes granulation, angiogenesis
    v. Hemostasis
5. **Indications**
    i. *Trauma wounds*:
        a. Open: Exposed bones/joints
        b. Soft-tissue trauma
        c. Degloving injury
    ii. Pressure ulcers
    iii. Diabetic ulcers
    iv. *Surgical wounds*: → Dehisced / → Closed
    v. Venous insufficiency ulcers
    vi. Skin flaps and grafts
    vii. Mx of laparotomy
    viii. Burns
6. **Contraindications**
    i. Necrotic tissue with eschar
    ii. Untreated OM
    iii. Unexposed fistulas
    iv. Malignant wounds
    v. Exposed NV bundle
    vi. Exposed anastomotic site
    vii. Clotting disorders (risk of bleeding)
7. **Technique**

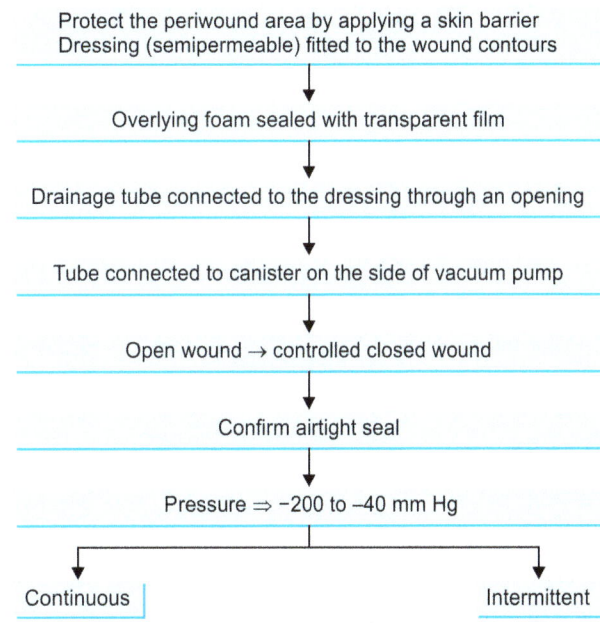

Dressing changed twice/week

8. **Side effects**
    i. Wound infection by anaerobes
    ii. Toxic shock syndrome
    iii. Bleeding
    iv. Ingrowth of granulation tissue into foam
    v. Pain
    vi. Maceration and pressure damage
9. **Recent advances**

Combination therapy:
    i. Incorporating bioactive factors
    ii. Antimicrobial silver
    iii. Platelet gel

RADIOFREQUENCY ABLATION

I. GOAL

1. To induce thermal injury to the tumor tissue by electromagnetic energy deposition.

2. Patient is a part of closed loop circuit which includes an:
   i. RF generator
   ii. Electrode needle
   iii. Large dispersive electrode (ground pads)

II. PROCEDURE

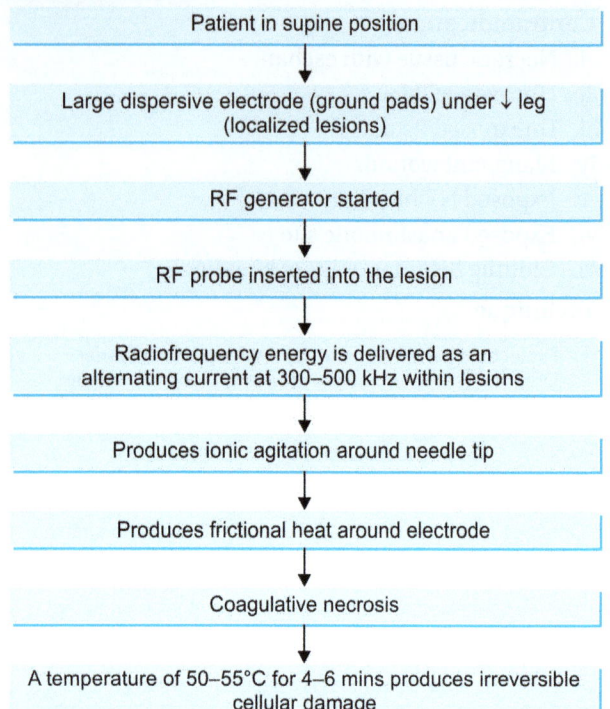

III. TYPES

1. Monopolar
2. Bipolar

Monopolar	Bipolar
• Circuit is completed inside the patient (patient is a part of circuit)	• Completed with the lesion
• Grounding pads (+)	• No
• Multiple lesions cannot be treated at same time	• Can be ablated at same time
• Arrhythmias (+)	• (−)

IV. ELECTRODE BLADE DESIGNS (FIG. 8)

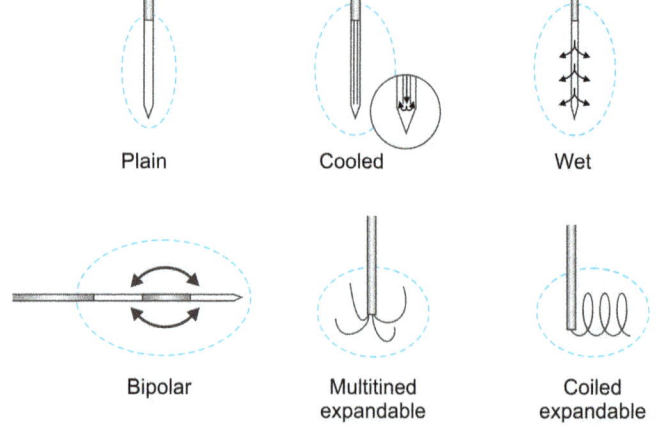

V. USES

1. Osteoid osteoma
2. RFA ablation of genicular nerves (medial, lateral) → For pain relief in OA knee → Effects for 6 months
3. RFA annuloplasty → for treatment of discogenic back pain

OZONE THERAPY

I. INTRODUCTION

1. Alternative medical technique that increases oxygen in the body through the introduction of O_3 (Ozone)
2. O_3: Highly unstable soluble gas with great oxidizing activity.
3. Mixture of O_3 and O_2 in a ratio of 0.1–5% O_3 and 95–99.5% O_2

II. MECHANISM OF ACTION

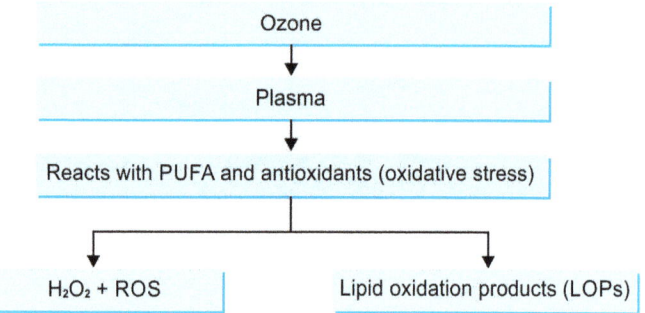

1. Sudden rise in H_2O_2 concentration
2. Rapid transfer into blood cells
3. Nuclear – erythroid – 2 – related factor activation (NRF-2)
4. ↑ Antioxidant activation → Free radical scavengers
5. ROS + LOPS react with WBCs

   Formation of proteins, cytokines, red blood cells

   ↑ tissue oxygenation
6. O_3 stimulates anti-nociceptive apparatus

   Raises pain threshold → Recovery of muscles and joint function.
7. Neoangiogenesis → ↑ blood supply
   i. Antimicrobial.
   ii. Immune modulating → Anti-inflammatory
   iii. Immune stimulating

III. APPLICATIONS

1. Musculoskeletal tissue repair:
   i. O_2 → ROS → Immediate effect
      → LOP → Late effect
      ↓
      Stimulate neurotransmitters, metabolism, hormones, CNS and endocrine
   ii. ↑IL-8 → Migration of leukocytes into tissues
       ↓
       Phagocytosis of bacteria and necrotic tissue of ulcers
   iii. PDGF, TGF-β
2. Adhesive capsulitis:
   i. Intra-articular O_3 inj.
   ii. ↑ROM, ↓Pain, better muscle relaxation
3. Hip bursitis
4. OA knee: Periarticular, intraarticular or SC injection
   Reduces degenerative process
5. Carpal tunnel syndrome: Indirect vessel mediated decompression of nerve roots.
6. Partial supraspinatus tear
7. Subacromial bursitis
8. Lumbar facet joint syndrome
9. Cervical disc herniation.
10. Chronic LBA
    ↓
    Proteoglycans oxidized → Osmotic pressure ↓
    ↓
    Volume of NP shrinks.
11. RA
12. Fibromyalgia
13. LSS

IV. CONTRAINDICATIONS

1. Pregnancy: Mutagenic risk
2. Hyperthyroidism
3. Severe anemia
4. Thrombocytopenia
5. CVS instability
6. Patient on ACE inhibitors

V. SIDE EFFECTS

1. O_3 toxicity
2. Gas embolism.
3. Pulmonary edema
4. Myocardial infarction
5. Muscle tears
6. Tendon ruptures
7. Hypersensitivity

VASCULARIZED FIBULA GRAFT

I. INTRODUCTION

Vascularized bone grafts allow living bone tissue (autograft) to be transplanted to an adjacent (pedicle) or remote (free) location and survive by maintenance and restoration of blood flow due to microvascular anastomosis.

II. ADVANTAGES AND BIOLOGY

1. Vascularity intact → Immediately viable (remain alive)
2. Does not undergo "Creeping substitution" or resorption as blood supply intact (no osteopenia), therefore decreased incidence of stress fracture.
3. Incorporates into adjacent host bone via 2° bone healing.
4. ↑ Mechanical strength, structural integrity.
   ↓
   Immediate stability
5. Rapid union, bone hypertrophy in response to applied stress over time.
6. Biomechanical fibula bears only 15% axial load across ankle → Minimal consequences on weight bearing.
7. Restoring longitudinal growth by inclusion of proximal growth plate → pediatrics (distal radius).
8. Revascularizing adjacent necrotic bone.
9. Improving local blood supply in scarred soft tissue beds.
10. Composite tissue loss reconstruction in single procedure → inclusion of skin, muscles, tendon and nerves.
11. Union even in bone damaged by chemotherapy and irradiation.

III. INDICATIONS (FIG. 9)

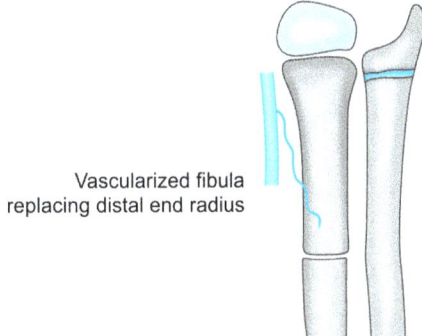

Vascularized fibula replacing distal end radius

Segmental bone defects (> 6–8 cm)	Biological failure of bone healing
• Traumatic bone loss	• ON hip
• Tumor resection	• Congenital pseudarthrosis tibia
• Osteomyelitis	• Persistent NU
• Infected nonunion	• Spinal fusion (TB spine)
	• Joint arthrodesis
	• Femur neck fracture

IV. PRINCIPLES AND TECHNIQUE

1. Preserve distal 5 cm fibula → avoids subsequent ankle instability and deformity.

2. Endosteal blood supply → Nutrient artery branch of peroneal artery.
   ↓
   Enters posterior fibular cortex at the junction of proximal 1/3rd and distal 2/3rd.
3. Preserve the multiple segmental musculoperiosteal vessels.
4. Usage → Isolated vascular bone graft
   → Osteomuscular flaps
   → Osteocutaneous flaps

Technique

1. Longitudinal incision over lateral aspect of fibula
   ↓
2. Superficial dissection → PL (anterior) and soleus (posterior)
3. Diaphysis circumferentially exposed preserving periosteum and its blood supply (marbled appearance)
4. Deep circumferential dissection → PL (anterior) and FHL (posterior)
5. Inter muscular septum divided protecting the peroneal artery and vein
6. Fibula osteotomized proximally and distally
7. Stabilization at recipient site and the microvascular anastomoses **(Fig. 10)**

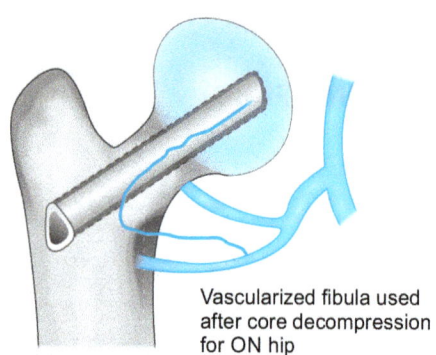

Vascularized fibula used after core decompression for ON hip

V. CONTRAINDICATIONS

1. Absence of vessels at donor or recipient site
2. PVD
3. DVT
4. Ankle instability, pain

VI. COMPLICATIONS

A. Early
i. Uncontrolled bleeding at fracture site
ii. Vessel thrombosis → Graft failure
iii. Torsion of vascular pedicle
iv. Inadequate peroneal pedicle length
v. Donor site morbidity

B. Late
i. Delayed union
ii. Stress fracture
iii. Infection

INTRAMEDULLARY NAILING– RECENT ADVANCES

I. PROXIMAL FEMORAL NAIL A2 (PFN–A2)

1. Indicated in intertrochanteric and subtrochanteric fractures
2. Insertion of PFNA: II blade compacts the cancellous bone → provides additional anchoring and rotational stability **(Fig. 11)**.

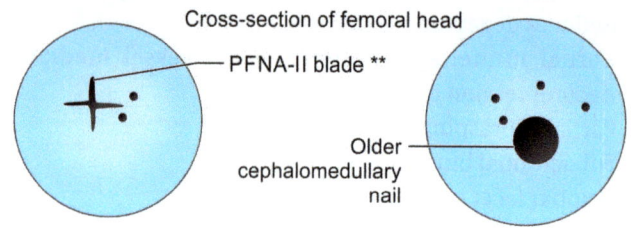

3. Higher cut out resistance
4. Larger surface → Maximal compaction and hold in osteoporotic bone

II. TRIGEN INTERTAN (FIG. 12)

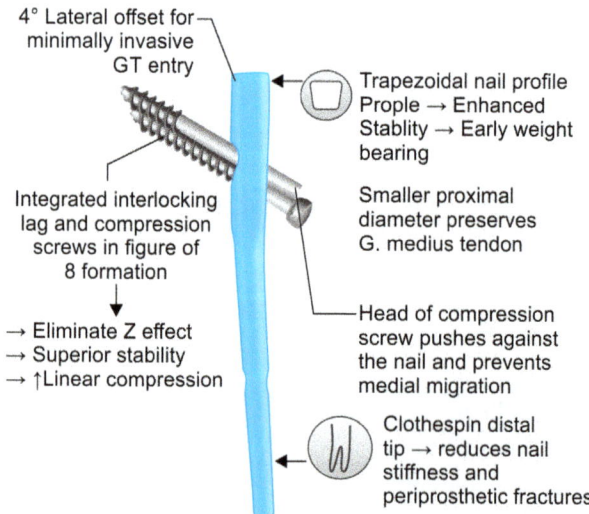

Indications
i. Intertrochanteric
ii. Subtrochanteric
iii. Femoral shaft fractures

III. TITANIUM ELASTIC NAILING SYSTEM (FIG. 13)

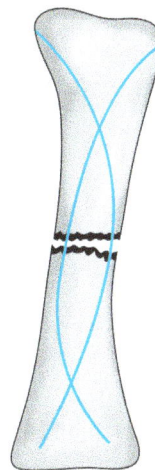

a. Mostly indicated in pediatric pts.
   i. Diaphyseal and certain metaphyseal fracture
   ii. Subcapital humerus fracture
   iii. Epiphyseal fracture (e.g., radial neck)
b. Adult patients
   i. Clavicle osteosynthesis
   ii. Forearm
   iii. Humerus fractures
c. TENS are bent and inserted
   ↓
   3-point fixation → Translational, bending and axial stability
d. Maximum divergence between 2 TENS at fracture site.

IV. EXPERT TIBIA NAIL

1. Indication → Proximal tibia fracture. Distal tibia fractures.
2. Multidirectional interlocking screws → Maintain alignment and stability in short proximal and distal tibia segments.
3. End cap achieves angular stability between proximal oblique screw and nail.

V. MULTILOC NAILING SYSTEM

1. For proximal humerus fractures.
2. Preserves hypovascular supraspinatus foot – print
3. Blunt screw tip → ↓ risk of 2° perforation
4. Suture holes → attachment of rotator cuff
5. Countersunk screw heads → ↓ Impingement.

VI. ACUMED FIBULAR ROD SYSTEM

1. Fibular plating → Hardware irritation, deep wound infection (elderly, diabetics)
2. Fibular rod system → Minimally invasive
   → Slot for syndesmotic screw
   → Good fracture stability

VII. REAMER IRRIGATOR ASPIRATOR

1. ↓ Intramedullary pressure
2. ↓ Fat embolism
3. ↓ Heat generation
4. ↓ Infected tissue

VIII. ANTIBIOTIC COATED IM NAIL WITH GROWTH FACTOR → rBMP

1. 2 layers of polymer on nail.
2. Superficial → Antibiotic nanoparticles.
3. Deep → Growth factor nanoparticles.

IX. COMPOSITE IM NAILING SYSTEM

1. Titanium alloys → High rigidity
   ↓
   Nail bears majority of load
   ↓
   Stress shielding effect
2. Hybrid composite of carbon fiber/epoxy
   ↓
   Decreased stress shielding

X. NAVIGATION

Conventional manual entry and locking
↓
Trial and error
↓
↑ Fluoroscopy exposures. Multiple bone drills. Surgical navigation → Laser guided robot reduces the above.

XI. DRUG ELUTING HEPARINIZED TITANIUM (Ti)

Surgical of Ti nail functionalized with heparin
↓
Gentamycin and BMP-2 sequentially attached to heparinized surface.

XII. INTRAMEDULLARY BONE STENT

1. Radial expansion → Circumferential stress at fracture site
2. Longitudinal contraction → Restores fracture.

XIII. INTRAMEDULLARY BONE TRANSPORT

Nonunion → Bone defect.

RECENT ADVANCES IN THR

RECENT ADVANCES AND IMPLANTS

1. **Short stem hip replacement (Proxima) (Fig. 14)**

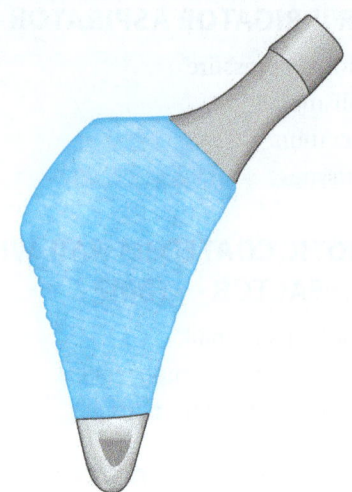

   i. Preserves more bone than THR
   ii. Prerequisites: Bone stock intact.
       Resurfacing unsuitable.
       ↓
       Extensive disease in head (ON)
   iii. Shaft → Not reamed.
   iv. Neck portion preserved.
       Soft tissue dissection
       Large diameter head → ↓ Dislocation

2. **Hip resurfacing:** (Write from SAQ)
3. **Dual mobility THR (Fig. 15)**

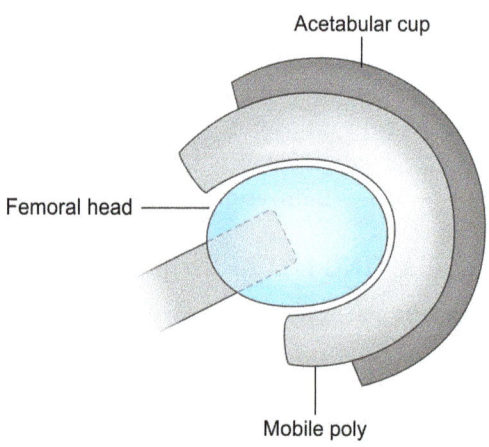

   i. ↓ Rate of dislocation.
   ii. ↑ ROM before impingement
   iii. ↓ Wear
   iv. Indications:
       a. Non-compliant patient → Dementia, alcohol
       b. Tumors
       c. ↑ Joint laxity
       d. Elderly

4. **Minimally invasive THR**

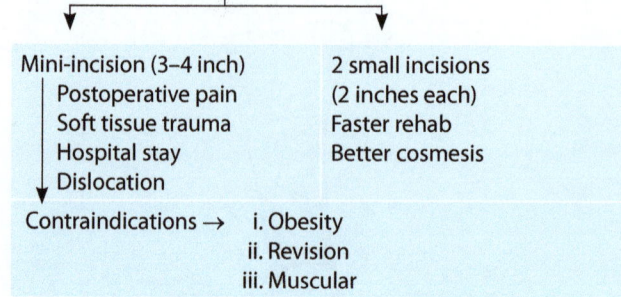

   Contraindications →
   i. Obesity
   ii. Revision
   iii. Muscular

5. **Direct anterior approach** → Bikini incision
   i. Best cosmesis
   ii. No disruption of short ER → ↓ Dislocation
   iii. Incision → 2 cm distal and lateral to ASIS. Sartorius and TFL plane
   iv. Femur approached by hyperextension, adduction and external rotation
   v. Disadvantage → Steep learning curve

6. **Robotic THR**
   i. MAKO system—most popular (Stryker)
   ii. 3D plan based on preoperative CT
   iii. Accurate bone preparation using robot assisted reamers
   iv. Better placement of implant
       ↓
       ↓ LLD, better offset, COR of hip

7. **3D printed implants:** Useful especially in revision cases with bone loss or tumor surgeries.

8. **Oxynium on poly bearing**
   Oxynium → Oxidized zirconium
   ↓
   Metallic alloy with ceramic surface
   ↓
   Wear resistance, without brittleness, chipping, and sweaking

9. **S-ROM stem**
   i. Modular femoral component
   ii. Stem and neck
   iii. Adjust anteversion, neck length and offset
   iv. Useful in cases of dysplasia

10. **M-L Taper hip prosthesis**
    Slim anteroposterior dimension
    ↓
    Preserves bone stock while providing M-L stability

VISCOSUPPLEMENTATION

I. INTRODUCTION

Injection of exogenous hyaluronic acid into diarthrodial joints.

II. PROPERTIES

1. Hyaluronic acid → High viscosity polysaccharide
   ↓
   Glycosaminoglycan (GAG)
   ↓
2. Produced naturally by β cells of the synovial membrane.
3. Under physiological conditions, it behaves as a salt → Sodium hyaluronate
4. Acts as a →
   i. Lubricant
   ii. Shock absorber

III. MECHANISM OF ACTION

1. Biomechanical
   i. Promotes better force distribution
      ↓
   ii. Decreased pressure on joint
      ↓
   iii. Recovers the rheological properties of the synovial fluid.
2. Biochemical
   i. Diminishes the gene expression of
      ↓
   ii. Cytokines and other enzymes associated with progression of OA
      ↓
   iii. Decreased prostaglandin and intra-articular metalloproteinase concentration.
   iv. Stimulates production of hyaluronic acid by synoviocytes
3. Analgesic
   → Diminishes nerve impulse and sensitivity of nociceptive nerve ends.
4. Chondroprotective
   Stabilizes the cartilaginous matrix
      ↓
   Stimulates chondrocyte proliferation.
5. Collagen
   Collagen type II and aggrecan production
      ↓
   Diminishes degradation of type II collagen.

IV. SOURCE

Exogenous HA

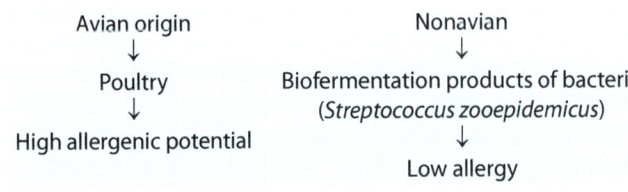

Molecular weight =   Low = 0.5×10^6 D
                     High = 6×10^6 D

V. INDICATIONS

1. Osteoarthritis → knee (early stages)
   i. Recovers viscoelastic properties
   ii. Analgesia
   iii. Improves function and regenerate cartilage
2. After knee arthroscopy
   Anti-inflammatory and analgesia.

VI. TECHNIQUE (FIG. 16)

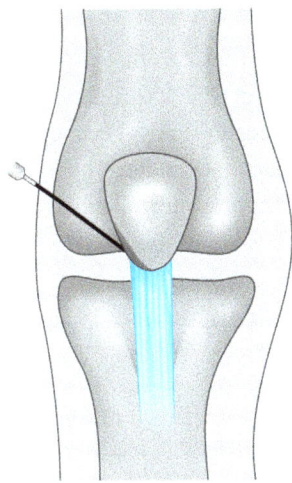

1. Under AAP, in OT
2. Sterile needle inserted lateral to patellar tendon (1 cm) and 1cm above lateral tibial plateau
3. Knee in extension
4. Needle directed 30° from the anterior knee surface vertical midline toward the intraarticular joint space

VII. RESULTS

1. Results take → 6–12 weeks to act
2. Effect lasts for 6 months after which the injection can be repeated
3. More effective than IA steroids
   ↓
   First 4 weeks not superior to steroids
   ↓
   Combination increases initial results of viscosupplementation

VIII. ADR

1. Effusion
2. Arthralgia
3. Pseudosepsis → Aseptic synovitis with warmth and large joint effusion.

IX. DISADVANTAGES

1. Efficacy uncertain: Contradictory reports in literature
2. Costly

STEM CELLS

I. INTRODUCTION

1. *Stem cells:* Undeveloped and undifferentiated biological cells capable of proliferation, self-renewal, conversion to differentiated cells and regenerating tissues.
2. Defined by its ability of **self-renewal**
   ↓
   Asymmetric division
   Restricted to one germ layer.
3. *Totipotent:* Cells that can develop into any cell type of human body along with forming placental cells
   → Only zygote (fertilized egg) is truly totipotent.
4. *Pluripotent:* Cells that can develop into cells of all 3 germ layers (ectoderm, mesoderm, endoderm)
   → Embryonic stem cells: Not used.
   Tumorigenesis ↔ Ethical concerns.
5. *Multipotent:* Cells that can develop into multiple lineages of a single germ layer.

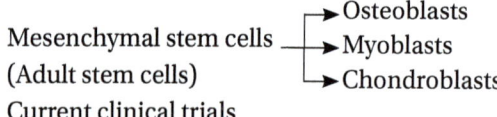

Mesenchymal stem cells → Osteoblasts, Myoblasts, Chondroblasts
(Adult stem cells)
Current clinical trials

II. APPLICATIONS

1. **Spinal cord injury**

   i. Background

   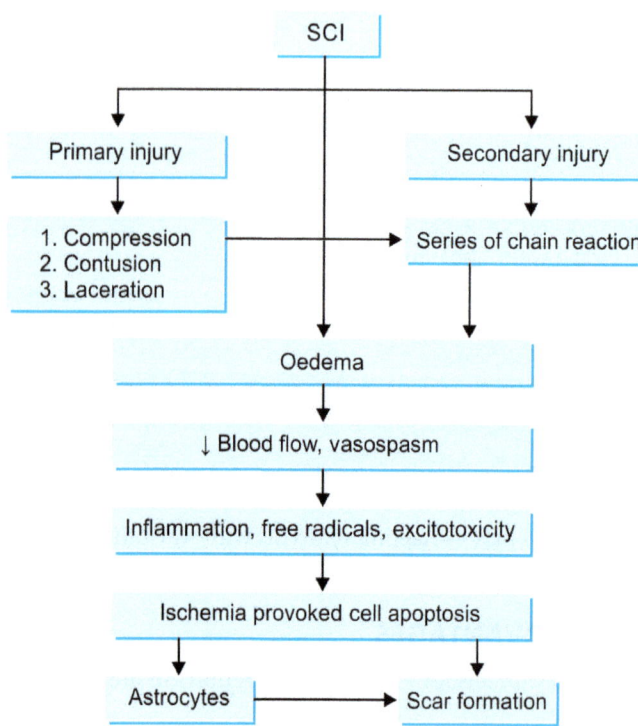

   ii. Rationale

   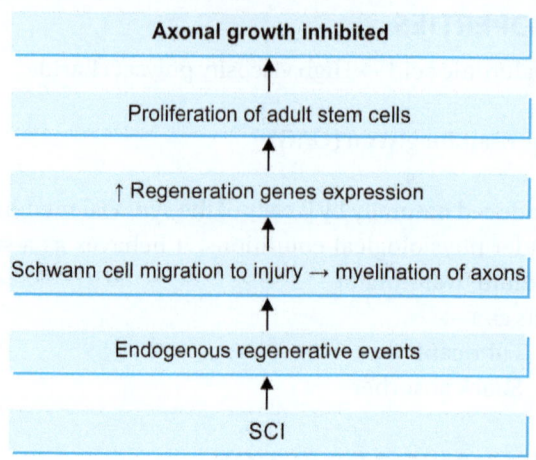

   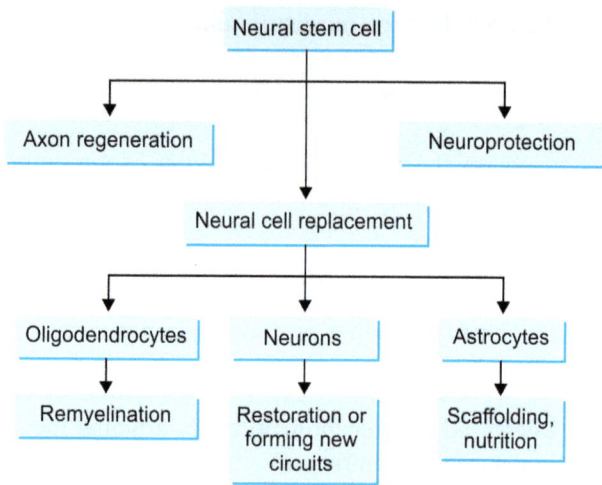

   iii. Administration route → Intrathecal
                              Intramedullary.

Intrathecal	Intramedullary
• ↓ Invasive	• ↑ Invasive
• ↑ No. of stem cells	• ↓ Stem cells needed
• (Homing) travel to site of injury ↓ Subarachnoid adhesions are barrier	• ∴ ↑ Effective
	• ↓ Side effects:
	– Intramedullary hemorrhage
	– CSF leakage
	– Additional injury

   iv. **Timing**
       Acute: <3 days.
       Chronic: >12 months
       Subacute: 3–12 months
       ↓
       Best stem cell survival.

   v. **Evaluation**
       a. Neurologic improvement
       b. ADL
       c. Electrophysiological studies
       d. Diagnostic MRI → Diffusion tensor imaging

vi. **Future prospects**
   Spinal cord synthetic scaffolds impregnated with stem cells.
vii. **Source of MSCs**

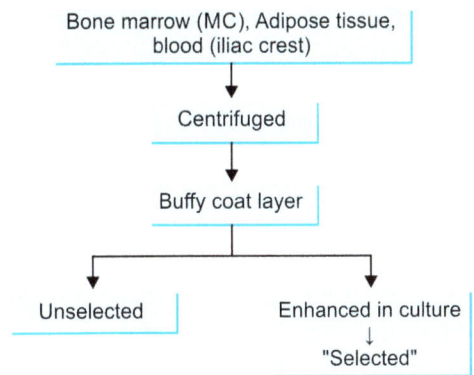

viii. **MOA**

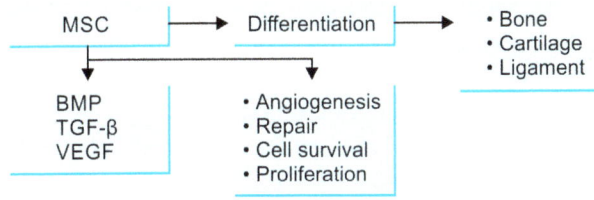

2. **Trauma and bone defects** → trauma and tumour.

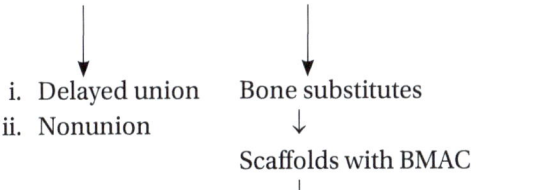

   a. No shortage
   b. ↓ Risk infection
   c. No donor site morbidity
3. **Spinal fusion**
4. **IVD degeneration**
   Percutaneous stem cell injection
   ↓
   i. ↑ Proteoglycans
   ii. Disc height maintained
5. Peripheral nerve injuries
6. Focal cartilage damage
   Autologous stem cell implantation
7. OA → MSC inhibit catabolic activity of MMP
8. HTO → Better osteointegration
9. Future → biologic arthroplasty
   3D printed scaffolds with MSC → Osteochondral grafts.
10. ON → Along with core decompression.
11. Wound healing - Open facture, Diabetes.
12. Bone tendon interface and tendon healing
    MSC → ↑ Sharpey fibers
    i. ACL, Menisci
    ii. Rotator cuff injuries
    iii. Retrocalcaneal bursitis
    iv. TA
13. Pediatric orthopedics
    i. Osteogenesis imperfecta: Systemic injection
       ↓
       ↑ Bone mass and growth.
    ii. Physeal injuries
14. Osteoporosis → ↑ trabecular bone and ↑density
15. Muscular dystrophies
    Muscle derived stem cells prevent conversion of muscles → fibrous tissue.

BIOABSORBABLE IMPLANTS

I. DEFINITION
Implants that are degraded in a biological environment, with the breakdown products being incorporated into normal cellular physiological processes or being excreted by the body.

II. RATIONALE
Developed to address issues with conventional non-absorbable implants including:
1. Migration
2. Growth disturbance
3. Rigidity
4. Radiopacity/interference with other imaging modalities
5. Infection
6. Need for implant removal operations

III. TYPES AND PROPERTIES
1. Bioabsorbable implants use polymers known as alpha-polyesters or poly (alpha-hydroxy) acids. *Namely:*
   i. **Poly lactic acid (PLA)**
      a. Molecular weight: 180,000–530,000 Da
      b. Melting point 174°C
      c. Slowest rate of degradation
      d. PLLA-Poly L lactic Acid (Levorotatory isomer) used most extensively as it retains the original strength the longest.
   ii. **Poly glycolic acid (PGA)**
      a. Molecular weight: 20,000–145,000 Da
      b. Melting point 230°C
      c. Intermediate absorption
   iii. **Polydioxanone (PDS)**
      a. Fastest degrading polymer (smallest molecular weight)
      b. May be absorbed completely by 6 months
2. These materials are used either as homopolymers/copolymers with each other → Improves the mechanical and degradation properties.

3. Degradation rate and thereby mechanical strength is affected by numerous factors:
   i. Molecular weight of the polymer
   ii. L/D isomers
   iii. Amorphous/crystalline form
   iv. Co-polymers with different properties
   v. Porosity
   vi. Loading conditions and local vascularity
   vii. Sterilization method

IV. DEGRADATION AND ELIMINATION

1. Principle route of elimination → Respiration
2. To a smaller extent → Urine and feces
3. Degradation occurs by:
   i. Hydrolysis (predominantly)
   ii. Non-specific enzymatic action (to a lesser extent)
   Mechanism of degradation and elimination

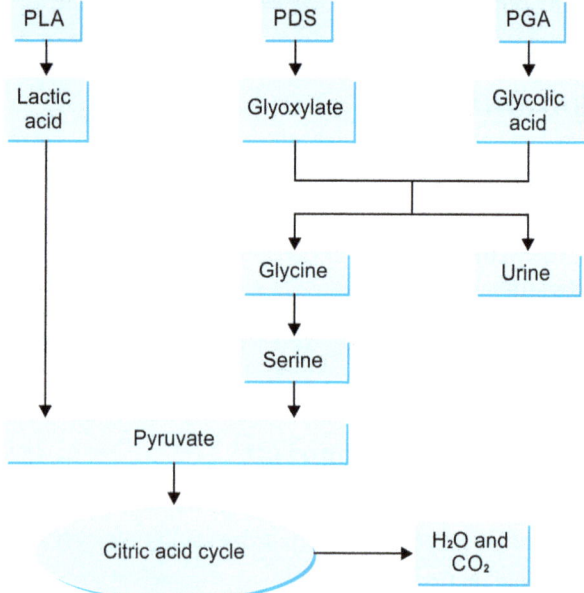

V. ADVANTAGES

1. Limit stress shielding (less stiff than conventional metallic implants) → ↓ osteopenia
2. Gradually apply load as they degrade → stimulate bone healing by Wolff's law
3. No interference in postoperative imaging
4. No need for a second procedure for implant removal
5. Can be antibiotic releasing, enabling use as antibiotic delivery devices/preventing postoperative infections
6. Can be used in locations where conventional implants cannot, e.g., intra-articularly, across growth plates

VI. DRAWBACKS

1. Inadequate stiffness: Weak compared to a metallic implant
2. Needs a period of immobilization
3. Low modulus of elasticity: Screws back out
4. High cost

VII. COMPLICATIONS

1. Delayed inflammatory reaction/sterile inflammatory foreign body reaction
   i. Erythematous, fluctuant swelling suddenly develops over healed wound
   ii. Mean interval between surgery and reaction has 12 weeks
2. Failure of fixation
3. Postoperative wound infection
4. Host tissue reaction-osteolysis, synovitis, hypertrophic fibrous encapsulation

VIII. CLINICAL APPLICATIONS

1. Bioabsorbable suture anchors
2. Bioabsorbable meniscus repair arrow: All inside meniscus repair
3. Osteochondral fracture fixation
4. Pediatric-fixing of physeal fractures, pediatric implants- no need of removal
5. Bioabsorbable mini plates for hand and foot surgery
6. Bioabsorbable spinal cages and anterior cervical plates

TRANEXAMIC ACID IN ORTHOPEDICS

I. INTRODUCTION

1. Antifibrinolytic agent
2. Prevents excessive blood loss in major orthopedic surgeries
   i. Spine → Scoliosis
   ii. Joint Replacement → Hip and knee arthroplasty (Primary and Revision)
3. Reduces ongoing blood loss if given early on in cases of polytrauma (CRASH – 2 trials)

II. MECHANISM

1. Analog of amino acid lysine
2. Reversibly binds on 4 to 5 lysine receptors on plasminogen. Prevents plasminogen to plasmin formation

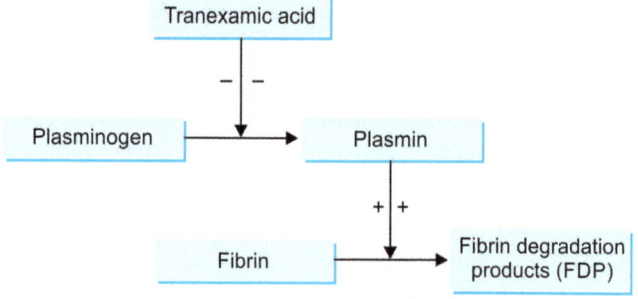

3. Fibrin is not broken down to FDP, thus reducing bleeding,

III. MODE OF ADMINISTRATION

1. Intravenous → 15 mg/kg
2. Oral
3. Intra-articular → 3 g

IV. SIDE EFFECTS

1. Blurring of vision
2. Seizures
3. Renal effects
4. Allergic reactions
5. Rapid infusion → Hypotension

V. CONTRAINDICATIONS

1. DVT/PE within 1 year
2. Patient on anticoagulants
3. CKD patients
4. Allergy

DAY CARE SURGERY

I. INTRODUCTION

1. Daycare surgery, also known as outpatient surgery, office-based surgery, same day surgery or ambulatory surgery does not require an overnight hospital stay.
2. Patient → Admitted, operated upon and discharged home on the same calendar day.
3. Usually, a stay of 4–6 hours is required but with more complex surgical procedures, longer stays may be required.

II. FACTORS

Patient related	Surgery related
• Young • Motivated • Compliant to postoperative protocol	• Postoperative care must be specific but is neither intensive nor prolonged and will not lead to unexpected admissions to the hospital • The risk of intra and postoperative blood loss should be low • Duration less than 90 min • Postoperative pain easily controlled • During the surgery there should not be unnecessary tissue traction, tension, manipulation, minimal ischemia and complete hemostasis.

III. INDICATIONS

A. Minimally Invasive

1. Local hydrocortisone injection
2. Joint aspiration
3. Needle biopsy
4. Skeletal traction

B. Endoscopic Procedures

1. Discectomy
2. Arthroscopy: Diagnostic/therapeutic
3. Epidural injection

C. Open Procedure

1. *Trauma:*
    i. Fracture fixation (Radius-Ulna)
    ii. External fixator application
    iii. Implant removal
2. *Infective:*
    i. Incision and drainage
    ii. Wound wash
3. *Open biopsy:* Infection, tumor
4. *Excision biopsy:* Bursa, ganglion, lipoma
5. *Contracture release:* Polio, cerebral palsy
6. *Soft tissue release:* Carpal tunnel syndrome, trigger finger, tenosynovitis
7. UKR, TKR

IV. ADVANTAGES

1. More economical for the patient in comparison to inpatient surgery.
2. Earlier mobilization.
3. Reduced risk of cross-infection.
4. Pre-booked date and less likely to be cancelled.
5. Shorter waiting lists and lesser uncertainty of a long wait.
6. Easier domestic arrangements.
7. Minimal disruption of patient's personal life.
8. Earlier return to the normal environment.
9. Avoidance of disruptive nights in hospital wards.
10. Less loss of time at work.
11. Less psychological disturbances in children and elderly patient.
12. Increased revenue generation for the hospital.

V. CONTRAINDICATIONS

Patient and surgical factors that are relative contraindications to outpatient TJA	
Patient or surgical factor	Comments
Patient factors	
Advanced age	Patients 75 years of age at risk for complications and readmission
ASA physical status	Increased risk for readmission after TJA in patients who are ASA physical status > III
Cardiac disease	Not well studied in outpatient TJA
COPD	Increased risk for postoperative pulmonary complications

Contd...

Contd...

Patient or surgical factor	Comments
Smoking	Impaired wound healing; increased risk for periprosthetic infection; increased risk for postoperative pulmonary complications
Chronic kidney disease or urinary retention	Increased risk for postoperative complications; risk for delayed discharge and Foley catheter placement
Chronic liver disease	Increased risk for postoperative complications
BMI > 35 kg/m²	BMI >40 kg/m² associated with postoperative complications; many centers use lower cutoff
Poorly controlled diabetes mellitus	HbA1C >8% associated with worse outcome
Hyper- or hypocoagulability	Management of anticoagulants challenging
Anemia	Increased risk for infection and delayed discharge
Parkinson's disease	Increased risk for falls
Opioid tolerance, alcohol abuse postoperative pain may be more difficult to control history, substance abuse history, severe anxiety or depression	Postoperative pain may be more difficult to control
Surgical factors	
Bilateral surgery	Pain and ambulation may be too difficult
Revision surgery	Longer duration of surgery and potentially greater postoperative pain
Bleeding disorder History of DVT/PE	

NAVIGATION AND ROBOTICS

I. INTRODUCTION

1. Computer navigation surgery systems monitor progress and provide surgeons with real time data for surgical procedures.
2. Used pre, during and post-surgery.

II. RATIONALE FOR USE

1. Improving surgical planning.
2. ↑ Accuracy of planned surgery.
3. Handling compromised situations—like improving the consistency of surgery in MISS.
4. Pedicular screw placement → ↓ canal penetration
5. Improving the undefined procedures—like the revision cases where most of the local landmarks are absent but overall alignment can be assessed by the computed systems.
6. Complicated fractures have comminution and the restoration of weight-bearing columns is difficult → restored using the computed systems.
7. Deformity correction → Hex Ilizarov → Taylors spatial frame → connected to software.

Joint Arthroplasties

1. Assessing joint irregularities and joint biomechanics.
2. To monitor the accuracy of the bone cuts.
3. Plan the component placement in advance.
4. To make recommendations on ligament balancing (TKA), vertical and horizontal offsets, acetabular version and inclination (THA).
5. Measure the intraoperative placement of the components in real-time.
6. Assess the postoperative alignment/placement with respect to (w.r.t.) preoperative plan.

III. ADVANTAGES

1. Restore accurate limb alignment.
2. Increase the survival of implanted joint → Secondary to better placement.
3. Constant guidance and monitoring during surgery.
4. Reduce the risk of complications related to implant fitting.
5. Secondary assistance during MISS procedures.
6. Decreased hospital stay
7. Record keeping of the surgery for later analysis.
8. No radiation during surgery.
9. Intraoperative range of motion analysis to achieve maximum function.

IV. DISADVANTAGES

1. Increased blood loss
2. Increased operative time
3. Increased risk of general complications like fat embolism, infection, atelectasis, etc., due to prolonged surgery
4. Cost
5. High learning curve (First 3 complications can be reduced at a high volume center)

V. WORKING

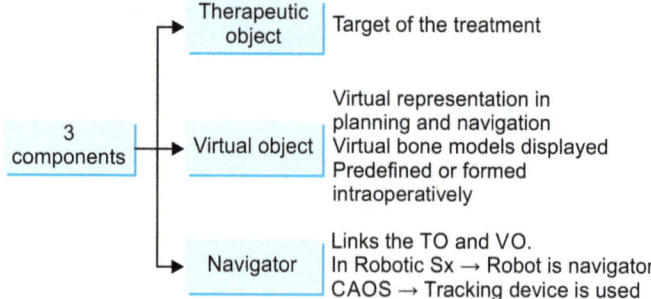

1. Navigator is the central element of CAOS → establishes a 3D coordinate system.
2. Localized the current orientation of surgical instruments (End effectors).
3. End effectors maybe → Passive (Navigation/CAOS), semiactive or active (Robots).
4. The navigation systems → many cameras → track surgical instrumentation, bony geometry and alignment.
5. Positioned above the patient and communicate with instruments and bony landmarks through light-emitting diodes (LEDs) or infrared rays.
6. The surgeon always has the option to override the information given by the computer.

Robotics "Forced Labor"

A machine that automatically carries out various tasks, requires little or no assistance from outside and can be programmable.

Two categories: (1) Haptic (or tactile or surgeon-guided) and (2) Autonomous system.

1. **Haptic:** Requires surgeon's continuous input for efficiently performing and completing surgery. The surgeon uses or drives the robot to perform an operation.
   UKR application:
   i. Surgeon's participation is must to complete UKR.
   ii. 3D computer model of the knee is prepared with the use of computed tomography (CT) scans preoperatively, which forms the basis of preoperative planning.
   iii. Based on this, surgeon marks the bony surfaces of femur and tibia during operation.
   iv. After taking the knee through a full range of motion, the flexion-extension gaps assessed, component size and implant placement finalized and a cutting zone is created for the robot. Preoperative planning and templating process forms the base for the system's algorithm.
   v. By viewing the 3D model of the knee on the monitor, the surgeon accurately manipulates the burr and resects the bone.
   vi. Forced controlled tip of the rotating burr cannot resect the bone outside the predefined cutting space.
   vii. The safety system automatically stops the burr when the surgeon goes beyond the cutting zone.
   viii. Smaller incisions, short recovery and rehabilitation time, hence can be performed as an outpatient procedure.
2. **Autonomous**
   Autonomous systems differ from the above by having more independency.
   After the operative site is approached by the surgeon, he sets up the machine and then engages the robot, which completes the remaining task, without the help of a surgeon.

ISOKINETIC EXERCISES

I. INTRODUCTION

1. Resistance training exercises are done to increase muscle strength → exercises cause muscles to contract against an external resistance.
2.

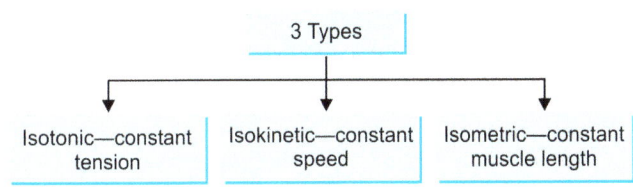

3. 'Iso' – same, 'kinetic' – speed
4. Isokinetic exercise involves muscle contractions at a constant speed throughout the entire range of motion.
5. Unlike isotonic exercises where the resistance varies with joint angle, isokinetic exercises employ specialized equipment that provides accommodating resistance, ensuring that the resistance matches the force exerted by the muscle at any given point in the range of motion.
6. This allows for maximal muscle activation across the entire movement, minimizing stress on joints and reducing the risk of injury.
7. ∴ It is also known as accommodating variable-resistance exercise.
8. It is an effective form of endurance and strength training, being carried out with the help of specialized machines → Dynamometers
9. Useful in Rehabilitation phase, and is considered to be much safer in rehabilitation of muscle and ligament injuries.
10. Machines used have the following components:
    i. Computer system
    ii. Dynamometer
    iii. Attachment for body parts – wrist, elbow, knee

II. TYPES

1. Concentric-concentric
2. Concentric-eccentric
3. Eccentric-eccentric

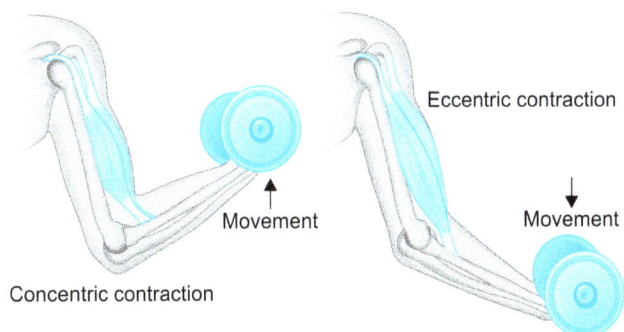

III. ADVANTAGES

1. The controls are preset → ∴ Patient cannot over exercise and there are no jerky movements
   ↓
   Less muscle strain and soreness
2. Prevents future injuries → As it ↑ balance by increasing strength and flexibility.
3. Muscles are trained throughout the entire range of motion – in a controlled and even manner.
4. Data obtained during exercise can be quantified and studied.
5. Monitors the response to treatment.
6. Useful in training targeted muscles.
7. Patient recovery:
   i. Athletes after injury
   ii. Athletes after surgery
   iii. Stroke patients

IV. DISADVANTAGES

1. Type of exercise movement does not reflect actual functional performance tasks.
2. High Cost
3. Availability is less
4. Specialized machines require space.
5. Requires trained professionals for carrying them out.

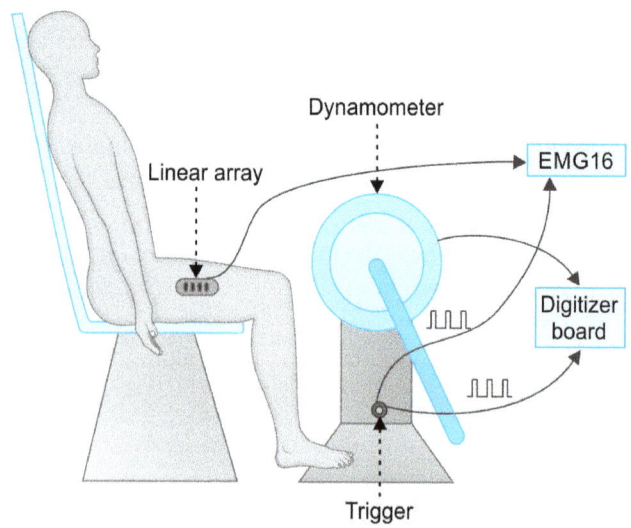

Fig. 2: Instrumentation architecture

TENS THERAPY (TRANSCUTANEOUS ELECTRICAL NERVE STIMULATION)

I. INTRODUCTION

1. Transcutaneous Electrical Nerve Stimulation delivers electricity across the intact surface of the skin to activate the underlying nerves.
2. Simple, non-invasive modality used for analgesia.

II. PRINCIPLES OF NERVE FIBER ACTIVATION

1. Initial stimulation of non-nociceptive nerve fibers like A-alpha, A-beta fibers which have low threshold of stimulation causing tingling.
2. This is followed by activation of A-delta and C- fibers causing pain
3. Low intensity current with pulse duration 50–500 μs stimulates larger diameter fibers (A-beta) without activation of smaller diameter fibers (A-delta and C).
4. Pulse duration more than 500 μs activates small diameter fibers.

III. TYPICAL FEATURES OF TENS

Pulse wave form	• Monophasic • Symmetric biphasic • Asymmetric biphasic
Pulse amplitude (adjustable)	1–50 mA
Pulse duration	50–500 μs
Frequency	1–200 Hz
Pulse patterns	• Continuous • Burst
Channels	• Single • Double

IV. TYPES

	Conventional TENS (High)	Acupuncture-like TENS (Low)	Brief Intense TENS
Physiological intervention	To activate large diameter non-notious afferent to elicit segmental analgesia	To produce muscle twitch to activate small diameter motor affrent to elicit extra segmental analgesia	To activate small diameter noxious affrents to elicit peripheral nerve blockade and extra segmental analgesia
Clinical technique	Low intensity /High frequency at site of pain to produce strong but comfortable sensation	High intensity/ Low frequency over muscle or Acupuncture points to produce strong but comfortable contraction	High intensity/ High frequency to produce maximum parathesia
Duration of stimulation	30 minutes	No more than 20 minutes	No more than 5 minutes

V. BIOPHYSICAL EFFECTS

1. Primary use is to control pain through Gate Control Theory
2. May produce muscle contractions.

3. Mechanisms of action:
   a. High TENS → Activates A-delta fibers.
   b. Low TENS → Releases B-endorphins.
   c. Brief-Intense TENS → Noxious stimulation to active C fibers.

VI. INDICATIONS

A. Relief of Acute Pain
1. Physical trauma- fracture ribs, minor medical procedures
2. Postoperative pain
3. Orofascial pain
4. Dental procedures

B. Relief of Chronic Pain
a. Low back pain
b. Arthritic pain: RA, OA
c. Myofascial pain
d. Neuropathic pain—trigeminal neuralgia, phantom pain, post-herpes pain
e. Cancer pain
f. CRPS (complex regional pain syndrome)

C. Non-analgesic effects
1. Neuromuscular stimulating effects
2. Fecal and urinary incontinence
3. Post-chemotherapy
4. Improving blood flow
5. Wound healing
6. Fracture healing
7. Raynaud's disease

VII. ELECTRODE PLACEMENT
1. Directly over painful sites: Trigger points
2. Dermatomes, Myotomes
3. Acupuncture points
4. Spinal nerve roots
5. May be crossed or uncrossed
6. Horizontal or vertical

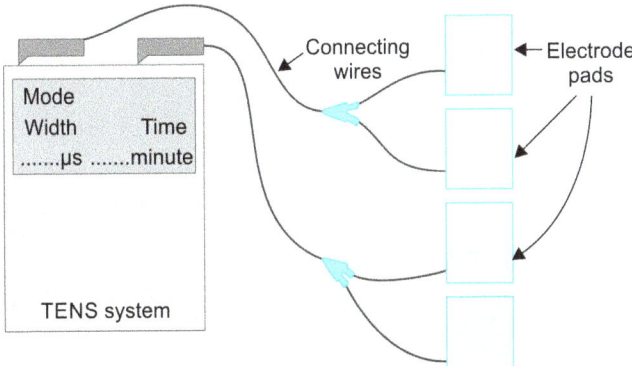

VIII. CONTRAINDICATIONS
1. Pacemakers
2. Cardiac conditions—arrhythmia
3. Over carotid sinus (vasovagal reflex)
4. Malignancy
5. Pregnancy
6. Active infections, Skin conditions
7. Areas over impaired or absent sensation
8. Neurological conditions: Epilepsy, stroke
9. Non-cooperative patients

IX. PRECAUTIONS/SIDE EFFECTS
1. Dysesthesia
2. Contact dermatitis
3. Autonomic reactions—nausea, dizziness, fainting

OT LIGHTS

I. INTRODUCTION
1. A well illuminated operative field is an absolute necessity for the operating surgeon for the best surgical outcome as well as for patients' safety.
2. OT lights are specifically designed to enable the surgical team to focus exclusively on the operation.
3. Majority of the OT lights operate with LED (light-emitting diode) → Use less energy to produce crisper and cooler illumination.

II. IDEAL CHARACTERISTICS OF OT LIGHT

A. Illumination
1. Ideal illumination at the center of 1m distance from light source: 120,000–160,000 Lux.
2. Illumination should be uniformly distributed to reduce the glare related eye strain.

B. Color Temperature (K)
1. It is the perceived coolness or warmth of light measure in Kelvin.
2. 4500K - day light (ideal light for human eye), 5500K - Bright sunlight
3. Modern day LED lights use → 4500K
4. Some LEDs can adjust color temperature → facilitating tissue differentiation.

C. Shadow Dilution
1. Ability of the surgical light to minimize the effect of obstructions.
2. Due to heads of surgeons in the operating field, there are chances of shadows being formed which reduces the effectivity of the light quality.

3. Shadows are influenced by the surface of the light source, how light is guided towards the field and the number of light sources.
4. More light beams improve the shadow dilution, improving the visibility of the surgical field.
5. An absence of cast shadow or coloured shadow is described as perfect shadow dilution.

D. Color Rendering Index (CRI)

1. CRI measures the ability of the light source to reveal various true colors at the operating field.
2. High CRI—indicates more colors can be differentiated and appreciated at the surgical fields when the light is on.
3. Low CRI—indicates colors cannot be differentiated in the surgical field. That is all the tissue colors appear as the same as color of the lighting source
4. Ideal OT light CRI: 85–100 (Natural daylight CRI = 100)

E. Depth of Illumination/Volume

1. Surgeons need illumination in three dimensions.
2. Merging several light patches—which are active at the same time at different heights create a uniform volume of light.
3. The best surgical light will have the highest volume of light at the cavity, even when the light is positioned more than one meter away from the surgical site.

F. Central Illuminance (Ec)

1. Illuminance (measured in Lux) at 1m distance from the light emitting surface in the light field center.

G. Light Field Diameter

1. Light field diameter, D10 refers to the diameter of light field around the light field center, ending where the illuminance reaches 10% of central illuminance (Ec).
2. D50 refers to the diameter of light field around the light field center, ending where the illuminance reaches of 50% of Ec.
3. Ideally, the D50 diameter should be at least 50% of D10.

H. Backup Possibility

1. In case of interruption of the power supply, the light should be restored within 5 seconds with at least 50% of the previous Lux intensity, but not less than 40,000 Lux.
2. Within 40 seconds the light should be completely restored to the original brightness.

III. PARTS OF THE OT LIGHT

1. <u>False roof ceiling</u> - is made at the intended position above the OT light. It usually will be present right above the OT Table.
2. <u>Main point (mount)</u> - is fixed to the false roof ceiling by screws, the mount acts as the center fixed point to which the stem gets attached.
3. <u>Stem</u> - is attached to the mount. It can be rotated 360° according to the need.
4. <u>Arms</u> - Stem is attached to various arms of the LED lights or the Camera screen. Number of arms depend upon the light system being used.
5. Arms can be rotated by 210° and moved up and down by 45°.

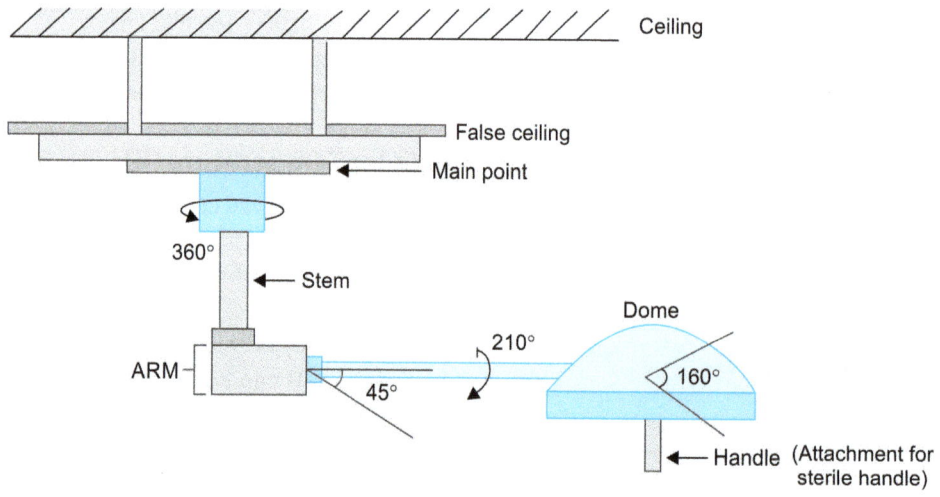

6. <u>Dual light system</u>
   i. One main light of 160,000 Lux and one satellite 120,000–1,40,000 Lux
   ii. Most commonly in general OT including orthopedic OT.

7. <u>Triple light system</u>
   i. One main light of 160,000 Lux and two satellites of 140,000 Lux.
   ii. Used in Cardiac OT.

8. Camera mounted OT light
    i. The third arm of the OT light will be connected to the monitor which displays the live video recording of the surgery being carried out.
    ii. Used in live surgery demonstration and recordings.
9. Dome - of the OT light is the rounded structure over which the LED lights are placed. This can be rotated by 160° by use of the handle.
10. Handle:
    i. Connected to the dome through which the surgeon can adjust the position of the light.
    ii. A sterilized detachable handle can be connected to this fixed handle. This enables the surgeon to adjust light intra-op without worrying about the sterility.

IV. RECOMMENDATIONS ON HOW TO USE LED LIGHTS

1. Positioning the light heads of the dome approximately 1m from the surgery field to improve the shadow dilution and best surgery field illumination.
2. Level of concentration of surgeon is enhanced by using an illumination similar to daylight - prevents the melatonin production which otherwise causes fatigue/exhaustion.
3. Start of the surgery day with 50% of intensity of the light.

EVIDENCE-BASED MEDICINE

1. Evidence-based medicine (EBM) is a scientific method that involves judicious and reasonable use of current data and evidence to improve healthcare decisions about individual patients.
2. It combines clinical experience and patient values with the best available research data.
3. There are 5 main steps for applying EBM to clinical practice:
    i. Formulating a clinically relevant question
    ii. Conducting a search for the best evidence
    iii. Critically appraising the evidence
    iv. Applying the evidence
    v. Evaluating the performance of EBM
4. EBM begins with a clinical question → an issue which the healthcare provider addresses with the patient.
5. Once the clinical question is identified, relevant scientific evidence related to the question, including study outcomes and opinions, is sought.
6. Differentiating the strength of data is important. For example, expert opinions are not as robust as a well conducted study, which is not as reliable as a set of well conducted RCTs.
7. ∴ Data should be graded based on its relative strength, with stronger evidence given more weight in clinical decision making.
8. EBM is commonly classified into 6 levels:
    i. Level IA: Meta-analysis of well-conducted RCTs, providing strong clinical evidence. Combined results enhance overall strength.
    ii. Level IB: Single well-conducted RCT, considered a gold standard in clinical medicine.
    iii. Level IIA: Well-designed non-randomized controlled study, with potential bias due to lack of randomization.
    iv. Level IIB: Case-control or cohort study, addressing clinical questions where randomized studies are not feasible or ethical.
    v. Level III: Non-experimental studies, including case series or poorly designed case-control/cohort studies.
    vi. Level IV: Expert opinions from respected authorities based on clinical experience.
9. Healthcare workers must apply their professional, clinical experience to interpret and apply the scientific evidence effectively to individual patient cases.

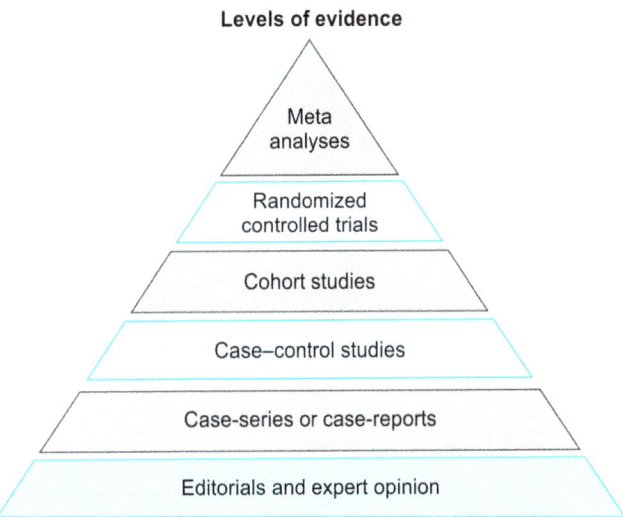

Index

Page numbers followed by *f* refer to figure.

A

Abdominal compartment syndrome 89
Abduction 57
   limitation of 51
Abrasion
   arthroplasty 103
   chondroplasty 23
Abrasive 94
Abscess 261
   bone collapse 144
   epidural 146
Acceptable closed reduction criteria 305
Acetabular 90
   cup, bearing surfaces for 92
   dysplasia 50
   fracture 98, 100, 271
   index 52, 86, 194
   labrum 88
   retroversion 86
   rim 88
   roofline 51
   tear drop 52
Acetabulum, superior 86*f*
Achilles
   displaces 315
   tendon
      lengthening 204
      rupture, risk of 184
      tendonitis 183
Achondroplasia 144, 196
Acromial stress fractures 174
Acumed fibular rod system 401
Acupuncture-like transcutaneous electrical stimulation 410
Acute hemolytic transfusion reactions 32
Acute lung injury, transfusion-related 32
Adam's forward bending test 149
Adamantinoma 225
Adduction 99
Adductor
   advancement 298
   tenotomy 194
Adenocarcinoma 248
Adhesive 94
   capsulitis 399
Adipose tissue 225
Adjacent segment disease 143, 160
Adverse drug reactions 10
Agility training 109
Airway obstruction 320

Aitken 44
Akin osteotomy 182
Albee's operation 119
Albumin 31
Alderman's gait 30
Alendronate 9, 83, 205
Allen classification 283
Allis sign 51
Allograft 23, 241, 242
   meniscus 115
Allopurinol 202
Alpha-angle 51
Amelia 18
Amino acid
   lysine, analog of 406
   sequence 18
Aminoglycosides 200
Amniocentesis 67
Amputation 41, 65, 241, 340
   aims of 340
   level of 341
   principles of 340
Analgesia 100
Analgesic 403
Anaphylactic reactions 32
Anemia 408
Aneurysmal bone cyst 227, 228
   evolution of 229
Angiography, pulmonary 34
Angiosarcoma 225
Angle calculation 149
Angular deformities 60, 63
Anhidrosis 141
Ankle 27, 175, 185, 193, 332
   deformities of 185
   foot orthosis 181, 184
   injuries 309
   management of 195
   sprain 308
Ankylosing spondylitis 144
Annulus fibrosus 137
Anorexia 238
Ant-eater sign 179
Anterior abdominal incision 160
Anterior cruciate ligament tear 105
Anterior hip dislocation 274
   Epstein classification of 274
Anterior interosseous nerve 351
Anterolateral ligament reconstruction 104
Antibiotics 338
   coated intramedullary nail 401

Anticoagulant therapy 35
Antifibrinolytic agent 406
Antituberculous drugs 262
Apatite 25
Apleys grinding test 113
Apparent equinus 192
Appendicular skeleton 17
Arcuate sign 106, 111
Arms 412
Arnold–Hilgartner grading 204
Arthritis
   end-stage 187
   inflammatory 124, 125
   medial sided 110
   mutilans 222
   post-traumatic 308
Arthrodesis 50, 204, 224, 241, 243
   failed limited 213
   triple 180
Arthrodiastasis 50
Arthrofibrosis 108, 112
   fear of 107
Arthrogram 53, 54, 302
Arthropathy
   hemophilic 202
   inflammatory 26, 180, 183
   progressive 121
Arthroplasty 34
Arthroscopic 121, 180
   anatomy 164
   capsule release 169
   debridement 100, 116, 292
   repair 292
   staging 168
   subchondral drilling 121
   transtibial technique 110
Arthroscopy 113
   diagnostic 165
Arthrotomy 80
Articular cartilage 20, 103, 104, 122
   over glenoid 165
Aseptic loosening 96, 126
ASIA impairment scale 278
Aspiration 116
Aspirin 35
Atelectasis 155
Athetoid 191
Atlantoaxial joint 131
Atlanto-occipital joint 131
Atrial fibrillation 10
Attitude 344

Atypical insufficiency fracture 10
Autograft 241, 242
   fascial material 115
   strut 261
Autoimmune disorders 18
Autologous cartilage implantation 103
Autologous chondrocyte implantation 23
Autologous transfusion 33
Autonomous systems 409
Axial skeleton 16
Axon 343

B

Baclofen 193, 386
Bado classification 266
Bakers cyst 116
Bankart lesion injury 165
Bankart repair 167
   bumper effect of 167f
Bare spot 165
Barlow's test 51
Basilar invagination 190, 198
Bed sores, prevention of 385
Below knee
   amputation 342
   cast 310
Bending moments 300
Benediction hand 351
Bennet and Rolando fractures 292
Beta-angle 51
Biceps brachii
   long head of 163
   rupture, long head of 171
Bigliani classification 169
Bioabsorbable implants 405
   use polymers 405
Biochemical theory 36
Biomechanics 77, 137, 362
Biophysical effects 410
Biopsy 223, 228
Bisphosphonates 8, 9, 50, 83, 205
Bladder
   abnormalities 140
   management 385
Bleeding disorder 248, 408
Blocks sodium channels 158
Blood
   components 30
   supply 47, 60, 131, 137, 288, 306
      effect 376
   transfusion, hazards of 32
   vessels 225, 341
Blount's staple epiphysiodesis 360
Blue sclera 189
Blumensaat's line 118
Body
   fluids, aspiration of 34
   heart-shaped 131
Bohler's angle 314
Bone 60, 122, 130, 225, 249, 341
   angina 122

bank 339
biopsy 227
cement 229, 231, 337, 338
   implantation syndrome 338
classification of 225
cyst 6, 122
defects 164
deformities, correction of 206
density, high 122
destruction, palpation of 226
development of 15
formation 7
fragility 189
grafting 91, 155, 160, 389
   techniques 84
healing 18, 20
   biological failure of 399
   types of 18
infection 248
islands of 97
joint 10
lengthening 241, 243
lesions 244
loss, severe 213
marrow aspirate 84
mass 7
matrix, demineralized 387
mechanical axis of 62
morphogenic protein 50, 389
pain 246
peg epiphysiodesis 58
plates 378
quality of 98
resorption 7
scan 205, 228, 246, 255, 327, 334
scintigraphy 334
stabilization 252
stock, preservation of 126
substitutes 387
transport, internal 364
tumors 225, 241
   benign 225
   malignant 225
turnover markers 7
Bony
   bruising 111
   deformities 184
   destruction 228
   fragment 312
   procedures 69, 194
   reconstruction 365
   resection 198
Book test 352
Bosworth fracture 311
Botulinum 386
   toxin 193, 195
Bounce home test 113
Boutonniere deformity 222
Bowel management 386
Boyd's amputation 65
Boyd's technique 353
Brachial plexus 346

Brachialis sign 304
Brachioradialis 352
Bridge therapy 220
Broden's view 315
Bronchospasm 338, 393
Brooker's classification 369
Brown tumor 6, 12
Bruner's rules 37
Bryant's traction 376
Budapest diagnostic criteria 368
Buford complex 165
Bulbocavernosus reflex 278
Bunnel methods 319
Bursitis 287
   retrocalcaneal 183
Bursoscopy 165
Buttress plate 378

C

Cadaveric donors 339
Caffey's hypothesis 47
Calcaneal fractures 314
Calcaneocuboid excisional arthroplasty 69
Calcaneofibular ligament 308
Calcaneoplasty 184
Calcaneovalgus foot 70
Calcaneum 67, 314
Calcific tendinitis 169
Calcitonin 8, 206
Calcium 8
   absorption 1
   excretion 1
   functions of 2
   metabolism 1
   preparations 1
   pyrophosphate 25
Calf
   muscles 199
   pain 179
   tenderness 34
Cam lesion 85f
Campanacci 230
Canadian C-spine rule 286
Canal stenosis 140
Cancellous bone 42
Capanna-morphologic subgroups 228
Capitellar shear fractures 76
Capsular incision, Z-shaped 101
Capsuloligamentous structures 163
Caput ulna syndrome 222
Carcinoembryonic antigen 246
Card test 352
C-arm 329
Carotid sheath 134
Carpal biomechanics 293
Carpal instability 293
   dissociative 293
   overview of 293
Carpal row, proximal 207
Carpal tunnel syndrome 206, 307, 399

Cartilage 20, 225
   bilayer of 137
   defects 21, 395
   injuries 21, 121
Cauda equina syndrome 145, 246, 277
Cavus 69
   foot 187
Cell
   biology 122
   counts 25
Cement, types of 338
Cementing
   techniques, evolution of 338
   zones of 96f, 339f
Central articular disc 292
Ceramic-on-polyethylene 92, 93
Cerebellar lesion 191
Cerebral dysfunction 37
Cerebral palsy 187, 190
Cervical disc herniation 399
Cervical extension 140
Cervical rib 216
   resection 216
Cervical spine 140, 218
   anatomy 130
   injuries 282
   lateral mass fixation for 151
Cervical spondylosis 138
Champagne glass pelvis 197
Chance fracture 281
Chandler's disease 81
Charcot's arthropathy 187
Charcot's joint 180
Charnley's original tech 338
Cheilectomy 50
Chemical
   burns 38
   examination 26
   sympathectomy 368
Chemotherapeutic agents 239
Chest 3
   injuries 319
   pain 94
Chevron osteotomy 124, 183
Chiari osteotomy 46
Chicken-wire calcification 233
Childress test 113
Cholesterol 25
Chondral injuries 106
Chondroblastoma 225, 232
Chondroid tissue 228
Chondrolabral junction 85
Chondrolysis 57
Chondromyxoid fibroma 225
Chondroplasties 73
Chondrosarcoma 225, 233, 234
Chordoma 225
Chromatolysis 343
Chromosome 195
Chronic degenerative tear 169
Chronic monteggia, management of 268
Chronic regional pain syndrome 367

Clamshell orthosis 65
Clavicle
   complete absence of 196
   osteotomy 198
Claw
   hand 352
   toes 41, 185, 186f
Cleidocranial dysostosis 195
Clindamycin 338
Clodronate 9
Clostridium histolyticum collagenase 210
Coagulation
   disorder, hereditary 202
   pathway 202
Codman's triangle 235
Colchicine 202
Colistin 338
Collagen 18, 112, 403
   relaxation of 68
   vascular disease 248, 339
Colles' fracture, complications of 307
Color rendering index 412
Combined ligamentous injuries 110
Compartment pressure monitoring 39
Compartment syndrome 38
Composite intramedullary nailing system 401
Compression
   fractures 281, 299
   plate 379
   role of 379
Compressive bandages 204
Congruence angle 119
Continuous passive motion 108
Conus medullaris 145
   syndrome 277
Conventional transcutaneous electrical stimulation 410
Cooling system 394
Cord 209, 347
   involvement 260
   lateral 347
   posterior 347
   pretendinous 210
Core
   biopsy 227
   decompression 83, 83f
Coronal pedicle angle 151
Coronary ligaments 112
Corrective valgus derotational osteotomy 60
Corrosion 92
Corrosive wear 94
Cortex erosions 235
Cortical avulsion fracture 106
Cortical bone 42
Corticosteroids 25, 200, 202, 220
Cosmesis 240
Costoclavicular space 215f
Costotransversectomy 262f
Cotton wool skull 205
Cover-up test 62

Coxa
   breva 59
   profunda 86
   valga 307
   vara 56, 59, 196, 307
      developmental 59
Cozen' test, provocative 209
Crepitus 117
Crossover sign 86
Cryoablation 247
Cryotherapy 117
Crystal
   arthritis 26
   arthropathy 183
   examination 25
Cuff-tear arthropathy 173
Cushing's syndrome 82
Cyclops lesion 108
Cysts 113
   congenital meningeal 144
   hemophilic 204
Cytokines, inflammatory 122

D

Dactinomycin 239
Damage control orthopedics 324
Dangerous hypocalcemic tetany 12
Dantrolene 386
   sodium 193
Darrach procedure 292
Day care surgery 407
Dead space management 252
Deafness 189
Debris 92
Deep circumferential dissection 400
Deep sulcus sign 106
Deep vein thrombosis 34
Deferasirox 33
Deferoxamine 33
Deformity 4, 122, 149, 160, 176, 179, 344
   correction 261
      indications 64
      principles of 64
   mild 183
   moderate 183
   severe 183
   source of 62
Degenerative disc disease 159, 395
Degenerative spine disease, spectrum of 138
Degradation 406
Delayed extravascular hemolytic reactions 32
Delbet classification 306
Deltoid
   lengthening of 172
   retensioning of 172
Dennis classification 281
Denosumab 8, 10, 147
Dense collagen rich scar 209
Dental crowding 196

Dentinogenesis imperfecta 189
Depomedrol 202
Dequervain's tenosynovitis 211
Desmoplastic fibroma 225
Destot sign 269
Diabetes mellitus 180, 408
Diarthrodial joints 131
Diazepam 386
Dickson-Diveley procedure 187f
Diffuse idiopathic skeletal hyperostosis 144
Dihydrofolate reductase 219
Disc
   degeneration theory 142
   function of 137
   herniation 138
   prolapse 146
   space narrowing 140, 145
Discoid meniscus 115
Dislocation 80, 102, 275
Distal
   fragment cortices 330f
   radius 305
   ulna 305
Distraction test 162
Dome osteotomy 124
Dorsal angulation 305
Dorsiflexion 213
Drawer test
   anterior 166
   posterior 110, 166
   posterolateral 111
Drehmann sign 57
Drugs 8, 201
   eluting heparinized titanium 401
Duchenne muscular dystrophy 198
Dugdale method 124
Dupuytren's contracture 18, 209
Dupuytren's diathesis 209
Dural tear 156
Durkan's test 208
Durotomy 142
Dwyer osteotomy 69
Dysbarism-Caisson's disease 82
Dysfunctional angular deformity 65
Dysphagia 141
Dysplasia 99
Dystonia 191
Dystrophies 199
Dystrophin gene 199

E

Early graft failure 108
Eccentric bony outgrowth 240
Ecchymosis 314
Edema 34, 111
Egawa test 352
Ege's test 113
Ehlers-Danlos syndrome 18

Elastic
   cartilage 20
   modulus 42
Elasticity, Young's modulus of 41
Elbow 301, 335
   recurvatum 185
   terrible triad of 290
Electrical
   stimulation 65, 357
   therapy 386
Electrode
   blade designs 398
   placement 411
Electrodiagnostic studies 344
Electrolyte disturbance 32
Electromyography 344
Elimination 406
Emergency splints 377
Empty-notch sign 106
Enchondroma 225, 234, 240
End plate sclerosis 140
Endochondral ossification 16
   pathologic activation of 122
Endocrine
   imbalance 120
   myopathies 248
Endoneural tubes 343f
Endoneurium 343
Endoprosthetic replacement 241, 242
Endoscopic procedures 407
Endosteal scalloping 234
Enneking staging system 226
Enoxaparin 35
Enthesopathy 183
Epicondylitis, lateral 208
Epidural steroids 158
Epineurium 343
Epiphyseal abnormalities 120
Epiphyseal drilling 50
Epiphysiodesis 360
Epiphysis 49
   sclerosis of 48
Equinocavovarus 195
Equinovalgus 176
Equinus 41, 69, 195
Erb's management 349
Erb's palsy 349, 350
Erectile dysfunction 386
Erythromycin 338
Erythropoietin 33
Ethylene oxide 340
Etoposide 239
Evan's calcaneal lengthening osteotomy 180
Evertor insufficiency 185
Ewing's sarcoma 225, 234, 238, 260
Ex vivo gene therapy 395
External beam radiotherapy 247
External fixator 124, 382
External rotation 99, 184

   recurvatum test 111
Extra-articular tenodesis 104
Extrusion 138
   index 86

F

Facet
   arthrosis 140
   fragments 315
   joints 131
Failed back syndrome 161
Failure to thrive 3
Fanconi syndrome 2
Farmer's procedure 65
Fascia
   closure of 102
   lata 100
Fasciculation 344
Fassier-Duval rods 190
Faster rehabilitation 125
Fat
   embolism 36
   microglobulinemia 37
Fatigue 94
Fatty infiltration 170
Febrile nonhemolytic reactions 32
Femoral bone reservation 89
Femoral epiphyseal-diaphyseal angle 57
Femoral head 82f
   bearing surfaces for 93
   fractures 100
   resection 100, 194
Femoral neck
   fracture 87, 89
      nonunion 90
   osteoplasty of 59
   short 59
Femoral segment 44, 45
Femoral tunnel placement 108
Femoroacetabular impingement 84, 100
Femur 62
   fractures, pediatric neck of 305
   head 44
      fracture 275, 276
      lateral subluxation of 49
   tumors, proximal 242
Ferguson classification 283
Fibrillations 344
Fibrin
   clot 115
   gel 392
   glue 157
Fibroblasts align 209
Fibrocartilage 20
Fibrocytes predominant 209
Fibromyalgia 218, 393
Fibro-osseous tunnel beneath 177
Fibrosarcoma 225, 248
Fibrous cortical defect 225

Fibrous dysplasia 236
Fibula grafting 83*f*
Fibular hemimelia 45, 358
Figure of 8 sign 86
Fine needle aspiration cytology 227
Finger 218
   deformities 221
   stiffness 308
Finkelstein test 212
Fixation technique 152
Fixator, stiffness of 383
Flail chest 322
Flat foot 180
   adult acquired 180
   deformities, end-stage 187
Flat panel detector 329
Fleck sign 312
Flexible flat foot 180
Flexion
   deformity 184
   extension views 140
   space, balancing of 127
Flexor tendon
   injuries 295
   reconstruction 297
   repair 297
Floating elbow 304
Fluid
   composition, normal 26
   removal 397
Fluorosis 144
Fondaparinux 36
Foot 175, 184, 185, 193, 332, 335
   arches 175
      analogy of 176*f*
   congenital anomaly of 67
   deformity 75, 185, 186, 195
      chronic progressive 180
   flat 27
   management of 195
Forearm derotational osteotomy 72
Forefoot abduction 179
Fowler's tenodesis 353
Fracture 164, 204, 272
   anterior wall 272
   classification of 292
   configuration 90
   displacement classification 302
   dynamization of 326
   elementary 272
   femoral 98
   fixation, failure of 91
   healing 395
   impending 229
   line, primary 315
   location 304
   management of 206
   multiple 189, 190
   pathological 228, 301
   pattern 273
   pelvis 268
   periprosthetic 94, 97
   recurrent 65
   site of 98
   subchondral 49
   surgical management of 8
Fragile opaque teeth 189
Fragmentation 48
Frank pseudoarthrosis 65
Freeze dried allograft 340
French technique, modified 68
Fresh frozen
   allografts 339
   plasma 31
Friction 93
Friedreich's ataxia 187
Froment's sign 352
Frozen shoulder 168
Fulkerson's osteotomy 120

G

Gage's sign 49
Gait 27, 30, 62, 192
   abnormal 57
   analysis 28
   antalgic 30
   circumduction 30
   crouch 192
   hamstring 30
   hand-to-knee 29, 30
   jump knee 192
   mechanism 178
   pathological 29
   sensory 30
   short limb 30
   shuffling 30
   stiff knee 192
   stomping 30
   training 385
   Trendelenburg 29, 29*f*, 57, 77, 99, 189
   waddling 197
Galeazzi sign 51
Galeazzi test 45
Gallow's traction 376
Gamekeeper's thumb 222, 298
Gardner well tongs 134
Gartland classification 303
Gas gangrene 325
Gastrocnemius 195
Gastrosoleus muscle, wasting of 183
Gate control theory 410
Gaucher's disease 6
Gene therapy 105, 200, 394
General vertebral column anatomy 133
Genetic defect 67
GeneXpert 260
Gentamycin 200, 338
Genu
   recurvatum 30, 118
   valgum 118
   varum 197
Germ cell abnormalities 235
Germline 394
Giant cell 230
   reparative granuloma 228
   tumor 229
Gibson interval 100
Gillquist view, modified 104*f*
Glenohumeral instability, types of 165
Glenohumeral joint 163
Glenohumeral stability, mechanics of 163*f*
Glenoid 165*f*
   cavity 163*f*
   component loosening 173
   labrum 163
      humeral avulsion of 167
Gluteus medius 101
Glycosaminoglycan 403
Godfrey's sign 110
Gout 200
Gower's sign 199
Gradually progressive disorder 50
Graft
   complications 142
   fixation 108
   malpositioning 108
Graft-versus-host disease 32
Gram stain 26, 325
Grass, blade of 205
Grauer classification 285
Great toe sesamoids 328
Greater trochanter 100, 101
Grey Turner sign 269
Gross motor function classification scale 191
Growth 60, 191
   disturbances 184
   factors 389
   modulation 63
      indication of 63
   phases of 63
Gurd's criteria 37

H

Haglund deformity 183
Hallux valgus 181, 181*f*
   angle 182
Hamada and Fukuda classification 170
Hammer toe 185
Hampton's hump 34
Hamstring tendon graft harvesting 107
Hand 335
   coolness of 216
   deformities of 221
   foot genital syndrome 18
Hangman's fracture 284
Hard callus 19
Hardcastle classification 311

Hardware failure 143
Hawkins classification 313
Head 3, 49
   neck offset ratio 86
Healed fusion, fracture of 213
Heart disease, congenital 198
Heel cord contractures 179
Heel off 28
Heel strike 27
Hemangioma 225, 260
   painful aggressive 153
Hemarthrosis 118, 202
Hematoma 146
   epidural 159
   formation 19
Hemicallostasis 124
Hemiparesis 192
Hemivertebra 17
Hemochromatosis, iatrogenic 33
Hemodilution, acute normovolemic 33
Hemophilia 202
Hemorrhage, retroperitoneal 269
Hemothorax 323
Henry and Thorburn classification 210
Heparin 35
Herndon hump 57
Heterotopic ossification 87, 89, 90, 97, 368
High medial nerve palsy 352
High tensile strength 137
Hilgenreiner's epiphyseal angle 59
Hilgenreiner's line 51, 52
Hindfoot
   abnormalities 183
   parallelism 68
   valgus 179
Hip 27, 45, 77, 91, 193, 218, 331, 335
   arthrodesis 92, 100, 194
   arthroscopy 87, 276
   biomechanics 77
   bursitis 399
   deformities, management of 194
   developmental dysplasia of 50
   dislocation 274-276
   disorders 75
   external rotation of 274
   Ganz surgical dislocation of 100
   hemiarthroplasty 92
   incongruous 56
   internal rotation of 274
   joint 79, 369
      degenerative disease of 99
   pain 83, 99, 100
   painful dislocated 194
   resurfacing 402
      arthroplasty 89
   sacrificing 83, 84
   safe surgical dislocation of 100
   soft tissue of 97
   surgery 369
   tuberculosis of 256, 256f
Histiocytosis 6
Holden's classification 366

Holding test 117
Homan's sign 34
Hormone
   effect 21
   replacement therapy 8
   theory 56
Horner's syndrome 141, 347
Hueter-Volkmann law 60
Hughston classification, modified 111
Humeral head, articular surface of 165
Humeral stem loosening 173
Humerus fracture, lateral condyle of 301
Humpback deformity 294
Hyaline cartilage 20
Hyaluronic acid 403
Hybrid fixator 364
Hydroxychloroquine 219
Hypercalcemia 246
   management of 245
Hyperextension 221
Hyperintense signal 111
Hyperparathyroidism 82, 246
Hyperplasia, angiofibroblastic 208
Hypertension 180
Hyperthermia, malignant 248
Hyperviscosity syndrome 245
Hyponatremia 95
Hypotension, normal 386
Hypothermia 32
Hysteresis 137

I

Ibandronate 9
Idiopathic chronic bone remodeling
   disorder 204
Iliopsoas inflammation 263
Iliotibial band contracture 118
Ilizarov ring fixator 124
Illumination, depth of 412
Immobilization 110
   external 190
Implant placement 63
Implantable penile prosthesis 386
In situ pins 58
Indian Hedgehog signaling molecule 122
Indomethacin 202
Induction 396
Infections 32, 260
   acute hematogenous 95
   chronic 95, 365
   deep 95
   sites of 256f
   source of 249
   spread of 250f
Inflammation 19, 121, 202
Injury 164
   degree of 343
   displaced 76
   mechanism of 266, 268, 299, 304, 309, 315

   neurovascular 96
   traumatic 138
Insall-Salvati index 118, 118f
Instability 122, 142, 163
   degree of 165
   inferior 166
Interferential therapy 396
Intermeniscal ligaments 112
Intermetatarsal angle 182
Internal disc disruption 138
Interscalene triangle 215
Intersection syndrome 212
Intervertebral disc 130, 137
Intervertebral foramen 131
Intra-articular epiphysis 253
Intra-articular fracture 122, 382
Intra-articular fusions 79
Intra-articular gene therapy 395
Intra-articular pressure 163
Intra-articular steroid injection 117
Intracarpal row instability 293
Intradiscal electrothermotherapy 156
Intramedullary bone
   stent 401
   transport 401
Intramedullary nailing 400
Intramedullary rods 190
Intramembranous ossification 15
Intraoperative cell salvage 33
Intrauterine pressure therapy 67
Intravertebral vacuum phenomenon 153
Intrinsic plus 221
Iron overload 33
Irritability 3
Ischemia 120
Isokinetic exercises 409
   types of 409
Isolated vascular bone graft 400

J

Jaipur foot 374
Jaundice 37
Jaw anomalies 198
Joint 3, 131
   arthroplasties 408
   atraumatic remodeling of 68
   debridement 103
   development of 16
   disease, inflammatory 24
   distraction 50
   dysplasia 122
   effusion 118
   filler 113
   infection 248, 249
   interphalangeal 221
   intervertebral 131
   involvement 218
   line tenderness 120
   orientation 62
   pain 393

reduction force 77
space narrowing 24, 100
stabilization of 185
subaxial 131
uncovertebral 131
Jones fracture 317

K

Kaeding-Miller stress fracture classification system 327
Kager's triangle 318
Keblish approach 129
Keller's procedure 183
Kessler methods 319
Kidney disease, chronic 408
Kienbock's disease 213, 214
Kiloh-Nevin syndrome 351
King's classification 148f
Kirkaldy-Willis theory 144
Kite's view 68
Klien's line, failure of 57
Klippel-Feil syndrome 17, 71, 197, 198
Klisic test 51
Klumpke's management 349
Klumpke's paralysis 349, 350
Knee 27, 45, 103, 218, 331, 335
　ankle foot orthosis 29f
　arthroscopy 103
　deformities, management of 194
　disorders 75
　effusion in 117, 120
　flexion 127
　　test 62
　immediate swelling of 106
　intra-articular pathologies of 103
　motion 127
　osteoarthritis of 121
　pain 57
　　persistent 112
　posteromedial corner of 104f
　rotational alignment of 127
　stiffness 122
Kocher's criteria 255
Krackow methods 319
Kummel disease 153
Kuwada classification 318
Kyphoplasty 152, 153, 156
Kyphosis 3, 197
　angle 140
　congenital 75

L

Lacertus fibrosis thickening 351
Lachman's test 106
Laminar air flow 390
Laminectomy 160
Laminoplasty 141
Laminotomy 160
Langerhans cell histiocytosis 153
Lapidus procedure, modified 183
Laprade anatomic reconstruction 112
Laryngeal nerve palsy, recurrent 141
Lasers 393
Lateral femoral
　circumflex artery 306
　condyle, posteromedial aspect of 105
Lautenbach method 252
LCWO 125
Leffert classification 347
Leflunamide 220
Leg 335
　length discrepancy 97
Lesions, multiple 246
Lever arm, failure of 30
Lhermitte's sign 140
　reverse 140
Lichtman classification 215
Ligament 131
　abnormal 215
　reconstruction 298
　subaxial 131
Ligamentous laxity 50
Ligamentum
　flavum 133
　teres 88
Light field diameter 412
Lignocaine 158
Limb 3, 99
　dangerous 340
　length discrepancy 358
　　calculation 359
　lengthening 358, 360, 361
　mechanical axis of 62
　salvage 241
　　surgery 241
　shortening 360
Limp 57
Lindberg syndrome 212
Lipid lowering agents 83
Lipoma 225
Liposarcoma 225
Lisfranc injury 311
Lisfranc joint 311
Liver disease, chronic 408
Load and shift test 166
Local antibiotic therapy 252
Local pedicle vascular bone graft 84
Locking plate 381
Long bone fracture 189
Lordotic curve 131
Lordotic lumbar spine 151
Low back pain 160
Low median nerve palsy 351
Low molecular weight heparin 35
Low ulnar nerve palsy 352
Lower leg alignment 126
Lower limb
　alignment 62
　axes of 126f
　myotomes 140
Lubrication 94
Lumbar 134, 136
　canal stenosis 144
　facet joint syndrome 399
　lordosis, loss of 145
　spinal stenosis, etiological classification of 144
　spine 136
　stenosis 197
　vertebrae 132
Lunate
　dislocation 294
　geometry 214
Luschka uncinate process 131
Lymphadenopathy, regional 248
Lymphoma 225, 238, 247, 260
Lytic lesion 230

M

Macrodeformation 397
Madelung deformity 210
Madura foot 264
Magerl technique 152
Malalignment test 62
Malignant transformation 241
Malrotation 305
Mannerfelt syndrome 222
Marfan's syndrome 18
Masquelet technique 364
Matrix metalloproteases, increased secretion of 122
Maudsley's test 209
Mayfield classification 294
Mayo procedure 183
McBride procedure 182f
McMurrays test 113
Meary's angle 70
Mechanical theory 36, 56
Medial compartment bone loss 124
Medial cord 347
Medial femoral circumflex artery 306
Medial longitudinal arch 175, 175f
　parts of 175f
　progressive collapse of 181
Medial meniscus 112
Medial opening wedge 124
Medial plantar nerve 178f
Median nerve 350
　compression sites for 351
　compressive neuropathy of 206
　dysfunction 307
　innervates 351
　palsy 351
Megaprosthesis 242
Mehta's angle 147
Membrane stabilization 158
Menelaus method 359
Meningocele 17
Meniscal allografts 105
Meniscal cysts 113, 116
Meniscal detachment 115

Meniscal regeneration 105
Meniscal repair 114
   augmentation 105
Meniscal scaffolds 105
Meniscal tear 103, 115
Meniscal transplantation 115
Meniscectomy 114
Meniscus 112
   bucket handle tear of 331*f*
   trephination 115
Merle D'Aubigne light bulb 84, 84*f*
Meromelia 18
Meropenam 338
Mesenchymal stem cells 404
Mesothelioma 248
Metabolic bone disease 4, 334, 339
Metacarpophalangeal joint flexion 353
Metal sensitivity 90
Metal-on-polyethylene 92, 93
Metaphyseal cysts 49
Metaphyseal vessels 306
Metaphysis, flaring of 190
Metastasis 226
Metastatic disease 153
Methotrexate 219
Methylmethacrylate, polymers of 337
Methylprednisone 158
Meyer's quadratus femoris 84
Microabrasions 121
Microdiscectomy, microscopic 155
Microfractures 22
Microsvasculature free fibular grafting 65
Microwave ablation 247
Midfoot, columns of 311
Milch classification 302
Mill's maneuver 209
Miller Warner classification 112
Milwaukee bracing 148
Minimally invasive
   spine surgery 155
   surgery 125
   video-assisted surgical intervention 103
Miosis 141
Mirel's score 246
Mitchell procedure 183
Mitosis 234
M-L taper hip prosthesis 402
Mobile bearing 126
Monoarticular arthritis 254
Monosodium urate 25
   crystals 201
Monteggia fracture 266
Monteggia lesions 76
Morel Lavallee lesion 286
Morning stiffness 209, 218
Moro's reflex 192
Mosaic pattern appearance 205
Mosaicplasty 103
Moseley chart 360
MOWO 125
Mucin clot 26
Multiagent chemo treatment 236
Multiligamentous knee injuries 109

Multiloc nailing system 401
Multiple blood transfusions 33
Multiple myeloma 6, 9, 153, 225, 243, 246, 260
Multiple septa traverse 230
Munchmeyer's diseases 369
Muscle 169, 341
   activation latencies 105
   atrophy 170
   attachment for 132
   biopsy 248
   disorders, chronic 344
   fibers, loss of 199
   fibrosis of 344
   imbalance 184
   pains 10
   pull distracts fracture 380
   spasm 184
   splitting 155
   tone 191
   wasting 99, 117
   weakness 248
Muscular dysfunction 99
Muscular dystrophies 248
Mycetoma 264
Mycobacteria growth indicator tube 260
Mycobacterium tuberculosis 258
Myelin 343
Myelogram 162
Myelomeningocele 17
Myelopathic signs 140
Myelopathy 139, 198
   classification of 140
Myerson classification 311
Myodesis 341
Myoelectric prosthesis 373
Myofascial plane 393
Myofibroblasts 209
   proliferation 209
Myoplasty 341
Myositis ossificans 369
Myotomes 140
Myotonia 199

N

Nades principles 251
Natural growth, characteristics of 63
Necrosis 234
Negative pressure wound 397
Neoplasm 287
Nerve 341
   blockade 368
   conduction
      studies 343
      velocity 344
   fiber activation, principles of 410
   injury 164, 344
      proximal 346
   repair 345
   root 131, 132
      blocks 158
   stimulation 368

   transfer 346
Neural compression, degree of 146
Neural decompression 261
Neural elements 143
Neuralgia, intercostal 155
Neuroblastoma, metastatic 238
Neurofibroma 225
Neurofibromatosis 2
Neurofibrosarcoma 225
Neurogenic bladder 370
Neurological deficit 261, 269
Neurolysis 345
Neuromuscular disease 187
Neuropathic claw foot 186
Neuropathy, peripheral 244
Neuropraxia 344
Neutralization 378
Nissl's granules, loss of 343
Nitrogen
   absence of 9
   presence of 9
Nodule 209
   formation 209
Noncontact pivoting injury 105
Nonfixation healing 115
Nonimmunologic reactions 32
Nonoperative adjunctive methods 357
Non-ossifying fibroma 225
Nora's lesion 240
Notochord remnant 137
Nuclear medicine 34
   scans 333
Nucleolar swelling 343
Nucleus pulposus 137
Nurick classification 140
Nutritional deficiency 207
Nutritional rickets 4

O

O' Donoghue, unhappy triad of 105
Obstetric paralysis 349
Obturator
   neurectomy 371
   sign 255
Occipitoatlantoaxial ligament 131
Ochsner's clasp test 351
Ocular inflammation 10
Odontoid fracture 285
Olecranon fracture 190
Oligohydramnios 71
Open reduction 55, 276
   and internal fixation 270, 293, 313
Orthobiologics 104, 389
Orthopedic 406
   diseases 189
   manifestations 202
   radiology 329
   traction in 375
Ortolani test 51
Osgood-Schlatter disease 206
Osinski reflex 278

Ossification centers 301
   appearance of 76
   fusion of 76
Osteitis
   circumscripta 205
   deformans 204
   fibrosa generalisata 5
Osteoarthritis 395
   hip 99
Osteoblast differentiation 195
Osteoblastoma 225
Osteochondral autograft transplantation 23
Osteochondritis dissecans 120
Osteochondroma 225, 234, 239
Osteoconductivity 387
Osteocutaneous flaps 400
Osteogenesis 387
   imperfecta 18, 153, 189
Osteogenicity 261
Osteoid 228
   osteoma 216, 225, 231, 334
Osteology 304
Osteoma 225
Osteomalacia 4, 6, 334
Osteomuscular flaps 400
Osteomyelitis 6, 238, 247, 249
   acute 249, 251
   chronic 251, 252
Osteonecrosis 81, 153, 176, 307
Osteopenia 190
Osteophytes 7, 145
   formation 122, 140
Osteoporosis 5, 9, 89, 144
Osteosarcoma 225, 235
Osteotomy 58, 84
   reduction and fixation of 102
   wedge, size of 124
Ottawa ankle rules 308, 310
Overgrowth 359
Ozone therapy 398

P

Packed red blood cells 31
Paget's disease 6, 9, 97, 144, 153, 204, 246
Paget–Schroetter syndrome 215
Pain 57, 91, 99, 122, 170, 202, 327
   abdominal 95
   acute 155, 411
   chronic 41, 198, 411
   generator theory 179
   management 204
   minimal 180
   neuropathic 386
   radicular 143
Paley's classification 64
Palmar carpal displacement 211
Palmaris longus tendon graft 298
Pamidronate 190
Parachute reflex 192

Paralysis, residual 184
Paralytic intrinsic muscle 366
Paralytic polio
   features of 184
   natural history of 184
Parathyroid hormone 11
Parkinson's disease 408
Parosteal osteochondromatous proliferation 240
Parosteal osteomyelitis 240
Pars interarticularis 132, 151
Patella
   abnormal excessive passive lateral displacement of 118
   recurrent dislocation of 117
Patellar
   clunk syndrome 103
   fracture 108
   tendon bearing cast 374
Patellofemoral arthrosis 110
Patellofemoral joint 104
   mechanics 128
Pavlik disease 53
Pediatric
   compartment syndrome 39
   diaphyseal forearm fractures 304
   forearm fractures 305
   fractures 299
   orthopedics 44
Pedicle screw 150
   insertion 151
Pellegrini-Stieda lesion 106
Pelvic
   obliquity 193
   osteotomies 55
   ring stable 269
Pemberton's osteotomy 55
Pen test 351
Pencil in cup deformity 222
Percutaneous core needle 235
Pericardial tamponade 322
Perilunate dissociation 294
Perineurium 343
Periosteal flap 24
Periosteal reaction 226, 235
Periosteum 299
Peripheral nerve injuries 343
Perkins line 52
Permeative growth pattern 235
Peroneal nerve injury 112
Perthes disease 47, 100, 334
Perthes lesion 167
Pes anserinus 120
Pes cavus 176
Pes planus 176, 179
Petechial rash 37
Phalen's test 208
Phemister epiphysiodesis 360
Phenol 386
Phlegmasia
   alba dolens 34
   cerulea dolens 34

Phocomelia 18
Physical therapy 123, 171, 368
   exercises 385
   role of 160
Physis 60
Piezoelectric effect 335
Pigmented villonodular synovitis 222
Pin fixator, components of 383
Pipkin's classification 275
Pipkin's sign 117
Pistol grip deformity 85*f*
Pivot shift test 106
Plantar
   concavity protects 175
   nerve, lateral 178*f*
Plastic deformation 304
Platelet 31
   rich plasma 31, 104, 390
Plica syndrome 116
Pneumothorax 155, 320
Pointing index 351
Poliomyelitis 186
Poly glycolic acid 405
Poly lactic acid 405
Polydactyly 73
Polydioxanone 405
Polyethylene 92, 126
Polymerase chain reaction 260
Polymethacrylate 337
Polytrauma 323
Ponseti method 68
Popliteal artery injury 110
Popliteal fossa 110
Popliteal hiatus 104
Positive dial test 110, 111
Positive fovea sign 292
Post-childhood hip disorders 89
Posterior atlanto-occipital membrane 131
Posterior cruciate ligament injury 109
   classification 110
Posterior hip dislocation 274
   Thompson and Epstein's classification of 274
Posterior interosseous nerve 354
Posterior ligamentous complex 281
Posterior malleolus fractures 310
Posterior sag sign 110
Posterior talofibular ligament 308
Posterior tibial
   nerve 178*f*
   tendon insufficiency 180
Posterolateral corner injury 110
Post-polio residual paralysis 184
Postradiation sarcoma 247
Post-surgery psychosis 95
Post-tourniquet syndrome 38
Pott's spine 6
   surgical management of 261
Prednisone 202
Preoperative autologous transfusion 33
Primigravida 71
Primitive mesenchymal cells 238

Progressive deformity, causes of 184
Progressive muscle dystrophy, Walton's classification of 198
Prosthesis 65, 372
    basic features of 342
    semi-constrained 173
Prosthetic joint infection 95
Protein 26
Protrusio acetabuli 86, 190, 237
Protusion 138
Proximal femoral
    focal deficiency 44
    nail A2 400
Proximal femur 253f, 328
    blood supply of 90
    normal trabeculae of 6f
Proximal fragment cortices 330f
Proximal radius 253f
Pseudoarthrosis 143, 160, 358
Pseudogout 144
Pseudomeningocele 157, 347
Pseudomonas 32
Pseudotumor
    hemophilic 204
    osseous 204
Psoas abscess 263
Ptosis 141
Pulmonary embolism 34, 38
Pulse
    amplitude 410
    duration 410
    patterns 410
    wave form 410
Pulvinar hypertrophy 50
Pure muscular dystrophy 198
Purtscher's retinopathy 37
Pyrexia 37

Q

Q-angle 118, 118f, 128f
Quadriceps 109, 206
    active test 110
    atrophy 113
    gait 29
    snip 129
    strengthening 119
    V-Y plasty 129
    wasting 120

R

Rachitic cat back 3
Radial head 290
    osteochondral fractures 76
Radial nerve 353
    supplies 354
Radiation
    hazards 330
    reduction 330
    therapy 224

Radiculopathy 139
Radiocapitellar joint dislocation 266
Radiofrequency ablation 397
Radionuclide therapy 247
Radiotherapy 247
Radioulnar joint dislocation, proximal 266
Radioulnar synostosis 72
    congenital 72
Raloxifene 8
Ratliff classification 307
Raynaud's phenomenon, unilateral 216
Reamer irrigator aspirator 391, 401
Reflexes 192
Regimental badge sign 166
Rehabilitation, postoperative 108
Reimer's migration index 52, 194
Renal aplasia 198
Renal tubular acidosis 2
Reperfusion syndrome 38
Respiratory insufficiency 37
Restores bone stock 125
Resuscitation 270
Retinal hemorrhages 37
Retinoblastoma, hereditary 235
Retrocalcaneal bursitis 183
Retropectoralis minor space 215f
Reverse shift test 111
Reverse shoulder arthroplasty 172
    evolution of 172
Reverse total shoulder arthroplasty 171
Reversible nerve blockade 158
Rhabdomyolysis 38
Rheumatoid 26
    arthritis 100, 103, 144, 217, 219, 221, 395
    cervical spondylitis 218
    hand 221
    nodules 222
Rhizomelic shortening 196
Rib 17
    hump 185
    vertebral angle difference 147
Rickets 2
Rifampicin 338
Rigault superomedial border 197
Ring positioning 363
Risedronate 9, 205
Robot-assisted and computer navigation 126
Robotic total hip replacement 402
Rolando fracture 293
Romosozumab 8
Roots 347
Rotation
    angulation, center of 124
    instant centers of 126
Rotational deformity, correction of 194
Rotator cuff 163
    arthropathy 169
        Hamada and Fukuda classification of 170

    disease 169
    muscles encircle 172
    repair 171
    tears 164, 169
Row carpectomy, proximal 295
Roy-Camille technique 152

S

Sacroiliitis 334
Sagittal facet theory 142
Salter's osteotomy 55
Salter-Harris fracture 240
Salvage osteotomies 56
Samilson and Binder criteria 171
Scalene muscles 215
Scalenectomy, anterior 216
Scaphoid
    fracture 212
    tubercle 207
Scapholunate dissociation 294
Scaphotrapeziotrapezoid arthritis 212
Scapula 196
    winging of 344
Scapular notching 174
Scapular spine fractures 174
Scarf osteotomy 183
Schmorl's nodes, painful 153
Sclera 189
Scoliosis 3, 75, 146, 147, 156, 193, 198
    congenital 198
    degenerative 144, 145
    management of 200
    neuroparalytic 185
    Research Society 146
Screw fixation 58
Scurvy 12, 18
Seddon classification, Tsuge modification of 366
Segmental bone defects 399
Selective dorsal rhizotomy 193
Self-compressing plate 379
Sensory 278, 351, 354
    disturbance, regional 162
    loss 41, 351
    test 208
Sentinel sign 269
Septic arthritis 26, 218, 253, 335
Septic joint 255
Septic reactions 32
Sequestrectomy 252
Sequestrum, types of 253
Serology 219
Seroma 287
Sexual health 386
Shallow trochlea 119
Shenton's line 52
Shock
    cardiogenic 35
    neurogenic 279
    types of 324

Shoe wear pain 183
Short neck 198
Short stem hip replacement 402
Short wave diathermy 395
Shoulder 163, 332, 335
    abduction test 140
    arthroscopy 164
    dislocation, recurrent 163, 164
    hypermobility of 196
    instability 163
    level of 149
Silver procedure 182
Silverskoid test 193
Single heel rise test 181
Sinus excision 261
Skeletal
    deformity 189
    development of 15
    fluorosis 14
    maturity 149
    muscle healing 395
    reconstruction 241
    traction 134, 273, 375
Skin
    flaps 340
    traction 375, 377
Slipped capital femoral epiphysis 56
Small cell osteosarcoma 238
Small spinal canal, congenital 144
Smith technique 353
Smooth fracture surfaces 91
Socket 342
Soft
    procedures 193
    tissue 215
        allografts 340
        balancing 126
        contractures, correction of 185
        defect 252
        dissection 80, 81
        palpation of 269
        sarcomas 241
        shadow 248
        swelling 204
Somatosensory-evoked potentials 157
Somerville-transverse bikini incision 79
Southwick slip angle 57
Spasticity, treatment of 193
Spica cast 54
Spina bifida 74
    occulta 17, 196
Spinal canal stenosis 197
Spinal cord
    injury 276, 404
    involvement 246
Spinal deformities 197
Spinal fusion 395, 405
    anterior 150
    methods 159
Spinal infections 144
Spinal orthoses 374

Spinal pseudoarthrosis 153
Spinal shock 278
    characteristics of 278
Spinal stabilization 261
Spinal stenosis 156
Spinal tuberculosis, pathogenesis of 258
Spinal tumor syndrome 260
Spine 3, 130, 190, 193, 247, 259, 331
    deformity 189
Spinous process 130, 132
Spondylolisthesis 142, 144, 159
    degenerative 145
Spondylolysis 142
Spondylosis 138
Sprengel deformity 197, 198
Spur sign 272
Spurling's sign 140
Staheli's shelf osteotomy 56
Stanmore classification 165, 165*f*
Staphylococcus aureus 254
Startle reflex 192
Static encephalopathy 190
Steel
    blanch sign of 57
    brown modification of 46
Steel's procedure 46
Stem cell 389, 404
    therapy 389
    transplantation 245
Sterilization, Rigault 340
Sternum 17
Steroids 158
    injection 116
Stiffness 99, 218
Stone procedure 183
Stoppa approach, modified 273
Strain 41
Stress 41, 137
    fracture 326, 334
    risers 97
    shielding 95, 242, 338
Stretching exercises 180
Stromelysin 122
Strontium 247
Stryker notch view 167
Stulberg grading 49
Subacromial bursitis 399
Subacromial impingement 169
Subpatellar crepitus 118
Subscapularis, fibers of 171
Subtalar arthrodesis 180
Subtrochanteric bow 45
Sucking chest wound 320
Sulcus
    angle 119
    test 166
Sulfasalazine 219
Sulphapyridine 219
Superficial abrasions 38
Superficial tenderness 162
Superior laryngeal nerve palsy 141

Supracondylar fracture humerus 302
Supracondylar humerus fracture 365
Supracondylar osteotomy 204
Supraspinatus 171
    tear, partial 399
    tendon retraction 170
Surgery 285
    complications of 208
    indications of 261, 281
    principles of 222, 241, 261
    timing of 185
    types of 79
Surgical decompression 196, 279
Surgical excision 370
    management of 226
Surgical sympathectomy 368
Surprise test 166
Suture anchor repair 184
Swelling 218, 301
    activity induced 122
Swing phase 28
Syme's amputation 65, 342, 342*f*
Syndactyly 18
Synovectomy 100, 103, 204, 224, 257
Synovial biopsy 103
Synovial cell sarcoma 247
Synovial chondromatosis 100
Synovial fluid
    analysis 24, 26, 201
    crystals, characteristics of 25
    features, normal 24
Synovial plicae 116
Synovioma 247
Synovitis 169
Synovium 122
Syphilis 339

T

Tachycardia 37
Talectomy 70
Talipes cavus 186
Talocalcaneal angle 68
Talofibular ligament, anterior 308
Talus 175
    blood supply of 176, 176*f*
    force of 315
    neck fractures 313
    superior articular surface of 175
Tardieu test 192
Tarsal coalition 178, 179*f*, 187
Tarsal sinus 177
Tarsal tunnel syndrome 177
Tear 113
    classification of 113
    mechanism of 113
    partial thickness 170
    pattern 114
    peripheral 292
Tectorial membrane 131
Temporary neurological deficit 159

Tenderness 110, 118, 218
Tendoachilles
   lengthening 180
   tendon rupture 318
Tendon 222
   adhesions 297
   chronic inflammation of 211
   healing, phases of 296
   injury 308, 335
   transfers 69, 346
   transplantation 120
Tennis elbow 208
Tensile lateral surface 328
Tension 321
   band 380
      principles 380
Tensioner standard wire tensioner 363
Tensioning device 379
Teriparatide 8, 83, 206
Terry Thomas sign 294
TFCC injury 291
   degenerative 292
   traumatic 292
Thallium 334
Thermotherapy 386
Thessalys test 113
Thomas test 99
Thomas traction splint 377
Thompson and Epstein's classification 274
Thoracic 282
   aortic disruption 323
   discectomy 155
   instability, White and Punjabi's checklist for 281
   outlet syndrome 215
   spine 135
   vertebrae 131
      peculiarity of 131
Thoracolumbar injury 279
   classification and severity score 281
Thoracolumbar kyphosis 197
Three strike rule 241
Thrombocytopenia, sudden 37
Thromboembolic disease 385
Thrombolytic therapy 35
Thromboprophylaxis 35, 36
Thumb 222
   adduction 353
   reconstruction of 73
   spice splint 298
Thurston-Holland fragment 302
Tibia 62, 328
   bone varus angle 124f
   congenital pseudoarthrosis of 64
   pseudoarthrosis of 358
   vara 65
Tibial hemimelia 358
Tibial osteotomy, high 123
Tibial plateau 124
Tibial torsion, external 118
Tibial tubercle 119, 206
   osteotomy 129

Tibial tunnel placement 107
Tibialis posterior motor weakness 181
Tibiofemoral arthritis, contralateral 125
Tibiofemoral subluxation 124
Tile's classification 269
Tiludronate 9
Tinel's sign 178, 208, 343, 347
Tissue
   debridement 252
   survival 39
Titanium 42
   alloys 401
   elastic nailing system 401
Tizanidine 193, 386
Tobramycin 338
Toes 218
Tonnis classification 100
Torsional injuries 299
Torticollis 71, 198
Total hip arthroplasty 84, 91, 285
   bearing surfaces in 92
Total hip replacement
   complications of 94
   evolution of 92
Total joint arthroplasty 204
Total knee arthroplasty 224
Total knee replacement 126
   contraindications of 128
Total wrist arthrodesis 295
Tourniquet paralysis 38
Tourniquet test 208
Toygar's angle 318
Trabecular destruction 214
Traction
   injury 347
   neuropraxia 89
Tranexamic acid 406
Transcutaneous electrical nerve stimulation
   therapy 410
   typical features of 410
Transgluteal approach 80
Transtibial tunnel drilling 108
Transverse arch 175, 175f
Transverse carpal ligament release 208
Trapezium 207
Trapezoid cross section 380
Trash lesions 75, 76
Trauma 34, 122, 249, 266, 343
   wounds 397
Trendelenburg gait 29, 29f, 57, 77, 99, 189
Trethowan's sign 57
Trevor's disease 240
Triamcinolone 158
Triangular metaphyseal fragment 60
Triceps 354
   surae insufficiency 185
Trident hands 196
Trigen intertan 400
Triphasic bone scan 334
Triplanar instability 268
Triple arthrodesis 70, 187, 187f

Trochanteric osteotomy 59
Trochlear dysplasia 119
   assessment 118
   Dejour classification of 119
Trochlear grove 104
Trochleoplasty 119
Trueta's hypothesis 47
Trunks 347
T-score 7
Tuber angle 314
Tuberculosis
   paraplegia 261
   pathogenesis of 258
   spine 258
Tuberculous paraplegia, classification of 260
Tuberosity fragment 315
Tumor 71, 155, 260, 332
   bulges 230
   markers 246
   osseous 216
Tuning fork 208
Typical cervical vertebrae 130

U

Ulna, fracture of proximal 266
Ulnar diaphyseal shortening 292
Ulnar
   nerve 352
   osteotomy 268
Ulnar paradox 352
Upper limb 185
   dermatomes of 17f
   myotomes 140
   tension tests 140
Uric acid, serum 201
Urinary hydroxyproline 205
Urinary retention 408
Urine calcium 62

V

Vacuum devices 386
Valgus
   deformity 65, 184
   intertrochanteric osteotomy 91
   osteotomy 50
   redirectional osteotomy 194
   stress test 110, 111
Van Nes rotationplasty 46
Vancomycin 338
Varus
   derotational femoral osteotomy 50
   extension osteotomy 50
   stem 97
   stress test 110, 111
Vascular anatomy 112
Vascularized fibula graft 399
Vastus lateralis 101
Vaughan-Jackson syndrome 222
Venous foot pumps 35

Venous thromboembolic events 142
Venous thromboembolism 34, 97
Ventilation perfusion ratio 34
Vertebral artery 142
  injury 142
  passes 130
Vertebral body 130
  compression fracture 152
Vertebral canal 144
Vertebral collapse 245
Vertebral column 17
  anatomy of 130
Vertebral foramen 130, 131
Vertebral rotation 149
Vertebroplasty 152, 156
Vicker's ligament 210
Video-assisted lumbar surgery 155
Video-assisted thoracic surgery 154, 155
Viral infection, hypothesized 205
Virchow's triad 97
Viscosity 338
Viscosupplementation 389, 402
Vitamin
  D 8
    deficiency 2, 4
    dependent rickets 3, 4
    disorders 2
    metabolism 2
  E doping 93
  K antagonist 36
Volar, congenital dyschondrosis of 210
Volkmann's fragment 310

Volkmann's ischemic contracture 41, 365
Von Rosen view 52

W

Waddell nonorganic signs 162
Waddling gait 197
Wafer procedure 292
Waldenstrom's sign 255
Walton's classification 198
Warfarin 36
Wassel classification 73
Weakness 170
Web space contracture 210
Weight 378
  bearing 123
  loss 100, 238
Weinstein monofilament test 208
Wiberg lateral center edge angle 52, 86
Wilbourn's classification 216
Wilson's method 58
Wilson's test 120
Windblown deformity 194
Winter's formula 147
Wolff's law 20
Woodward procedure 198
Wormian bones 190, 196
Wound
  care 297
  complications 94, 142, 188
  contraction 397

Wrist 218, 222, 332, 335
  arthrodesis 213
  arthroplasty 222
  level of 206
  stiffness 308

X

Xanthine oxidase enzyme 202
Xiphisternum 359
X-ray
  chest 196
  lateral 294
  skull 196

Y

Yellow ligament 133
Yergason test 171
Youm's index 214
Yount procedure 200

Z

Zancolli's capsulodesis 353
Zancolli's classification 366
Zein alcoholic solution 229
Zig-zag deformity 222
Zirconium metal alloy 93
Zoledronic acid 9, 83, 205
Z-score 7
Zygophyseal joints 132

EU GSPR Authorised Reprsentative
Logos Europe, 9 rue Nicolas Poussin
1700, La Rochelle, France
Phone: +33 (0) 6 67 93 73 78
E-mail: contact@logoseurope.eu